INFECTIOUS DISEASES

text and color atlas

SECOND EDITION

A Slide Atlas of Infectious Diseases, based on the contents of this book, is available. In the slide atlas format the material is split into volumes, each of which is presented in a binder together with numbered 35mm slides of each illustration. Each slide atlas volume also contains a list of abbreviated slide captions for easy reference when using the slides.

Further information can be obtained from:

Gower Medical Publishing, Middlesex House
34–42 Cleveland Street, London W1P 5FB

Gower Medical Publishing
101 5th Avenue, New York, NY 10003, USA

Nankodo Co Ltd
42–6 Hongo 3-Chome, Bungkyo-ku, Tokyo 113, Japan

INFECTIOUS DISEASES

text and color atlas

SECOND EDITION

W. Edmund Farrar MD, FACP

Professor of Medicine and Microbiology
Medical University of South Carolina
Charleston, South Carolina, USA

Martin J. Wood FRCP

Consultant Physician
East Birmingham Hospital
Birmingham, UK

John A. Innes BSc, FRCP, FRCP (Ed.)

Consultant Physician
East Birmingham Hospital
Birmingham, UK

Hugh Tubbs MBBS, MRCS, MSc, DCH, FRCP

Consultant Physician and Senior Lecturer
North Staffordshire Hospital Centre
Stoke-on-Trent, UK

Gower Medical Publishing • London • New York

Distributed in USA and Canada by:

J B Lippincott Company
East Washington Square
Philadelphia
PA 19105
USA

Distributed in UK and Continental Europe by:

Gower Medical Publishing
Middlesex House
34–42 Cleveland Street
London W1P 5FB
UK

Distributed in Australia and New Zealand by:

Harper and Row (Australia) Pty Ltd
PO Box 226
Artarmon
NSW 2064
AUSTRALIA

Distributed in Southeast Asia, Hong Kong, India and Pakistan by:

Harper and Row (Asia) Pte Ltd
37 Jalan Pemimpin 02-01
Singapore 2057

Distributed in Japan by:

Nankodo Co Ltd
42-6 Hongo 3-chome
Bunkyo-ku
Tokyo 113
JAPAN

British Library Cataloguing in Publication Data
Infectious Diseases. – 2nd ed.
    I. Farrar, W.E.
    616.9

Library of Congress Cataloging-in-Publication Data is available on request.

ISBN 0–397–44718–3

© Copyright 1992 by Gower Medical Publishing,
34–42 Cleveland Street, London W1P 5FB, England.
The right of W. Edmund Farrar, Martin J. Wood, John A. Innes and Hugh Tubbs to be
identified as the authors of this work has been asserted by them in accordance with the
Copyright, Designs and Patents Act 1988.
All rights reserved. No part of this publication may be reproduced, stored in a retrieval
system or transmitted in any form or by any means electronic, mechanical, photocopying,
recording or otherwise, without prior written permission of the publisher.

Setting & page make-up on Apple Macintosh˙.
Text set in New Century Schoolbook; captions set in Helvetica.
Originated in Hong Kong by Mandarin Offset Ltd.
Produced by Imago Productions (FE) PTE Ltd.
Printed in Singapore.

Project manager:	Stephen McGrath
Design:	Ian Spick
	Judith Gauge
	Anne-Marie Woodruff
Illustration:	Ian Spick
	Judith Gauge
	Anne-Marie Woodruff
	Lee Smith
	Dereck Johnson
Index:	Nina Boyd
Production	Susan Bishop
	Adam Phillips
Publisher	Fiona Foley

PREFACE

The purpose of this book is to provide a comprehensive account, in words and pictures, of infectious diseases. The emphasis is on clinical appearances but many illustrations of radiology, gross and microscopic pathology and pathogenic microorganisms are also included. In selecting material for inclusion in this book we have concentrated on the needs of physicians and other clinical workers, but there is also much which will be of interest to clinical microbiologists.

We hope that the book will be useful as an aid to the recognition and diagnosis of infectious disease, and that it will also facilitate an understanding of the pathogenesis of a wide variety of infections. The book is also intended to provide a source of visual material for those teaching the subject of infectious diseases.

We have tried to do justice to both rare and common infectious diseases, and to include illustrations of important common conditions which some might not think worth photographing. Our aim has been to include most infectious diseases of global importance, since what may seem a somewhat obscure condition to the reader in one part of the world may be of great significance in another country or continent.

ACKNOWLEDGEMENTS

This collection of slides could not have been assembled without the generous collaboration of many friends and colleagues in various parts of the world. We wish to express here our appreciation to all of them; the sources of individual slides are given in the captions.

Large groups of slides or other special help (or both) were provided by the following individuals: Dr J. Douglas Balentine, Dr J. R. Cantey, Dr Alan N. Carlson, Dr R. Duncan Catterall, Dr J. Clay, Dr Michael B. Cohen, Dr John T. Cunningham, Dr Joel K. Curé, Dr Christopher Edwards, Dr Benjamin K. Fisher, Dr Paul D. Garen, Professor Alasdair M. Geddes, Dr Gordon R. Hennigar, Dr. Thomas W. Holbrook, Dr H. Preston Holley, Ms Mary Jenkins, Dr R. Duren Johnson, Dr Stewart Knutton, Professor Harold P. Lambert, Dr David A. Lewis, Dr J. Newman, Dr Sidney Olanskey, Dr Lawrence C. Parrish, Ms A. Elena Prevost, Dr Eleanor S. Sahn and Dr T. F. Sellers, Jr.

Irene Burr prepared portions of the manuscript with much patience and expertise.

At Gower, Stephen McGrath, Ian Spick, Zak Knowles and Fiona Foley deserve special thanks for their patience, cooperation and commitment.

Finally, we thank Carver, Stephanie, Janet and Diana for their essential support and encouragement in this effort.

WEF
MJW
JAI
HT

Charleston, Birmingham and Stoke-on-Trent, 1991.

PICTURE ACKNOWLEDGEMENTS

We are grateful to the authors of the following books for allowing us to reproduce their illustrations in *Infectious Diseases*. (The first figure reference is from *Infectious Diseases;* the number in parentheses refers to the original publication).

Gordon AG, Lewis BV. *Gynaecological Endoscopy.* London: Chapman and Hall, 1988: 7.88 (4.7).

Hoffbrand AV, Pettit JE. *Clinical Haematology Illustrated.* Oxford: Pergamon Medical Publications, 1982: 13.33 (16.7); 13.34 (16.14).

Ioachim HL. *Pathology of AIDS.* New York: Gower Medical Publishing, 1988: 14.1 (I 1.3A); 14.7 (II 2.26); 14.8 (II 2.25); 14.11 (II 4.3); 14.15 (II 5.74); 14.16 (II 5.44); 14.17 (I 3.1); 14.18 (II 5.49); 14.19 (II 5.80); 14.22 (I 3.5); 14.25 (I 9.1); 14.28 (II 5.76); 14.29 (II 5.77); 14.37 (II 5.8); 14.38 (II 4.60); 14.41 (I 7.4); 14.42 (I 7.5); 14.44 (II 9.47); 14.46 (II 9.61); 14.48 (II 9.64); 14.49 (II 6.1); 14.50 (II 3.2).

Misiewicz JJ, Bartram CI, Cotton PB, Mee AS, Price AB, Thompson RPH. *Atlas of Clinical Gastroenterology.* London: Edward Arnold, 1987: 4.4 (2.48); 4.9 (2.49); 4.35 (6.26); 4.51 (6.17); 4.53 (6.16); 4.58 (9.7); 4.59 (9.2); 4.68 (9.41); 4.70 (9.36); 4.71 (9.40); 4.72 (9.43); 4.73 (6.22); 4.78 (5.38); 4.79 (5.39); 4.84 (5.36); 4.85 (5.37); 4.86 (5.34); 4.92 (9.16); 4.95 (9.17); 4.98 (9.13); 4.99 (9.14); 4.106 (6.1); 4.126 (6.15); 4.133 (6.13); 4.137 (6.4); 4.142 (6.8); 4.144 (6.9); 4.149 (6.6); 4.150 (6.11 RIGHT); 4.156 (6.12); 5.15 (17.11); 5.16 (17.16); 5.17 (17.14); 5.18 (17.13); 5.19 (17.12); 5.20 (17.19); 5.21 (17.20); 5.23 (19.13); 5.24 (19.14); 5.30 (17.22); 5.31 (17.21); 5.48 (17.54); 5.49 (17.52); 5.50 (17.53); 5.54 (17.56); 5.60 (20.43); 7.62 (13.37); 7.65 (13.38); 7.80 (13.36).

Morse S, Thompson S, Moreland A. *Atlas of Sexually Transmitted Diseases.* New York: Gower Medical Publishing, 1989: 7.21 (9.9); 7.68 (3.22); 7.81 (10.35); 7.19 (6.30).

Perkin D, Rose FC, Blackwood W, Shawdon HH. *Atlas of Clinical Neurology.* London: Baillière Tindall, 1986: 3.47 (9.50); 3.49 (13.9); 3.55 (9.48); 3.90 (9.30); 3.129 (2.11); 3.140 (2.9 LEFT).

Spalton DJ, Hitchings RA, Hunter PA. *Atlas of Clinical Ophthalmology.* Edinburgh: Churchill Livingstone, 1984: 12.3 (4.40); 12.25 (4.27); 12.38 (4.11); 12.40 (4.12); 12.47 (4.45); 12.50 (4.47); 12.51 (4.48); 12.53 (4.49); 12.56 (4.52); 12.57 (4.43); 12.62 (10.41); 12.64 (10.42); 12.73 (14.55):

Weiss MA, Mills SE *Atlas of Genitourinary Tract Disorders.* New York: Gower Medical Publishing, 1988: 6.3 (10.5); 6.16 (6.18); 6.22 (9.9); 6.47 (17.14); 6.49 (15.17).

CONTENTS

CONTENTS

THE HEAD AND NECK

1

GINGIVOSTOMATITIS

Host defences against infection of the mouth are extremely complex. The normal oral flora includes over one hundred bacterial species, many anaerobic, whose presence contributes to protection against disease by the production of bactericidal substances, by the depletion of nutrients and by their influence on oxygen tension. The flow of saliva provides secretory IgA, peroxidase, which interacts with thiocyanate ions in food and hydrogen peroxide produced by commensal bacteria, lysozyme and lactoferrin, which chelates the iron required for bacterial metabolism. Other salivary proteins may inhibit the adhesion of bacteria to teeth or mucosal surfaces. The rapid turnover of oral epithelium also helps to remove bacteria which have adhered to epithelial cells. Polymorphonuclear leucocytes which are able to phagocytose bacteria, enter the oral cavity in the saliva and by diapedesis through capillary walls.

Vincent's infection

Vincent's infection (acute necrotising ulcerative gingivitis) is a periodontal infection generally seen in young adults. Risk factors include poor oral hygiene, debility and possibly emotional stress. The infection causes ulceration of the gingiva, particularly in the interdental areas; necrosis of the epithelium may produce a pseudomembrane in which fibrin, bacteria and leucocytes are caught up (Fig. 1.1). Bleeding is common and the lesions are very painful. In more severe cases there is regional lymphadenopathy, fever and malaise. Sometimes the infection spreads to involve the tonsils, a development which causes intense painful dysphagia (Vincent's angina). Bacteriological investigation reveals mixed infection with treponemes, such as *Borrelia vincenti*, and fusobacteria (Fig. 1.2). The infection responds rapidly to treatment with a short course of metronidazole, but attention should also be given to dental hygiene and any correctable cause of debility once the acute illness has settled down.

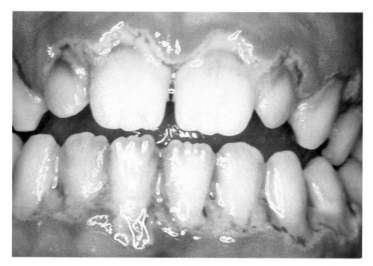

Fig. 1.1 Acute necrotizing ulcerative gingivitis (Vincent's infection). Ulceration of the gingival margin spreading into the gums.

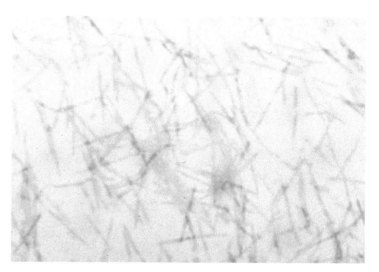

Fig. 1.2 *Fusobacterium*, a genus of gram-negative anaerobic bacteria common in the mouth, here seen as delicate rods with tapering ends.

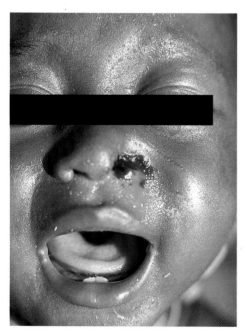

Fig. 1.3 Noma. An early lesion showing destruction of nostril and inflammatory swelling below the left cheek.

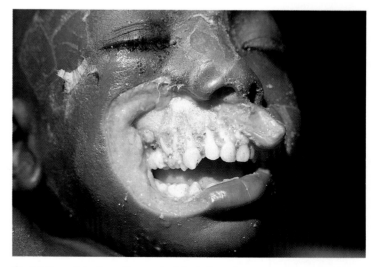

Fig. 1.4 Noma. Late stage with necrosis of cheek, lips and gum.

Noma

Noma (cancrum oris) is a severe, locally destructive oral infection seen in children debilitated by malnutrition or other chronic disease. It is found only in poorer parts of Africa, South America and Asia. Like Vincent's infection it is caused by a mixture of spirochaetes and fusiform anaerobic bacteria, and it may begin with a small ulcer of the gingiva. The lesion spreads rapidly to produce gangrene of the lips, cheeks and jaw (Figs 1.3 & 1.4).

Treatment with metronidazole or penicillin controls the infection but the ultimate outcome depends on the disability caused by tissue destruction and on the scope for relieving the underlying cause of the child's ill health.

Herpes simplex

Primary infection

Gingivostomatitis is the commonest clinical manifestation of primary infection with Herpes simplex virus, type 1 (HSV 1). Rare in infancy because of passive immunity from the mother, it reaches its peak incidence between the ages of 1 and 5 years. The incidence then drops in later childhood before rising again to a second, though much lower peak in early adult life. Man is the only source of the infection and the usual mode of transmission is through contaminated saliva. The virus can frequently be isolated from asymptomatic individuals and so the source of infection is not always clinically apparent. Direct contact with an infected person, often by kissing, seems to be important; airborne transmission is less likely to occur. About 80% of non-immune subjects exposed to infected material themselves become infected.

The illness starts with systemic features of fever and irritability followed by the appearance of inflammation of the gingiva. Vesicles appear on the tongue, gingiva, lips, buccal mucosa and hard palate; they are soon deroofed to form shallow ulcers which may coalesce (Figs 1.5 & 1.6). The lesions are very painful, bleed easily and are often covered by a greyish black membrane. Vesicular lesions may also appear on the skin surrounding the mouth (Fig. 1.7), and additional lesions may develop at sites such as the nose, eye, fingernails (Fig. 1.8) and perineum, presumably

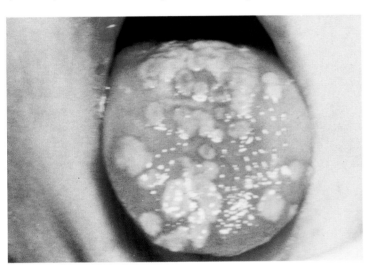

Fig. 1.5 Herpes simplex. Numerous shallow ulcers filled with white exudate on the tongue of a young child with primary herpes simplex infection.

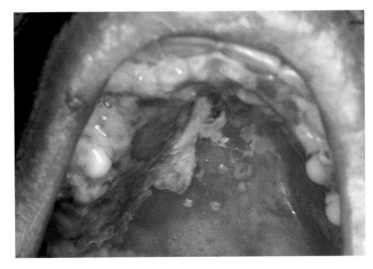

Fig. 1.6 Primary herpes simplex. Ulceration of palate and gums.

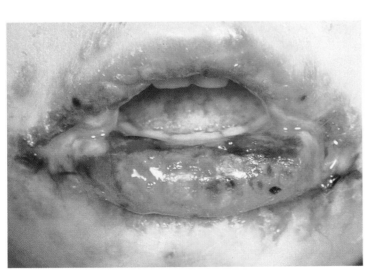

Fig. 1.7 Herpes simplex. Vesicular lesions on the skin of the upper and lower lips and cheeks of a child with primary herpes simplex infection.

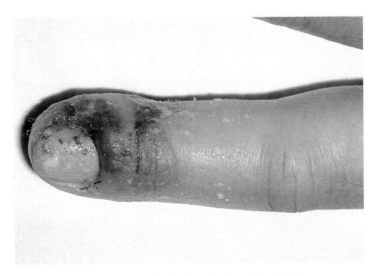

Fig. 1.8 Herpetic whitlow. Primary infection of a nail bed in a child with simultaneous primary herpes simplex infection of the mouth, often mistaken for bacterial paronychia.

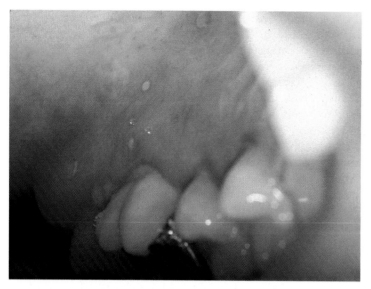

Fig. 1.9 Herpetic stomatitis. Oral ulceration following sexual transmission of HSV 2, showing buccal lesions in the mouth of a woman infected through orogenital contact.

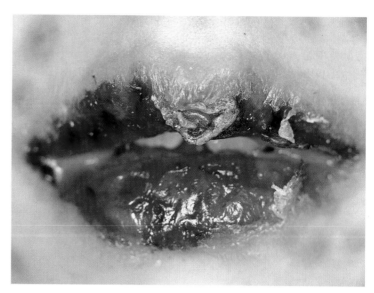

Fig. 1.10 Stevens–Johnson syndrome. Ulceration of the lips with surrounding skin affected by erythema multiforme.

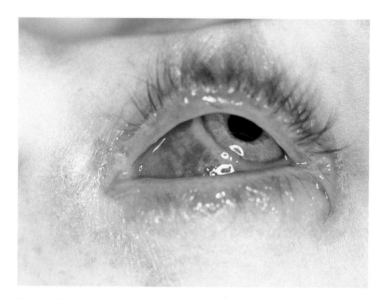

Fig. 1.11 Conjunctival inflammation in Stevens–Johnson syndrome.

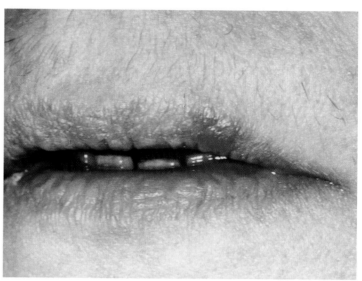

Fig. 1.12 Herpes simplex. Groups of vesicles on the mucocutaneous margin of the lip. These are typical of the early stage of recurrent disease.

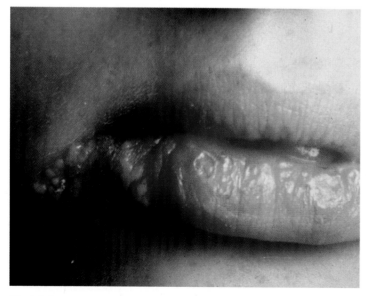

Fig. 1.13 Herpes simplex. Later stage of recurrent disease showing pustule formation and scabbing.

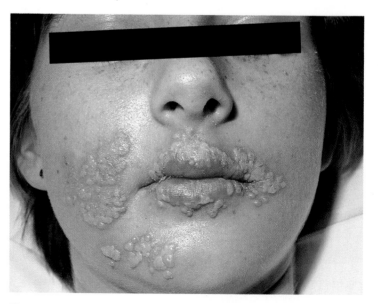

Fig. 1.14 Herpes simplex. Severe example of recurrent disease.

by autoinoculation. Accompanying the local lesions there may be regional or generalized lymphadenopathy and splenomegaly. There may be lymphocytosis of the peripheral blood and biochemical evidence of mild hepatitis.

Primary infection of the mouth may also be caused by HSV 2 (herpes genitalis) (Fig. 1.9).

The diagnosis can be confirmed by isolating HSV from the saliva or by the examination of biopsies. However, the clinical appearance and age of the patient is usually enough to allow a confident diagnosis to be made. The main cause of confusion in older patients is Stevens–Johnson syndrome, which produces a similar appearance of the lips and mouth (Fig. 1.10). However, in Stevens–Johnson syndrome there is often inflammation of other mucous membranes and a generalized skin eruption of erythema multiforme (Fig 1.11)

The illness is generally a self-limiting one with resolution after 10–14 days. The main clinical problems are with the control of pain, the maintenance of good oral hygiene and the provision of an adequate intake of fluids, by the intravenous route where necessary. In severe cases rapid improvement may follow the use of intravenous acyclovir. Specific viral complications are uncommon although occasional cases of herpetic encephalitis follow immediately after primary gingivostomatitis.

Secondary infection

Following primary infection, HSV migrates to the sensory nerve ganglion of the affected dermatome and persists there indefinitely in latent form. At a later date the virus becomes reactivated, migrates down the sensory nerve and causes a painful local skin eruption close to the site of the original primary infection. These reactivations occur in about 45% of subjects who had an oral primary lesion. In addition, many people who never have secondary herpetic lesions intermittently shed the virus from the mouth.

Reactivation of latent herpetic infection may be provoked by fever, sunlight, trauma to the sensory nerve nucleus and possibly psychological stress. Hormonal factors are presumably involved in the regular recurrences experienced by some women during menstrual periods. In general the risk of reactivation declines with increasing age.

The commonest site of recurrent HSV 1 infection is the lip, particularly the mucocutaneous junction (Figs 1.12, 1.13 & 1.14). In spite of the extensive intra-oral involvement seen in primary lesions, secondary lesions within the mouth are very rare except in patients with HIV infection, among whom atypical recurrences of herpes simplex infection are seen (Fig. 1.15).

Other sites of secondary lesions are the nose and the skin of the cheeks or chin. The first sign of reactivation is a tingling sensation of the skin for about 24 hours. This is followed by the eruption of vesicles which rupture after 1–2 days to leave an area of ulceration. The lesion is painful but less so than in primary herpetic infection.

Treatment with oral or topical acyclovir may shorten the illness if it is started at an early stage. Oral acyclovir is also effective for prophylaxis in patients who experience frequent recurrences.

Intra-oral Herpes Varicella–Zoster

Chicken pox (see Chapter 11) often causes a sparse eruption of vesicles within the mouth, particularly on the palate (Fig. 1.16). These are soon deroofed by abrasion from the tongue or food, leaving a number of small ulcers. Herpes varicella–zoster virus is shed from these lesions into the mouth and is probably important as a source of infectious secretions which spread the disease by the airborne route.

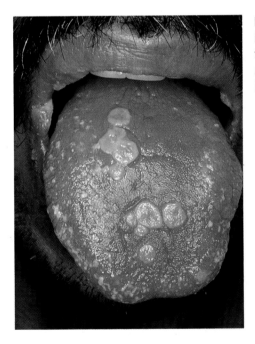

Fig. 1.15 Recurrent HSV1 infection. Ulceration of the tongue in a patient with AIDS. By courtesy of Dr B. K. Fisher.

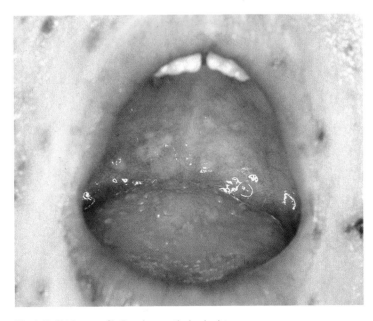

Fig. 1.16 Chicken pox. Shallow ulcers on the hard palate.

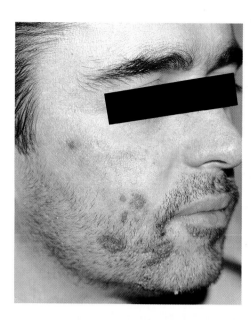

Fig. 1.17 Shingles. Rash involving maxillary division of the trigeminal nerve.

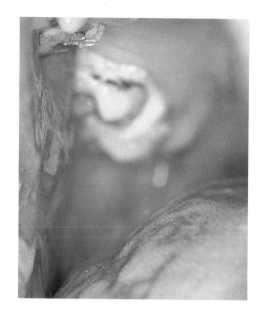

Fig. 1.18 Shingles. Ulceration of buccal mucosa with purulent exudate (same patient as Fig. 1.17).

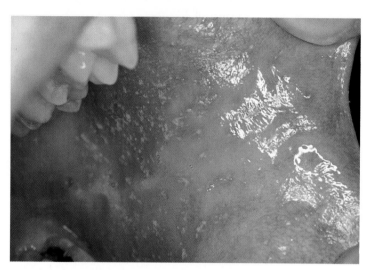

Fig. 1.19 Measles, with Koplik's spots on the buccal mucosa. This is an unusually severe case, enough to cause considerable discomfort when feeding.

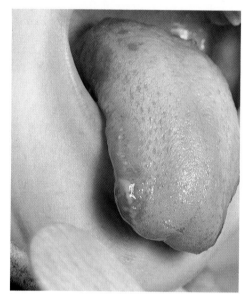

Fig. 1.20 Hand, foot and mouth disease. Ulceration of the tip of the tongue.

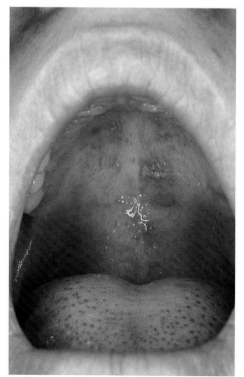

Fig. 1.21 Hand, foot and mouth disease. Ulcers on the hard palate and tongue.

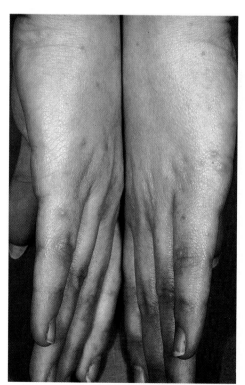

Fig. 1.22 Hand, foot and mouth disease. Lesions on hands in the same patient as Fig. 1.21.

Shingles (see chapter 11) produces intra-oral lesions when it affects the maxillary division of the trigeminal nerve. The condition always affects the overlying skin as well. Typical symptoms are pain followed by the appearance over the buccal mucosa of irregular vesicles which rapidly develop into shallow ulcers. The ulcers are surrounded by a rim of hyperaemic mucosa and may be covered by a thin grey film of exudate (Figs 1.17 & 1.18).

Measles

Measles (see Chapter 11) always affects the buccal mucosa with generalized hyperaemia which gives it a bright red, velvety appearance. In addition Koplik's spots (Fig. 1.19), tiny white lesions similar to damp grains of salt on the mucosa opposite the premolar teeth may be seen in many cases. These are highly specific for measles and, as they tend to precede the development of the exanthem, they may allow an early diagnosis to be made.

Hand, foot and mouth disease

This condition is characterized by the appearance of ulcers in the mouth and a maculopapular or vesicular rash on the hands and feet. It is caused by infection with coxsackie virus (usually type A16 but occasionally other types) and often appears in small outbreaks within families. It incubates for 4–7 days and generally affects young children. The painful oral lesions are ulcers or vesicles distributed anteriorly on the lips, palate, tongue and buccal mucosa (Figs 1.20, 1.21 & 1.22). Systemic features and lymphadenopathy are absent and recovery is uneventful.

Candidiasis

Candida species growing in the budding yeast form are normally found in small numbers among the commensal flora of the mouth, large bowel and vagina. The most common species is *Candida albicans,* which behaves as an opportunistic pathogen. The size of the Candida population is kept in check by several host defence functions, including the presence of normal bacterial commensal flora, which secrete antifungal substances and compete for nutrients. Healthy subjects may be affected by oral candidiasis when treated with broad spectrum antibiotics. Other conditions predisposing to candidiasis include the use of systemic corticosteroids or other immunosuppressive drugs, the use of inhaled corticosteroids for asthma, diabetes mellitus and depression of cell-mediated immunity. Trauma to the gingiva from ill-fitting dentures may increase the above risks. In addition, chronic candidiasis associated with skin infection is seen in hypoadrenalism, hypoparathyroidism and a number of inherited immunological disorders such as DiGeorge syndrome and chronic familial mucocutaneous candidiasis.

The most common appearance (pseudomembranous candidiasis) is of a white, curd-like exudate applied to the buccal or gingival mucosa, the palate, the posterior part of the tongue and sometimes the pharynx (Fig. 1.23). The exudate is easily displaced revealing the erythematous and sometimes bleeding mucosa below. Swabs taken in this way usually show yeast forms and pseudohyphae made up of strands of elongated cells and hyphae penetrating the epithelium. The organism can be cultured on Sabouraud's agar (Fig. 1.24).

Other clinical varieties include atrophic candidiasis, which appears as a flat red lesion on the tongue or palate, and angular cheilitis.

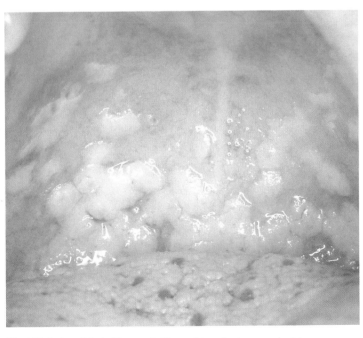

Fig. 1.23 Oral candidiasis. Plaques of white exudate on the tongue and palate.

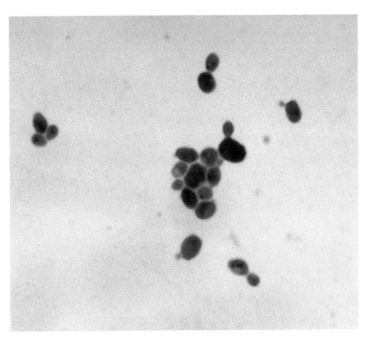

Fig. 1.24 *Candida albicans.* Smear from culture on Sabouraud's medium showing the yeast from of the oval gram-positive structures. In clinical specimens of a mixture of yeast and mycelial forms is often seen.

Oral candidiasis is a particularly common feature of AIDS and AIDS-related complexes (Fig. 1.25). It is often the earliest clinical sign of HIV infection and may persist for months. Oesophageal infection frequently coexists and causes painful dysphagia.

Oral candidiasis is treated by removing any of the above predisposing factors, where this is possible. In some cases this is all that is required – if not then local treatment with lozenges of nystatin or amphotericin should be used. If oral candidiasis is particularly persistent in patients with immunodeficiency, treatment with oral fluconazole is indicated. The regular use of chlorhexidine mouthwashes may help to prevent oral candidiasis in patients at risk of infection.

Oral hairy leucoplakia

Hairy leucoplakia is a fixed white lesion of the oral mucosa seen in patients with HIV infection. It is most commonly found on the lateral margins of the tongue, where it may have a corrugated pattern with vertical ridges. It can spread to cover any extent of the tongue either as a single or as multiple lesions (Fig. 1.26). Histological examination shows benign epithelial hyperplasia (Fig. 1.27), and the presence of Epstein–Barr virus in affected cells has been demonstrated by a number of techniques (Fig. 1.28). Treatment is unnecessary as the condition seldom causes symptoms.

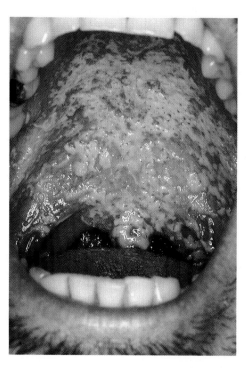

Fig. 1.25 Oral candidiasis. Severe infection in a patient with AIDS.

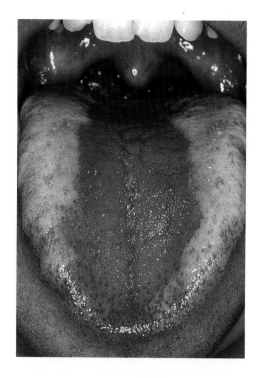

Fig. 1.26 Hairy leucoplakia. Typical distribution of white discolouration along the edges of the tongue.

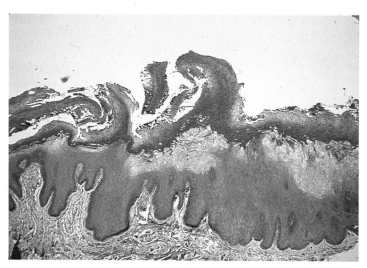

Fig. 1.27 Hairy leucoplakia. Histological appearance showing hyperkeratosis and vacuolation of clumps of prickle cells. There is little subepithelial inflammation. By courtesy of Dr M. B. Cohen.

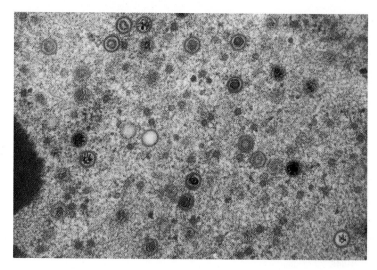

Fig. 1.28 Hairy leucoplakia. Electron micrograph showing intranuclear Epstein–Barr virus particles. ×100 000. By courtesy of Prof. J. S. Greenspan.

PHARYNGOTONSILLITIS

A wide variety of bacteria and viruses are capable of causing pharyngeal infection. The interpretation of microbiological studies is difficult, because for many organisms that can be pathogens at this site there are nasopharyngeal carrier states in which no harmful effects can be detected. The nature of the balance between commensal and pathogenic function is poorly understood in many instances but presumably involves specific immunity and the prescence of other bacterial species which may exert some kind of antimicrobial effect.

The most common infective causes are group A β-haemolytic streptococci, adenoviruses, enteroviruses and influenza, parainfluenza and Epstein–Barr viruses. Generally speaking it is not possible to determine the cause of pharyngotonsillitis by inspection. All relevant organisms can cause signs of acute inflammation extending over the pharynx or tonsils. However, there are some local and distant features which favour one or another group of organisms.

Streptococcal tonsillitis

Group A β-haemolytic streptococci are the most common bacterial cause of tonsillitis and account for 25–30% of all cases. There is a wide range of clinical severity, from mild inflammation with little systemic disturbance to an acute disabling fever accompanied by severe dysphagia, intense local inflammation and tender local lymphadenopathy. The tonsils may be deep red in colour and partially covered with a thick yellowish exudate (Fig. 1.29).

The diagnosis of streptococcal tonsillitis can only be made with certainty by identifying the organism in samples taken from the throat (Fig. 1.30). The importance of doing so depends on the approach to treatment, bearing in mind the risk of non-infective complications such as rheumatic fever and acute glomerulonephritis. Any one of three approaches can be used:

• Treat all cases of tonsillitis with an antistreptococcal antibiotic without investigation. This ensures that all patients who might benefit from such treatment will do so, including those with undiagnosed diphtheria, and it extends this benefit to those cases with false negative cultures of throat swabs. However, it unnecessarily exposes two-thirds of patients to the risk of drug toxicity.

• Take a throat swab and wait for the result before prescribing an antibiotic for confirmed streptococcal disease. This represents the ultimate degree of economy in drug use, but assumes that the only important action of antibiotic treatment is to prevent rheumatic fever (and possibly glomerulonephritis) – treatment within the first week of acute infection seems to be enough to prevent these risks. However, there is some evidence that the symptoms of streptococcal tonsillitis improve more rapidly when an antibiotic has been given and the personal and economic value of this effect should not be underrated. Moreover, while the patient is still harbouring viable streptococci he/she is able to transmit the infection to others.

• Take a throat swab from all patients, start antibiotic treatment and discontinue it if the result of the culture is negative. This seems to be the most beneficial approach where circumstances permit.

Attempts to speed up diagnosis by the identification of streptococci in tonsillar exudate by Gram stain of a direct smear have been uniformly unsatisfactory. However, rapid results can be obtained with methods which detect group A β-haemolytic streptococcal antigens in throat swab material. A number of kits are now available employing either latex agglutination or enzymic techniques, usable outside the laboratory and giving results within an hour.

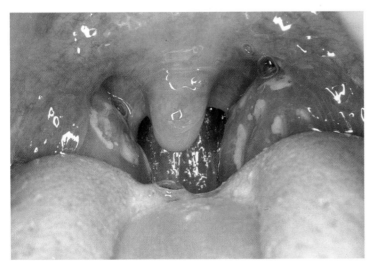

Fig. 1.29 Streptococcal tonsillitis. Intense erythema of the tonsils and surrounding tissue with a creamy-yellow exudate.

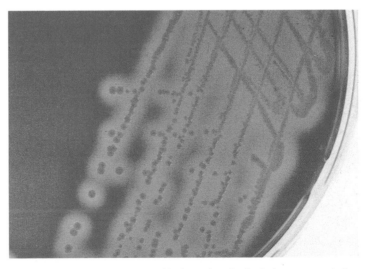

Fig. 1.30 *Streptococcus pyogenes* on a blood agar plate. Small colonies are surrounded by a clear zone of β-haemolysis.

Scarlet fever

Certain strains of *Streptococcus pyogenes* produce an erythrogenic toxin which causes scarlet fever in susceptible subjects (see chapter 10). Examination of the mouth reveals, in addition to the local effects on the tonsils, abnormalities of the tongue. Initially the tongue is covered by a white exudate through which the papillae project (the white strawberry tongue – Fig. 1.31). Later the exudate is shed to reveal bright red inflammation of the underlying tissue (the red strawberry tongue – Fig. 1.32).

Anaerobic tonsillitis

Anaerobic tonsillitis is a rare but severe condition characterized by necrosis and by spread of infection. Initially this spread takes place locally, but if it involves the jugular vein metastatic spread may result in septic embolization of the lungs, joints and central nervous system. The most commonly isolated organism is *Fusobacterium necrophorum*.

Peritonsillitis

Peritonsillar cellulitis and abscess (quinsy) are important complications of sore throat. Their onset is marked by an increasing intensity of painful dysphagia, the development of trismus and, frequently, radiation of pain to the ear. On examination the patient is febrile and has tender enlargement of the tonsillar lymph nodes. The anatomy of the fauces is distorted by swelling of the peritonsillar tissues, often obscuring the tonsil itself, and the soft palate and uvula are displaced to the opposite side (Fig. 1.33). There may be an area of marked reddening over the abscess itself, indicating that it is close to discharging into the oral cavity. The condition is almost always unilateral.

Microbiological sampling of peritonsillar abscesses yields a mixed growth of predominantly anaerobic organisms, particularly *Bacteroides melaninogenicus* and *Fusobacterium* species. *S. pyogenes* is isolated in about 25% of cases. Treatment is by surgical drainage where an abscess has developed and by appropriate antibiotics. Penicillin is usually effective but if penicillin-resistant

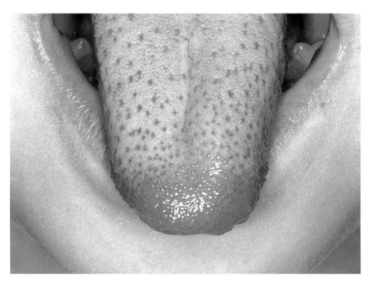

Fig. 1.31 White strawberry tongue.

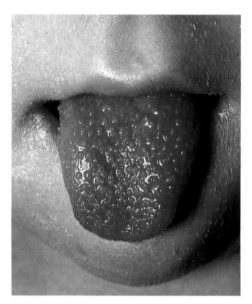

Fig. 1.32 Scarlet fever. Red strawberry tongue. The white coating has peeled off to reveal the deep red tongue with its projecting papillae.

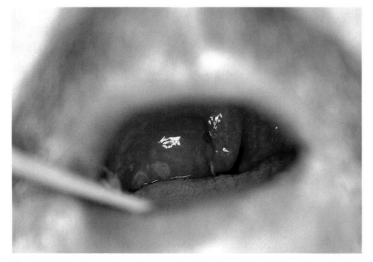

Fig. 1.33 Peritonsillar abscess. Gross swelling of the tissues in front of the right tonsil with displacement of the uvula to the left. Trismus prevents the patient from opening the mouth fully.

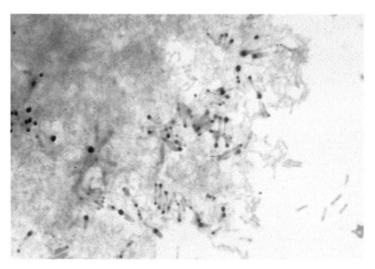

Fig. 1.34 *Corynebacterium diphtheriae*, here seen as straight or slightly curved green rods. The volutin granules stain black with this method. Albert's stain.

anaerobes are present metronidazole should be added or clindamycin substituted.

Diphtheria

Diphtheria is caused by infection with *Corynebacterium diphtheriae*, a gram-positive bacillus (Fig. 1.34) which produces an extremely potent exotoxin. Its clinical features arise partly from the local inflammatory effect at the site of implantation and partly from the distant effects of the toxin on the heart and the nervous system. Most cases appear in children and affect the upper respiratory tract, but in tropical and subtropical countries skin infections also occur. Transmission is usually by airborne spread of respiratory droplets but skin infection may spread by direct contact. Asymptomatic carriers, particularly those who harbour the organism in the nose, are an important source of infection.

The disease, which incubates for 2–6 days, is one of gradual onset with systemic features becoming more

severe over a period of up to a week. These include low grade fever, headache, weakness and vomiting. Local symptoms of pain in the respiratory tract may be surprisingly mild, especially in children.

Infection limited to the nose causes a purulent nasal discharge, sometimes blood stained, but significant amounts of toxin are seldom absorbed from this site. Similarly, toxin absorption is usually slight in infection limited to the surface of one or both tonsils.

More severe effects are expected where the infection spreads to involve the pharynx and larynx. The affected mucosa is covered by a thick, firmly adherent membrane, dirty brown or green in colour (Fig. 1.35) and made up of bacteria, desquamated epithelial cells, leucocytes, fibrin and blood. It can be dislodged only with difficulty and if this is done the tissue below bleeds. The presence of such a membrane in the larynx or trachea can cause respiratory embarrassment (Fig. 1.36). Local lymph node enlargement is common and the surrounding oedema of the subcutaneous tissues may cause a 'bull neck' appearance (Fig. 1.37). From the pharynx and larynx enough toxin may be absorbed to produce serious complications. These are first seen in the heart towards the end of the first week of the illness. They may take the form of circulatory collapse caused by a direct toxic effect on the myocardium, tachyarrythmias or conduction defects. ECG changes are common and myocarditis is associated with elevated serum levels of glutamic oxalacetic transaminase.

Neurological complications arise somewhat later as a result of toxic demyelination. The first sign comes in the third week with the development of palatal palsy which causes difficulty in swallowing and an abnormal tone of the voice. In the fourth week ocular and facial paralysis may develop, and by the seventh week signs of pseudobulbar palsy may appear. Paralysis of the limbs or respiratory muscles is rare.

The laboratory diagnosis of diphtheria starts with the isolation of a corynebacterium from specimens taken from the site of infection. It is then necessary to distinguish it by biochemical tests from other diphtheroid organisms and to determine if it has the capacity to produce toxin by

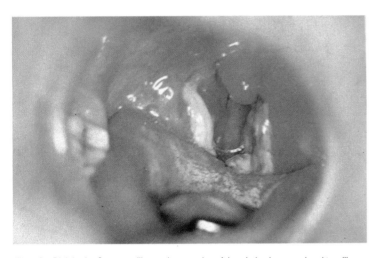

Fig. 1.35 Diphtheria. Gross swelling and congestion of the whole pharyngeal and tonsillar area. A dirty white exudate covers the tonsils and is spreading to the posterior pharyngeal wall. By courtesy of Dr K. Nye.

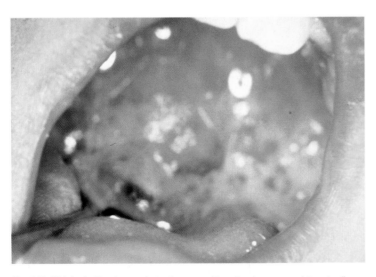

Fig. 1.36 Diphtheria. Respiratory obstruction caused by extensive grey exudate extending over the whole pharyngeal area and obscuring the normal anatomical features.

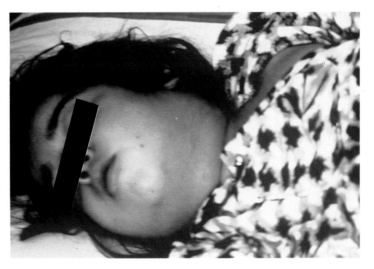

Fig. 1.37 Diphtheria. 'Bull neck' appearance found in severe cases with periglandular oedema extending from cheek to clavicle.

guinea pig inoculation or by immunoprecipitation (Elek's test).

Treatment for suspected diphtheria must proceed without waiting for laboratory confirmation of the diagnosis. Diphtheria antitoxin is given in a dose of 20 000–100 000 units intravenously after a preliminary intradermal test for hypersensitivity. An antibiotic (usually penicillin or erythromycin) is given to relieve the local lesion and to prevent further production of toxin. In laryngeal diphtheria a tracheostomy may be required to maintain the airway and, where there is a risk of cardiotoxicity, cardiac monitoring with provision for any necessary therapeutic interventions should be performed. Rarely, in cases of pharyngeal diphtheria, necrosis of the soft palate may be severe enough to cause perforation (Fig. 1.38).

Meningococcal Infection

Meningococcal infection is spread by the respiratory route and appears to be able to cause mild pharyngitis which in some cases is a prelude to septicaemia. The pharyngitis itself has no clinical distinguishing features but in meningococcal septicaemia the petechial rash which is present in about half of the cases may occasionally involve the mucous membranes of the mouth (Fig. 1.39).

Infectious mononucleosis

Epstein–Barr virus (EBV) is a member of the herpes virus group. It has the specific ability to infect B lymphocytes which undergo blast transformation and are stimulated to produce antibody. Viral DNA is incorporated into the genome of the cell and the infection of the B cell line persists indefinitely. B cell stimulation provokes a vigorous immunological response in which T lymphocytes proliferate, suppressing and destroying some of the infected B cells. It is this proliferation of T cells that is responsible for the presence of 'atypical' mononuclear cells in the peripheral blood (Fig. 1.40) and causes the acute lymphadenopathy and splenomegaly found in some patients. Eventually the T cell response eliminates almost all of the infected B cells and the illness subsides. However, a small number of infected B cells persists in the lymphoid tissue of the oropharynx and possibly the salivary glands.

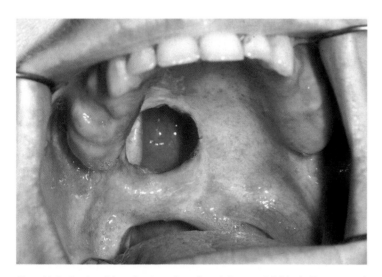

Fig. 1.38 Perforation of the soft palate, a late effect of pharyngeal diphtheria. By courtesy of Dr C. J. Meryon.

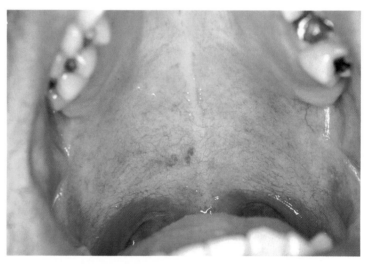

Fig. 1.39 Meningococcal septicaemia. Petechiae on the hard palate.

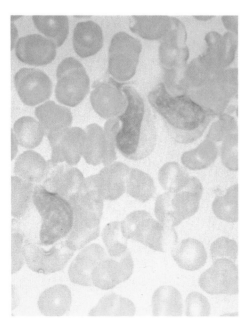

Fig. 1.40 Blood film showing atypical lymphocytes in infectious mononucleosis.

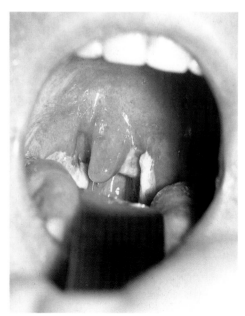

Fig. 1.41 Infectious monucleosis. Swollen tonsils and uvula with a white exudate. There are petechiae on the soft palate.

Lifelong latent infection follows and, although recurrence of symptoms is unusual, intermittent salivary excretion of EBV over long periods is well documented.

EBV infection induces a range of diseases in man. Its clinical manifestations depend to a considerable extent on the age of the patient when first infected. Where infection is acquired in early childhood no distinctive illness is produced. However, during adolescence and early adult life infection causes the syndrome of infectious mononucleosis in about 50% of susceptible subjects. Epidemiological observations show that in countries where domestic overcrowding is common and hygiene is poor, 90% of children have serological evidence of EBV infection by the age of 2 years. However, in Western countries many children remain susceptible until teenage, when the major method of spread seems to be by kissing.

The characteristic features of infectious mononucleosis are fever, tonsillitis, generalized lymphadenopathy, splenomegaly and hepatitis. The fever persists for about 2 weeks and is associated with general malaise and fatigue, although the patient does not look severely ill. The tonsils are enlarged, often to a very marked degree, and covered with a white exudate (Fig. 1.41). Superficial lymphadenopathy is common and is most often seen in the neck (Fig. 1.42). The glands, which are soft and mobile, are not usually painful and there is no surrounding inflammatory reaction. Splenomegaly can be detected clinically in about 50% of patients and is greatest towards the end of the first week of illness. Clinical hepatomegaly is less common although biochemical tests of liver function are usually abnormal. A mild erythematous macular rash is occasionally present for 1–2 days in the early stages; where treatment has been given with ampicillin a vasculitic maculopapular eruption almost always follows. (This is a temporary susceptibility and does not imply that the patient is also allergic to penicillin.)

Complications of infectious mononucleosis include haemolytic anaemia, thrombocytopenia, meningoencephalitis, Guillain–Barré syndrome, mononeuritis (Fig. 1.44) and transverse myelitis. Splenic rupture has occasionally been reported, and in small children with excessive enlargement of pharyngeal lymphoid tissue, asphyxia has occurred (Fig. 1.45).

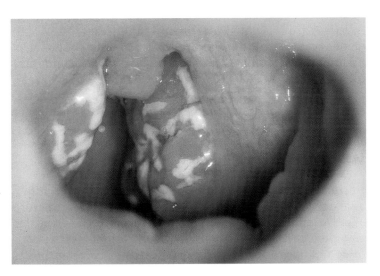

Fig. 1.42 Infectious mononucleosis. Gross tonsillar enlargement with a white exudate.

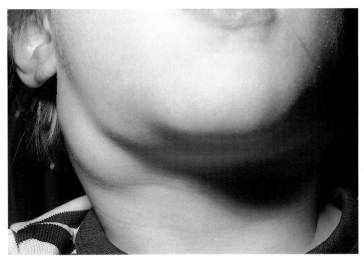

Fig. 1.43 Infectious mononucleosis. Cervical lymphadenitis with no visible sign of acute inflammation.

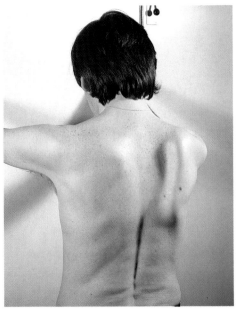

Fig. 1.44 Infectious monucleosis. Wing scapula caused by paralysis of the nerve to serratus anterior.

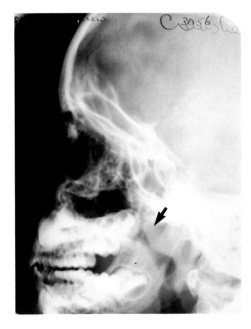

Fig. 1.45 Infectious mononucleosis. Lateral x-ray showing narrowing of the posterior nasal airway (arrowed) by enlarged lymphoid tissue.

Fatal cases of EBV infection are rare but have been observed in kindreds with an X-linked recessive immune defect known as Duncan's Disease. In male members of affected families EBV infection may cause a fulminant illness with only B lymphocyte proliferation and the development of a lymphoma-like condition. (Unlike a true lymphoma, the B lymphocyte proliferation is polyclonal.) In other cases the infection seems to wipe out all the B lymphocytes and agammaglobulinaemia follows.

Laboratory diagnosis of infectious mononucleosis starts with the examination of a film of peripheral blood. Absolute lymphocytosis is found and there will be large numbers of 'atypical' mononuclear cells. In most patients with symptomatic infection with EBV the serum contains a heterophile antibody capable of agglutinating sheep red cells. This antibody can be detected by the Paul–Bunnell test or by one of the rapid screening slide tests derived from it. Heterophile antibody is not usually present in subclinical infection with EBV. A number of other infections, such as cytomegalovirus and toxoplasmosis may induce similar changes in the blood film, but without heterophile antibody.

Occasionally the appearance of heterophile antibody is delayed or absent and the specific diagnosis then depends on the demonstration of EBV-specific antibodies. Antibodies to viral capsid antigen (VCA) are detectable in the form of IgG and IgM. They appear early and are almost always present by the time symptoms are present. IgG to VCA persists indefinitely and its presence only confirms EBV infection at some time in the past. IgM to VCA lasts for only 4–8 weeks and its detection confirms recent EBV infection. Antibody to early antigen (EA) is slower to appear (3–4 weeks after onset) and can be found in only 70% of cases. Antibody to Epstein–Barr nuclear antigen (EBNA) also appears late (3–4 weeks) but it can reliably be detected in all infections. Thus the demonstration that it is present in convalescent but not in acute serum confirms recent EBV infection.

There is no specific treatment for infectious mononucleosis. Corticosteroid therapy is often used where asphyxia is threatened, for haemolytic anaemia and for severe thrombocytopenia but there is little information on their efficacy.

EBV is consistently be recovered from biopsy specimens of Burkitt's lymphoma in African patients (Fig. 1.46). There is strong epidemiological evidence that other environmental influences may also be important with EBV as cofactors in the causation of the tumour.

Herpangina

Herpangina is an uncommon disease found in children aged 2–10 years. Its main features are fever, painful dysphagia, abdominal pain and vomiting. Examination of the throat reveals a small number of lesions over the tonsils, soft palate, pharynx and anterior tonsillar pillars. These lesions start as vesicles but soon rupture to form shallow ulcers (Fig. 1.47). It is caused by infection with Coxsackie A virus (several serotypes).

Pharyngoconjunctival fever

Adenovirus infections, particularly with serotypes 3 and 7, often affect the eye as well as the throat. The syndrome of pharyngoconjunctival fever starts with moderately severe systemic symptoms of fever, malaise, myalgia and headache. Pharyngeal involvement appears next, ranging in extent from isolated ulceration of the palate (Fig. 1.48) or pharynx to painful bilateral exudative tonsillitis. It is associated with follicular conjunctivitis, which is bilateral in a quarter of cases. Corneal involvement has been reported. Outbreaks of this syndrome occur during the summer months and may be associated with swimming pools. The incubation period is about 8 days.

Epiglottitis, Croup and Laryngitis

Patients presenting acutely with stridor, respiratory embarrassment, hoarseness and pain in the throat require rapid diagnostic assessment to determine the need for emergency treatment. The condition is commonest in children and may be the result of epiglottitis, severe tonsillitis (particularly in infectious mononucleosis), peritonsillar or retropharyngeal abscess, croup, diphtheria, tracheitis, foreign body aspiration, angioedema or congenital abnormalities.

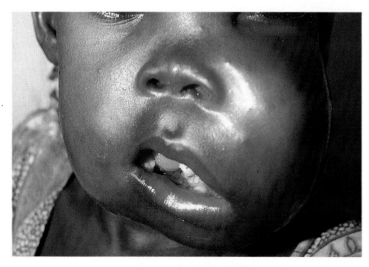

Fig. 1.46 Burkitt's lymphoma. A tumour of the jaw in an African child.

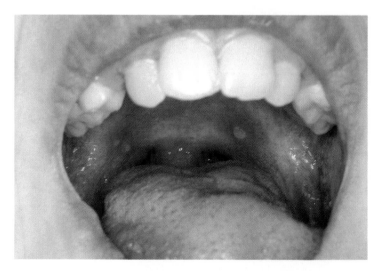

Fig. 1.47 Herpangina. Ulceration of the palate and the anterior pillar of the tonsil.

ACUTE EPIGLOTTITIS

Acute epiglottitis is a dangerous illness which may cause death by asphyxia. It is most often seen in children aged 2–4 years and is more common in boys. Cases are also described in adults. The causative organism is almost always *Haemophilus influenzae* type b, and most cases are associated with bacteraemia. This type of haemophilus has a capsule of mucopolysaccharide which helps it to resist phagocytosis and favours the development of invasive disease. Rarely, other organisms such as *Streptococcus pneumoniae*, *Staphylococcus aureus* and other *Haemophilus* species have been isolated from blood cultures during acute epiglottitis. Clusters of cases have been described, but the risk of disease in susceptible contacts is low. The strain of *H. influenzae* that causes epiglottitis appears to be different from that which causes meningitis and mixed 'outbreaks' do not seem to occur.

The inflammation begins on the anterior surface of the epiglottis and spreads to involve other supraglottic structures (but not the vocal cords or trachea). This is a critically narrow part of the respiratory tract, and in children especially the calibre of the airway is rapidly diminished. Inflammatory exudate and laryngeal spasm may aggravate the respiratory embarrassment.

Typically the patient presents with high fever, sore throat and pain (of short duration) on swallowing. Within 24 hours (often much less), respiratory difficulty is evident. Inspiratory stridor and hoarseness develop, and as breathing becomes more difficult the patient adopts a sitting position with the head held forward and the mouth open. He may be unable to swallow his saliva, which drips from the mouth. The temperature is high and the child looks toxic and agitated.

The diagnosis in advanced cases is clear from the above symptoms and signs. Immediate treatment is required to secure the airway and this must be arranged promptly while keeping to a minimum any disturbance to the patient. Endotracheal intubation should be carried out in an operating theatre by an experienced team which should include an otolaryngologist, a paediatrician and an anaesthetist. If intubation is impossible, tracheostomy should be carried out.

Clinical diagnosis is more difficult in early cases and in adults. However, if acute epiglottitis is suspected, the patient should be taken to the operating theatre and the throat examined with preparations in place to proceed with intubation if necessary. All patients also require parenteral antibiotic treatment. This should be started with a third generation cephalosporin such as ceftriaxone, or with a combination of ampicillin and chloramphenicol given at 6-hourly intervals. Chloramphenicol levels in the serum should be monitored; the drug may be stopped if testing shows that the organism recovered from the patient is sensitive to ampicillin. Antibiotic treatment should be continued for one week and the patient can usually be extubated after three days.

A lateral neck x–ray examination has been recommended in cases where the diagnosis is in doubt (Fig. 1.49). However, such x–rays are not easy to interpret and time should never be lost in carrying out this investigation where the patient already has signs of respiratory difficulty.

Croup

Croup is an acute febrile illness with stridor, hoarseness and cough. It is a disease of young children, most cases occurring in the age range 3 months to 3 years. It is more common in boys. The central pathological feature is subglottic obstruction of the trachea by inflammation of the mucosa. This is the narrowest part of the child's main airways and, encircled by the cricoid cartilage, it cannot expand outwards. Most cases of croup are caused by infection with parainfluenza virus, especially type 3. Respiratory syncytial virus causes a small proportion of cases and influenza A virus makes a variable contribution to the total of cases depending on its prevalence in the community at large. Cases caused by influenza A virus tend to be more severe. Other agents reported as causes of croup are influenza B virus, rhinoviruses, adenoviruses, enteroviruses and *Mycoplasma pneumoniae*.

The illness usually begins with upper respiratory symptoms of rhinitis and sore throat. After two or three days symptoms worsen with the development of a barking cough, inspiratory stridor and dyspnoea. These features tend to be worse at night and they fluctuate in severity

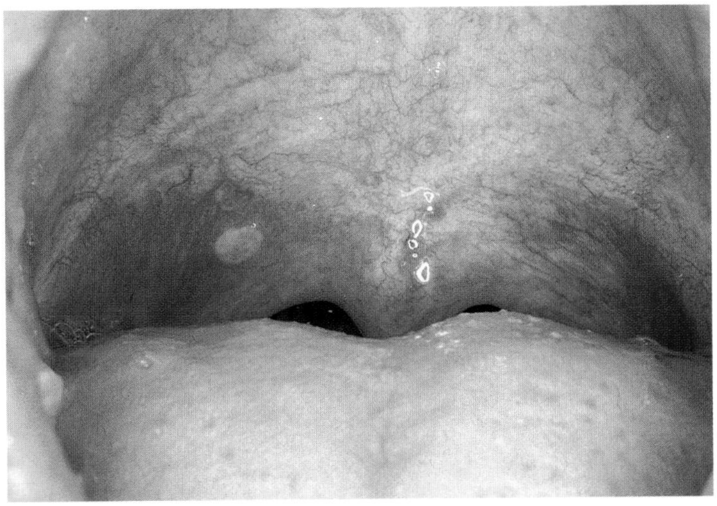

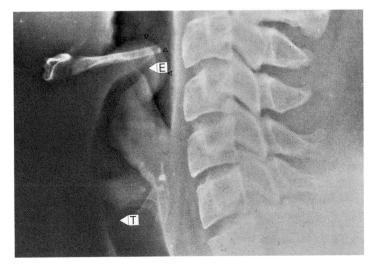

Fig. 1.48 Pharyngoconjunctival fever. Lesions of the palate due to infection with adenovirus type 3.

Fig. 1.49 Acute epiglottitis. Lateral radiograph of the neck showing the tracheal air shadow (T), and rounded swollen tissue shadow of the enlarged epiglottis (E).

over a number of days. In severe cases the chest wall retracts during inspiration and the respiratory rate rises to about 40 per minute. With increasing fatigue, the child's respiratory efforts eventually decline and ventilatory failure follows. The tempo of deterioration in severe cases of croup is significantly slower than in epiglottitis – when endotracheal intubation has to be performed it is generally because of exhaustion and a gradual deterioration in ventilation rather than an immediate risk of asphyxia.

The diagnosis depends largely on recognition of the above clinical pattern. Radiographic examination of the neck may show narrowing of the subglottic trachea, a more dependable investigation than in epiglottitis. Virus isolation from specimens of tracheal aspirate and throat washings is frequently successful. The most common problem in differential diagnosis the distinction of croup from epiglottitis. Of simple clinical observations, the most useful are the very rapid onset, severe systemic toxicity and dysphagia which are found in epiglottitis, and the prodromal upper respiratory symptoms and barking cough which are found in croup.

Treatment is supportive. There are no suitable antiviral agents and bacterial superinfection is uncommon. Nursing the patient in a humidified atmosphere is conventionally advised but the value of doing so is unknown and there is a danger that the paraphernalia required will frighten the child and make nursing more difficult. In severe cases, monitoring of respiratory rate and arterialized capillary blood gas tensions give the best guide to progress and greatly help in the decision on whether supplemental oxygen or assisted ventilation is needed. Conflicting experience has been reported with the use of inhaled aerosolized racemic epinephrine and intramuscular dexamethasone.

RHINITIS AND SINUSITIS

The common cold

The common cold is a syndrome of nasal obstruction, sneezing, nasal discharge and minor systemic disturbance found in patients of all ages and in all parts of the world. A wide variety of viruses can cause the condition but the commonest agents are the rhinoviruses, (up to 50% of cases) and coronaviruses (15–20% of cases) (Fig 1.50). Infection with respiratory syncytial virus, influenza virus, parainfluenza and adenoviruses may also cause limited disease of this kind in some subjects.

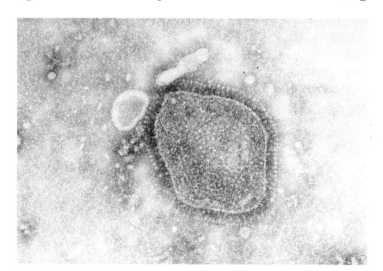

Fig. 1.50 The coronavirus is pleomorphic in appearance, 80–169nm in diameter, with projections called peplomers on the surface.

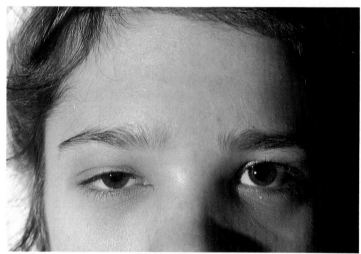

Fig. 1.51 Acute frontal sinusitis with swollen left eyelid.

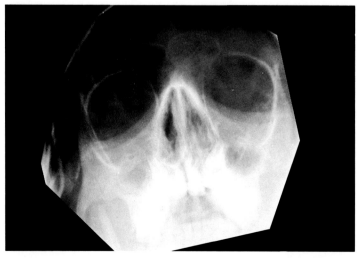

Fig. 1.52 Acute sinusitis. Radiograph showing opacification of left frontal sinus (same case as Fig. 1.51).

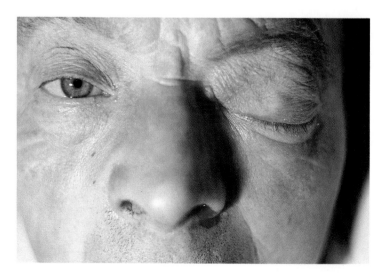

Fig. 1.53 Rhinocerebral mucor mycosis. Bloodstained nasal discharge with left sided ptosis and proposis. By courtesy of Dr J. Snape.

Acute sinusitis

The paranasal sinuses (maxillary, ethmoidal, frontal and sphenoidal) develop from invagination of the nasal mucosa during intrauterine life and undergo expansion and pneumatization during childhood. They are lined with pseudostratified ciliated columnar epithelium which also contains goblet cells and mucous glands. The mucus is transported to the sinus ostia by ciliary action and through the ostia it discharges into the nose. Normally it is not possible to recover microorganisms from the sinuses.

Acute sinusitis develops when the action of the cilia is impaired and/or the sinus ostia are narrowed. The most common cause of these abnormalities is the common cold in which ciliary clearance is reduced and the ostia may be blocked by mucosal swelling. Acute sinusitis is reported to complicate about 0.5% of cases of the common cold. Additional risk factors include anatomical abnormalities of the nasal septum and turbinates, nasal polyps and allergic inflammation. Bacterial growth then occurs within the sinuses and symptoms of acute infection develop. In a small proportion of cases, infection enters the maxillary

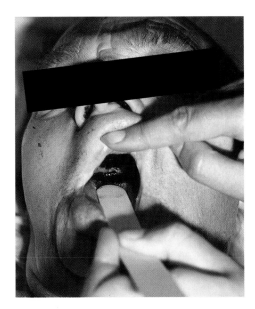

Fig. 1.54 Rhinocerebral mucor mycosis with infarction of the hard palate. By courtesy of Dr J. Snape.

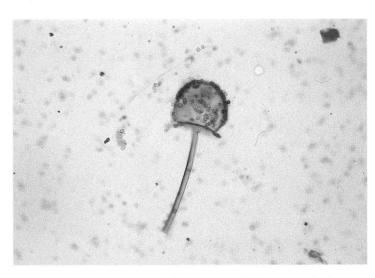

Fig. 1.55 Rhinocerebral mucor mycosis. Sporangiospore of *Rhizopus oryzae* (family Mucoraceae) isolated from the patient in Fig. 1.54. By courtesy of Dr J. Snape.

sinuses by direct spread from an apical abscess of an adjacent tooth.

The most common sites of acute sinusitis are the maxillary sinuses. Several studies have examined the microbiology of community-acquired maxillary sinusitis by sinus puncture; they have found that the great majority of cases are associated with infection with *Streptococcus pneumoniae* (about 40%) or *Haemophilus influenzae* (about 30%). These figures are similar in children and adults. Where the infection has spread from a dental abscess, mixed anaerobic organisms such as bacteroides, fusobacteria and anaerobic streptococci are usually present. Nosocomial sinus infection in patients with trauma or prolonged nasal intubation is generally caused by aerobic gram-negative bacilli – the same group of organisms may be isolated from cases of acute sinusitis in patients with Kartagener's syndrome, cystic fibrosis and the immotile cilia syndrome.

The clinical features of acute sinusitis are pain, localized according to which sinus is involved, sometimes accompanied by nasal discharge and fever. In a few patients there will be tenderness or even erythema and swelling over the infected sinus (Fig. 1.51) and, in the case of maxillary or frontal sinusitis, it may be possible to demonstrate impaired transillumination.

Sinus aspiration is the definitive method of confirming acute infection but it is not generally performed because of the discomfort it causes and the risk of complications such as bleeding and osteomyelitis. Radiography is a simpler alternative and is reliable where the film shows opacification of a sinus (Fig. 1.52) or the presence of an air–fluid level. Computerized tomography provides an alternative and highly accurate method of visualizing the sinuses.

The treatment of acute sinusitis consists of the use of a suitable antibiotic and measures to correct (if possible) any physical barrier to the normal drainage of the sinus. The antibiotic is usually selected initially on empirical grounds; agents such as amoxycillin and cotrimoxazole are effective in the majority of cases. Failure of response to treatment is an indication for sinus puncture, particularly if the patient has risk factors for unusual forms of infection.

Acute sinusitis may be complicated by spread of pyogenic infection to neighbouring structures, such as the facial bones, the brain or the orbit (see Chapter 12). These are very dangerous developments and their onset is generally marked by the appearance of much more severe systemic disturbance in addition to the local effects of the extended infection.

Fungal Sinusitis

Fungal sinusitis is rare but has been reported in diabetics and following maxillary trauma. It is generally associated with invasion of the nasopharynx and central nervous system. The fungi involved are members of the family Mucoraceae and the condition is known as rhinocerebral mucor mycosis. The clinical presentation is usually acute with headache, fever, bloodstained nasal discharge and periorbital oedema (Fig. 1.53). Extension of the infection leads to mucosal necrosis (Fig. 1.54), proptosis and cranial nerve palsies. The diagnosis is made by isolation of the fungus from cultures (Fig. 1.55).

INFECTIONS OF THE EAR

Otitis externa

The peculiar anatomical characteristics of the skin of the ear are important in determining the features of otitis externa. Firstly, the skin of the auditory canal and auricle is very tightly applied to the underlying bone and cartilage. This leaves little room for soft tissue swelling and when skin infections do occur they quickly become very painful. Secondly, the cartilage of the ear depends on the perichondrium for its blood supply. Damage to the perichondrium may therefore lead to necrosis of the underlying cartilage. Thirdly, the skin of the auditory canal contains glands which secrete cerumen which protects it from microorganisms. If the cerumen is removed, infection is more likely.

The commonest organisms isolated from otitis externa are *Pseudomonas aeruginosa* (about 70% of cases) and *Staphylococcus aureus* (about 15% of cases). Manipulation of the external ear is painful and the auditory canal contains purulent exudate (Fig. 1.56). Treatment should begin with careful toilet of the auditory canal. In mild cases treatment with a topical antibiotic or 0.25% acetic acid solution is sufficient. Severe cases should be treated with an appropriate systemic antibiotic.

Malignant Otitis Externa

Elderly patients with diabetes mellitus are susceptible to an aggressive form of external otitis caused by *P. aeruginosa*. It begins as does normal otitis externa and spreads at first through clefts in the cartilage (Fig.1.57). It then involves the periauricular tissues, the parotid gland, the temperomandibular joint, the soft tissues at the base of the skull and the temporal bone. Osteomyelitis spreads and the seventh, ninth, tenth, elventh and twelvth cranial nerves are destroyed. Thrombosis of the jugular vein and the lateral sinus may follow. Treatment is with surgical debridement and topical and parenteral antipseudomonal antibiotics. Mortality is high, particularly where cranial nerve damage has already occurred.

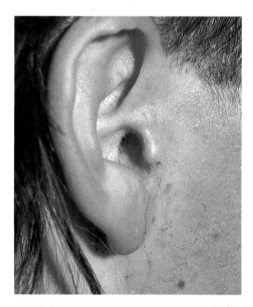

Fig. 1.56 Acute otitis externa. An inflamed auditory canal with purulent exudate.

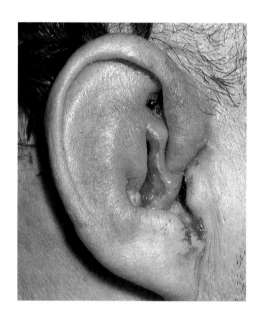

Fig. 1.57 Malignant otitis externa. Early appearance showing dusky erythema over the cartilaginous parts of the external ear. There is a bloodstained discharge from granulation tissue on the floor of the auditory canal.

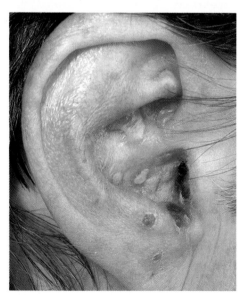

Fig. 1.58 Ramsay Hunt syndrome. Vesicles on the auricle and in the external auditory canal.

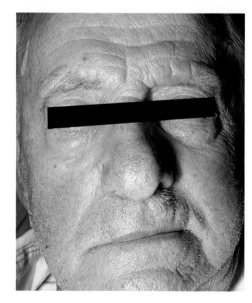

Fig. 1.59 Ramsay Hunt syndrome. Paralysis of the right facial nerve following shingles of the external ear.

Ramsay Hunt syndrome

Herpes varicella–zoster infection of the geniculate ganglion, when it reactivates, causes an unusual variety of shingles known as the Ramsay Hunt syndrome. Its features include a vesicular rash of the ear, lower motor neurone paralysis of the facial nerve, loss of taste sensation over the anterior two thirds of the tongue, a vesicular eruption on the anterior pillar of the fauces and hyperacusis caused by paralysis of the stapedial nerve. These effects are always unilateral and not all may be manifest in all patients.

The first symptom of the condition is usually pain in the ear. After a short interval a vesicular rash appears on the auricle (Fig. 1.58) within the auditory canal and, rarely, on the tympanic membrane. Sometimes there is also shingles of one of the upper cervical dermatomes (herpes occipitocollaris). Facial palsy follows and may persist for several weeks (Fig. 1.59). Vesicular eruption within the mouth is rather uncommon and the disturbance of taste sensation is seldom noted by the patient.

Acute otitis media

Acute bacterial otitis media is one of the commonest infections of young children. The highest attack rates are seen in the age range 6–18 months. Recurrent attacks at a later age are most common in those who have suffered in infancy. The pathogenesis of the condition depends on infection and on mechanical or functional disturbance of the middle ear or eustachian tube. Most attacks are preceded by symptoms of viral upper respiratory infection.

Partial blockage of the eustachian tube, followed by absorption of oxygen in the middle ear cleft, produces a negative pressure which may suck nasopharyngeal commensal bacteria from the nasal end of the eustachian tube into the ear. Bacteria may also reach the middle ear through lymphatic channels. The organisms most commonly responsible for acute otitis media are *Streptococcus pneumoniae*, *Haemophilus influenzae* and *Branhamella catarrhalis*.

The clinical features of acute otitis media are variable and depend to a great extent on the age of the patient. In infants fever, irritability, vomiting and diarrhoea are most common while in older children and adults ear pain, often severe, dominates the picture. There may be a purulent discharge from the ear and mastoid tenderness. Hearing loss can be demonstrated by laboratory testing in almost all cases but is not often noted by the patient. Preceding upper respiratory symptoms are frequent.

On examination the tympanic membrane appears dull red in colour and is either immobile or bulging outwards (Figs 1.60 & 1.61). If the drum has perforated, there will be purulent material in the external canal and this will have to be removed before the drum can be inspected fully. The patient may also show signs of upper respiratory infection and there may be features of meningeal irritation. Spread of infection to the mastoid air cells may cause swelling and tenderness of the mastoid process (Fig. 1.62).

Diagnostic tympanocentesis is seldom practised in acute otitis media and an empirical choice of antibiotic therapy must be made, based on the knowledge of likely pathogens and their local pattern of drug susceptibility. In the past ampicillin and amoxycillin have been adequate but with

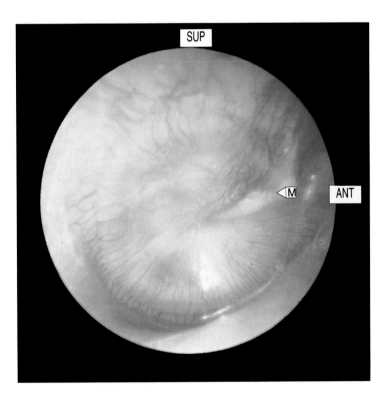

Fig. 1.60 Acute otitis media. Early stage showing mild injection of the drum (D), especially in the region of the malleus (M). By courtesy of Dr M. Chaput de Saintonge.

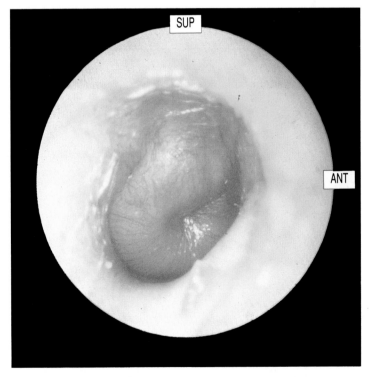

Fig. 1.61 Acute otitis media. Advanced stage showing bulging of the drum (B) on both sides of the malleus (M), which is obscured. By courtesy of Dr M. Chaput de Saintonge.

the rising incidence of β-lactamase-producing *Haemophilus influenzae* and *Branhamella catarrhalis* in some localities the best choice may be a cephalosporin, a combination of trimethoprim and sulfamethoxazole or a combination of amoxycillin and clavulanic acid. A response is usually seen within 72 hours and treatment is continued for 10–14 days. Therapy with antihistamines and decongestants has not been shown to be beneficial.

Tuberculous Otitis Media

Tuberculous infection may reach the middle ear by spread up the eustachian tube from the pharynx or by blood-borne spread from a primary lesion elsewhere. It generally presents as chronic otitis media with intermittent aural discharge. The tympanic membrane may have multiple perforations and the mastoid air cells are usually involved (Fig. 1.63). Attempts to isolate the organism from the discharged material are usually unsuccessful and the diagnosis is often delayed until histological examination of currettings is undertaken. The condition responds to conventional antituberculosis treatment.

Actinomycosis

Actinomyces are filamentous gram-positive bacteria which cause chronic suppurative infection with a tendency to sinus formation. These infections are locally invasive and readily cross tissue planes. The organisms are to be found in the normal oral flora and infection of the face usually develops against a background of dental trauma or infection. Most cases are caused by *Actinomyces israelii* (Fig. 1.64).

Cervicofacial actinomycosis generally presents as an indurated swelling over the lower border of the mandible. It grows slowly and is relatively painless. Eventually suppuration takes place and it discharges through a sinus to the exterior or to the oral cavity (Figs 1.65 & 66). Untreated, the infection extends locally to involve the bones of the face and the base of the skull. The salivary glands and tongue may also be invaded.

The organism may be isolated from abscesses and material discharging from sinuses. Typically the pus contains yellow-coloured, gritty clumps of organism, known as 'sulphur granules', visible to the naked eye and under the microscope (Fig. 1.67).

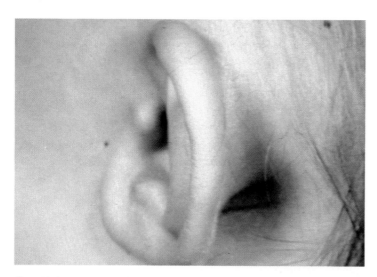

Fig. 1.62 Acute mastoiditis. Oedema of the skin and subcutaneous tissue – the ear is pushed downwards and forwards but the skin fold behind the auricle is preserved.

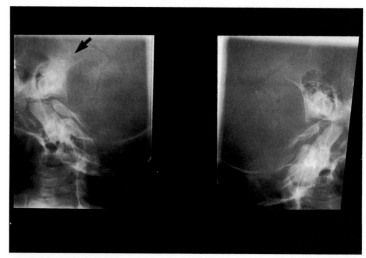

Fig. 1.63 Tuberculous otitis media. Radiograph of mastoid air cells showing opacification on the affected (arrowed) side.

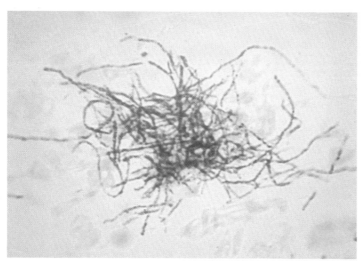

Fig. 1.64 Actinomycosis. Gram stain from an actinomycotic lesion showing gram-positive branching filaments of *Actinomyces israelii*. By courtesy of A. E. Prevost.

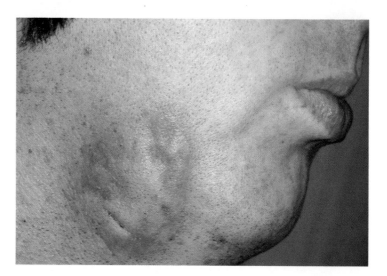

Fig. 1.65 Cervicofacial actinomycosis. Erythema and induration of the skin overlying odontogenic infection. By courtesy of Mr C. J. Meryon.

The infection responds to prolonged treatment with penicillin or tetracycline, initially given parenterally. Surgical measures may also be needed for the treatment of persistent sinuses or the removal of necrotic material.

INFECTIONS OF THE PAROTID GLAND

Mumps

Mumps is an illness of worldwide distribution, principally affecting children and spread by airborne droplets of infected saliva. Infection is followed by lifelong immunity but only in 60–70% of cases does it cause disease. There is no animal reservoir and chronic carriage in humans has not been observed. The infection incubates for 2–3 weeks.

The commonest manifestation of mumps is salivary gland enlargement. The parotid gland is most often affected and in 75% of cases both sides are involved. Other salivary glands may be involved but less frequently and seldom without parotitis. Enlargement of the parotid gland is painful and accompanied by high fever, but there is no suppuration. The swelling fills the space between the mastoid and the angle of the jaw, extending forward over the cheek. Typically it displaces the lobe of the ear laterally (Figs 1.68 & 1.69). The orifice of the parotid duct within the mouth appears prominent and inflamed but there is no purulent discharge. The gland reaches its maximum size within 2-3 days and then returns quite rapidly to normal. Salivary gland enlargement often takes place sequentially and as each gland becomes affected the temperature may rise again.

Although mumps is by far the most common cause of febrile nonsuppurative parotitis, other viruses have been identified as the cause of similar disease including parainfluenza type 3, coxsackie and influenza A. This probably accounts for reported instances of second attacks of mumps. It is not normally necessary to call upon the laboratory to confirm the diagnosis of mumps but where this is needed the virus can be isolated from saliva and urine. Serological testing is also available but there may be cross-reaction with parainfluenza which, like mumps virus, belongs to the paramyxovirus group.

While salivary gland enlargement is the most common manifestation of mumps virus infection, there are many

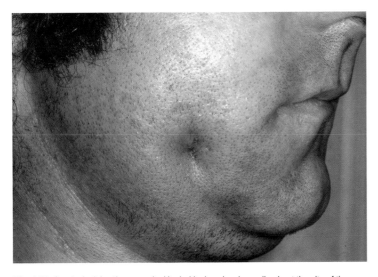

Fig. 1.66 Cervicofacial actinomycosis. Healed lesion showing a dimple at the site of the previously discharging sinus. By courtesy of Mr C. J Meryon.

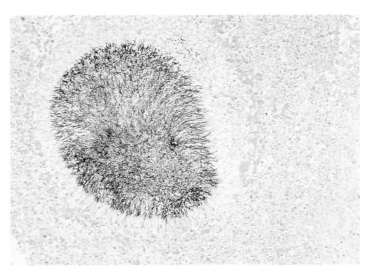

Fig. 1.67 Actinomycosis. Histological appearance of the 'sulphur granule' (bacterial aggregation) in tissues.

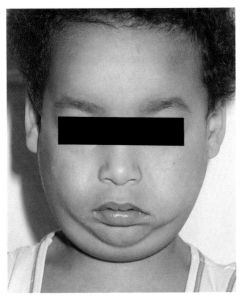

Fig. 1.68 Mumps. Bilateral parotid and submandibular gland enlargement displacing the ear lobes laterally.

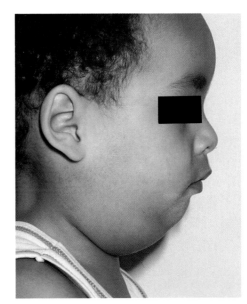

Fig. 1.69 Mumps. Lateral view showing enlargement of salivary glands.

others including meningitis, encephalitis, deafness, pancreatitis, epididymo-orchitis and oophoritis, which are potentially more serious and which may occur with or without salivary gland involvement (see later chapters).

Pyogenic parotitis

Acute pyogenic infection of the parotid gland is favoured by conditions which slow down the passage of secretions along the slender length of the parotid duct. These include calculi, plugs of mucus, starvation, dehydration and pre-existing disorders of the gland which reduce the amount of secretions. It seems likely that infection reaches the gland by retrograde flow along the duct; however, more than 90% of infections are with *Staphylococcus aureus*, far from the most common potential pathogen among the mouth flora. Haematogenous spread of infection to an abnormal parotid gland is also possible.

The clinical emergence of acute pyogenic parotitis takes place against the background of whatever pre-existing abnormality has rendered the condition likely. Extreme tenderness is commonly present along with enlargement of the gland and erythema of the overlying skin (Fig. 1.70). Massage of the gland, where this is tolerable, may cause the extrusion of pus at Stensen's duct (Fig. 1.71). In neglected cases abscess formation occurs and the infection may discharge through the skin of the cheek (Fig. 1.72). The organism can be recovered from this material and often from blood cultures.

Treatment is with a parenteral antistaphylococcal antibiotic such as flucloxacillin or as directed by the isolation of other pathogens. Measures should be taken to correct predisposing factors where possible. Surgical treatment is occasionally needed to deal with abscesses or calculi.

Cervical lymphadenitis

Cervical lymphadenitis is commonplace with many infections causing pharyngotonsillitis, including in particular streptococcal, adenovirus and Epstein–Barr virus infection, diphtheria and peritonsillar abscess. In these conditions the pharyngotonsillar condition dominates the clinical picture and the diagnosis depends on assessment of the primary site of infection.

Isolated cervical lymphadenitis presents a different problem and is associated with a rather more sinister list of diagnoses of which a few arise from infections. In general it is reasonable to observe enlarged but undiagnosed cervical lymph nodes for up to three weeks before seeking a definitive diagnosis by biopsy, assuming that there are no strong pointers to a particularly urgent cause. This philosophy is based on the assumption that if the gland is malignant, the condition is already beyond radical cure unless it is a haematological malignancy, in which case, if there is no other clue to the diagnosis, a short delay of this order will make no difference to the outcome.

Tuberculosis

Tuberculous cervical lymphadenitis is the commonest form of nonrespiratory tuberculosis, accounting for one-third of such cases in white patients and one-half in Asians (Fig. 1.73). It may result from tonsillar primary infection where contaminated raw milk is the vehicle of infection, but more often it arises from lymphatic spread from a pulmonary primary complex, either by way of the mediastinum or across the pleural space (Figs 1.74 & 1.75). Occasionally primary infection of the conjunctiva may be the source with spread to the preauricular nodes and beyond (Figs 1.76, 1.77 & 1.78).

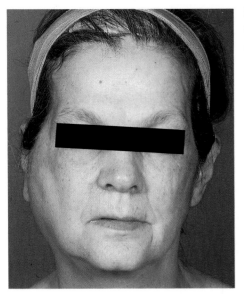

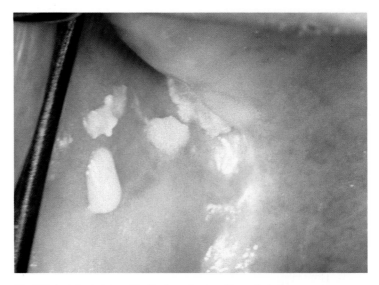

Fig. 1.70 Acute bacterial parotitis with unilateral parotid swelling.

Fig. 1.71 Acute bacterial parotitis. Pus is exuding from Stensen's duct.

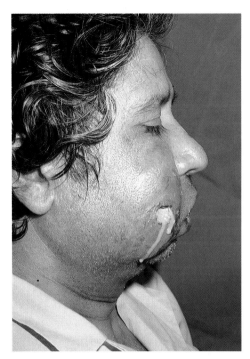

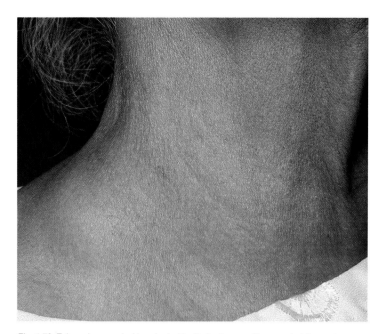

Fig. 1.72 Acute bacterial parotitis. Advanced disease with an abscess discharging to the exterior in a patient with diabetes mellitus.

Fig. 1.73 Tuberculous cervical lymphadenitis. Early disease with no acute inflammatory features.

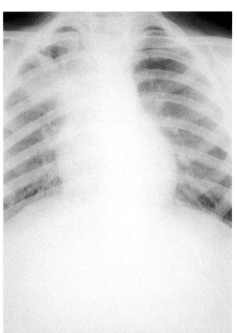

Fig. 1.74 Primary tuberculosis. Chest radiograph showing primary complex in right upper lobe.

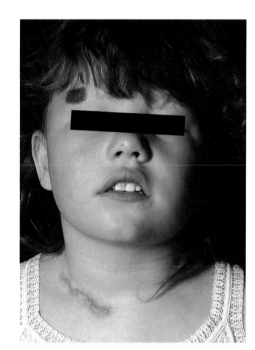

Fig. 1.75 Tuberculous cervical lymphadenitis. Inflammation has spread to the surrounding tissues and a cold abscess is discharging to the exterior (same patient as Fig. 1.74).

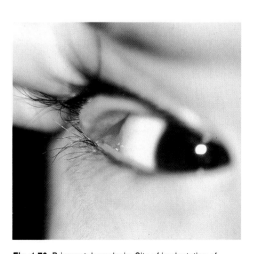

Fig. 1.76 Primary tuberculosis. Site of implantation of infection beneath the upper eyelid. The patient shared a bed with a sister who had open pulmonary tuberculosis.

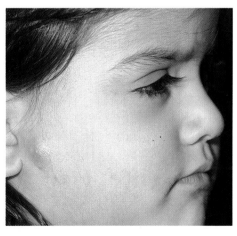

Fig. 1.77 Primary tuberculosis of the conjunctiva. Enlargement of the preauricular lymph node, from which *Myocabaterium tuberculosis* was isolated.

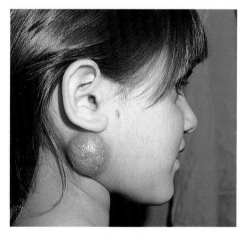

Fig. 1.78 Tuberculous cervical lymphadenitis. Infection has spread to the cervical glands.(Same patient as in Figs 1.76 & 1.77.)

The usual clinical presentation is a lump in the neck without any associated symptoms. Usually it has increased in size over a number of weeks and is only slightly painful. In long–standing cases there may be signs of fluctuation and the overlying skin may be red. Once suppuration has advanced to this extent, discharge to the exterior is almost inevitable.

The diagnosis should be confirmed by histological (Fig. 1.79) and microbiological examination of biopsied material. The tuberculin skin test is almost always strongly positive. A negative test throws serious doubt on the diagnosis whatever the histological features may be.

Conventional antituberculosis treatment is ultimately effective in curing the infection although in 25% of cases signs of continuing inflammation emerge during the first few months of treatment.

Atypical mycobacterial infection

Pathogenic mycobacteria other than *M. tuberculosis* are found in various sources in the human environment including soil, dust, water and animals. Their geographical distribution is uneven and the prevalence of human infections varies widely from region to region. The method of transmission of these organisms to humans is not well understood but probably includes inhalation, ingestion and direct inoculation into the skin.

Cervical lymphadenitis is usually caused by the species *M. scrofulaceum* and *M. avium–intracellulare* and is found most often in young children. Submandibular and submaxillary nodes are the commonest site and the condition presents with the gradual enlargement of a gland over a number of weeks. The swelling is only slightly tender and suppuration and discharge are unusual (Fig. 1.80). Systemic disturbance is absent or minimal and there are usually no other clinical features.

The diagnosis is generally made when the lump is biopsied. The histological picture is similar to that of tuberculosis and the precise aetiology can only be determined by culture of the organism. Where material is not available for culture, an indication of the likely cause may be given by skin testing. A negative tuberculin test in a

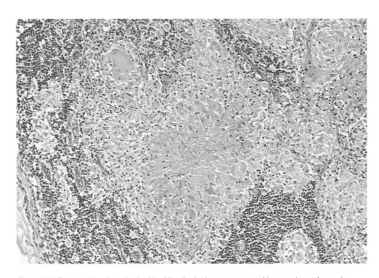

Fig. 1.79 Tuberculous lymphadenitis. Histological appearance with granuloma formation, giant cells and caseation.

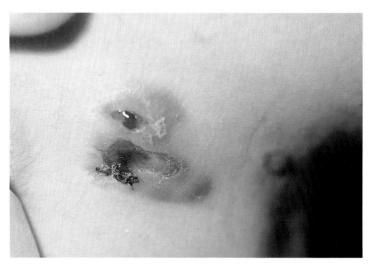

Fig. 1.80 Atypical myobacterial infection. Lymphadenitis and skin involvement by *Mycobacterium avium* in a healthy young child.

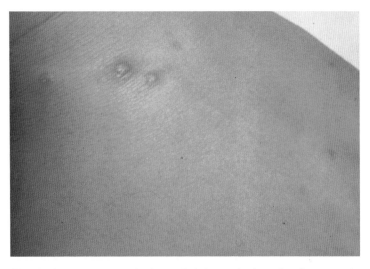

Fig. 1.81 Cat scratch disease: showing papular lesions at site of scratches. By courtesy of Dr. T. Sellers, Jr.

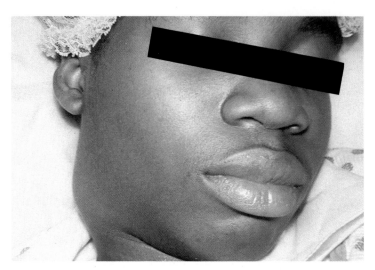

Fig. 1.82 Cat scratch disease. Large cervical lymph nodes in a drowsy patient with complicating encephalitis. By courtesy of Dr. T. Sellers, Jr.

child who is in a low risk group for tuberculosis suggests atypical infection. In some cases positive reactions may be obtained using the counterpart of tuberculin prepared from atypical mycobacteria.

Surgical excision is probably all that is required for the treatment of atypical mycobacterial lymphadenitis in otherwise healthy children. There is no clear evidence of benefit from chemotherapy and multiple drug resistance is common.

Cat scratch disease

Cat scratch disease is believed to be caused by infection with an as yet incompletely characterized bacterium. It has been most widely reported in North America where it is most common in young adults during the winter months.

Its characteristic feature is tender localized lymphadenopathy, usually persisting for 1–2 months. The most frequently affected sites are the upper limb and the head and neck (Fig. 1.81). In about 50% of the cases the glands become fluctuant and the overlying skin is discoloured. There is a strong association with preceding cat scratch in the area of drainage of the lymph nodes and in about 50% of cases a primary skin lesion can be recognised at the site of inoculation (Fig. 1.82). An atypical variety is one cause of Parinaud's syndrome and presents with preauricular lymphadenitis. About two-thirds of patients with cat scratch disease have mild systemic symptoms.

The diagnosis depends on the histological appearance of the lesion, the history of contact with a cat and the exclusion of other pathology.

The condition is self-limiting but successful antibiotic treatment with aminoglycosides has recently been reported.

Toxoplasmosis

Members of the cat family are the definitive hosts of the intracellular protozoon *Toxoplasma gondii*. Oocysts produced in the cat intestine are excreted in the faeces and develop into an infectious form. Other mammals, including man, may then be infected by ingesting food contaminated by cat faeces. Inside the gut, trophozoites develop and cross the intestinal epithelium before being disseminated through the lymphatics or the blood stream. Any cell may be infected; intracellular multiplication and cell death follows. Immunity develops and eventually the infection is localized and overcome. However, some organisms escape destruction by forming tissue cysts, particularly in muscle and brain. The disease may then be transmitted if the animal's infected tissues are later consumed, raw or undercooked, by another mammal.

Serological surveys show that most human infections acquired after birth are unrecognised. The usual clinical manifestation is superficial lymphadenopathy, usually in the neck. One or more groups of lymph nodes may be involved and the signs of acute inflammation are usually absent. Occasionally there are accompanying symptoms of fatigue and malaise and the illness may persist with fluctuating severity for weeks or months.

Complications of acquired toxoplasmosis are rare in healthy subjects but include involvement of the eye, heart and brain. Acute infection during pregnancy carries a serious risk of fetal involvement.

The diagnosis of acute toxoplasmosis can be confirmed by isolation of the organism from cultures of tissue specimens or buffy coat, by serological tests or by histological examination (Fig 1.83).

No treatment is required for uncomplicated infection in healthy subjects unless they are pregnant, in which case spiramycin should be given.

Acute suppurative lymphadenitis

Acute suppurative lymphadenitis of the neck in the absence of a detectable primary source of infection is occasionally seen in young children. The commonest sites are the glands of the submandibular areas and the anterior

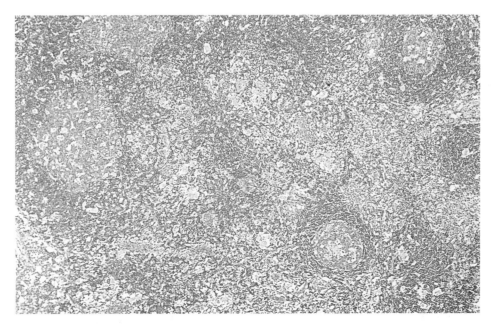

Fig. 1.83 Toxoplasmosis. Histology of lymph node showing follicular hyperplasia and clusters of epithelioid histiocytes in germinal centres. By courtesy of Dr C. W. Edwards.

triangle. Most are caused by infection with *Staphylococcus aureus* or, less frequently, *Streptococcus pyogenes*. Clinically the illness presents with fever and rapid enlargement of the affected gland over a few days (Fig. 1.84). Fluctuation often develops and if untreated the abscess discharges spontaneously through the skin (Fig. 1.85).

Infection of developmental cysts

Branchial cysts are either developmental abnormalities of the first or second branchial pouches or the result of epithelial inclusions in lymph nodes. They are lined with epithelium and most have lymphoid tissue in their walls. Clinical presentation is usually in the third decade of life and about 15% are infected when first observed. The most common position is the upper third of the left side of the neck, anterior to the sternomastoid muscle (Fig. 1.86). Treatment is by surgical excision.

Thyroglossal duct cysts arise from remnants of the thyroglossal duct which embryologically connects the thyroid gland to the posterior end of the tongue. They are subcuta-

neous midline cysts usually around the level of the hyoid bone, moving with swallowing and protrusion of the tongue (Fig. 1.87). The commonest age of presentation is 5 years. In 5% of cases the cysts are tender and enlarge rapidly as a result of infection (Fig. 1.88).

DEEP NECK SPACE INFECTIONS

Retropharyngeal space infections

The retropharyngeal space lies between the prevertebral fascia and the buccopharyngeal fascia and extends from the base of the skull to the superior mediastinum. Infections arise in this site either by lymphatic spread to the retropharyngeal lymph nodes from infected adenoids or nasopharynx, or as a result of trauma.

The retropharyngeal lymph nodes atrophy after the age of 4 years; most infections of the retropharyngeal space that spread from the upper respiratory tract are seen in children below this age. Typically the illness begins with nasopharyngeal symptoms followed by the development of more severe systemic symptoms, high fever, dysphagia,

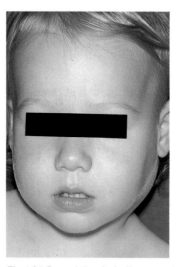
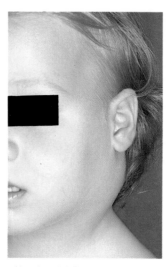

Fig. 1.84 Pyogenic lymphadenitis at an early stage of lymph node inflammation.

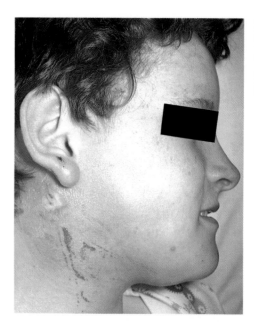

Fig. 1.85 Pyogenic lymphadenitis. Discharging abscess of postauricular gland following infection at the site of ear piercing.

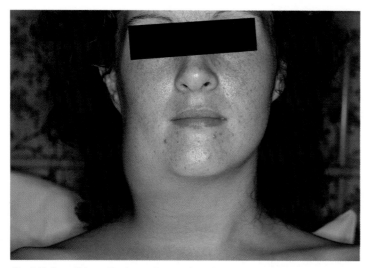

Fig. 1.86 Branchial cyst. Tender swelling anterior to the sternomastoid muscle with oedema of the surrounding soft tissue.

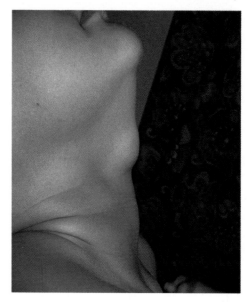

Fig. 1.87 Thyroglossal duct cyst. Subcutaneous swelling in midline, closely related to the hyoid bone.

dyspnoea and neck stiffness. Physical examination may be difficult but it may be possible to see the posterior pharyngeal wall bulging forwards. Lateral x-rays of the neck confirm the widening of the retropharyngeal space. In adults similar infection is usually the result of trauma.

Treatment is by surgical incision of the abscess and administration of appropriate antibiotics.

Prevertebral Space Infection

The prevertebral space lies behind the prevertebral fascia and in front of the vertebral bodies. It extends along the whole length of the spine. Infections in this space are usually secondary to haematogenous osteomyelitis of the vertebrae (Fig. 1.89). Prevertebral space infection in the neck produces clinical features similar to those of retropharyngeal infection.

Treatment is guided by the same principles but the choice of antibiotic is likely to be different in view of the bony source of the infection. Instability of the spine requires attention on its own merits.

Submandibular space infection

There are two components of the submandibular space – the sublingual space superiorly and the submaxillary space inferiorly. They are vulnerable to infection by direct extension from the lower jaw, particularly following dental sepsis. Infection may also follow compound fractures of the mandible and lacerations of the floor of the mouth.

Infection of the sublingual space usually arises from the anterior teeth and spreads within the space on both sides, pushing the floor of the mouth upwards.

The submaxillary space is infected from the lower third and fourth molar teeth. There is swelling lateral and inferior to the body of the mandible but the floor of the mouth is not affected (Fig. 1.90).

The sublingual and submaxillary spaces intercommunicate. Infection starting in one compartment may spread to the other, leading to a highly dangerous condition known as Ludwig's angina. It presents with rapidly extending indurated cellulitis beginning below the jaw and in the floor of the mouth, pushing the tongue upward (Fig. 1.91).

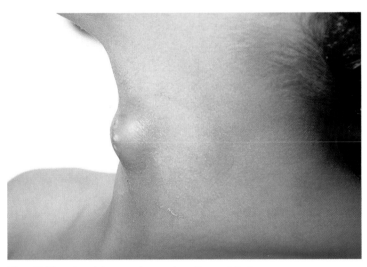

Fig. 1.88 Thyroglossal duct cyst. Presentation with acute infection.

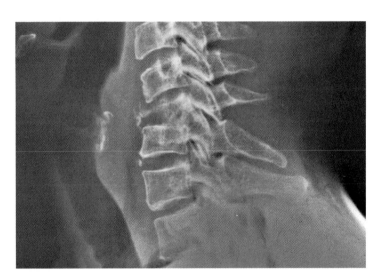

Fig. 1.89 Prevertebral abscess. Lateral radiograph of the neck showing abnormally deep soft tissue shadow between the trachea and the cervical vertebrae. The body of C5 is destroyed by osteomyelitis.

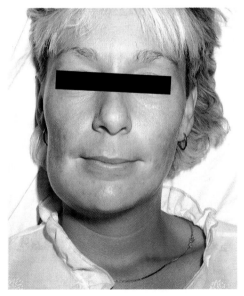

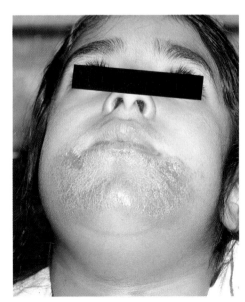

Fig. 1.90 Submaxillary space infection, the result of spread from dental abscess.

Fig. 1.91 Ludwig's angina. The patient had lacerated the underside of the tongue on her teeth during a dystonic reaction to prochlorperazine.

As the condition worsens the mouth is held open and the patient may have difficulty in eating, speaking and breathing. The infection spreads to the neck and causes supraglottic oedema which threatens asphyxia (Figs 1.92 & 1.93). High fever and severe systemic toxicity are the rule.

Treatment is initially by securing the airway either by tracheostomy or endotracheal intubation. Broad spectrum antibiotic cover should be employed until the infecting agents have been identified (Fig 1.94). Abscess formation is rare and surgical drainage is seldom indicated.

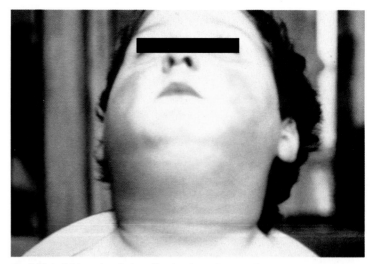

Fig. 1.92 Ludwig's angina. Patient with a hugely swollen neck. The swelling involves the whole of the sublingual and submandibular spaces. The overlying skin is tender and hot.

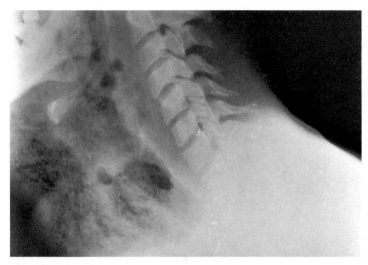

Fig. 1.93 Radiograph of the neck showing gas formation in anaerobic cellulitis. By courtesy of Dr T. F. Sellers, Jr.

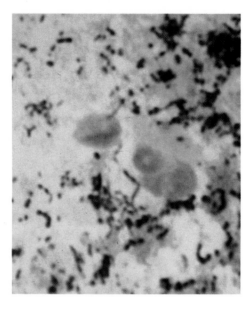

Fig. 1.94 Ludwig's angina. Gram stain smear of pus – a few pus cells are seen and a large number of bacteria, mostly gram-positive cocci. By courtesy of Dr V. E. Del Bene.

2
LOWER RESPIRATORY TRACT

Below the larynx there is normally no microbial population. This sterility is maintained by host defences which are both anatomical and immunological.

The physical barriers to infection include the filtering and humidifying action of the nose, the presence of gag and cough reflexes, the respiratory excursion of the lungs, the patency of the airways, the production of bronchial mucus of normal quality and in normal amounts, and the expulsion of that mucus (and whatever may be caught up in it) by ciliary function. Immunological defence mechanisms include the production of specific circulating or secretory antibody, the presence of cell-mediated immunity and the function of alveolar macrophages.

Failure or absence of any of these provisions renders the subject vulnerable to respiratory infection. In some instances the damage caused to the respiratory defence mechanisms by one infection itself renders the patient susceptible to superinfection with other organisms.

BRONCHITIS

Acute bronchitis

Among previously healthy subjects, acute bronchitis is generally the result of infection with a respiratory virus to which they have no specific immunity. The most common organisms are influenza viruses A and B, parainfluenza viruses 1, 2 and 3, *Mycoplasma pneumoniae*, adenovirus and respiratory syncytial virus. Bronchitis is also a constant feature of measles and pertussis.

Cigarette smokers are particularly likely to suffer from acute bronchitis because of the excessive amounts of bronchial mucus that they produce (Fig. 2.1), because the action of their cilia is abnormal and because, in some, part of the normal bronchal epithelium has undergone squamous metaplasia (Fig. 2.2). In these patients *Haemophilus influenzae* or *Streptococcus pneumoniae* can almost always be isolated from the sputum, although the initial infection may have been caused by one of the respiratory viruses mentioned above. Where the patient has already received antibiotic treatment, there may be an overgrowth of coliform organisms normally found in the bowel.

The main clinical feature is cough productive of sputum which is usually purulent and is occasionally tinged with blood. In addition there may be wheeze and breathlessness. Systemic features are variable but usually minor.

The histological appearance is of submucosal infiltration with acute inflammatory cells, desquamation of the ciliated epithelium and an intrabronchial exudate of fibrin, pus cells and blood (Fig. 2.3).

Acute bronchitis is a self-limiting condition; where it occurs in normal subjects there is little evidence that antimicrobial treatment is effective. However, in patients with pre-existing chronic bronchitis or with asthma, acute bronchitis with purulent sputum should be treated with an oral antibiotic effective against *H.influenzae* and *S. pneumoniae*.

Whooping cough

Children with whooping cough have widespread tracheobronchitis but most do not have pneumonia. Indeed, one of the hallmarks of the disease is the contrast between the frighteningly severe prolonged coughing bouts and, in infancy, apnoeic attacks and the general wellbeing of the patient between episodes. The lungs, however, may be affected: diffuse pneumonia may be seen, sometimes as the presenting feature of the illness, and lobar or

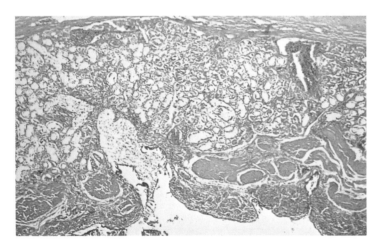

Fig. 2.1 Chronic bronchitis. Histological appearance showing hypertrophy of smooth muscle and proliferation of mucous glands. By courtesy of Dr C. W. Edwards.

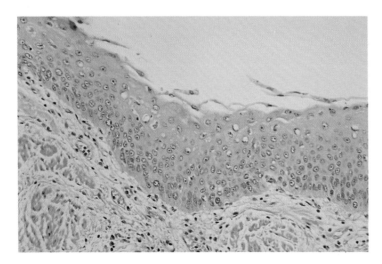

Fig. 2.2 Squamous metaplasia. The normal ciliated columnar epithelium of the bronchial tree has been replaced by squamous epithelium. By courtesy of Dr C. W. Edwards.

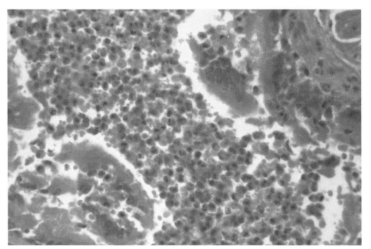

Fig. 2.3 Acute bronchitis. Histopathology showing lumen of affected bronchus filled with a mass of polymorphonuclear leucocytes with some red cells. H & E stain.

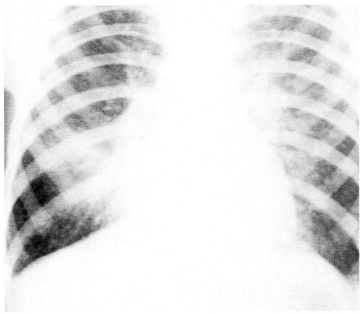

segmental collapse is not uncommon. Fig. 2.4 shows the chest radiographs of a child with whooping cough. The posteroanterior view shows diffuse and patchy shadowing together with a more prominent shadow in the distribution of the right middle lobe. Collapse of the right middle lobe is clearly seen in the lateral view.

Frenal ulcer is an uncommon but well recognised complication of whooping cough (Fig. 2.5). The frenum of the child's tongue is eroded by the frequent gagging and vomiting which follows coughing bouts. It heals uneventfully.

Acute bronchiolitis

This syndrome of fever accompanied by cough and respiratory distress is found almost exclusively in infants as a result of infection with respiratory syncytial virus (RSV). Its incidence shows a regular seasonal effect with most cases occurring in January or February (Fig. 2.6).

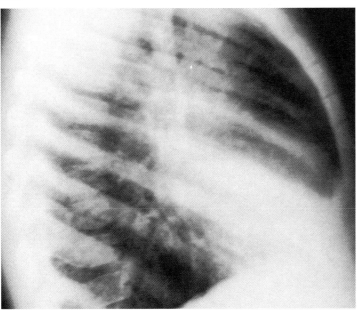

Fig. 2.4 Whooping cough. Chest radiographs showing patchy consolidation and collapse of the right middle lobe.

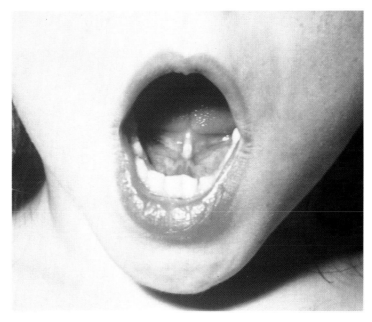

Fig. 2.5 Frenal ulcer in whooping cough. By courtesy of Dr G. D. W. McKendrick.

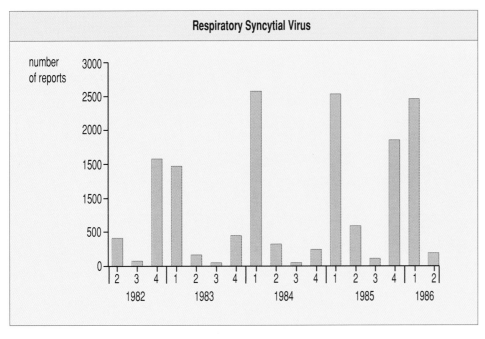

Fig. 2.6 Acute bronchiolitis. Seasonal variation in quarterly reports of isolation of respiratory syncytial virus in England and Wales. Redrawn from CDSC data.

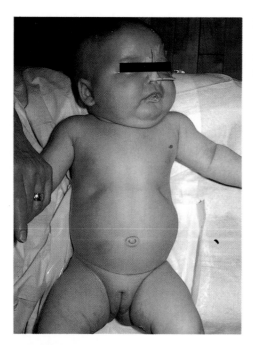

Fig. 2.7 Acute bronchiolitis. Prominent intercostal retraction indicating lower airway obstruction.

The illness begins with several days of upper respiratory symptoms followed by cough, tachypnoea, wheeze and intercostal muscle retraction (Fig. 2.7). Radiographic features usually include hyperinflation of the lungs (Fig. 2.8) and interstitial infiltrates caused by atelectasis: peribronchial thickening and consolidation and collapse, particularly of the upper lobe of the right lung, are also seen (Fig. 2.9). The diagnosis may be confirmed rapidly by immunofluorescent staining of secretions aspirated from the pharynx (Fig. 2.10). The histological appearance is shown in Fig. 2.11.

Second attacks of RSV infection can occur and, although they are not usually as severe as the initial attack, they may play an important part in the spread of outbreaks.

PNEUMONIA

Viral pneumonia

All of the respiratory viruses that cause acute bronchitis

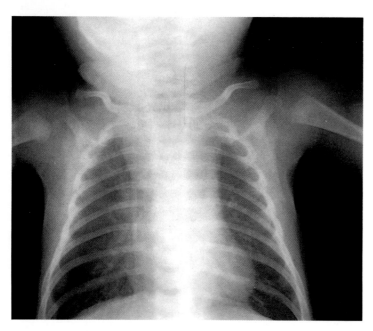

Fig. 2.8 Acute bronchiolitis. Early radiographic appearance – flat diaphragms and hyperlucent lower lung fields indicate hyperinflation.

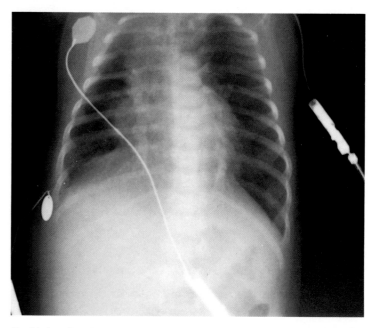

Fig. 2.9 Acute bronchiolitis. Radiograph taken in later stage of disease with collapse of right upper lobe and congestive cardiac failure (note enlarged liver).

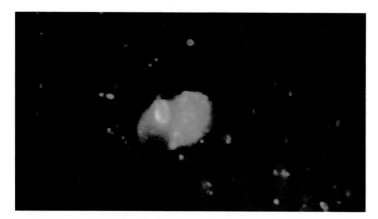

Fig. 2.10 Acute bronchiolitis. Immunofluorescent preparation from the nasopharynx. Cells infected with respiratory syncytial virus fluoresce bright green. By courtesy of Prof. H. Stern.

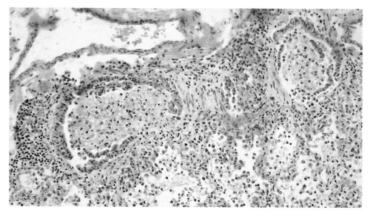

Fig. 2.11 Acute bronchiolitis. Autopsy appearance of lung, showing lymphocytic peribronchiolar infiltration with necrosis of the epithelium and obstruction of the lumen by inflammatory cells, sloughed epithelium and mucus. There is also pneumonitis of the surrounding lung. By courtesy of Dr C. W. Edwards.

may also cause pneumonic consolidation. If the infection is in a previously healthy subject, there are often no distinctive features of pneumonia and its presence may be detected only because a chest x-ray has been taken: viruses rarely cause severe pneumonia in such patients and when this happens it is often difficult to rule out the additional presence of bacterial infection. Immunosuppression renders patients much more susceptible to severe viral pneumonia.

The clinical features of viral pneumonia generally include mild to moderate constitutional disturbance accompanied by cough which is often unproductive. In severe cases there may be dyspnoea and cyanosis but the physical signs in the chest are often less than would be expected from the radiographic extent of the disease. Pleuritic pain is an uncommon feature.

Measles pneumonia

Among the commonest examples of severe viral pneumonia in healthy subjects is that associated with measles (in countries where that infection is still prevalent). In developed countries, pneumonia is its most frequent fatal complication and among the immunosuppressed severe pneumonia is a common feature of measles infection. Histologically it is characterized by interstitial infiltration with mononuclear cells and multinucleate giant cells (Fig. 2.12). The chest x-ray usually shows lobular consolidation irregularly distributed through both lungs (Fig. 2.13). Measles and its complication can be prevented by active immunization, which is normally performed between the ages of 12 and 15 months, though in tropical countries it may be necessary to bring this age range forward by 3 months to give the best results. Unimmunized children exposed to a case may be protected by active immunization if this is given within 3 days of first exposure. Otherwise they may be protected by passive immunization with normal human immunoglobulin.

Varicella pneumonia

Pneumonia is rarely seen in healthy children with chicken pox. However, in adults and in those of any age with immunosuppression, pneumonia is more common and sometimes severe. Signs of pulmonary involvement usually appear during the evolution of the rash accompanied by cough and tachypnoea. The chest radiograph (Fig. 2.14) shows widespread infiltration with nodules of variable size and shape. Histologically the bronchial epithelium contains intranuclear inclusion bodies (Fig. 2.15). Following recovery from varicella pneumonia, the x-ray may remain abnormal with nodular calcification sparsely distributed over the lung fields.

Patients with pneumonia caused by varicella-zoster virus should be treated with intravenous acyclovir.

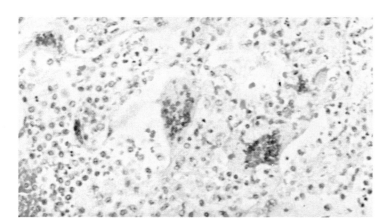

Fig. 2.12 Measles pneumonia. Histology showing mononuclear cell infiltration and multinucleate giant cells. H & E stain.

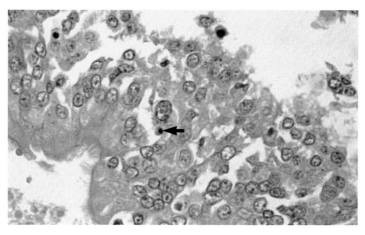

Fig. 2.13 Measles pneumonia. Chest radiograph showing widespread lobular opacities.

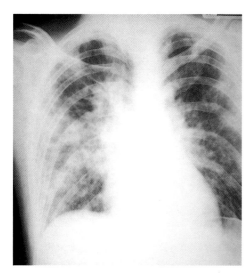

Fig. 2.14 Chicken pox pneumonia. Chest radiograph showing widespread patchy infiltrates throughout both lungs in a patient with Hodgkin's disease.

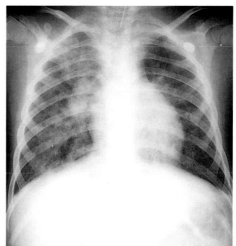

Fig. 2.15 Chicken pox pneumonia. Histological section of bronchial epithelium showing intranuclear inclusions (arrowed). By courtesy of Dr C. W. Edwards.

Cytomegalovirus pneumonia

Cytomegalovirus (CMV) infection in postnatal life generally produces either subclinical infection or a syndrome resembling infectious mononucleosis. The respiratory tract is not an important site of disease in previously healthy subjects. In patients with severe immunosuppression, however, CMV may affect the lungs. The problem is greatest among transplant recipients, who may also suffer graft rejection.

Clinically, the illness in transplant recipients is characterized by fever, nonproductive cough, dyspnoea and hypoxia, the symptoms generally developing over a period of two weeks or less. The radiographic abnormality of the lung in cytomegalovirus pneumonia tends to be interstitial rather than alveolar, with very fine, hazy shadowing in the middle and lower zones, giving a 'ground glass' effect. Definitive diagnosis is difficult because of the uncertainty over the interpretation of CMV isolation from respiratory secretions or urine. Often there are other potential pathogens from the same sources and the most reliable method is lung biopsy. Cytomegalovirus pneumonia is characterized histologically by the presence of the 'owl's eye' inclusion body (Figs 2.16 & 2.17).

Cytomegalovirus is also isolated quite frequently from bronchial washings obtained from patients with AIDS. There is some doubt in such cases about the significance of this finding: there is almost always another likely pathogen identified in the patient's lungs and the presence of cytomegalovirus seem to lack prognostic significance. The suggestion has been made that, in the lung, an inflammatory reaction to cytomegalovirus requires a greater immune response than can be mounted by AIDS patients.

Herpes simplex pneumonia

As with cytomegalovirus, pneumonia caused by herpes simplex virus (HSV) is virtually confined to patients with immune suppression or other severe generalized illness such as alcoholism or burns. The radiographic effect of herpes simplex pneumonia is variable but generally consists of multifocal, nodular, interstitial infiltrates. Monoclonal antibody techniques can be used to identify HSV in samples obtained through the bronchoscope by washing or brushing. The gross appearance at autopsy (Fig. 2.18) shows extensive consolidation with areas of haemorrhage. However, as with other forms of viral interstitial pneumonia, the appearances are nonspecific.

A histological section of a lung affected by herpes simplex pneumonia (Fig. 2.19) shows a large bronchus with intense subepithelial infiltration with inflammatory cells. Within the lumen there is also irregular proliferation of mononuclear cells. In the characteristic cell of HSV infec-

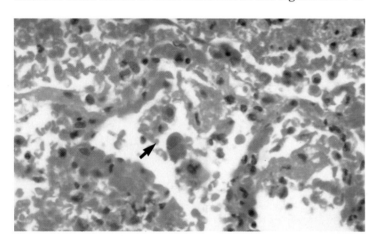

Fig. 2.16 Cytomegalovirus pneumonia. Histology showing congestion and infiltration of alveolar walls and owl's eye cell (arrowed) in alveolar space. H & E stain.

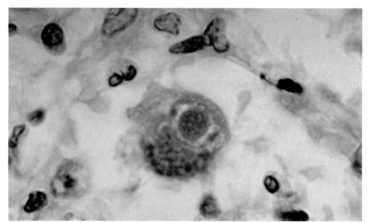

Fig. 2.17 Cytomegalovirus pneumonia. Higher power magnification of owl's eye cell with cytomegalovirus inclusion. H & E stain.

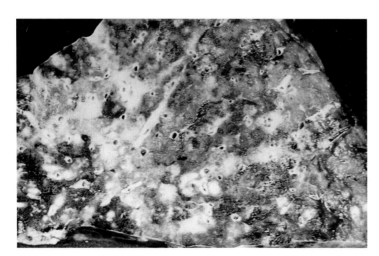

Fig. 2.18 Herpes simplex pneumonia. Gross appearance of affected lung at autopsy showing areas of extensive consolidation with haemorrhage.

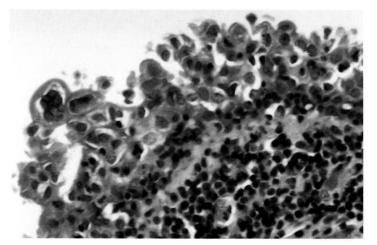

Fig. 2.19 Herpes simplex pneumonia. Histological section of lung showing large bronchus with subepithelial infiltration and irregular proliferation of mononuclear cells. H & E stain.

tions, the nuclear material is displaced to the periphery by an eosinophilic intranuclear inclusion body. Treatment of herpes simplex pneumonia is with intravenous acyclovir.

Bacterial pneumonia

Bacterial pneumonia may be divided into those cases occurring in healthy subjects who are exposed to a virulent organism to which they have no pre-existing immunity, and those which occur in patients who already have some deficiency of host defences. The first group includes most cases of pneumonia caused by *Streptococcus pneumoniae* and *Legionella pneumophila*. Pneumonias with broadly similar clinical features are also caused by *Mycoplasma pneumoniae*, *Chlamydia psittaci* and *Coxiella burnettii*. They are generally acquired in the community. Lung infection in patients with poor host defences includes bronchopneumonia, aspiration pneumonia and lung abscess. The causative organisms are often of lesser virulence and include aerobic and anaerobic organisms from the upper respiratory tract and, in some cases, from the bowel. Several different species of organism may be present in one infection.

Pneumococcal pneumonia

Streptoccocus pneumoniae is the commonest cause of com-

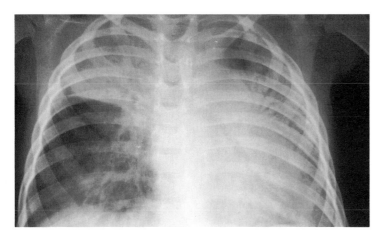

Fig. 2.20 Pneumococcal pneumonia. Chest radiograph showing lobar consolidation affecting both lungs. An air bronchogram is easily seen in the left middle zone.

munity-acquired pneumonia in previously healthy persons. Most cases are sporadic but outbreaks have been reported among military recruits, South African coal miners and the islanders of Papua/New Guinea. Pneumococcal infection is commoner in patients with absent splenic function, either because the organ has been removed or because it has suffered infarction (especially in sickle cell disease). Increased susceptibility is also found in patients with Hodgkin's disease, chronic lymphocytic leukaemia and myeloma. The immunological deficiency in these groups of patients involves difficulty with the initiation of antibody production or with the clearance of bacteria from the bloodstream. Often they present with early features of pneumococcal septicaemia alone, but in some cases lobar pneumonia may develop.

The illness, which is of acute onset, is characterized by severe systemic symptoms such as high fever, rigors, prostration and, sometimes, headache and delirium. These are followed shortly by pleuritic chest pain, cough and breathlessness. The appearance of cold sores caused by HSV around the lips or nose (see Fig 1.12) is a common development as the rest of the illness unfolds, but it is not specific for infections with *S. pneumoniae*. In a small number of patients with pneumococcal pneumonia, meningitis is also present.

The chest x-ray generally shows an alveolar pattern of consolidation in a single lobe, but sometimes more than one lobe is affected (Fig. 2.20) and in a few cases the disease is confined to a single pulmonary segment. The persistence of fever after the first 48 hours of treatment is often a sign of the development of empyema. During convalescence, radiographic improvement lags behind clinical recovery and it may well be 6 weeks before the x-ray returns to normal. Radiographic resolution is slowest in the elderly and in cases where the lingular segments of the left upper lobe are affected.

The diagnosis is most reliably made by the isolation of the organism from blood culture, but this is successfully achieved in only 30% of cases. In the remainder the diagnosis may be supported by the finding of large numbers of *S. pneumoniae* in purulent sputum (Fig. 2.21) or by the identification of pneumococcal antigen in sputum, blood or urine (Fig. 2.22). The Quellung reaction permits rapid diagnosis of pneumococci in sputum by the use of specific antisera or mixtures of antisera which, when

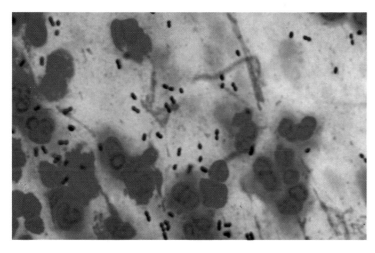

Fig. 2.21 Pneumococcal pneumonia. Preparation of sputum showing predominance of pneumococci mostly as lanceolate diplococci. Gram's stain. By courtesy of Dr J. R. Cantey.

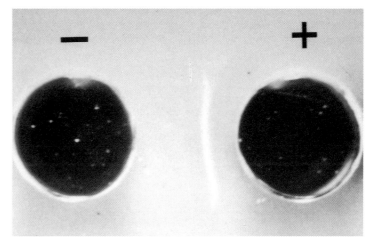

Fig. 2.22 Pneumococcal pneumonia. Counterimmuno-electrophoresis for detection of pneumococcal antigen showing line of precipitation.

added to a slide of the organism allows easy identification of the swollen bacterial capsule (Fig. 2.23). The white cell count in the peripheral blood is high with neutrophilia, and plasma levels of acute phase reactants rise. The shunting of blood through consolidated parts of the lung leads to arterial hypoxaemia, while at the same time hypocapnia results from the increased respiratory rate caused by fever and pleuritic pain.

The histological appearance is of a profuse intra-alveolar exudate containing neutrophil polymorphonuclear leucocytes, red cells and fibrin (Fig. 2.24). At autopsy the cut surface of affected parts of the lung is said to resemble liver (hepatization). Patients who recover generally do so completely, with resolution of the exudate and return of the pulmonary structure to normal.

The prevention of pneumococcal pneumonia in high-risk groups has been attempted by active immunization with a polyvalent vaccine containing antigens from those strains of the organism most often incriminated in septicaemias. This is fairly successful in previously healthy subjects such as military recruits, but less so in patients with haematological malignancy. Where elective splenectomy is to be undertaken, immunization should precede the operation but is still worth doing in patients who have already had their spleen removed. The risk of pneumococcal infection seems to be greatest in the first few years following the operation, and in this group the addition of prophylactic antibiotic therapy with daily penicillin for 2–3 years should be considered.

Atypical Pneumonia

The above description is traditionally regarded as 'typical' of acute pneumonia. When an acute, community-acquired, pneumonic illness presents with a different pattern of features it may be referred to as 'atypical'. This term has come to mean a condition associated with pulmonary parenchymal infection, occurring in previously fit subjects and dominated by mild to moderate systemic symptoms of more gradual onset. Cough, often unproductive, may be the only respiratory complaint.

The organisms most often responsible for atypical pneumonia are *Mycoplasma pneumoniae*, *Legionella pneumophila*, *Coxiella burnetti* and *Chlamydia* species.

Mycoplasma pneumonia

Mycoplasma pneumoniae is second in frequency to *S. pneumoniae* as a cause of community-acquired pneumonia in healthy subjects. Most cases are sporadic but outbreaks do occur, and the incidence of the illness shows a cyclical pattern with peaks at intervals of three or four years in

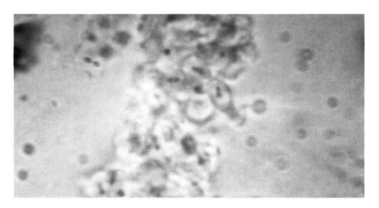

Fig. 2.23 Quellung reaction. The wide zone of pneumococcal capsular swelling is seen. By courtesy of Dr T. F. Sellers.

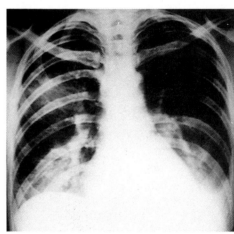

Fig. 2.25 Mycoplasma pneumonia. Chest radiograph showing patchy consolidation in several areas in both lungs.

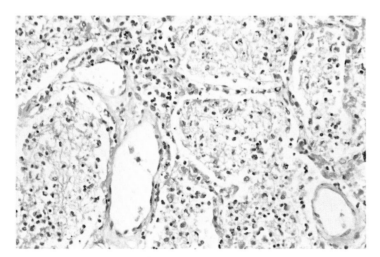

Fig. 2.24 Pneumococcal pneumonia. Histopathology showing inflammatory exudate filling alveolar spaces. H & E stain. By courtesy of Dr C. W. Edwards.

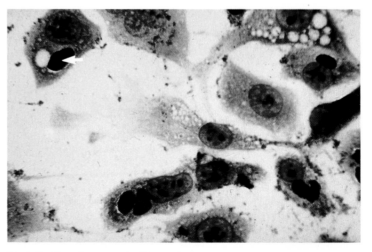

Fig. 2.26 *Chlamydia pneumoniae*. Tissue culture showing the organism as densely black-staining intracytoplasmic inclusions (arrowed). McCoy cells with cycloheximide. By courtesy of Dr G. Ridgeway.

the UK. Where clusters of cases appear in small communities, the individual cases tend to be separated by several weeks.

Mycoplasma predominantly infects children and young adults, and it may also cause acute infection of the middle ear, sinuses and bronchial tree. Its presentation is less abrupt than that of pneumococcal pneumonia and the illness is generally less severe. Complications are rare, though haemolytic anaemia has been described and there are associations with Stevens–Johnson syndrome and Guillain–Barré syndrome.

Physical findings in the chest are usually limited to the presence of localized crepitations without other indication of consolidation or pleural involvement.

The chest x-ray most often shows consolidation of one or more pulmonary segments (Fig. 2.25). Sometimes there is diffuse lobular involvement but pleural complications do not seem to occur. A specific aetiological diagnosis can be made by culturing the organism from sputum though few laboratories offer this as a routine service. Otherwise the diagnosis depends on serological testing for antibodies to the organism. In about 50% of cases cold agglutinins are present in the blood. These may first be detected when an attempt is made to prepare a blood film for examination. Cold agglutinins are uncommon in other conditions and their presence in the blood of a patient with pneumonia is strong presumptive evidence of infection with mycoplasma. The presence of cold agglutinins seldom manifests itself clinically but high titres are associated with haemolytic anaemia; occasionally it leads to arterial thrombosis. Other abnormalities of laboratory investigations are rare and nonspecific.

Mycoplasma infections are generally self limiting, but recovery is accelerated by the use of antibiotics such as erythromycin and tetracycline given for 2–3 weeks. Fatal cases are rare but have been recorded.

Psittacosis

Chlamydia psittaci is an organism intermediate in size between viruses and bacteria. It is an obligate intracellular parasite but it reproduces by binary fission and is sensitive to a number of antibiotics. It is acquired by environmental contact with birds which may themselves be sick or may be healthy carriers. The organism is present in the bird's droppings which dry and may then be inhaled by humans after dispersal by air currents. Infection in birds is not confined to those the psittacine (such as parrots); outbreaks in humans have been reported among workers in poultry farms.

As with other atypical pneumonias the illness generally starts as an undifferentiated fever of mild to moderate severity. Organ-specific symptoms such as cough, dyspnoea, abdominal pain, confusion and haematuria may follow and the pulmonary involvement may be come sufficiently extensive to cause respiratory failure.

The main clue to the diagnosis is the history of contact with birds. In severe cases there is almost always a history of close, indoor contact with birds, but in mild cases this may not be the case. Otherwise the specific diagnosis depends on serological testing. The chest x-ray may show almost any extent of lobular, segmental or lobar consolidation at one or more sites. Tests of liver function often reveal hepatocellular disturbance.

Psittacosis is potentially a very serious disease. In the first reported human outbreak, before the time of antibiotics, the mortality was 40%. Treatment should be given with tetracyclines or, in the case of intolerance, erythromycin.

TWAR pneumonia

During the mid-1980s serological surveys in the USA and Finland reported the existence of an unusual serotype of *Chlamydia psittaci* as a common cause of mild respiratory infection. This organism, initially known as TWAR (from the laboratory identifying letters of the first two isolates) but now designated *Chlamydia pneumoniae* (Fig. 2.26) differs from *C.psittaci* in its pattern of transmission and in the range of illness with which it is associated. It appears to be a human pathogen only and is transmitted from person to person by respiratory droplets. Infection may be subclinical or may cause respiratory symptoms which, although not usually severe, may persist for several weeks. Pneumonia, generally confined to a single pulmonary segment, is the commonest feature and pharyngitis with hoarseness is relatively frequent by comparison with similar infections caused by mycoplasma or viruses. Systemic symptoms are mild.

The diagnosis of infection with *C. pneumoniae* requires the use of a serotype-specific microimmunofluorescence test for detecting chlamydial antibody. Complement fixation tests alone do not distinguish between species or serotypes of *Chlamydia*. Studies carried out in university students have shown a 12% incidence of this form of infection in cases of pneumonia, the prevalence of past infection in blood donors in London has been reported at 21%.

The optimum form of treatment has not yet (on the serological evidence) been established. The organism is sensitive *in vitro* to both erythromycin and tetracycline, but results of treatment with erythromycin have been disappointing. Tetracycline, where not contraindicated, may be the best choice.

Q Fever

Q fever results from infection with *Coxiella burnetti*, an organism which causes apparently asymptomatic infection in farm animals such as sheep and cattle. It is present in their urine, faeces, milk and products of conception. The infection may be acquired by man as the result of drinking raw, infected milk, but it seems to be much more commonly acquired by inhalation of infected dust. Coxiellae are resistant to dehydration, and once they have been shed by the animal onto a field or farm building floor, they survive for long periods. They are dispersed by air currents and may infect humans so exposed in an apparently random manner. A number of outbreaks of Q fever have been reported, including some among subjects with no close association with farm animals or the countryside.

The diagnosis of Coxiella infection is made by serological testing, which is complicated by the fact that cultures of different maturity express different antigens on the cell surface. Fresh cultures express a surface antigen which is known as Phase II, whereas cultures of greater maturity express the Phase I antigen. This is of particular importance in determining whether a patient has gone on to develop chronic Q fever.

The illness caused by Q fever is rather more acute in onset than other forms of atypical pneumonia. The presenting symptoms are usually fever and headache, with cough being a minor and variable feature. In some cases the presentation is more suggestive of meningitis or encephalitis, but abnormalities of the CSF are rare.

Laboratory investigations at the start show no characteristic abnormality, though moderate disturbance of liver function is common. The chest x-ray usually shows isolated segmental consolidation. The definitive diagnosis is reached by demonstrating a rising titre of antibody to the Phase II Coxiella antigen in the serum. In some cases the rise in antibody titre is not detectable until several weeks after the onset of the illness.

Q fever responds to treatment with tetracyclines. The main concern is not over the initial pneumonic illness but with the possibility of the development of endocarditis several months later. This is associated with the appearance in the serum of antibodies to the Phase I antigen.

Legionnaires' Disease

The Legionellaceae are a family of fastidious, slow growing, aerobic, gram-negative bacteria of which *Legionella pneumophila* is the member most commonly found as a cause of human disease (Fig. 2.27). It occurs naturally in aqueous habitats. For disease to occur, a susceptible person must inhale an infected aerosol of sufficiently small particle size to penetrate to alveolar level. Outbreaks of legionnaires' disease have been caused by contamination of cooling water systems used in industrial premises or in air conditioning plant, of hot water systems in large buildings such as hotels and hospitals, of recreational pools and

of respiratory therapy equipment. Sporadic cases are most common in the late summer and autumn. The frequency of legionnaires' disease as a cause of community-acquired pneumonia varies between 2% and 15% in different studies.

Legionnaires' disease affects men more than women, and is most common in the 40–70 year age group. It is rarely found in children. The disease is more severe in smokers, alcoholics, diabetics and in immunosuppressed patients. Serological surveys show that some infections are subclinical, and that some give rise to a 'flu-like' illness known as Pontiac fever, in which pneumonia does not occur. The reasons for these different manifestations of the same infection are unknown.

The clinical features of legionnaires' disease overlap with those of other acute pneumonias and it is not possible to make a certain diagnosis on the strength of the clinical observations alone. However, there is a relatively high incidence of confusion and other neurological findings, diarrhoea and liver and renal dysfunction. These features, in a patient seriously ill with pneumonia and, particularly, with recent exposure to possible sources of legionella infection, make a diagnosis of legionnaires' disease much more likely.

Specific investigation of the cause of legionnaires' disease depends on direct identification of the organism by culture or immunofluorescent staining, or on the demonstration of a rising titre of antibody in the serum. In some cases the organism can be isolated from blood or expectorated sputum, but a higher yield of positive results has been reported from lung secretions obtained by transtracheal aspiration or bronchoalveolar lavage (Fig. 2.28).

A retrospective diagnosis may be made by serological testing using the indirect fluorescent antibody test. The rate at which specific antibody appears in patients with legionnaires' disease varies from less than a week to more than a month. It is therefore necessary to examine specimens taken not only during the acute and early convalescent stages but also in late convalescence (about 6 weeks)

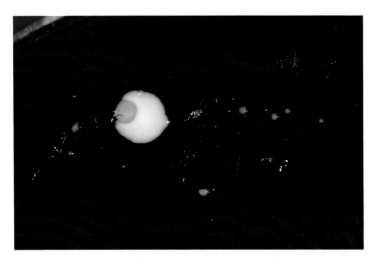

Fig. 2.27 Legionella pneumophila. White colonies easily identified on buffered charcoal yeast extract medium. By courtesy of Dr I. Farrell.

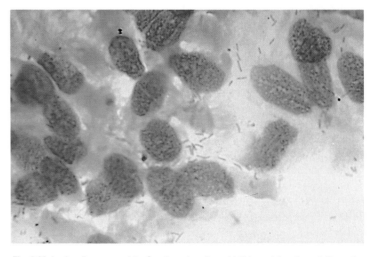

Fig. 2.28 Legionella pneumophila. Specimen from bronchial biopsy taken through fibreoptic bronchoscope in a patient with fulminant Legionnaires' disease. The organism can be isolated on selective culture media or by guinea pig inoculation. By courtesy of Dr S. Fisher-Hoch.

to ensure a maximum diagnostic yield.

Other laboratory investigations are likely to show moderate neutrophilia of the peripheral blood and, in about half of the cases, hyponatraemia. Proteinuria and evidence of hepatocellular disturbance are also seen. The chest x-ray appearance is somewhat variable, with segmental, lobar and nodular shadows all being reported. These may be restricted to one part of the lung, but in about one-third of cases more than one lung zone is affected (Fig. 2.29). Rapid deterioration of the chest x-ray appearance over the first few days seems to be particularly common in legionnaires' disease. Pleural effusions occasionally develop but are small. Radiographic recovery may be slow and there are reports of permanent lobar collapse and fibrosis in survivors of severe attacks.

Erythromycin has been used most widely for the treatment of legionnaires' disease. In severe cases it should be given intravenously and consideration should be given to the addition of another agent such as rifampicin. If erythromycin cannot be used, doxycycline is the recommended alternative. The reported mortality in cases admitted to hospital is 5–15% in previously healthy patients and 70% in the immunosuppressed. Fig. 2.30 illustrates the autopsy appearance of extensive pulmonary consolidation in a case of Legionnaires' disease.

Staphylococcal pneumonia

Nasal carriage of *Staphylococcus aureus* can be detected in about 30% of the population at any given time, and will occur at some time in about 80%. However, staphylococcal pneumonia is rare and is almost never found in previously healthy adults. It seems that in order for this organism to become established in the lungs there must be some pre-existing damage or susceptibility. The most common of these are influenza, measles, chronic bronchitis, bronchial obstruction, pulmonary surgery and cystic fibrosis. The condition is also seen more frequently in the very young.

Staphylococcal pneumonia in children is most common in the first 8 weeks of life and may be preceded by a viral respiratory infection. Patients or their close contacts often have minor staphylococcal skin infections. The condition of the child deteriorates rapidly with fever, non-productive cough, tachypnoea, signs of respiratory distress and circulatory collapse. The chest x-ray shows irregular patches of consolidation which progress rapidly and often become bilateral. Common complications include effusion, pneumatoceles (Fig. 2.31) empyema and pneumothorax. Septicaemia occurs in about a third of cases and may lead to metastatic infection of bone, soft tissue, meninges and pericardium.

Among adults staphylococcal pneumonia is most likely to be seen in the aftermath of an influenza virus infection, which may cause severe damage to the ciliated epithelium of the airways. It seems to be particularly likely in those who already have chronic disease of the lungs or heart. As in children the onset of the illness is marked by a dramatic deterioration in the patient's condition, usually with fever, rigors, cough, dyspnoea and pleuritic pain, often accompa-

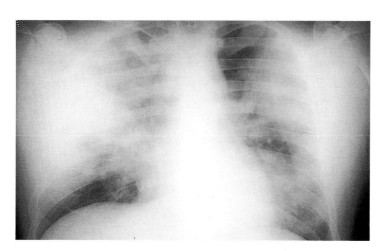

Fig. 2.29 Legionnaires' disease. Chest radiograph showing extensive consolidation affecting parts of all lobes of the lungs.

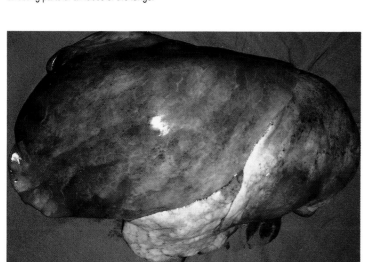

Fig. 2.30 Legionnaires' disease. Autopsy specimen showing consolidation of upper and lower lobes of right lung.

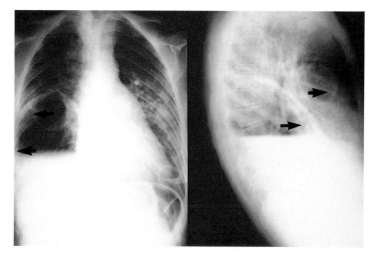

Fig. 2.31 Staphylococcal pneumonia. Posteroanterior and lateral chest radiographs of infant showing pneumatoceles (arrowed) in right middle and lower lobes and in left lower lobe.

nied by mental confusion and shock. The chest x-ray changes are similar to those described in children, except that pneumatocoeles are rarely seen. The diagnosis depends on the isolation of the organism from blood or from bronchial secretions (Figs 2.32 & 2.33). The sputum is often bloodstained and, when samples are available, the organism can readily be identified. Pleural fluid from effusion or empyema may also provide diagnostic specimens.

Wherever the clinical features and background of a case suggest staphylococcal pneumonia, parenteral treatment with at least one anti-staphylococcal antibiotic should be started immediately. Drainage of effusions, empyemas and abscesses should be carried out where necessary and ventilatory and circulatory support may be needed, although assisted ventilation adds to the risk of pneumothorax. Even with these measures the mortality from severe staphylococcal pneumonia has been reported to be about 40%.

Pneumonia caused by Enterobacteriaceae

Enterobactericeae are not normally able to establish themselves in the lower respiratory tract. When they are detected as a cause of pneumonia, there is almost always some defect of host defences which has permitted soiling of the lower airways with organisms already present in the mouth. This generally means two things: firstly, that there has been some circumstance such as prolonged hospital admission, broad spectrum antibiotic administration or immunosuppression, which has allowed the normal oropharyngeal flora to be replaced by enteric organisms; and secondly, that there is some physical defect in the patient's ability to evacuate foreign material from the bronchial tree. The latter may be the result of coma, neurological or structural abnormality of the larynx, impaired ability to cough, especially after thoracic or upper abdominal surgery, repeated vomiting or oesophageal regurgitation, structural abnormality of the bronchi, such as chronic bronchitis, bronchial carcinoma or bronchiectasis, and tracheostomy or endotracheal intubation. Several of these risk factors frequently coexist.

The condition takes the form of bronchopneumonia. Its onset may be marked clinically by little more than a mild fever, an increase in respiratory rate or a nonspecific deterioration in the general condition of a patient already ill for one of the reasons given above. The x-ray appearance

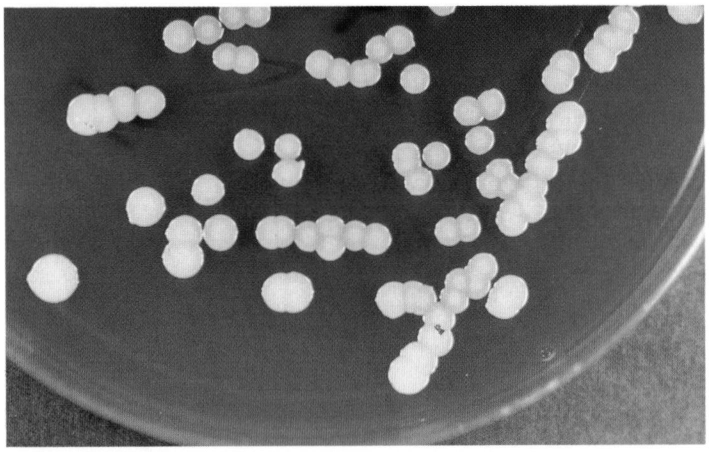

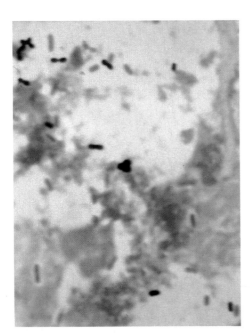

Fig. 2.32 *Staphylococcus aureus.* Blood agar plate showing large slightly yellow colonies with a clearly defined edge. There is no zone of haemolysis.

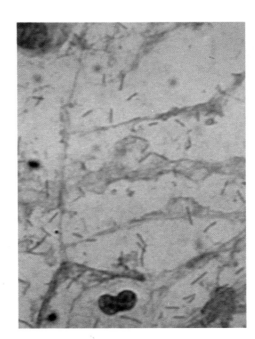

Fig. 2.33 *Staphylococcus aureus.* Gram stain of culture showing characteristic irregular clusters of gram-positive cocci. There are no spores or capsules.

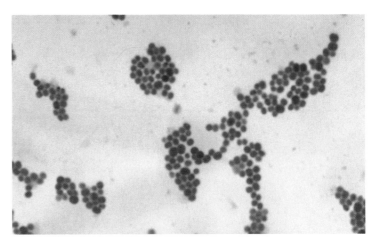

Fig. 2.34 Gram-negative pneumonia. Gram stain of sputum showing gram-negative bacilli and streptococci (which were anaerobic). Sometimes the clear zone of the bacterial capsule can be seen. By courtesy of Dr J. F. John, Jr.

Fig. 2.35 Gram-negative pneumonia. Gram stain of septum showing gram-negative rods of *Pseudomonas aeruginosa.* By courtesy of Dr H. P. Holley, Jr.

is that of irregular consolidation often involving the lower lobes of both lungs. Results of the examination of expectorated sputum are difficult to interpret because the sample may be contaminated by organisms from the mouth. More reliable specimens may be obtained, if indicated, by transtracheal aspiration or bronchoscopy. In view of the pathogenesis of this form of pneumonia it is not surprising that in many cases a mixed growth of organisms, including gram-positive and gram-negative aerobes and anaerobes, is obtained (Fig. 2.34). Of the Enterobacteriaceae, *Escherichia coli* is the most frequently identified, but similar infection may be caused by *Klebsiella*, *Proteus* and *Providencia* species. *Pseudomonas aeruginosa*, which belongs to the family Pseudomonadaceae, may also cause bronchopneumonia, especially in neutropenic patients (Fig. 2.35). Histologically the infection is multifocal, individual areas of inflammation being centred around small bronchi and gradually enlarging to produce a confluent zone of diseased lung (Fig. 2.36).

Treatment is by removal or counteraction, where possible, of any of the above risk factors and by an appropriate antibiotic or combination of antibiotics. The prognosis depends largely on the severity of the patient's underlying illness.

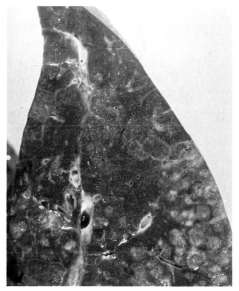

Fig. 2.36
Bronchopneumonia. Cut surface of postmortem lung showing areas of inflammation centred on small bronchi.

Klebsiella pneumonia

In addition to its ability to cause bronchopneumonia as described above, *Klebsiella pneumoniae* may occasionally cause a primary lobar pneumonia, though its occurrence is generally limited to subjects with debilitating diseases such as alcoholism or diabetes mellitus. The illness is a severe one, usually affecting the upper lobes and causing parenchymal destruction. Cavitation is common (Figs 2.37 & 2.38) and the patient may cough out large amounts of mucoid and bloodstained sputum.

Plague

Plague is caused by infection with *Yersinia pestis*, a small, pleomorphic, nonmotile gram-negative bacillus, whose pathogenicity seems to depend upon the production of exotoxin, endotoxin and an envelope protein known as Factor 1, which confers resistance against phagocytosis. The organism primarily affects mammals (especially rodents) and their fleas. Wild rodent plague is known to exist in western parts of the USA, in Africa, South America, the Middle East, Southeast Asia and in Indonesia. Cases occur in humans when they are bitten by infected fleas, when they are exposed to the carcasses of infected animals, for example while skinning rabbits, or when they inhale an infected aerosol. The first two mechanisms give rise to bubonic plague, which may be complicated by septicaemia and pneumonia. In turn these cases may be the source of person-to-person spread through infected aerosols, leading to epidemic pneumonic plague. Human pneumonic plague may also be acquired by aerosol inhalation in laboratory accidents.

Pneumonic plague incubates for a short time (2–4) days and then proceeds rapidly through a brief prodromal period of fever, headache and malaise to fulminant pneumonic features including cough, with bloodstained mucopurulent sputum, tachypnoea and dyspnoea. Disseminated intravascular coagulation often complicates the illness and without treatment most patients die within a few days.

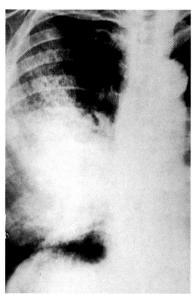

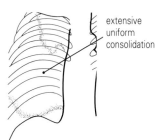

Fig. 2.37 Klebsiella pneumonia. Chest radiograph showing early stage with uniform consolidation in the right lung.

extensive uniform consolidation

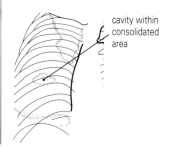

Fig. 2.38 Klebsiella pneumonia. Chest radiograph taken one day later than that in Fig. 2.37 showing abscess formation in the pneumonic area.

cavity within consolidated area

The diagnosis is confirmed by identification of the organisms in smears or cultures of sputum, blood (Fig. 2.39) or material aspirated from a bubo. The chest x-ray shows multifocal areas of consolidation of varying size (Fig. 2.40).

Where the clinical suspicion of pneumonic plague arises, treatment should be started immediately with streptomycin or tetracycline. Close contacts of cases of suspected pneumonic plague should also be given prophylactic treatment with tetracycline or a sulfonamide.

Tularemia

Francisella tularensis, the causative organism of human tularemia, is a small, gram-negative, nonmotile coccobacillus. Its natural reservoir is in wild animals (especially rabbits and hares) of the Northern Hemisphere, in the blood-sucking arthropods that feed on them, and in water and soil in their environment. Human infection usually arises from direct contact with infected animal carcasses, or from infected arthropod bites.

The clinical features of tularemia arise from inflammation at the site of implantation of the organism (usually the skin but occasionally the conjunctiva); regional lymphadenopathy and blood-borne dissemination cause prolonged systemic symptoms (the typhoidal form). Pulmonary complications are frequent and take the form of pneumonic consolidation of variable distribution and extent (Fig. 2.41). The diagnosis is usually made by serological testing: isolation of the organism requires animal inoculation and there is a significant risk of spread of infection within laboratories by infected aerosols. Streptomycin is the drug of choice with tetracycline and chloramphenicol as alternatives. Mortality in untreated tularemia is 5–15% but with treatment it falls to less than 1%.

TUBERCULOSIS

Primary pulmonary tuberculosis

Primary tuberculosis may occur at any epithelial site, but it is now most uncommon to find new cases of infection in organs other than the lung. The disease is spread by infected aerosols coughed out by persons already suffering from active pulmonary tuberculosis. Only those particles which are respirable to alveolar level penetrate far enough to be successfully implanted in the lung; larger particles are deposited in the upper respiratory tract or the bronchial tree and are expelled. In the susceptible subject, establishment of the infection provokes the development of a small area of inflammatory reaction (the Ghon focus) followed soon afterwards by spread to the regional lymph nodes. These two elements make up the primary complex.

Primary tuberculosis is often subclinical and where symptoms do occur they are mostly systemic in nature. Typical features include fever, anorexia and lethargy, sometimes accompanied by mild respiratory symptoms such as an unproductive cough. In a small proportion of cases the development of erythema nodosum provides an important clue to the diagnosis (Fig. 2.42). Otherwise, physical signs, other than fever, are likely to be few and nonspecific. Investigation of the patient should start with tuberculin skin testing (Fig. 2.43) which becomes positive

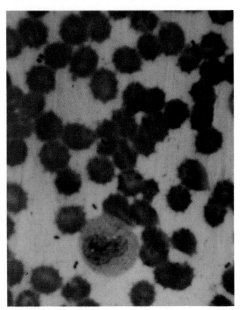

Fig. 2.39 Plague. Smear of peripheral blood from a patient with septicaemic plague showing bipolar forms of *Yersinia pestis*. Van Gieson stain. By courtesy of Dr J. R. Cantey.

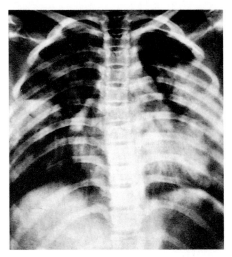
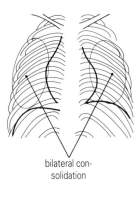

bilateral consolidation

Fig. 2.40 Pneumonic plague. Chest radiograph showing extensive bilateral consolidation. By courtesy of Dr J. R. Cantey.

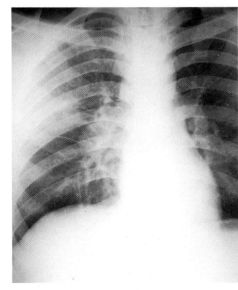

Fig. 2.41 Tularaemia. Radiograph showing patchy consolidation in the right upper and lower lobes. By courtesy of Dr T. F. Sellers, Jr.

3–10 weeks after aquisitition of the infection, unless there is some reason for cell-mediated immunity to be depressed. The most likely such reason is a preceding viral infection such as measles, which can itself contribute to the pathogenesis by rendering the patient more susceptible to tuberculosis. The chest x-ray may show either or both elements (lymphatic and parenchymal) of the primary complex (Figs 2.44 & 2.45). In young children the lymphatic element tends to be more evident and in adults, the pulmonary parenchymal part. In uncomplicated primary tuberculosis little sputum is produced and the isolation of the organism may require the examination of gastric washings taken first thing in the morning.

Most cases of primary tuberculosis heal with out treatment, but in about 10–15% of cases progression of the infection results in the appearance of disease over the fol-lowing two years. These complications may arise through spread of the infection with in the lung itself, by lymphatic spread or by bloodborne spread.

Progressive tuberculous pneumonia

This form of tuberculosis is found in adults and in adolescents, but very seldom occurs in younger children. It affects the upper parts of the lung first, spreading caudally as time goes on and usually involving the contralateral lung in a similar fashion at a relatively early stage. The upper parts of the lung seem to be more susceptible, through a combination of better ventilation and poorer circulation. Organisms may reach the upper parts of the lung either by haematogenous dissemination from the primary complex, or as a result of intrabronchial spread from the

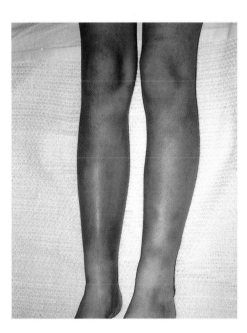

Fig. 2.42 Erythema nodosum. Tender raised nodules over the shins of a child with primary tuberculosis.

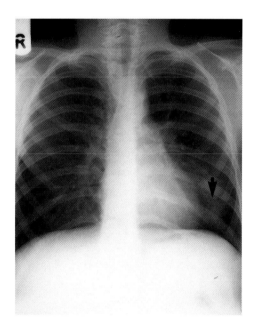

Fig. 2.44 Primary tuberulosis. Chest radiograph showing Ghon focus (arrowed) in lower zone of left lung.

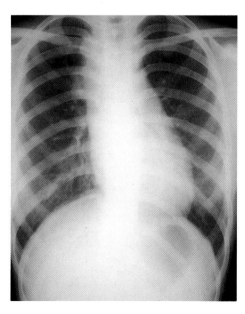

Fig. 2.45 Primary tuberculosis. Chest radiograph showing right hilar and paratracheal lymphadenopathy.

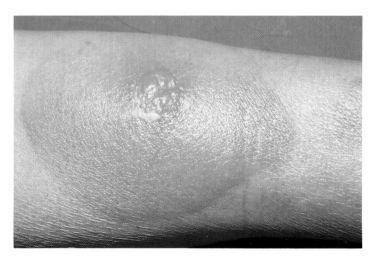

Fig. 2.43 Tuberculin test. Erythema and induration at site of intradermal injection of 5 tuberculin units in a child with primary tuberculosis. This is an unusually severe reaction. Mantoux method.

Ghon focus. Histologically there is granulomatous inflammation with caseous necrosis, coalescence of adjacent tubercles and rupture into the bronchial lumen (Fig. 2.46). As a result, such cases are likely to have sputum heavily contaminated with *Mycobacterium tuberculosis* (Fig. 2.47) and they will be infectious to others. Destruction of lung tissue is followed by fibrotic collapse and ultimately by calcification.

Clinically, progressive pulmonary tuberculosis presents as a subacute pneumonia with systemic and respiratory symptoms steadily worsening over weeks or a small number of months. Dominant symptoms include fever, sweating, weight loss, chest pain and productive cough, often with haemoptysis. Sputum examination for mycobacteria is likely to be positive both on a stained smear and on culture. The chest x-ray is always abnormal, advanced cases showing bilateral upper and middle zone irregular consolidation, often with cavitation and sometimes with lobar collapse or effusion (Figs 2.48 & 2.49). In early cases the disease may be localized, particularly to the apical or posterior segments of one upper lobe, and the opacities may have a soft or fluffy appearance (Fig. 2.50).

Without treatment this form of tuberculosis has a mortality of about 50% and a further 25% of cases go on to a chronic stage of alternating remission and relapse. However, excellent results are obtained from antituberculosis chemotherapy, the small number of failures being found in those cases where the patient was moribund by the time treatment was started.

Lymphatic spread

From the regional lymph nodes infection may spread by way of lymphatic vessels to the mediastinum, and beyond to supraclavicular and submandibular nodes in the neck or to retroperitoneal nodes in the abdomen. Infection may

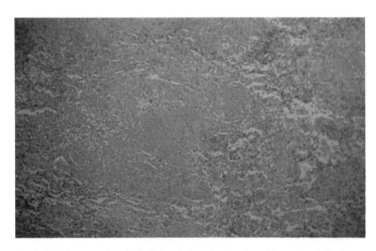

Fig. 2.46 Pulmonary tuberculosis. Histopathology showing dense inflammatory infiltration, granuloma formation and caseous necrosis. By courtesy of Dr R. Bryan.

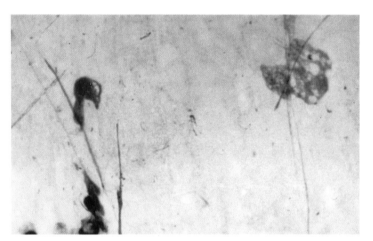

Fig. 2.47 Pulmonary tuberculosis. Preparation of sputum showing large numbers of pink-staining tubercle bacilli. Ziehl–Neelson stain.

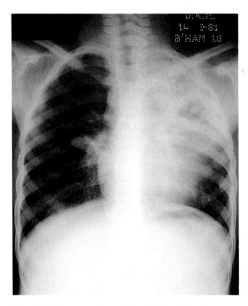

Fig. 2.48 Pulmonary tuberculosis. Chest radiograph showing consolidation and cavitation of left upper lobe.

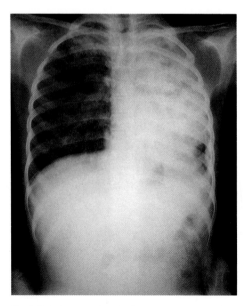

Fig. 2.49 Pulmonary tuberculosis. Chest radiograph showing extensive consolidation of the left lung with partial collapse. Less severe changes are seen on the right.

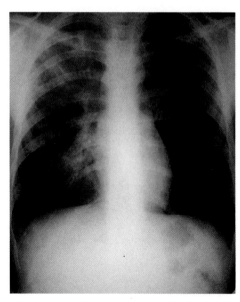

Fig. 2.50 Pulmonary tuberculosis. Chest radiograph showing early and limited pulmonary disease.

also reach the supraclavicular glands by spread across the pleural space from a subpleural Ghon focus in the upper lobe. Tuberculous mediastinal lymphadenopathy most often affects the paratracheal groups of glands. It may cause systemic symptoms but local symptoms are rare, only very occasional patients describing retrosternal pain. However, these glands may caseate and become necrotic, leading to the spread of infection through the bloodstream or to adjacent serous cavities (Figs 2.51 & 2.52). In the course of treatment of primary or lymphatic tuberculous it is quite common to observe new evidence of lymph node involvement. This does not necessarily mean that treatment is defective and in almost all cases a satisfactory outcome will be obtained without the need for alteration of the therapeutic regime.

Bronchial complications of primary tuberculosis.

The lymph nodes draining a segment or lobe of lung are arranged in a ring round the root of the relevant bronchus. If they become enlarged as part of a primary tuberculous complex they may compress the bronchus and obstruct it partially or completely. This is particularly seen in young children, possibly because of the narrow calibre of their airways and the immaturity of the cartilaginous elements of the bronchial walls. The most commonly affected bronchi are those of the middle lobe and the anterior segments of the upper lobes. Occasionally enlarged mediastinal glands compress the trachea or even the oesophagus.

These bronchial complications of tuberculosis, sometimes known as epituberculosis, seldom cause serious aggravation of symptoms and are usually detected by their effect on the chest x-ray. The commonest appearance is collapse of the affected segment or lobe (Figs 2.53 & 2.54), but in some cases partial obstruction allows persistent pyogenic infection in the distal part of the lung. In a few cases the bronchus is obstructed during expiration only, leading to

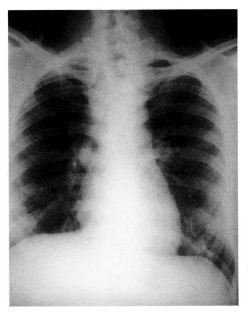

Fig. 2.51 Tuberculosis of mediastinal glands. Chest radiograph showing widening of superior mediastinum by enlarged right paratrachael lymph nodes.

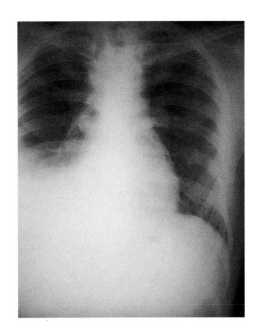

Fig. 2.52 Tuberculous pleurisy. Chest radiograph showing small right pleural effusion. Same patient as Fig. 2.51, x-rayed one week later.

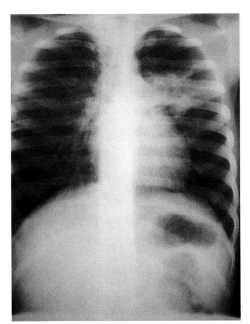

Fig. 2.53 Bronchial complications of tuberculosis. Posteroanterior chest radiograph showing collapse of anterior segment of left upper lobe.

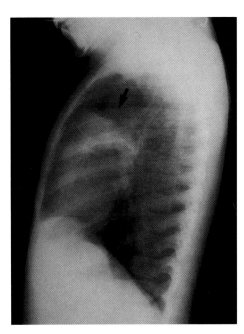

Fig. 2.54 Bronchial complications of tuberculosis. Lateral chest radiograph showing collapse of the anterior segment of the left upper lobe (arrowed).

overinflation of the affected lobe. This may be more easily detected by clinical examination unless radiographs are taken in both inspiration and expiration (Fig. 2.55).

The prognosis in epituberculosis is good unless the infection spreads from the lymph node to the adjacent bronchial epithelium, causing tuberculous endobronchitis. If this happens, later fibrosis may lead to bronchostenosis and localized bronchiectasis.

Tuberculous pleurisy

Tuberculous infection may reach the pleura by direct extension from a pulmonary lesion, through the blood stream or as the result of leakage of caseous lymph nodes at the hilum of the lung or in the mediastinum. Of these, the last is probably the usual cause of tuberculous pleurisy seen in older children and young adults 6–12 months after the acquisition of tuberculous infection. The discharge of even small amounts of tuberculous material into the pleural space is capable, in sensitized subjects, of provoking the effusion of large amounts of serous fluid, containing high concentrations of protein and moderate numbers of lymphocytes, but very few bacilli. Direct smear examinations of pleural fluid are very seldom positive for mycobacteria and attempts to culture the organism are successful in only about 40% of cases. A more fruitful method of investigation is by pleural biopsy, which shows characteristic features in up to 75% of cases (Fig. 2.56). The tuberculin test is almost always strongly positive – a negative test throws very serious doubt on the diagnosis. The condition is almost always unilateral and if an x-ray is taken after removal of the pleural fluid, the underlying lung usually appears to be normal.

Tuberculous pleurisy is a self limiting condition, but in untreated cases, pulmonary parenchymal tuberculosis follows within two years in about 15% of cases. Treatment, as for other forms of tuberculosis, is therefore indicated in all cases. The addition of corticosteroids for the first 3 months accelerates the rate of reabsorption of the effusion and may reduce the incidence of late pulmonary constriction from pleural fibrosis.

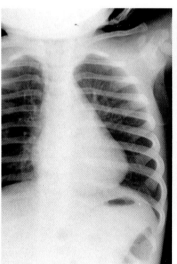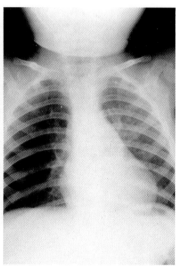

Fig. 2.55 Bronchial complications of tuberculosis. Chest radiographs taken in inspiration (left) and expiration (right), illustrating the effect of incomplete bronchial obstruction in preventing exhalation from the right lung. By courtesy of Dr P. Weller.

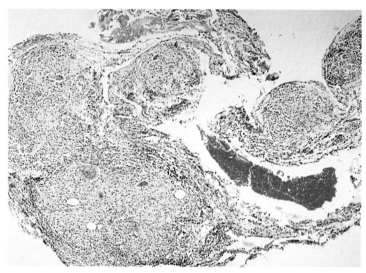

Fig. 2.56 Tuberculous pleurisy. Histology of punch biopsy showing noncaseating granulomata with multinucleate giant cells. By courtesy of Dr C. W. Edwards.

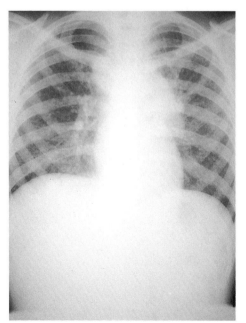

Fig. 2.57 Miliary tuberculosis. Radiograph appearance of diffuse uniform micronodular shadows evenly distributed throughout the lungs. Film also shows hilar and mediastinal lymphadenopathy.

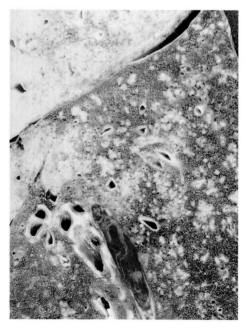

Fig 2.58 Miliary tuberculosis. Gross specimen of lung showing cut surface covered with white nodules, fairly uniform in size, which are miliary foci of tuberculosis. The adjacent lobe shows confluent consolidation.

Miliary tuberculosis

Bloodborne dissemination of tubercle bacilli is common after primary infection, probably arising from infected lymph nodes. In most cases this process is clinically silent but in a few it leads to overt miliary tuberculosis. The risk is greatest in the youngest children. About 90% of cases of overt miliary tuberculosis occur within a year of the acquisition of infection. The condition is marked by profound constitutional disturbance. Although the chest x-ray shows diffuse infiltration, respiratory symptoms are uncommon. Signs of meningitis are found in about 25% of cases.

The diagnosis depends on the appearance of the chest x-ray (diffuse micronodular opacities throughout both lungs – Fig. 2.57) the tuberculin test (generally positive unless the patient is already moribund) and the isolation of the organism. Samples of sputum and gastric washings are frequently positive, and positive results may also be obtained from bone marrow or urine, even in the absence of other signs of renal infection.

Without treatment miliary tuberculosis is always fatal (Fig. 2.58). However, as with most other forms of the disease, excellent results are obtained if treatment is started before the patient has become desperately ill.

Postprimary tuberculosis

Tubercle bacilli have the capacity to remain dormant, but viable, for long periods in healthy subjects. Where primary infection has healed spontaneously, a proportion of patients will continue to harbour organisms capable of causing disease in the future. Such reactivation to cause postprimary tuberculosis may occur in any organ, but it is most common in the lung. Reactivation is more likely to occur in patients with chronic disease causing general debility, such as alcoholism, malnutrition and diabetes mellitus, or with cellular immunodeficiency, particularly that caused by HIV infection. Immunosuppressant drug treatment has a similar effect and may be an indication for prophylactic chemotherapy in patients with a history of untreated tuberculosis in the past.

Postprimary pulmonary tuberculosis usually evolves slowly, and it is common for patients to report symptoms going on for several months before the diagnosis is made. The initial symptoms are usually respiratory, with persistent cough, purulent sputum sometimes containing blood, chest pain and eventually breathlessness. Later in the illness, systemic symptoms of fever, sweating, lethargy and weight loss also appear. The histopathology, anatomical distribution and radiographic features are the same as those described for progressive primary pulmonary tuberculosis but there may also be signs of previous, healed disease in the form of contraction of the upper lobes and calcification.

The diagnosis is made by bacteriological examination of sputum, but if none is available samples obtained by bronchoalveolar lavage may give positive results. The tuberculin test is likely to be positive, but less reliably so than in tuberculous disease which closely follows primary infection. Other investigations may yield a number of nonspecific signs of chronic disease such as normochromic, normocytic anaemia, hypoalbuminaemia and elevated serum levels of acute phase reactants.

When postprimary pulmonary tuberculosis reaches a far advanced stage, a second phase of dissemination may occur through the bloodstream or by the epithelial implantation of organisms coughed from the lungs. In this way secondary lesions may appear in the intestine and in the larynx. Laryngeal tuberculosis is usually a very late development associated with painful dysphagia, hoarseness and enhanced infectivity. Figs 2.59, 2.60 and 2.61 show the chest radiograph, lung and larynx of a patient who died within a day of presentation with far advanced postprimary pulmonary tuberculosis.

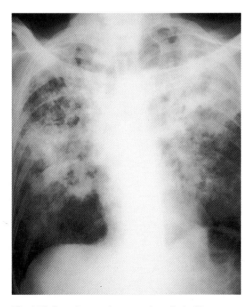

Fig. 2.59 Postprimary pulmonary tuberculosis. Chest radiograph showing far advanced disease.

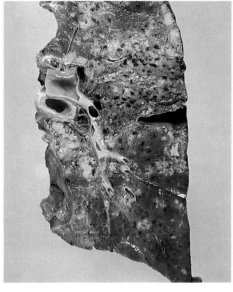

Fig. 2.60 Postprimary pulmonary tuberculosis. Autopsy appearance of lung (same patient as Fig. 2.59) showing extensive caseous necrosis, particularly of the upper lobe and the apical segment of the lower lobe.

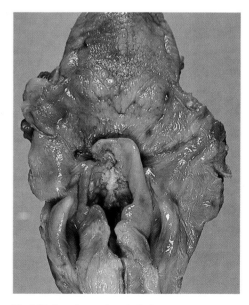

Fig. 2.61 Postprimary tuberculosis. Autopsy appearance of larynx. (Same patient as Fig. 2.59.)

Reactivation in immunosuppressed subjects

Where tuberculous infection reactivates in a patient with profound depression of cellular immunity, the clinical, radiographic and histopathological features may differ considerably from those described above. The disease is more likely to disseminate to other organs and its clinical presentation may be marked only by progressive constitutional disturbance. Histologically there may be little sign of granuloma formation or caseation, but lesions often contain large numbers of organisms. The chest x-ray usually does not show the features of overt miliary tuberculosis (described earlier) and cavitation seldom occurs. The tuberculin test is likely to be negative and the diagnosis depends on the identification of tubercle bacilli in bacteriological specimens or biopsies.

In HIV-infected subjects tuberculosis is particularly common. Among those who have previously had primary tuberculous infection and who have not received treatment, the rate of tuberculous disease is around 30%. Presumably most of this disease results from reactivation, and it is often discovered before the onset of severe immunodeficiency. When tuberculosis occurs in patients who already have other AIDS-defining conditions, the radiographic appearance is often surprisingly similar to that of primary disease in children (Figs 2.62 & 2.63).

OTHER BACTERIAL INFECTIONS

Atypical mycobacterial infection of the lung

Mycobacteria other than those which cause tuberculosis are widely distributed in the environment. They are saprophytes and are found particularly in soil and water. Some are capable of causing disease of the lungs, but only when there is preceding structural damage to the lung architecture, or severe deficiency of cell-mediated immunity. The species involved include *M.kansasii*, *M.avium*, *M.intracellulare* and *M.malmoense*. The diagnosis can only be made by isolation of the organism from cultures made from bronchial secretions or biopsy material. In general it is wise to require repeated isolation of such organisms, combined with radiographic deterioration or persistent symptoms, before embarking on treatment.

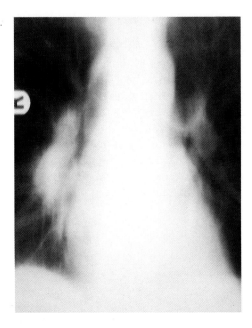

Fig. 2.62 Tuberculosis in AIDS. Anteroposterior tomogram of the right lung in a patient already profoundly immunosuppressed, showing enlarged hilar glands.

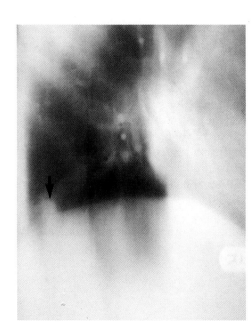

Fig. 2.63 Tuberculosis in AIDS. Lateral tomogram of the chest showing a peripheral lesion (similar to a Ghon focus) in the posterior basal segment of the lower lobe of the right lung (Same patient as in Fig. 2.62.)

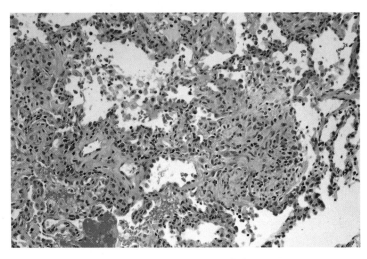

Fig. 2.64 *Mycobacterium avium* complex infection in AIDS. Chronic inflammatory infiltration of the lungs without granuloma formation. By courtesy of Dr M. B. Cohen.

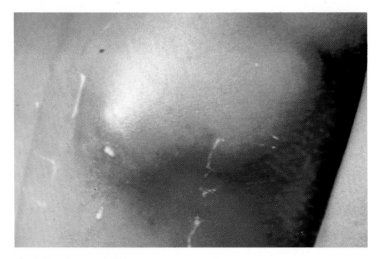

Fig. 2.65 Actinomycosis. Subcutaneous mass and sinus formation on the chest wall. By courtesy of Dr T. F. Sellers, Jr.

In patients with AIDS, infection with organisms of the *Mycobacterium avium* complex (MAC) are particularly frequent and may involve the bowel and lymph nodes as well as the respiratory tract (Fig. 2.64). In some cases the organism can be isolated from blood cultures. MAC infections in AIDS patients generally appear at a late stage in the illness. They cannot be cured and drug treatment is reserved for the palliation of severe constitutional disturbance associated with septicaemia.

Actinomycosis

Thoracic actinomycosis may affect the lungs, pleura, subcutaneous tissue or skin. The initial site of infection is often uncertain and the condition may evade diagnosis until a subcutaneous mass and eventually a discharging sinus develop (Fig. 2.65). The radiographic appearance is of pulmonary consolidation, sometimes multifocal and sometimes cavitated. The diagnosis is made by identifying the organ in the material discharging from a sinus or in surgical biopsies (Fig. 2.66).

Nocardiasis

The organisms causing these infections are aerobic actinomycetes. The most common human species is *Nocardia asteroides* and pulmonary infection takes the form of pneumonic consolidation, abscesses (Fig. 2.67), pleural involvement and empyema (Fig. 2.68). Solitary coin lesions are also seen. Many patients with nocardiasis have severe underlying disease and are immunosuppressed. The diagnosis may be made by the examination of stained smears of pus or sputum, which shows irregular or beaded, narrow, branching filaments (Fig. 2.69).

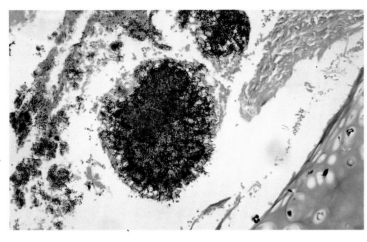

Fig. 2.66 Actinomycosis. Histological demonstration of black-staining organisms in bronchial biopsy. Grocott stain. By courtesy of Dr C. W. Edwards.

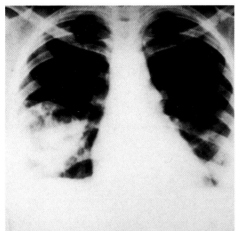

Fig. 2.67 Pulmonary nocardiasis. Radiograph showing a large rounded lesion in the right lower zone with multiple cavities. By courtesy of Dr T. F. Sellers, Jr.

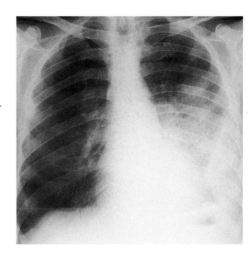

Fig. 2.68 Pulmonary nocardiasis. Radiograph showing consolidation in the lower lobe of the left lung and associate pleural effusion.

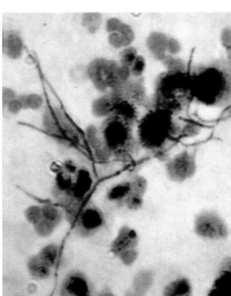
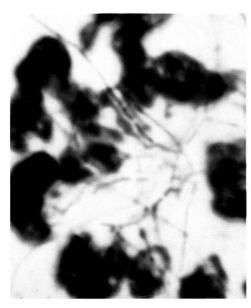

Fig. 2.69 Pulmonary nocardiasis. *Nocardia asteriodes* in sputum. Left: Acid-fast stain. By courtesy of Dr T. F. Sellers, Jr. Right: Gram's stain. By courtesy of Dr H. P. Holley.

FUNGAL INFECTION OF THE LUNG

Systemic fungal infections can be divided into those which occur in previously healthy subjects and those which are seen only in compromised hosts. The former include histoplasmosis, coccidioidomycosis, blastomycosis, cryptococcosis and paracoccidioidomycosis while the latter comprise pneumocystosis, aspergillosis, systemic candidosis and mucormycosis. All of these infections may involve the lung. Those in the opportunist group have a worldwide distribution, while the others are only encountered in restricted geographical areas.

Pneumocystis carinii pneumonia

Pneumocystis carinii (Figs. 2.70 & 2.71) is a fungus which has a predilection for mammalian lung. It is believed to be widely prevalent but it is not of sufficient pathogenicity to cause disease in healthy subjects. Infection is probably acquired at an early age in many people but, as long as their cellular immunity remains intact, no illness results. Profound disturbance of T-helper lymphocyte function, and perhaps of the function of alveolar macrophages, leaves the subject vulnerable to reactivation or acquisition of *P.carinii* and the development of pneumonia. This was first recognised in children with severe malnutrition and later in patients undergoing chemotherapy for leukaemia. However most experience of this form of pneumonia has come from the study of patients with HIV infection. *Pneumocystis pneumoniae* pneumonia (PCP) is the commonest first indicator for diagnosis of AIDS in untreated HIV positive patients in the Western World. Its development correlates closely with a count of CD4-positive lymphocytes (T helper cells) in the peripheral blood of less than 200/mm^3.

In HIV-positive subjects the onset of symptoms in PCP may be rapid, but where close observation is carried out symptoms can be seen to develop over a period of weeks or even months. The earliest symptom is an unproductive cough, followed by dyspnoea on exertion. Gradually these symptoms worsen, the cough becomes productive of purulent sputum, dyspnoea becomes apparent at rest and systemic symptoms of fever and malaise appear.

Clinical examination reveals sparse pulmonary crepitations and the patient may be febrile. Desaturation of the arterial blood with oxygen may already be evident but, if not, it can almost always be demonstrated on exercise by pulse oximetry. The chest x-ray is normal at the start of the illness, but in advanced cases (Fig. 2.72) it eventually shows diffuse, perihilar alveolar-type opacity. However, in some cases the x-ray shows non-specific localized consolidation, and where aerosolized pentamidine has been used for prophylaxis, infection may be confined to the apices of the lungs. The diagnosis may be supported by the demonstration of an abnormal gallium scan of the lungs or by an abnormal rate of clearance of DPHA from the lungs.

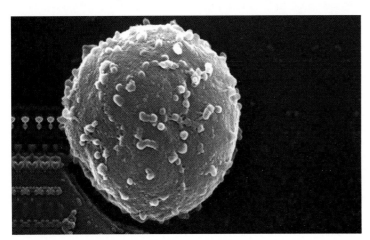

Fig. 2.70 *Pneumocystis carinii.* Cyst visualized by scanning electron microscopy. Platinum coated. ×15 000. By courtesy of Dr M. Forte.

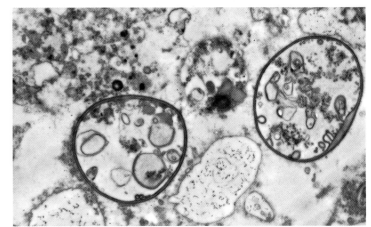

Fig 2.71 *Pneumocystis carinii.* Transmission electron micrograph of human *P. carinii* from lung tissue of a patient with AIDS. Uranyl acetate and Reynolds lead citrate. ×7 500. By courtesy of Dr M. Forte.

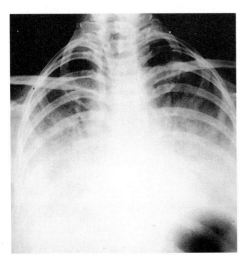

Fig. 2.72 *Pneumocystis carinii* pneumonia. Chest radiograph showing advanced disease with dense infiltrates in both lungs.

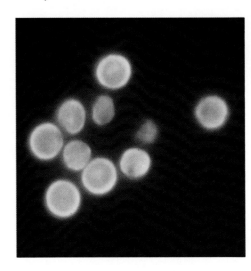

Fig. 2.73 *Pneumocystis carinii* pneumonia. Fluorescent monoclonal antibody stain of bronchoalveolar washings. By courtesy of Dr K. Nye.

The definitive diagnostic test is the identification of the organism in either sputum, bronchial washings (Fig. 2.73) or lung biopsies (Figs 2.74 & 2.75). In experienced hands these techniques are highly sensitive and specific for the examination of samples obtained by bronchial lavage; furthermore, in some centres almost equally good results have been obtained by the examination of induced sputum. The treatment of PCP is with high dose trimethoprim and sulfamethoxazole or with pentamidine, either intravenously or by inhalation. Recovery rates for either regime are 75–90%. However, after recovery there is a 30–40% risk of relapse during the following year. Prophylactic treatment is therefore indicated in patients who have recovered from a first attack of PCP or who have HIV infection and whose CD4 positive T lymphocyte count is less than 200/mm^3. This may take the form of monthly aerosolized pentamidine, daily trimethoprim/sulfamethoxazole or weekly dapsone.

Histoplasmosis

Classical histoplasmosis is caused by infection with *Histoplasma capsulatum* (Fig. 2.76), a dimorphic fungus normally found in soil particularly when contaminated by excreta from birds or bats. Human infection is most common in eastern and central parts of the USA, with other foci in Central and South America, parts of Africa and the Far East. Inhalation of spores leads to the establishment of disease in the lungs, with parenchymal consolidation and hilar lymphadenopathy. The infection may disseminate through the blood or within the lung, but spontaneous healing is the most likely outcome.

Most primary infections are subclinical and are detected only by the development of a positive histoplasmin skin test, but some cause symptoms such as fever, headache, cough and malaise. In a few cases erythema nodosum or erythema multiforme are observed. Rarely the respiratory symptoms become severe, with dyspnoea and cyanosis. Patients with acute pulmonary histoplasmosis often have a history of environmental exposure to likely sources of infection and small outbreaks sometimes occur. Rare sequelae include persistent lymphadenopathy with bronchial obstruction, fibrosing mediastinitis following caseous necrosis of lymph nodes, and pericarditis.

Attempts to isolate the organism in primary infection are seldom successful and the laboratory diagnosis usually depends on serological testing. Histoplasmin skin testing is unlikely to be helpful unless the patients previous skin test status is known. Moreover, histoplasmin skin testing may itself cause seroconversion. The chest x-ray shows one or more soft parenchymal shadows with enlargement of the hilar or mediastinal glands (Fig. 2.77). In a few

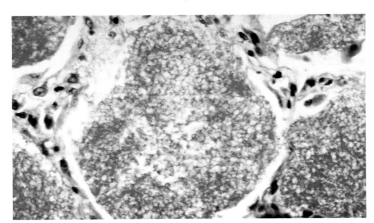

Fig. 2.74 *Pneumocystis carinii* pneumonia. Histopathology of transbronchial lung biopsy showing alveolar spaces filled with foamy material which is composed of a mass of pneumocystis organisms. H & E stain.

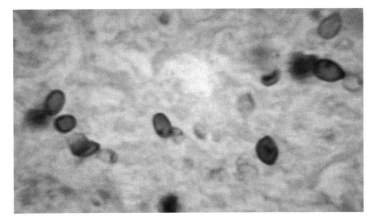

Fig. 2.76 Histoplasmosis. Histological section showing yeast form of *Histoplasma capsulatum*. Methenamine silver stain. By courtesy of Dr T. F. Sellers, Jr.

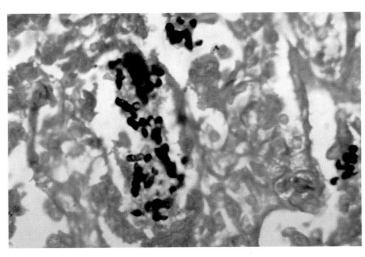

Fig. 2.75 *Pneumocystis carinii* pneumonia. Lung section showing densely staining clusters of cysts. Methenamine silver stain.

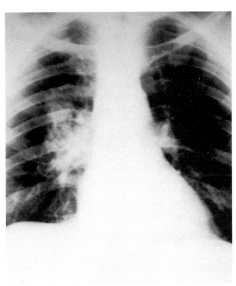

Fig. 2.77 Acute histoplasmosis. Chest radiograph of primary infection showing patchy infiltration and a prominent right hilar shadow. By courtesy of Dr T. F. Sellers, Jr.

cases late calcification takes place in the peripheral lesions, and they remain permanently visible on the x-ray (Fig. 2.78).

Chronic pulmonary histoplasmosis is most frequently recognised in middle-aged male patients in the USA. Many patients already have emphysema or are smokers. Common symptoms are cough with purulent and sometimes bloodstained sputum, weight loss and fever. The chest x-ray shows segmental lesions in the upper lobes often with fibrosis and cavitation (Fig. 2.79). Cavities may enlarge gradually, compressing the surrounding lung. The principle diagnostic difficulty is in distinguishing the condition from tuberculosis. The definitive test is sputum culture, although many samples may have to be examined before a single positive culture is obtained.

Progressive disseminated histoplasmosis may occur in previously healthy subjects but it is usually seen in infants, in the elderly and in immunosuppressed patients (Fig. 2.80). Chest x-rays may show nodular or micronodular pulmonary infiltrates and hilar lymph nodes may be enlarged.

Specific treatment for histoplasmosis with amphotericin B is not usually required in the acute pulmonary form, but it is indicated in chronic cavitary disease of the lungs and in progressive disseminated disease. Surgical treatment may be beneficial in fibrosing mediastinitis and pericarditis.

Coccidioidomycosis

Coccidioidomycosis is caused by infection with *Coccidioides immitis*, a fungus found in the soil of hot arid parts of the Americas (Fig. 2.81). Most cases are reported from the south western USA, but other areas of Central and South America are also affected. The organisms enter the body by inhalation and establish themselves in the lung. Outbreaks are sometimes recognised but most infections are subclinical.

The clinical features of acute pulmonary coccidioidomycosis are fever, malaise, cough and chest pains. The incubation period is 1–3 weeks and the condition may be accompanied by erythema nodosum (especially in women) and erythema multiforme (especially in children). The illness lasts 10–21 days and in the great majority of cases it resolves spontaneously. The chest x-ray shows pulmonary infiltration (Fig. 2.82) often accompanied by hilar gland enlargement or pleural effusion. The diagnosis can be made by serological testing. In a few patients, particularly pregnant women, the immunosuppressed and those with very high titres of serological markers, dissemination takes place. Treatment with amphotericin B is indicated when acute coccidioidomycosis is diagnosed in such patients.

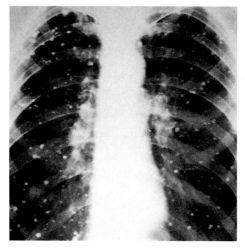

Fig. 2.78 Histoplasmosis. Chest radiograph showing scattered calcification in healed miliary lesions. By courtesy of Dr M. Pearson.

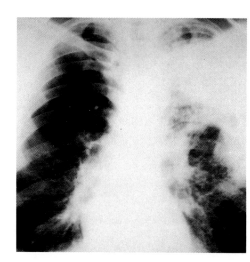

Fig. 2.79 Chronic histoplasmosis. Radiograph showing contraction of left upper lobe with multiple cavities. These features are very similar to those of chronic pulmonary tuberculosis.

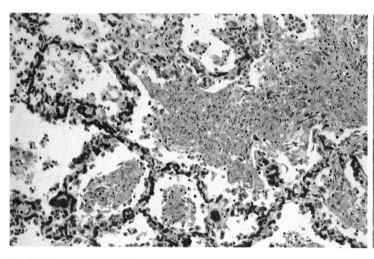

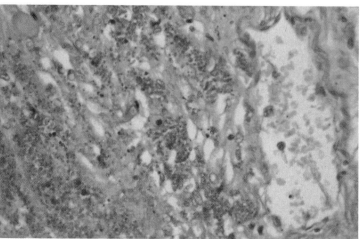

Fig. 2.80 Histoplasmosis in AIDS. Histopathology of lung infection. Left: Low magnification showing intra-alveolar exudate. Right: High magnification showing showing large numbers of magenta-staining organisms. By courtesy of Dr M. B. Cohen.

Chronic pulmonary coccidioidomycosis

In some cases of acute coccidioidomycosis the disease remains active within the thorax. This may give rise to solitary pulmonary nodules, thin walled cavities (usually in the upper half of the lung) or progressive pulmonary infiltration. Systemic symptoms such as fever may also be present. The diagnosis can sometimes be confirmed by recovering the fungus from sputum, and the patient's serological tests are usually positive. Chemotherapy is generally indicated for such cases and surgery may be required to establish the cause of solitary nodules (Fig. 2.83).

Aspergillosis

Pulmonary disease caused by fungi of the genus *Aspergillus* (Fig. 2.84) have a worldwide distribution. They are found particularly in soil and rotting vegetation. The organism produces spores which are carried on air currents and enter the body by inhalation, becoming implanted either in the lung or, occasionally, the paranasal sinuses. Disease is rare without some pre-existing condition such as immunosuppression or structural abnormality.

Aspergilloma

An aspergilloma is a ball of fungus (Fig. 2.85), which has grown in a cavity already present in the lung. Such cavities are usually the residue of healed tuberculosis although other causes such as sarcoidosis, histoplasmosis and bronchiectasis are occasionally found. The main symptom is cough and the main hazard to the patient comes from haemoptysis which is often recurrent and sometimes massive. Fever and other systemic symptoms

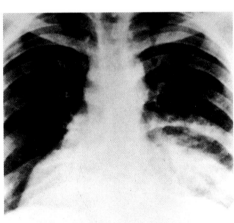

Fig. 2.81 Coccidioidomycosis. Histological section of lung tissue containing a spherule of *Coccidioides immitis*. H & E stain. By courtesy of A. E. Provost.

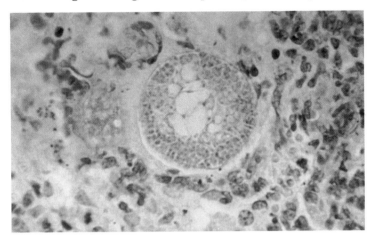

Fig. 2.82 Coccidioidomycosis. Chest radiograph showing right lower lobe consolidation. The appearance is nonspecific and could be produced by a number of pathogens.

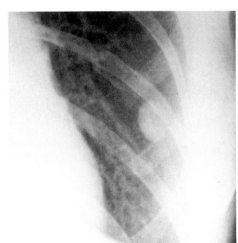

Fig. 2.83 Coccidioidomycosis. Chest radiograph showing solitary lung nodule.

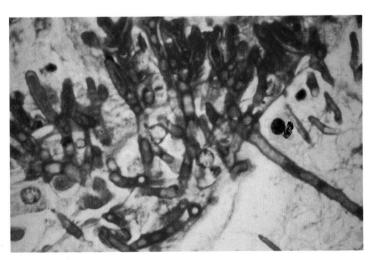

Fig. 2.84 Aspergillosis. Histological section of the lung showing wide non-septate hyphae of *Aspergillus* with acute angle branching. By courtesy of Dr T. S. J. Elliot.

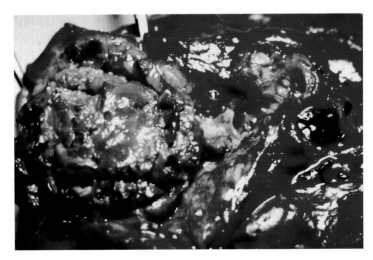

Fig. 2.85 Aspergilloma. Macroscopic appearance of fungus ball accupying a large pulmonary cavity. By courtesy of Dr V. E. Del Bene.

are unusual. The diagnosis is mainly a radiographic one. The x-ray shows a solid mass separated from the walls of the cavity by a crescent of air (Figs 2.86 & 2.87). When the patient is moved from the vertical to the horizontal position, the position of the mass within the cavity also moves. Sputum microscopy and culture are often positive for the organism (usually *A. fumigatus*) and the serum usually contains antibodies to aspergillus.

Surgery should be considered if the patient suffers from haemoptysis or has increasingly severe symptoms arising from chronic suppuration of the lung. Unfortunately in many cases the extent of pulmonary disease or the poor physical condition of the patient contraindicate operative intervention. Medical treatment is generally ineffectual but there have recently been promising reports of the use of long-term oral itraconazole.

Invasive aspergillosis

In patients with severe immunosuppression aspergillus may cause an acute disseminated illness of which pneumonia is the most frequent manifestation. The condition is most common in patients with acute leukaemia and cardiac or renal transplantation. The risk is greater in those with neutropenia, and those on cytotoxic and high-dose corticosteroid therapy. The main clinical features are fever and cough, with the development of pulmonary infiltrates (Fig. 2.88) which rapidly become larger and more numerous. The organism is difficult to isolate from sputum and the definitive diagnosis usually requires lung biopsy (Fig. 2.89). The condition is often fatal despite treatment with amphotericin B. Immunosuppressed patients may also suffer from mucosal ulceration caused by aspergillus (Fig. 2.90).

Allergic bronchopulmonary aspergillosis

This condition is seen in patients who have asthma, eosinophilia of the peripheral blood and sputum, and transient pulmonary opacities on x-ray (caused by the presence of plugs of mucus containing fungal hyphae which obstruct the bronchi). It is associated with immediate type hypersensitivity, as demonstrated by a positive skin prick test to aspergillus antigen or specific IgE in the serum. In

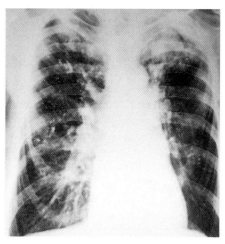
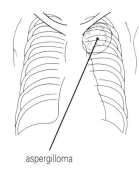

aspergilloma

Fig. 2.86 Aspergilloma. Chest radiograph showing fungus ball within cavity in the upper lobe of the right lung of a patient with old tuberculosis.

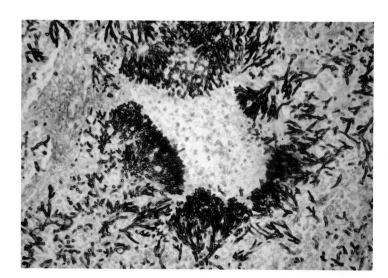

Fig.2.87 Aspergilloma. Tomogram of lung cavity containing fungus ball outlined by air space.

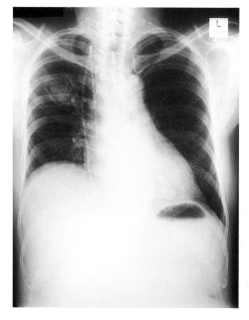

Fig. 2.88 Invasive aspergillosis. Chest radiograph showing early lesion in right lung. Patient with acute myeloblastic leukaemia. By courtesy of Dr C. Kibbler.

Fig. 2.89 Invasive aspergillosis. Histological section showing masses of branching fungal hyphae invading the lung parenchyma and blood vessels. Grocott stain. By courtesy of Dr C. Kibbler.

chronic cases permanent bronchial damage may lead to proximal saccular bronchiectasis. Antifungal treatment is ineffective and the mainstay of treatment is the use of corticosteroids and inhaled bronchodilators to suppress bronchial inflammation and to keep the airways as widely patent as possible.

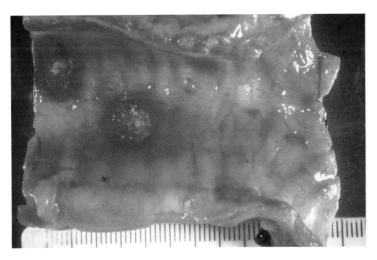

Fig. 2.90 Disseminated aspergillosis. Tracheal ulceration in an immunosuppressed patient. By courtesy of Dr T. S. J. Elliot.

LUNG ABSCESS

Abscess formation in the lung implies a combination of inflammatory exudate, local ischaemia and destruction of the normal architecture of the lung. These processes arise because of the pathological characteristics of specific organisms or through defects of host defences. Whatever their cause, lung abscesses are likely to give rise to prolonged fever, cough, purulent sputum and neutrophilia of the peripheral blood.

Where the infection has reached the lung by contiguous spread or through the bloodstream, the x-ray abnormality may be confined to a coin lesion or to a ring shadow containing a fluid level. In other cases, abscess formation occurs as part of a more widespread pneumonia. In this case it will be detected radiographically only if it has ruptured into a bronchus and become partly filled with air (Fig. 2.91). Pneumonias caused by certain specific organisms, notably *S. aureus* and *K.pneumoniae*, have a particular tendency to lead to abscess formation. This is especially seen in infants with staphylococcal pneumonia, in whom a large number of small abscesses, known as pneumatocoeles, may develop. They may enlarge rapidly as a result of coughing or crying; if they are located subpleurally there is a considerable risk of pyopneumothorax.

Abscesses caused by mixed bacterial flora

Most lung abscesses are nosocomial infections arising through a combination of lapses in host defences which allow soiling of the lower respiratory tract with upper respiratory flora and which prevent the clearance of such organisms by mucociliary action or coughing. These risk factors include coma, general anaesthesia, laryngeal incompetence, repeated vomiting, chronic upper respiratory sepsis and bronchial obstruction caused by tumours, inhaled foreign bodies and inspissated secretions.

The organisms present will be those found in the oropharynx, normally a mixture of aerobic, microaerophilic

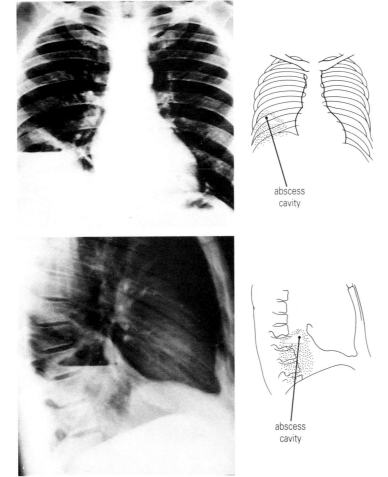

Fig. 2.91 Lung abscess. Chest radiographs, posteroanterior and lateral, showing abscess cavity in lower lobe of right lung.

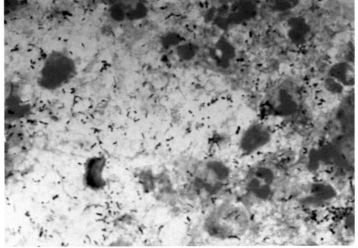

Fig. 2.92 Lung abscess. Gram stain of pus showing gram-positive cocci and various gram-negative and gram-positive rods. By courtesy of Dr J. R. Cantey.

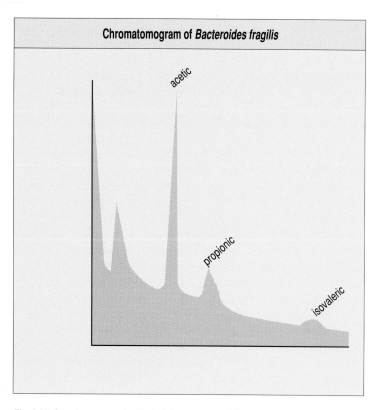

Chromatomogram of *Bacteroides fragilis*

acetic

propionic

isovaleric

Fig. 2.93 Gas chromatography. Typical chromatogram of *Bacteriodes fragilis* showing peaks of acetic, propionic and isovaleric acids. By courtesy of Dr V. E. Del Bene.

and anaerobic forms (Fig. 2.92). However, in patients who have been in hospital for some time or have received treatment with broad spectrum antibiotics, the normal oral flora may have been overgrown by commensals from the large bowel, and these may then cause sepsis in the lung. When anaerobic infection is present, the sputum is likely to be foul-smelling.

As these organisms are often of relatively low pathogenicity in the lung, abscesses of this kind often present in a gradual fashion; symptoms may be present for weeks before investigations are undertaken. Treatment involves correction, where possible, of the predisposing abnormality of host defence. Bronchoscopic examination is indicated to detect bronchial obstruction and may also be valuable in removing tenacious secretions and in obtaining reliable microbiological specimens, uncontaminated by upper respiratory flora. Mixed infections are common and care should be taken to examine specimens for anaerobic organisms. Gas chromatography is a useful adjunct in the diagnosis of anaerobic infections (Fig. 2.93). Large abscesses require surgical drainage but with smaller abscesses a trial of conservative treatment is reasonable. Associated pleural effusion and empyema are common (Fig. 2.94).

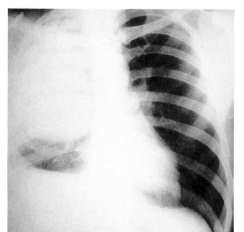

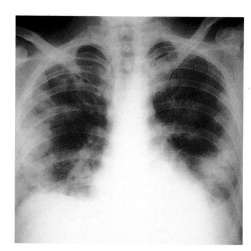

Fig. 2.94 Large encysted empyema of right lung with an additional small effusion. *Eikenella corrodens* was the major organism isolated.

Fig. 2.95 Haematogenous lung abscess. Chest radiograph showing multiple staphylococcal lung abscesses in a drug addict with tricuspid endocarditis.

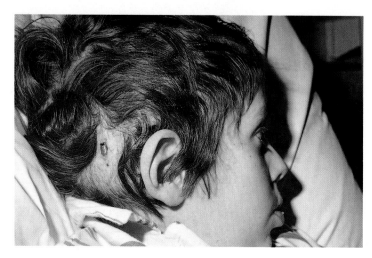

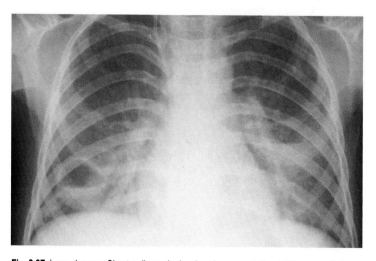

Fig. 2.96 Child with infected Spitz Holter valve.

Fig. 2.97 Lung abscess. Chest radiograph showing abscesses in the right lower and left middle zones. The ventriculoatrial shunt can be seen in the superior vena cava.

Haematogenous lung abscess

In general, septicaemia carries a low risk of the development of metastatic lung abscesses. A notable exception to this rule is where the septicaemia arises from endocarditis of the tricuspid valve. The responsible organism is usually *S. aureus* or occasionally *Candida albicans*, particularly in intravenous drug abusers. In the latter, multiple and bilateral small lung abscesses are common and there may also be empyema (Fig. 2.95). A similar appearance is seen in some cases of infection of ventriculoatrial shunts used for the relief of hydrocephalus (Figs 2.96 & 2.97).

Amoebic lung abscess

In the course of infection with *Entamoeba histolytica,* organisms may travel from the colon, through the portal vein, to the liver where an abscess may develop (usually in the right lobe). As the abscess enlarges it involves the diaphragm in the inflammatory process and eventually the infection may penetrate to the lung. Further suppuration at this site produces a lung abscess (Fig. 2.98) from which amoebic pus may be expectorated. In these cases serological tests for amoebic infection are almost always positive.

BRONCHIECTASIS

Bronchiectasis is a pathological condition in which the walls of bronchi are permanently damaged by persistent or recurrent infection. The main morbid anatomical features are as follows: alterations in the bronchial epithelium with squamous metaplasia or ulceration; variable widening of the bronchial lumen with production of cystic or saccular spaces (Fig. 2.99); infiltration of the bronchial wall with neutrophils; obliteration of side branches, peribronchial fibrosis; and the appearance of superficial anastomotic blood vessels linking the bronchial and pulmonary arterial circulations.

In order that these changes may occur there must be some pre-existing abnormality, either of the bronchial anatomy, or of the general resistance to pulmonary infection. This abnormality may be congenital, such as cystic fibrosis, the immotile cilia syndrome and hypogammaglobulinaemia. Others cases may be acquired: localized bronchiectasis may follow partial bronchial obstruction by tuberculous stenosis, chronically retained foreign bodies or benign tumours. It is possible that some cases of diffuse bronchiectasis result from widespread bronchial damage due to complicated viral or bacterial infection in early childhood. Other causes of bronchiectasis include allergic bronchopulmonary aspergillosis and chronic sarcoidosis.

Whatever the cause of bronchiectasis, involvement of the dependent parts of the lung is likely to lead to troublesome symptoms of recurrent bronchial and pneumonic infection, sometimes with the production of large volumes of purulent sputum, and with haemoptysis. In addition many patients have symptoms of chronic airways obstruction. Where there is persistent suppuration the general health of the patient may be poor.

The bacteriology of bronchiectasis is, in most cases, similar to that of chronic bronchitis and aspiration pneumonia. *H. influenzae* and *S. pneumoniae* are frequently present and, in hospitalized patients or following antibiotic treatment, resistant strains of Enterobacteriaceae are common. Among the exceptions to this rule are cystic fibrosis and allergic bronchopulmonary aspergillosis. In children with cystic fibrosis *S. aureus* is the most common pathogen, while in those patients who survive to late teenage persistent infection with *P. aeruginosa* is almost inevitable. In allergic bronchopulmonary aspergillosis microscopic examination of the sputum will demonstrate the hyphae of *A. fumigatus*, although other pathogens may affect the damaged lung.

In some cases the possibility of bronchiectasis may be suspected from examination of a plain chest x-ray. Common features include the following: irregular areas of consolidation, fibrosis and collapse; the presence of cystic

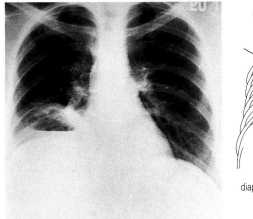
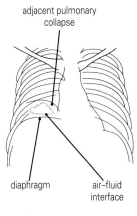
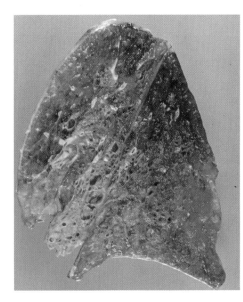

Fig. 2.98 Amoebic lung abscess. Chest radiograph showing an abscess cavity in the lower lobe of the right lung following contiguous spread of infection from a liver abscess. By courtesy of Dr B. Strickland.

adjacent pulmonary collapse

diaphragm

air–fluid interface

Fig. 2.99 Bronchiectasis. Macroscopic appearance of right lung showing dilated bronchi in fibrotic and partially collapsed middle lobe.

bronchial walls, seen as parallel lines radiating from the hila (Fig. 2.100). However, the plain x-ray does not allow the diagnosis to be made with certainty – for this purpose bronchography is required (Fig. 2.101). Computerized tomography of the chest is almost as good as bronchography and is much more acceptable to the patient who requires serial examination (Fig. 2.102).

Treatment is directed primarily at eliminating any predisposing factor where this is feasible. This may be successful in replacement therapy for congenital hypogammaglobulinaemia but there are few other causes which can be easily corrected. Otherwise, medical management consists of antibacterial chemotherapy as indicated by the sensitivity of the most abundant organisms isolated from the sputum, and physiotherapy in the form of postural drainage. In addition, reversible diffuse airway obstruction should be treated with a bronchodilator.
Surgical resection of the diseased area is some times indi-

cated where conservative measures have failed, but it is essential to carry out bronchography on both lungs to ensure that the disease is localized.

HELMINTH INFECTIONS

Hydatid disease of the lung

Hydatid disease is caused by the presence in the lung or other organs of the larval stage of the cestode *Echinococcus granulosus* (Fig. 2.103). The disease is widely distributed, and is particularly common in the Middle East and South America.

The mature adult form of *E. granulosus* inhabits the intestine of the dog and lays eggs which are excreted in the faeces. Ingestion of these ova by a secondary host, which is usually the sheep, but may be man, is followed by the development of oncospheres which penetrate the

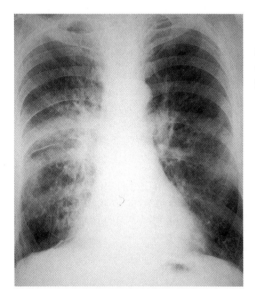

Fig. 2.100 Bronchiectasis. Plain chest radiograph showing irregular areas of collapse, consolidation and fibrosis.

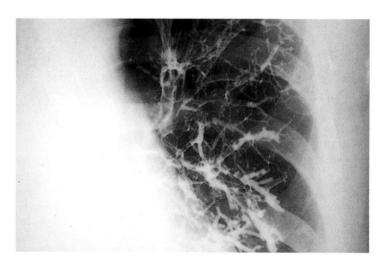

Fig. 2.101 Bronchiectasis. Bronchogram showing dilated, irregular bronchi in lingula and left lower lobe.

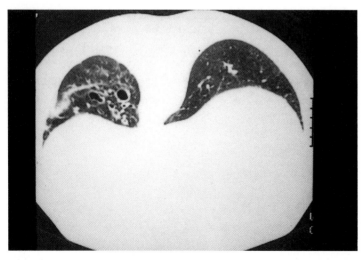

Fig. 2.102 Bronchiectasis. Computerized tomogram showing bronchial dilatation and pulmonary fibrosis.

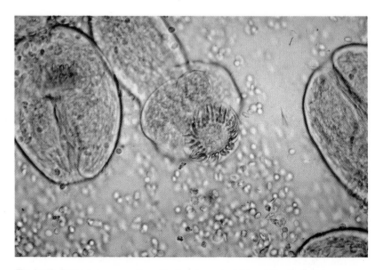

Fig. 2.103 *Echinococcus granulosus.* Scolices from a hydatid cyst showing both invaginated and evaginated hooklets and suckers. By courtesy of Prof. W. Peters.

the development of oncospheres which penetrate the mesenteric vessels and migrate through the blood stream to distant organs, particularly the liver and lungs. The oncosphere the develops into a cyst with two walls, an outer ectocyst and an inner germinal endocyst from which new larvae (scolices) develop in large numbers. The cyst is filled with fluid and gradually enlarges (Fig. 2.104), in some cases filling the whole of a hemithorax.

Hydatid cysts provoke very little inflammatory reaction and their pathological effects are generally the result of compression of the surrounding tissue as they expand. In the lung this may cause erosion of bronchi, blood vessels and the mediastinum leading to persistent bronchial infection or haemoptysis. The rupture of a hydatid cyst into a bronchus discharges watery fluid into the airways and may occasionally asphyxiate the patient. Usually the par-

tially evacuated cyst becomes the site of pyogenic infection and a lung abscess is formed. Rupture of a cyst into the pleural cavity is a serious development as it seeds the pleura with scolices from which a large number of new cysts may eventually develop. A similar situation may arise from the rupture into the pleural space of a hepatic hydatid cyst.

The diagnosis should be suspected in any patient who has lived in an endemic area and who presents with a persistent pulmonary or pleural lesion. In uncomplicated cases the cyst has a homogeneous appearance and a finely delineated margin (Fig. 2.105). Computerized tomography adds to the detail that can be detected in lung cysts (Fig. 2.106). Multiple lung cysts are present in about 20% of cases, and 10% also have liver cysts. If the cyst has partially ruptured (Fig. 2.107), the internal (laminated) mem-

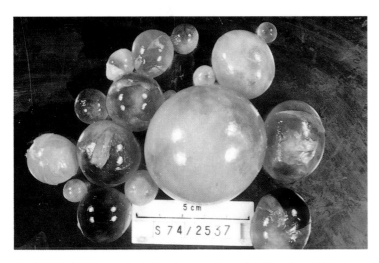

Fig. 2.104 Hydatid disease. Surgical specimen showing multiple thin-walled, fluid-filled cysts.

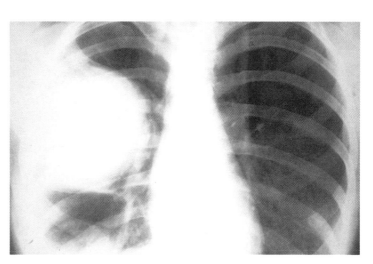

Fig. 2.105 Hydatid disease. Chest radiographs showing well-defined round lesion in middle zone of right lung.

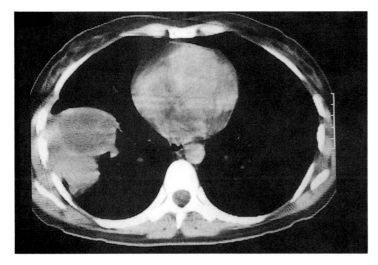

Fig. 2.106 Hydatid disease. CT scan of the thorax showing hydatid cyst of right lung.

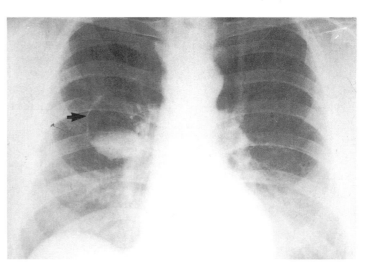

Fig. 2.107 Hydatid disease. Chest radiograph showing partially evacuated cyst (arrowed) in the middle zone of the right lung.

brane may collapse and be seen floating on fluid within the cysts (Fig. 2.108). Microscopic examination of the sputum may reveal scolices, hooklets or portions of cyst membrane in cases where rupture has occurred. Intradermal skin testing with fresh hydatid fluid (the Casoni test) is positive in 90% of cases and there is also a complement fixation test.

Where the infection is causing symptoms, treatment by surgical resection should be considered. Particular care must be taken to remove cysts intact – spillage of cyst fluid into body cavities may cause seeding of the tissues with large numbers of larvae. Perioperative treatment with praziquantel may help to prevent this complication. Where surgical treatment is not possible, drug treatment with mebendazole or albendazole may be effective.

Sometimes a cyst is found incidentally on a routine chest x-ray. In such cases it is reasonable to keep the patient under observation and defer treatment until the cyst enlarges or begins to cause symptoms.

Paragonomiasis

The lung fluke (*Paragonimus westermani* and other species) causes infection in humans through the ingestion of raw, or partially cooked, infected crabs or crayfish. Young worms penetrate the wall of the small bowel and migrate to the lungs. There they provoke an inflammatory reaction which eventually leads to abscess formation, cysts and fibrosis (Fig. 2.109). The patient may have haemoptysis and cough up large numbers of eggs which can be identified microscopically. The disease is most common in the Far East, with some cases also found in Africa, India and South America. Treatment is with praziquantel.

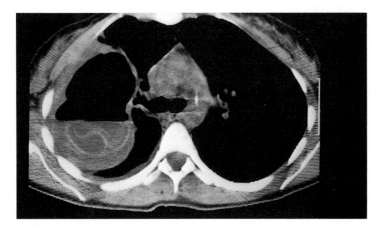

Fig. 2.108 Hydatid disease. Computerized tomogram showing ruptured cyst with internal membrane floating within cavity.

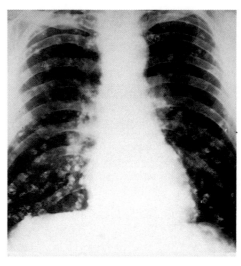

Fig. 2.109 Paragonomiasis. Chest radiograph showing multiple rounded lesions in both lung fields, many of them calcified.

3

THE NERVOUS SYSTEM

MENINGITIS

Meningitis is defined as inflammation of the meninges, usually but not always due to infection. Meningitis may be acute or chronic. Acute meningitis may be purulent (usually bacterial) or aseptic (usually, but not always, viral). Characteristic features of meningitis are stiff neck (Fig. 3.1), and other clinical signs of meningeal irritation and abnormalities of the cerebrospinal fluid, including pleocytosis (increase in the number of cells), elevation of the protein concentration and diminished glucose concentration. Fever, headache, mental obtundation and signs of cranial nerve dysfunction may also be present. In purulent meningitis the cells in the CSF are usually predominantly neutrophils, whereas in aseptic meningitis mononuclear cells usually predominate.

Aseptic meningitis

Aseptic (non-purulent) meningitis may be caused by a wide variety of agents, most commonly by viruses. With only a few exceptions, which are described below, the clinical picture provides few clues toward an aetiological diagnosis, but the epidemiological setting may be helpful in some cases. Most patients have headache, fever, stiff neck and photophobia. Distinction between viral and bacterial meningitis depends primarily upon examination of the cerebrospinal fluid. The CSF in viral meningitis usually contains from 50–500 leukocytes/mm³, predominantly lymphocytes. Early in the course of the disease there may be a predominance of neutrophils but within 12–24 hours there is usually a shift to a predominance of lymphocytes. The CSF glucose is normal (above 40mg/dl) in nearly all cases, but may occasionally be low in infections due to lymphocytic choriomeningitis, herpes simplex or mumps viruses. Protein concentration is usually elevated but is rarely above 200mg/dl.

Common viral causes of aseptic meningitis in industrialized countries are echoviruses, coxsackieviruses, herpes simplex virus and the human immunodeficiency virus. In developing countries polioviruses and lymphocytic choriomeningitis virus remain important. In immunocompro-

mised patients meningitis due to cytomegalovirus (Fig. 3.2) and adenoviruses, often with an associated encephalitis, is sometimes seen. Other infections which may be associated with the acute aseptic meningitis syndrome are leptospirosis, syphilis, tuberculous meningitis and cryptococcal meningitis, which are described below. Non-infectious (or presumed non-infectious) causes of this syndrome include carcinomatous involvement of the meninges, chemical irritation, Mollaret's meningitis, Behçet's syndrome, the Vogt–Koyanagi–Harada syndrome, sarcoidosis, lupus erythematosus and many drugs.

Enteroviruses are small RNA viruses which are distributed throughout the world . Most serotypes of echoviruses and coxsackieviruses are capable of causing aseptic meningitis. The most common serotypes associated with this syndrome have been echoviruses 4, 6, 9, 11, 16 and 30, and coxsackieviruses A7, A9 and B2-B5. In the northern hemisphere most cases occur in late summer and early fall. Attack rates are highest in children less than 1 year old, but meningitis due to these agents is also seen in older children and young adults. Pharyngitis and other symptoms of upper respiratory tract infection may be present. The disease may be biphasic in course, with signs and symptoms of meningitis occurring several days after the patient has apparently recovered from a non-specific viral illness. Specific aetiological diagnosis of enteroviral meningitis depends upon viral isolation, since serological diagnosis is impractical because of the large number of serotypes. Throat washings, stools and CSF should be cultured. If an agent is isolated its pathogenic role may be confirmed by demonstrating a rising titre of antibodies after infection. In areas where poliovirus infections are common, these viruses may cause an illness indistinguishable from that produced by echoviruses and coxsackieviruses. Very rarely, echoviruses and coxsackieviruses have caused the Guillain–Barré syndrome, transverse myelitis or a flaccid motor paralysis, which is usually milder than poliomyelitis and followed by complete recovery. A chronic, progressive meningoencephalitis may occur in immunocompromised individuals, especially those with X-linked agammaglobulinemia. Except for the vaccines against poliomyelitis, there are no specific vaccines or

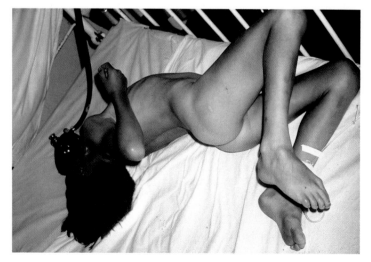

Fig. 3.1 Bacterial meningitis. Severe opisthotonos, due to spasm of muscles of neck, back and extremities.

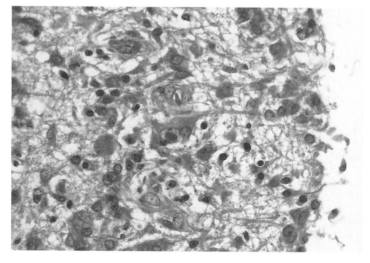

Fig. 3.2 Cytomegalovirus encephalitis. Subependymal cell containing large intranuclear Cowdry type A inclusion of CMV. H & E stain. By courtesy of Dr. P. Garen.

antiviral agents effective against enteroviral infections. A few cases of persistent enteroviral infection in immunocompromised individuals have responded to administration of immune globulin.

Mumps virus is a single-stranded RNA virus of the paramyxovirus family. Mumps is worldwide in distribution, occurring primarily in school-age children and adolescents. Although parotitis is the characteristic manifestation of mumps virus infection, involvement of the central nervous system is very common; up to 50% of individuals with mumps but without clinical evidence of meningitis exhibit pleocytosis in the CSF. Clinical meningitis occurs in 1–10% of individuals with mumps parotitis; only about half of patients with mumps meningitis have parotitis. Meningitis usually occurs a few days after the appearance of the parotitis, but may occur before or as long as 2 weeks after onset of parotitis. As with parotitis, the incidence is higher in men, and most cases occur in spring and summer. More serious disease of the nervous system, such as encephalitis, deafness, facial palsy, transverse myelitis, Guillain-Barré syndrome or poliomyelitis-like paralysis, occurs rarely. Specific laboratory diagnosis of mumps meningitis is rarely worthwhile but the virus usually can be isolated from saliva, and frequently from CSF, during the first week of illness. Diagnosis may be confirmed by demonstration of a rising titre of antibody in the serum.

The most serious form of disease of the nervous system caused by herpes simplex viruses is encephalitis (discussed below), usually due to type 1 virus, but type 2 virus can also cause meningitis. Meningitis is a common complication of primary genital herpes virus infection especially in women; up to 36% of women and 13% of men have headache, nuchal rigidity and photophobia. CSF pleocytosis is commonly found in those ill enough to have lumbar puncture. Meningitis also occurs as a component of disseminated infection in newborn infants of women with active genital herpes virus infection. Sacral radiculopathy, with sacral paraesthesias, urinary retention and constipation, or transverse myelopathy may also occur.

Human infection with lymphocytic choriomeningitis virus is associated with exposure to rodents and their urine. Most sporadic cases are attributed to contact with infected mice (Mus musculus), and all reported outbreaks have been traced to contact with infected Syrian hamsters. The clinical picture differs from that seen in the usual case of aseptic meningitis. Initially there is a non-specific febrile illness sometimes with a maculopapular rash and lymphadenopathy. This subsides, and is followed within a few days by onset of severe headache, elevated CSF pressure and occasionally papilloedema. Only a minority of patients exhibit signs of meningitis. Rarely orchitis, mild pericarditis or arthritis may occur. The second phase of the illness coincides with appearance of antibody, and may represent an immunological phenomenon. Diagnosis may be made by demonstrating a rise in antibody titre or by intracerebral inoculation of mice with blood or spinal fluid followed in 1 week by injection of endotoxin, which precipitates illness in infected mice. Except for prevention of contact between humans and rodents by community rodent control programs, there are no effective preventive measures against LCM infection.

Aseptic meningitis may occur during infection with the human immunodeficiency virus. It is a component of the acute retroviral syndrome, which occurs around the time of seroconversion, in approximately 25% of patients. An acute or subacute meningitis, lasting from days to months may also occur later in the course of HIV infection, with or without evidence of immunodeficiency.

In leptospirosis, aseptic meningitis is a common manifestation of the second or immune stage of the disease. Although leptospires may be found in the CSF during the first non-specific febrile stage of leptospirosis, they disappear during the second week with the appearance of serum antibody. CSF pleocytosis occurs in 80–90% of patients during the second week of illness and half of these will exhibit clinical signs of meningitis. A biphasic illness or history of contact with animals may provide clues to the diagnosis; otherwise the meningitis is non-specific in its manifestations. In the USA leptospirosis probably accounts for approximately 10% of cases of aseptic meningitis. The meningitis usually lasts only a few days (rarely 2–3 weeks) and virtually all anicteric patients recover. Specific diagnosis may be made by demonstration of leptospires in the blood or CSF during the first stage of the illness or in the urine during the second stage, or by retrospective demonstration of a rising titre of antibody. Since the prognosis is uniformly favorable in anicteric cases, antibiotic therapy is probably not indicated, but recent studies show that therapy with penicillins or tetracyclines is beneficial in severe cases of leptospirosis.

In syphilis aseptic meningitis may occur, especially during the secondary stage and may be the first manifestation of infection with Treponema pallidum. Papilloedema, cranial and peripheral neuropathies, mental deterioration and seizures occur more frequently in syphilitic than in viral meningitis. Although most cases occur during the first year after infection, meningitis may occur months or years later. Recent studies show that up to a third of patients with untreated primary or secondary syphilis have T. pallidum organisms present in the CSF, and both serum and CSF serological studies should be performed whenever syphilis is a possible cause of the aseptic meningitis syndrome. Older treatment regimens for neurosyphilis utilizing intramuscular penicillin may be inadequate; currently aqueous penicillin G, 12–24 million units per day (2–4 million units every 4 hours) given intravenously for 10–14 days, is recommended.

Bacterial meningitis

Bacteria causing meningitis usually reach the meninges via the blood stream. The 3 most common bacterial causes of meningitis outside the neonatal period (Streptococcus pneumoniae, Neisseria meningitidis and Haemophilus influenzae) all inhabit the mucosal surface of the nasopharynx, and meningitis is often associated with bacteraemia originating from this site. Pneumococcal meningitis also commonly occurs with pneumococcal pneumonia, and by direct extension from infection of the paranasal sinuses or via skull fracture with communication between the nasopharynx and the subarachnoid space. Multiplication of bacteria in the subarachnoid space results in intense vascular congestion and formation of a purulent exudate over the surface of the brain (Fig. 3.3) and spinal cord (Fig. 3.4), especially in the sulci (Fig. 3.5) and at the base of the brain. Microscopically the exudate is seen to consist of acute inflammatory cells (Fig. 3.6), in this case confined to the subarachnoid space, contained by the arachnoid membrane on the outermost surface and the pia mater on the innermost surface close to the cerebral cortex. Ventriculitis, due to multiplication of bacteria in the ventricular system, is often present (Fig. 3.7).

Bacterial meningitis often progresses rapidly and patients usually seek medical attention within 24 hours after onset of symptoms. Most patients have headache, signs of meningeal irritation and altered consciousness with or without focal neurological signs. Cerebrospinal fluid (CSF) usually exhibits an increased cell count (>1000/mm³), with predominance of polymorphonuclear leukocytes, increased protein concentration (>150 mg/dl) and decreased glucose concentration (<40 mg/dl). (If either papilloedema or focal neurological deficits are found on physical examination, lumbar puncture should be delayed until CT or MRI examination is performed, in order to exclude the presence of a mass lesion, with increased risk of herniation of the brain.) Gram stain of the sediment of centrifuged CSF will reveal organisms in nearly 90% of patients in whom bacterial cultures are positive (Figs 3.8 & 3.9). Prior antibiotic therapy reduces the yield of both culture and gram stain examination, but results of cell count, protein and glucose measurement are usually unaltered, unless the patient has received treatment for several days before examination of the CSF. In previously treated patients, counterimmunoelectrophoresis and latex agglutination tests may provide a specific aetiological diagnosis even though the culture is negative.

Meningococcal meningitis occurs most commonly in children and young adults. The infection is worldwide in distribution; most cases occur in winter and spring. *Neisseria meningitidis* is a bean-shaped, oxidase-positive (Fig. 3.10), gram-negative diplococcus which inhabits the mucosal surface of the human nasopharynx and is transmitted by respiratory secretions. Of the 9 serogroups of *N. meningitidis*, groups A, B, C and Y are responsible for most infections. Asymptomatic nasopharyngeal carriage of *N.*

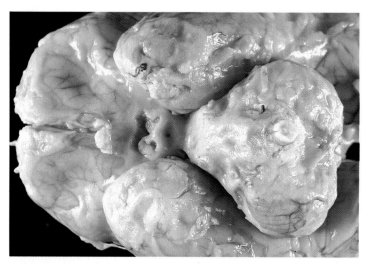

Fig. 3.3 Bacterial meningitis. Gross specimen with copious subarachnoid purulent exudate covering base of brain and enveloping brainstem and cerebellum. By courtesy of Dr P. Garen.

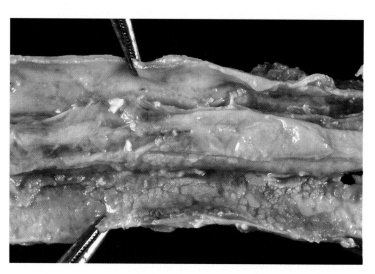

Fig. 3.4 Bacterial meningitis. Spinal cord obscured by thick subarachnoid purulent exudate in bacterial meningitis. By courtesy of Dr P. Garen.

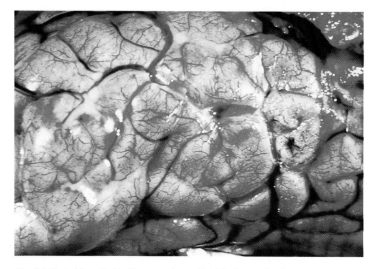

Fig. 3.5 Bacterial meningitis. Gross specimen of fresh brain revealing intense acute congestion of meningeal blood vessels and purulent exudate in sulci.

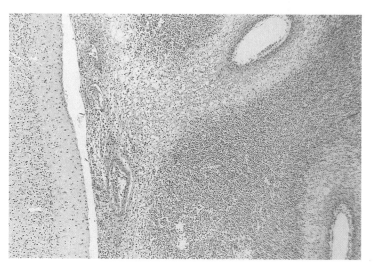

Fig. 3.6 Bacterial meningitis. Intense subarachnoid acute inflammatory exudate in bacterial meningitis. Note lack of involvement of underlying brain. H & E stain. By courtesy of Dr P. Garen.

meningitidis is much more common than clinical disease. The incidence of nasopharyngeal carriage varies greatly among different communities and at different times, and is not closely correlated with the incidence of meningitis. The duration of nasopharyngeal carriage ranges from a few weeks to more than 2 years, and after weeks or months often results in development of protective immunity against clinical illness. Concomitant viral or mycoplasmal respiratory infection may increase the likelihood of bacteraemic spread of the organism from the nasopharynx to the meninges. Except in young infants and the very old, meningococcal meningitis usually presents with headache, confusion and stiff neck. Focal neurological signs and seizures are less common in meningococcal meningitis than in meningitis due to *S. pneumoniae* or *H. influenzae*; this correlates with the rarity of focal cerebral involvement found at autopsy in fatal cases of meningococcal infection. Meningitis is often accompanied by an intense bacteraemia, with production of septic shock, petechiae and purpuric lesions on the skin, and widespread vascular lesions of internal organs including haemorrhagic infarction of the adrenal glands, renal cortical necrosis and disseminated intravascular coagulation.

Strains of *N. meningitidis* are susceptible to many antibiotics; most strains are susceptible to penicillin G and third generation cephalosporins such as cefotaxime and ceftriaxone, but overwhelming infection may result in death in spite of appropriate therapy. Rare strains of relatively penicillin-insensitive *N. meningitidis* have been found. At the present time, the treatment of choice is large doses of either penicillin G or a third generation cephalosporin given intravenously. Effective antibiotic therapy has reduced the case-fatality rate from more than 70% to less than 10%.

Nasopharyngeal carriage rates of *N. meningitidis* are greatly increased in household contacts of patients and in certain closed populations during epidemics, and household contacts have been shown to have a greatly increased attack rate of meningitis. Elimination of meningococci from most nasopharyngeal carriers can be achieved by administration of rifampin (600mg twice daily for 2 days). A quadrivalent vaccine containing polysaccharides of

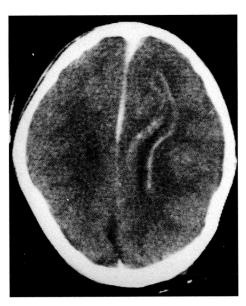

Fig. 3.7 Bacterial meningitis. CT scan showing enhancement of the ependyma of the right lateral ventricle as seen in the ventriculitis complicating bacterial meningitis. By courtesy of Dr G. D. Hungerford.

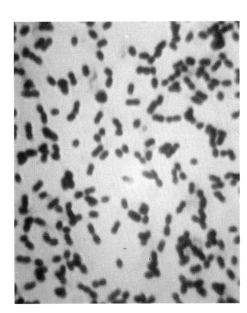

Fig. 3.8 Pneumococcal meningitis. Large numbers of gram-positive diplococci in cerebrospinal fluid with only a few fragments of degenerating polymorphonuclear leucocytes. Gram's stain. By courtesy of Dr T. F. Sellers, Jr.

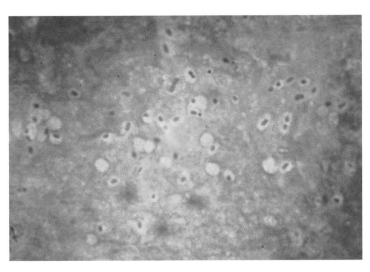

Fig. 3.9 *Klebsiella pneumoniae* meningitis. Gram stain of cerebrospinal fluid showing many heavily encapsulated gram-negative bacilli and much proteinaceous material. By courtesy of Dr V. E. Del Bene.

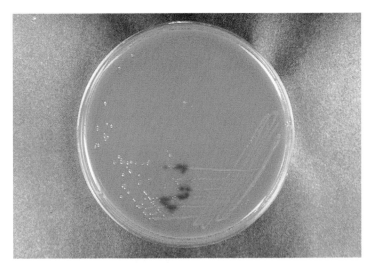

Fig. 3.10 *Neisseria meningitidis*. Oxidase test on chocolate agar. All members of this genus give a positive oxidase test. The reagent (tetramethyl-*p*-phenylendiamine hydrochloride) is spread over the plate. The colonies of Neisseria turn purple.

groups A,C,Y and W-135 is now available for immunoprophylaxis in epidemic situations. Children under the age of 2 years respond poorly to meningococcal vaccines, and there is no effective vaccine against group B strains.

Haemophilus influenzae is a small, gram-negative coccobacillus which inhabits the upper respiratory tract of humans. Most cases of meningitis are due to type b strains and occur in children under the age of 2 years; the disease is rare over the age of 6 years but occasional cases occur in elderly individuals. In spite of this age limitation, the attack rate is greater than that due to any other type of bacterial meningitis in the United States and many other countries. Onset of meningitis is often preceded by evidence of an upper respiratory infection. The clinical picture resembles that due to bacterial meningitis of any cause. Because it is a disease of young children, subdural effusion is a common complication (Fig. 3.11). Serious neurological sequelae persist in approximately half of the patients who recover. Approximately 20% of strains of *H. influenzae* produce a plasmid-mediated β-lactamase and are resistant to ampicillin. Standard therapy consists of chloramphenicol plus ampicillin, given intravenously in large doses. If the strain is found to be susceptible to ampicillin, treatment can be continued with ampicillin alone. Recent studies show that third generation cephalosporins such as ceftriaxone and cefotaxime are effective in the treatment of meningitis due to this organism. Administration of corticosteroids reduces the incidence of hearing loss in children with meningitis due to *H. influenzae*. Conjugant vaccines, consisting of type b polysaccharide complexed with either non-toxic diphtheria toxoid or *N. meningitidis* outer membrane proteins, are immunogenic in children aged 2 months or older and are recommended for routine use. For individuals with congenital or acquired hypogammaglobulinaemia, passive immunization may be achieved by intravenous administration of gamma globulin every 3 weeks. Chemoprophylaxis with rifampin is recommended for all household contacts (children and adults) where there are children (other than the index case) less than 4 years old;

such chemoprophylaxis is also recommended in nurseries and day-care centers. A patient returning from hospital to a household in which there are other young children should also receive rifampin in order to eradicate the nasopharyngeal carrier state.

Streptococcus (formerly *Diplococcus*) *pneumoniae* is a gram-positive coccus which typically appears as a lancet-shaped encapsulated diplococcus in clinical material (see Fig. 3.8). Pneumonia is the most common type of serious pneumococcal infection (see Chapter 2), but *S. pneumoniae* is also the most common cause of bacterial meningitis in adults over the age of 30. The disease is especially common in the very young and the very old, and in individuals who have predisposing factors such as sickle cell disease, asplenia, alcoholism, multiple myeloma, chronic lymphocytic leukaemia agammaglobulinaemia and concomitant endocarditis, pneumonia, sinusitis or otitis media due to *S. pneumoniae*. The organism may reach the meninges via the blood stream from a pneumonic focus or endocarditis, or by direct extension from infection in the paranasal sinuses or mastoid or through a skull fracture with communication between the nasopharynx and the subarachnoid space. The clinical picture and CSF profile are similar to those observed in other forms of bacterial meningitis. The incidence of coma and focal neurological deficits is relatively high in meningitis due to this organism, and the mortality rate is especially high in neonates and in adults over the age of 40. Depending upon geographic area, a variable proportion of strains of *S. pneumoniae* is relatively resistant to penicillin G (MIC ≥0.1µg/ml), so all clinically significant isolates should be tested for susceptibility to penicillin with oxacillin disks. Less commonly, strains resistant to ≥2µg/ml are encountered. Such highly-resistant strains were found initially in South Africa, but more recently they have been isolated in many other countries. Infections due to penicillin-susceptible strains may be treated with large doses of penicillin G given intravenously, but those due to more resistant strains should be treated with third generation cephalosporins such as cefotaxime or ceftriaxone. Patients allergic to penicillin may be treated

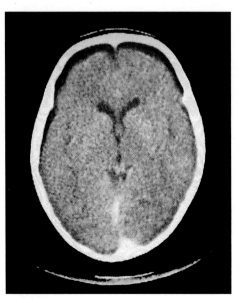

Fig. 3.11 Bacterial meningitis. CT scan showing subdural effusion in frontal region in a patient with meningitis due to *Haemophilus influenzae*. By courtesy of Dr G. D. Hungerford.

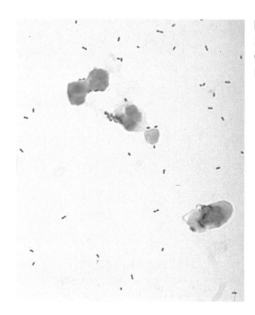

Fig. 3.12 Listeria meningitis. *L. monocytogenes* in CSF. Gram's stain. By courtesy of Dr K. Nye.

with chloramphenicol. A 23-valent vaccine containing capsular polysaccharides of the pneumococcal types most frequently involved in serious systemic infections is available, and is recommended for healthy adults over the age of 65 and several categories of adults and children at high risk for pneumococcal disease.

Meningitis due to gram-negative bacilli (excluding neonatal meningitis and infections caused by *H. influenzae*) has increased in frequency in recent years. Most cases occur in association with neurosurgical procedures, head trauma or bacteraemia originating from a distant focus. The organisms most frequently involved are *Klebsiella pneumoniae* (see Fig. 3.9), *Escherichia coli*, and *Pseudomonas aeruginosa*. The clinical picture resembles that seen in other forms of bacterial meningitis, except as it may be modified by the underlying condition of the patient. Introduction of the third generation cephalosporins has greatly improved the therapy of gram-negative bacillary meningitis. One of these agents should be given intravenously in maximum dosage, probably in combination with an aminoglycoside. If *P. aeruginosa* is suspected, ceftazidime should be selected. If for any reason a third generation cephalosporin cannot be used, the regimen should include an aminoglycoside given by the intraventricular route via an Ommaya reservoir as well as intravenously. Bacteriological and clinical response may be slow, and treatment should be continued for at least 10 days after the cultures of the CSF become negative. Acute or chronic meningoencephalitis occurs rarely in patients with brucellosis.

Listeria monocytogenes usually causes meningitis in neonates or in immunocompromised older children and adults. In neonates the source of the organism is the genital tract of the mother. The gram-positive rods found on culture of the CSF resemble diphtheroids (Fig. 3.12), and may be discarded as contaminants from the skin unless the clinician communicates the suspicion of meningitis to the laboratory personnel. A characteristic tumbling motility and β-haemolysis on blood agar aid in the correct identification of *L. monocytogenes*. Both ampicillin given in large doses intravenously plus an aminoglycoside and

trimethoprim-sulphamethoxazole have been used successfully in the treatment of listeria meningitis.

Bacterial meningitis occurring in the neonatal period differs in several respects from the disease seen in older children and adults. Signs and symptoms pointing specifically to meningeal infection may be lacking. A small number of polymorphonuclear leucocytes and an 'elevated' protein concentration may be present normally in the CSF of neonates and the glucose concentration may not be definitely abnormal even in the presence of infection. The most common infecting organisms are *E. coli*, group B streptococci, enterococci and *L. monocytogenes*, all components of the vaginal and perineal flora of the mother. Group B streptococci (*Streptococcus agalactiae*) cause two distinct types of meningitis in neonates. Early-onset meningitis occurs during the first 5 days of life, often within the first 24 hours, and is frequently associated with obstetric complications and/or prematurity. These infants exhibit signs of respiratory distress, lethargy, poor feeding, fever and jaundice, without signs of meningitis; the diagnosis can only be made by examination of the CSF. Late-onset meningitis appears between 7 days and 3 months after birth, at a mean age of approximately 3 weeks. Serotype III accounts for 95% of late-onset infections. This type of infection usually occurs in term infants and is rarely associated with maternal obstetric complications. These organisms are uniformly susceptible to penicillin G and this is the drug of choice when the aetiological diagnosis has been established. Most authorities recommend initial therapy with ampicillin plus an aminoglycoside for suspected neonatal group B streptococcal infection, because of the synergistic effect of this combination on these organisms.

Meningitis developing in patients who have ventriculoatrial or ventriculoperitoneal shunts represents another special case. Coagulase-negative staphylococci, *Staphylococcus aureus* and *Propionibacterium acnes*, presumably originating from the patient's skin, are the organisms isolated most frequently, with gram-negative bacilli and enterococci found occasionally. For cure of these infections it is usually necessary to remove the shunt and give appropriate systemic antimicrobial therapy. In a minority of patients, when the antibiotic susceptibilities of the infecting organism and circumstances allow intensive treatment with bactericidal agents given by both intravenous and intraventricular routes, it has been possible to eradicate the infection without removal of the shunt.

Recurrent episodes of bacterial meningitis may occur when there is a communication between the subarachnoid space and the paranasal sinuses, middle ear, nasopharynx or skin. Communication with the paranasal sinuses, middle ear or nasopharynx usually results from fractures of the cribriform plate (Fig. 3.13), paranasal sinuses or petrous portion of the temporal bone. There is often a history of head trauma, sometimes many years previously. In most cases the causative organism is *S. pneumoniae*, but other bacterial inhabitants of the upper respiratory tract are occasionally found. An investigation for the presence of CSF rhinorrhoea (Fig. 3.14) or otorrhoea should be carried out, by injecting either contrast material or a radioactive tracer into the lumbar subarachnoid space and testing

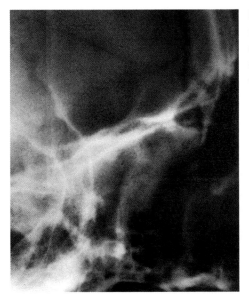

Fig. 3.13 Recurrent bacterial meningitis. Lateral skull film showing fracture through the cribriform plate. By courtesy of Dr G. D. Hungerford.

for its appearance in the nose or ear. Fluid from the nose may be tested for glucose content; this is a much lower in nasal secretions than in CSF unless meningitis with hypoglycorrhachia is present. Communication between the subarachnoid space and the skin may be associated with congenital defects such as cranial or lumbosacral midline dermal sinuses (Fig. 3.15) or meningomyelocoele. In these cases the infecting organisms are usually gram-negative bacilli. Any defects identified should be repaired surgically. Occasionally, recurrent meningitis results from a persistent parameningeal focus of infection; surgical drainage or removal of the lesion may be necessary. Very rarely episodes of recurrent meningitis due to intestinal bacteria have been associated with hyperinfection with *Strongyloides stercoralis*.

Tuberculous meningitis and tuberculoma

Tuberculous meningitis may occur as an isolated event, due to rupture of an asymptomatic cerebral tuberculoma into the subarachnoid or ventricular space, or it may be part of the picture of miliary (disseminated) tuberculosis. This latter situation prevails in approximately 75% of patients and evidence of tuberculosis outside the nervous system, most frequently in the lung, can usually be found. When meningitis results from rupture of a solitary subependymal tubercle the diagnosis depends upon findings in the CSF. The illness may begin acutely but more often the onset is insidious, with gradual development of headache, low-grade fever and signs of meningitis. The chronic meningitis (Figs 3.16, 3.17 & 3.18) is most marked

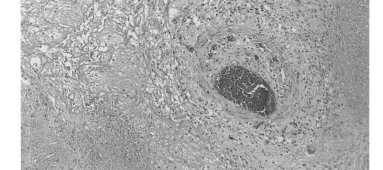

Fig. 3.14 Recurrent bacterial meningitis. Demonstration of cerebrospinal rhinorrhoea. By courtesy of Dr T. F. Sellers, Jr.

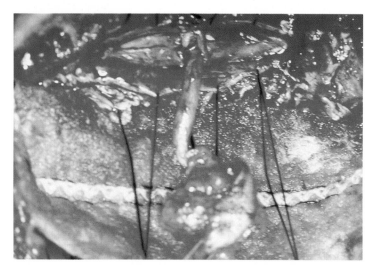

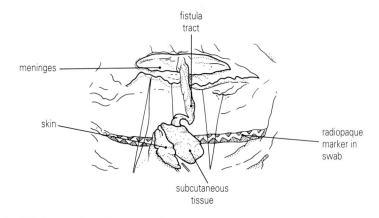

Fig. 3.15 Recurrent bacterial meningitis. Surgical photograph showing a well-defined fistula tract in the sacral region extending from skin to meninges. By courtesy of Dr P. Perot.

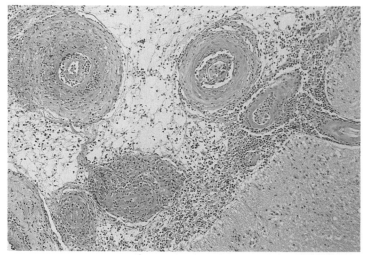

Fig. 3.16 Tuberculous meningitis with granulomatous inflammation. A meningeal vessel demonstrates partial occlusion and organization. Adjacent acute necrosis is apparent. H & E stain. By courtesy of Dr P. Garen.

Fig. 3.17 Tuberculous meningitis. Acute tuberculous meningitis with marked involvement of vessel walls and occlusion of smaller vessels. This vascular involvement can result in infarction. H & E stain. By courtesy of Dr P. Garen.

at the base of the brain (Fig. 3.19), and the thick gelatinous exudate often involves cranial nerves (Fig. 3.20) with production of cranial nerve palsies (Fig. 3.21). As the disease progresses the level of consciousness may be diminished and focal neurological deficits may appear. CSF examination typically reveals pleocytosis with 100–500 cells/mm³, with predominance of lymphocytes, elevated protein (100–500mg/ml), and glucose concentration which may be normal or diminished. Acid-fast bacilli are seen in stained smears of centrifuged CSF in less than a third of patients; the yield may be increased by repeated examinations and by staining the pellicle which forms in the CSF on standing in a test tube. Computed tomographic (CT) scanning may reveal the chronic basilar meningitis and tuberculomata within the brain (Fig. 3.22). Tuberculous meningitis may be treated with drug regimens effective in the treatment of pulmonary tuberculosis, such as isoniazid plus rifampin for 6 months, with pyrazinamide given during the first 2 months. If the level of consciousness is diminished or if focal neurological deficits are present, addition of corticosteroids for the first few

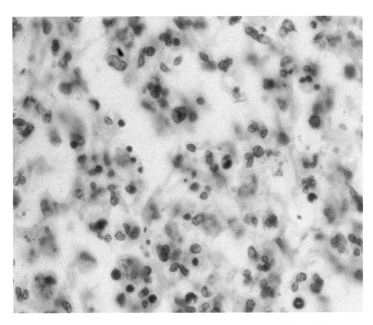

Fig. 3.18 Tuberculous meningitis. Inflammatory exudate containing multiple acid-fast rod-shaped bacilli. Kinyoun carbolfuchsin stain. By courtesy of Dr P. Garen.

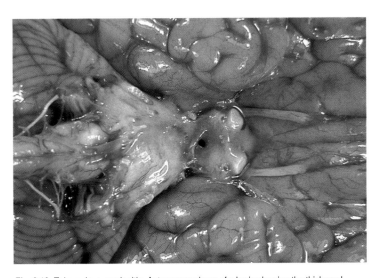

Fig. 3.19 Tuberculous meningitis. Autopsy specimen of a brain showing the thickened gelatinous basal meninges, especially thick in the region of the optic chiasma and over the pons.

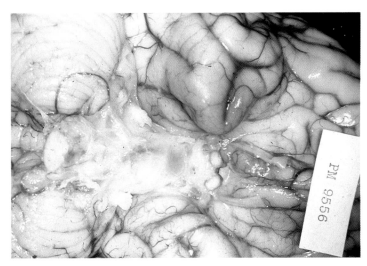

Fig. 3.20 Tuberculous meningitis. Autopsy specimen of the brain of a child showing a sheet of white exudate which encompasses and obscures the basal cranial nerves. By courtesy of Dr J. D. Balentine.

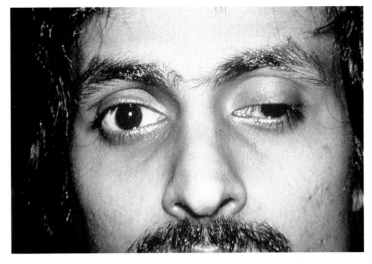

Fig. 3.21 Tuberculous meningitis. Cranial nerve palsies are fairly common. This patient's progress was generally satisfactory but he developed left III paralysis, shown here by ptosis and lateral deviation of the left eye caused by unopposed action of the lateral rectus.

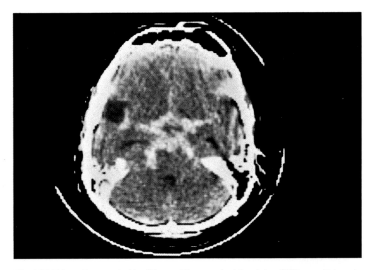

Fig. 3.22 Tuberculous meningitis: CT scan. The vessels of the circle of Willis are thickened and irregular due to contrast enhancement in the inflammatory tissue of the adjacent subarachnoid space. By courtesy of Dr J. Ambrose.

weeks of treatment may be beneficial. Since culture of the organism from CSF may require several weeks, it may be necessary to begin treatment empirically; clinical improvement after a week or 2 of therapy provides some support that the meningitis is due to *Mycobacterium tuberculosis*.

In the absence of meningitis, tuberculomata usually present as space-occupying lesions (Figs 3.23, 3.24 & 3.25), often with onset of seizures. CT scanning usually reveals

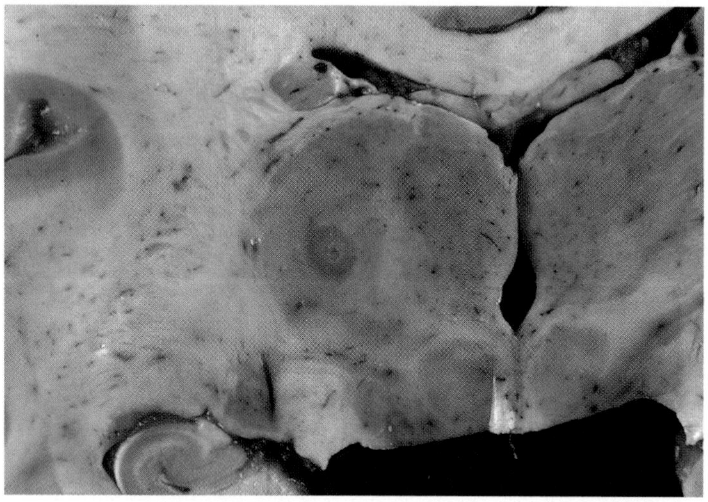

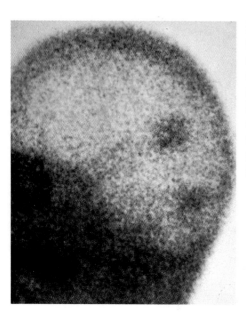

Fig. 3.23 Tuberculoma. Single tuberculous lesion with cavitating necrotic centre present in the thalamus. By courtesy of Dr P. Garen.

Fig. 3.24 Tuberculoma. Microscopic tuberculoma with central caseation and palisading granuloma. H & E stain. By courtesy of Dr P. Garen.

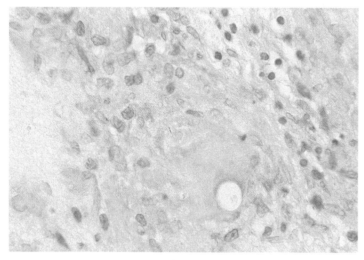

Fig. 3.25 Tuberculoma. Acid-fast bacillus in a granulomatous lesion. Kinyoun carbolfuchsin stain. By courtesy of Dr H. Whitwell.

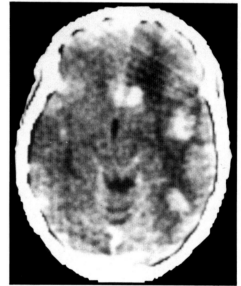

Fig. 3.26 Tuberculoma of the brain. CT scan showing multiple rounded lesions with surrounding oedema. The CT appearance of tuberculoma may be similar to that of pyogenic abscess, a fungal lesion or a meningioma. By courtesy of Dr J. Ambrose.

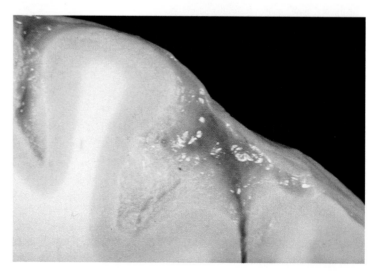

Fig. 3.27 Tuberculoma of the brain. Isotope scan showing two areas of abnormal contrast. The appearance is non-specific but the investigation provides useful information especially where CT scanning is not available. By courtesy of Dr E. Wolinsky.

Fig. 3.28 Cryptococcal meningitis. Cross-section of the frontal cortex revealing gelatinous material, which is the capsular material of the organism, in the sulci.

multiple avascular mass lesions surrounded by oedema (Fig. 3.26). Isotope scanning may reveal one or more areas of increased uptake (Fig. 3.27). When the diagnosis is known therapy with antituberculous drugs should be initiated and surgery avoided if possible, as fewer neurological sequelae result from medical therapy. Concomitant corticosteroid therapy may reduce cerebral oedema and result in improvement of symptoms. If the diagnosis is made by biopsy, no further excision should be performed and antituberculous therapy should be instituted.

Fungal meningitis

The yeast-like fungus *Cryptococcus neoformans* is by far the most important cause of fungal meningitis. Prior to the era of AIDS only about half of patients with cryptococcal meningitis were overtly immunocompromised; Hodgkin's disease, non-Hodgkin's lymphoma and high-dose corticosteroid therapy were the most common underlying conditions. Many apparently immunocompetent individuals exhibit defective cell-mediated immunity to *C. neoformans* following recovery from cryptococcal meningitis; whether these defects were present prior to the illness or represent a sequela of the infection is not known. Approximately 10% of patients with AIDS develop cryptococcal meningitis; the incidence is even higher in areas where the organism is especially abundant, such as the south east of the USA. Pathologically, there is a chronic meningitis, often with relatively little inflammatory reaction, as well as scattered cystic lesions comprised of fungal cells embedded in large quantities of the gelatinous polysaccharide capsular material, and distributed deeply within the sulci and in the brain substance (Figs 3.28, 3.29 & 3.30).

C. neoformans is worldwide in distribution and appears to be ubiquitous in nature. Humans acquire the organism by inhalation; pulmonary infection, though often inconsequential, is the initial pathogenetic event. The fungus has a special predilection for the meninges, and meningitis may occur as an isolated manifestation or as part of a disseminated infection. The illness often develops gradually with headache, irritability, impairment of memory and judgment and changes in behaviour. Temperature may or may not be elevated and signs of meningeal inflammation may be minimal or absent. Papilloedema and cranial nerve palsies are relatively common. Except in patients with AIDS, abnormalities are nearly always found in the CSF. Typically there is elevation in the opening pressure, lymphocytic pleocytosis, elevated protein and decreased glucose concentration. Cryptococci are seen on India Ink preparation in approximately 50% of patients. The large polysaccharide capsule of the organism, surrounding the refractile cell wall, gives *C. neoformans* a highly distinctive appearance (Figs 3.31 & 3.32). Cryptococcal polysac-

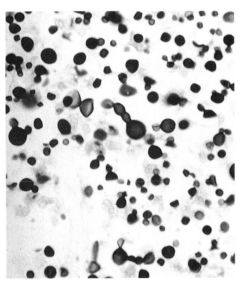

Fig. 3.29 Cryptococcal meningitis. *Cryptococcus neoformans* in exudate within the subarachnoid space. The apparent empty space between the organisms is capsular material. Methenamine silver stain.

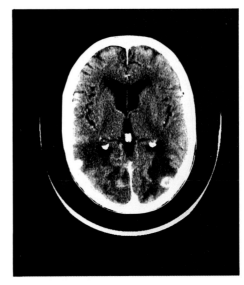

Fig. 3.30 Cryptococcal meningitis. CT scan showing multiple enhancing lesions in the brain, surrounded by oedema. By courtesy of Dr J. Curé.

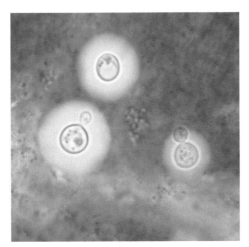

Fig. 3.31 Cyptococcal meningitis. India ink preparation of CSF sediment demonstrating the prominent capsule of the organism. Note the highly refractile cell wall and internal structure of the yeast. By courtesy of A.E. Prevost.

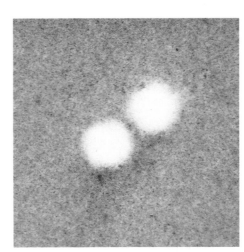

Fig. 3.32 Lymphocytes in CSF sediment. Note that these cells lack the prominent refractile cell wall and internal structure seen in *Cryptococcus neoformans*. India ink preparation. By courtesy of Dr J. R. Cantey.

charide antigen is detectable in CSF in 85%, and if serum is also tested for antigen it will be found in approximately 95% of patients.

In patients with AIDS the signs of inflammation in the CSF are drastically diminished: cell count, protein or glucose concentration may be normal in half the patients, and in 20% all three parameters are normal. India ink exami-

nation is positive in up to 85% of patients with AIDS, and cryptococcal antigen can be demonstrated in the CSF in nearly every case. Culture of the CSF yields the organism in virtually all cases, and the organism can often be cultured from other sites such as blood, sputum, urine, faeces or biopsy material.

The standard regimen for treatment of cryptococcal meningitis is the combination of amphotericin B, given intravenously, plus 5-fluorocytosine (flucytosine), administered orally, for at least 6–10 weeks. In patients with AIDS, suppressive treatment with amphotericin B, administered intravenously once weekly for the rest of the patient's life, is relatively effective in preventing recurrence, which is otherwise common. Fluconazole, an antifungal azole, which is well absorbed after oral administration, has also been shown to be very effective in preventing recurrence, although it is not very effective in the treatment of cryptococcal meningitis.

Meningitis due to *Coccidioides immitis* (Fig. 3.33) is virtually limited to individuals living in or travelling through desert areas of the south-western USA, Mexico and Central and South America where this fungus is endemic, although a few cases have resulted from exposure to fomites originating in the endemic area. Coccidioidal

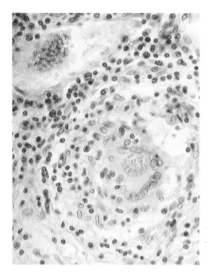
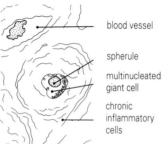

Fig. 3.33 Coccidiodial meningitis. Granulomatous meningitis due to *Coccidioides immitis* showing a multinucleated giant cell containing a spherule of the organism with many endospores. Periodic acid–Schiff stain.

blood vessel

spherule

multinucleated giant cell

chronic inflammatory cells

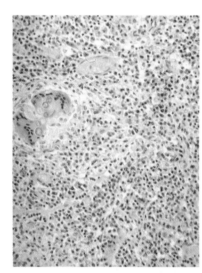
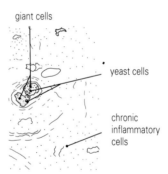

Fig. 3.34 North American blastomycosis. Granulomatous meningitis with multinucleated giant cells containing *B. dermatitidis*. H & E stain.

giant cells

yeast cells

chronic inflammatory cells

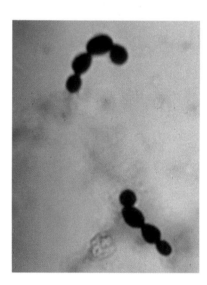

Fig. 3.35 Disseminated candidiasis. Gram stain of CSF sediment showing typical morphology of *Candida albicans*. By courtesy of A. E. Prevost.

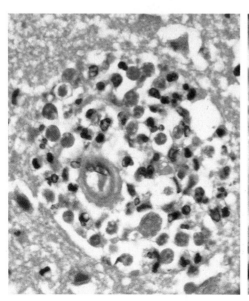
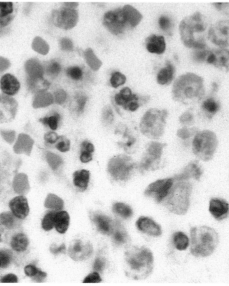
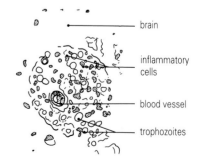

Fig. 3.36 Primary amoebic meningoencephalitis. Left: Section of brain showing trophozoites of *Naegleria fowleri* and inflammatory cells in a Virchow-Robin space from a fatal case in an eight-year-old child. Right: Higher power showing the large rounded trophozoites scattered among inflammatory cells. H & E stains. By courtesy of Dr S. Conradi.

brain

inflammatory cells

blood vessel

trophozoites

meningitis may occur as part of a generalized infection or may represent the only extrapulmonary site of disease. The illness may be extremely indolent with headache and only minimal signs of meningeal irritation for a long period of time. Examination of the CSF reveals a mononuclear (or rarely eosinophilic) pleocytosis, elevated protein and decreased glucose concentration. Specific aetiological diagnosis is usually made by mycological or serological diagnosis of pulmonary or disseminated coccidioidomycosis, or by finding antibody or the organism in the CSF. Successful treatment of coccidioidal meningitis is very difficult to achieve. Most cures have required combined systemic and either intraventricular or intrathecal administration of amphotericin B for 1 or 2 years; some authorities recommend continuation of treatment for the lifetime of the patient. The new azole agents, intraconazole and fluconazole, may simplify the therapy of this disease.

Rarely, meningitis may be caused by other invasive fungi, such as *Histoplasma capsulatum, Blastomyces dermatitidis* (Fig. 3.34) or *Candida albicans* (Fig. 3.35), usually as part of a disseminated infection.

Parasitic meningitis

Eosinophilic meningitis may be produced by invasion of the central nervous system by larval or adult forms of several different species of helminths, including *Angiostrongylus cantonensis* (the rat lung worm), *Gnasthostoma spinigerum* (a human hookworm), *Bayliscaris procyonis* (the raccoon ascarid), *Cysticercus cellulosae* and *Paragonimus westermani*. The diagnosis may be suggested on immunological and clinical grounds, by serological testing or occasionally by finding the organism in the CSF. Treatment is the same as that for infection outside the nervous system.

A rare cause of meningoencephalitis is infection with the free-living amoeba *Naegleria fowleri*. This organism is found worldwide in warm fresh water. Most patients have a history of swimming in fresh water shortly before onset of the illness. After nasal inoculation the amoebae evidently penetrate the submucosal nervous plexus and the cribriform plate to reach the olfactory bulbs and frontal lobes of the brain. There is haemorrhagic necrosis of the olfactory bulbs and contiguous areas of the brain, and eventual development of a diffuse meningoencephalitis and purulent leptomeningitis. The *Naegleria* trophozoites are found in the olfactory nerves and around blood vessels in the brain (Fig. 3.36) and and associated myocarditis may also be seen. The earliest symptom is often alteration in taste or smell. This is followed by abrupt onset of fever, headache, nausea and vomiting, nuchal rigidity and alteration in consciousness. Most patients progress rapidly to coma and death within a week. Examination of CSF reveals changes characteristic of purulent meningitis: neutrophilic pleocytosis, elevated protein and diminished glucose concentration. Motile trophozoites can usually be found in a wet mount of CSF (Fig. 3.37). Only two patients are known to have survived primary amoebic meningoencephalitis; both received high-dose systemic and intrathecal therapy with amphotericin B; one also received systemic and intrathecal miconazole and systemic rifampin and sulfisoxazole.

Another rare form of amoebic infection of the nervous system is a focal encephalitis due to several species of *Acanthamoeba (Hartmannella)* in immunocompromised patients. In these patients granulomatous skin lesions are present prior to the development of the necrotizing granulomatous lesions in the brain (Fig. 3.38). Brain biopsy is the only method available for making this diagnosis during life. Most cases have been fatal and little is known about therapy. Antimicrobial susceptibility tests have given variable results; pentamidine, ketoconazole, miconazole, and 5-fluorocytosine appear to be more active than amphotericin B against this organism.

ENCEPHALITIS

Encephalitis is inflammation of the brain parenchyma, nearly always a response to invasion by microorganisms, primarily viruses. Frequently there is concomitant meningitis, so the disease is usually a meningoencephalitis. Depression of consciousness ranging from lethargy to coma, focal neurological deficits and seizures are relatively common.

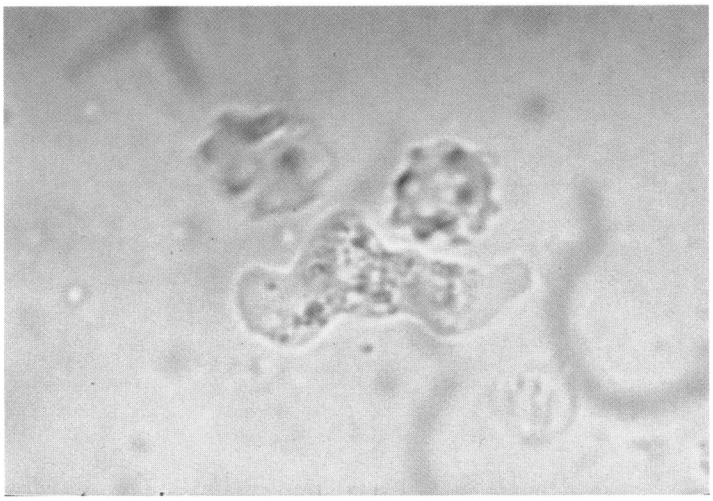

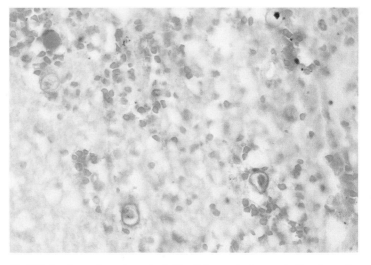

Fig. 3.37 Amoebic meningoencephalitis. Wet mount of CSF sediment showing motile *Naegleria fowleri* from a fatal case in an 8-year-old child. By courtesy of A. E. Prevost.

Fig. 3.38 Acanthamoeba meningoencephalitis with haemorrhagic necrosis. Organisms with thick irregular capsules and central basophilic nucleus. H & E stain. By courtesy of Dr P. Garen.

Rabies

Rabies is a severe viral encephalitis which is nearly always fatal. The virus can infect virtually all mammalian species. Because of geographical isolation, animal control measures and/or quarantine practices, it is absent from many countries including the United Kingdom, Japan, several Scandinavian countries and Australia. Where domestic animal rabies has not been adequately controlled, dogs account for 90% of reported human cases. In areas where rabies in domestic animals is well controlled, such as the USA, Canada and many countries of western Europe, dogs account for less than 5% of human cases. Cats and certain species of domestic livestock also cause a small proportion of human infections, but a vast reservoir exists in wild mammals. Species which are important in the causation of human rabies in various parts of the world include skunks, raccoons, foxes, wolves, mongooses, jackals and insectivorous and vampire bats. The incidence of human rabies is high in India, the Philippines and many countries in Africa. Most human cases result from bites but well-documented transmission has also occurred via scratches, contamination of mucous membranes with infected saliva, corneal transplantation from a donor with rabies and inhalation of aerosolized virus in bat caves and in laboratories working with the virus.

The incubation period is usually from a few days to 3 months. A small proportion have onset of illness between 3 months and 1 year, and rarely the incubation period may last from 1–5 years or even longer. During most of the incubation period the virus multiplies locally near the site of inoculation, possibly within muscle cells. The virus then spreads via peripheral nerves to the central nervous system, and by the time symptoms have occurred has travelled outward via efferent pathways to most tissues of the body, including the salivary glands. When symptoms appear approximately half of the patients have pain or paraesthesia at the inoculation site, but otherwise the manifestations are non-specific and include fever, malaise, fatigue, headache and anorexia. Within a few days neurological manifestations supervene; these may include apprehension, anxiety, agitation, irritability, insomnia, hyperactivity, disorientation, hallucinations, bizarre behaviour, seizures, nuchal rigidity and paralysis. Hyperactivity and delirium are usually intermittent, alternating with periods of orientation and relative calm. Hydrophobia (spasms of the pharynx and larynx provoked by attempts at drinking or even the sight of water) or aerophobia (similar effects produced by blowing air on the face of the patient) occur in approximately 50%. A few patients die during this period, but most go on to develop progressive paralysis and eventually coma. Only three patients are known to have recovered from rabies, all during the 1970s. Although most cases of human rabies occurring during the last 20 years in the United States and certain other industrialized Western countries have received intensive supportive care, there have been no additional survivors and the disease must still be considered virtually 100% fatal. Expert intensive care does prolong the period of survival. Potentially fatal complications include respiratory failure, progressive refractory hypoxaemia, seizures and cardiac arrhythmias.

A history of exposure to rabies virus and a typical clinical picture, especially if hydrophobia and/or aerophobia are present, strongly suggests the diagnosis. Most patients with rabies develop high titres of serum antibody, but individuals who have been immunized with the potent modern human diploid cell vaccines may develop titres as high as those seen in clinical rabies. In such patients determination of antibody levels in the cerebrospinal fluid may be valuable, since high titres of antibody in the CSF are seen only in clinical disease. The virus has been isolated antemortem from saliva, brain tissue, CSF, urine sediment, and tracheal secretions, and postmortem virus isolation has been obtained from many other tissues of the body. Specific immunofluorescent staining of rabies virus may be accomplished using brain biopsy specimens, corneal impressions or skin biopsy. Histological examination of brain tissue from human cases typically shows perivascular inflammation in grey matter, neuronal degeneration and, in 70–80% of cases, Negri bodies, which are round or oblong eosinophilic cytoplasmic inclusions which often contain basophilic spots (Figs 3.39 & 3.40). Immunofluorescent staining of Negri bodies is more sensitive than conventional histological techniques.

Because treatment of rabies is so unsatisfactory, correct post-exposure prophylaxis is extremely important. The

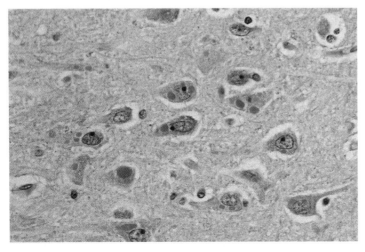

Fig. 3.39 Rabies. Multiple cytoplasmic Negri bodies in hippocampal pyramidal neurons. H & E stain. By courtesy of Dr P. Garen.

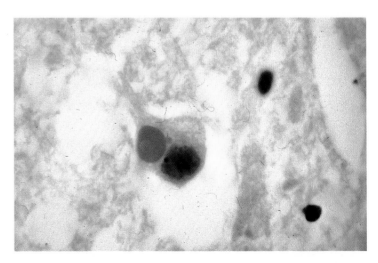

Fig. 3.40 Rabies. Histological section of brain showing a Negri body. H & E stain

physician faced with the decision of whether or not to treat a potential rabies exposure should obtain specific, current recommendations dealing with this issue *and follow them to the letter*. Generally speaking, optimal post-exposure prophylaxis includes thorough cleansing of the wound to its deepest extent using a 20% soap solution, active immunization with human diploid cell vaccine, administered intramuscularly in the deltoid region as five 1ml doses given on days 0, 3, 7, 14 and 28, and a single dose of human rabies immunoglobulin (20IU/kg), up to half infiltrated around the site of exposure and the remainder given intramuscularly in the gluteal region or anterolateral aspect of the thigh. Individuals at high risk from rabies because of occupation, residence or travel may receive pre-exposure prophylaxis consisting of three 1ml doses of human diploid cell vaccine given intramuscularly in the deltoid region on days 0, 7 and 21 or 28. Chloroquine phosphate given for malaria chemoprophylaxis may interfere with the development of the antibody response to rabies vaccine.

Herpes simplex encephalitis

Herpes simplex encephalitis is a rare complication of herpes simplex infections, but herpes simplex virus (HSV) is one of the most common causes of sporadic acute viral encephalitis in the USA and many other countries. Unlike most other types of infection due to this virus, encephalitis does not seem to be more common in immunocompromised individuals, except perhaps in those with HIV infection. Most cases are due to type 1 virus (HSV-1) but cases occurring during the neonatal period may be due to type 2 virus (HSV-2), acquired from the mother with genital herpes infection. The virus apparently reaches the brain via neural routes during active primary or recurrent infection. Pathologically the infection produces a necrotizing haemorrhagic encephalitis which most commonly involves the temporal lobes (Figs 3.41, 3.42 & 3.43). Clinical features often include fever, headache, behavioural disorders, difficulty in speaking and focal seizures. A relatively characteristic feature is olfactory hallucinations. Examination of the cerebrospinal fluid usually reveals moderate elevation of the protein concentration, normal glucose and moderate pleocytosis with both mononuclear and polymorphonuclear leukocytes. EEG, computed tomographic (CT) scanning (Fig. 3.44) and magnetic resonance imaging (MRI – Figs

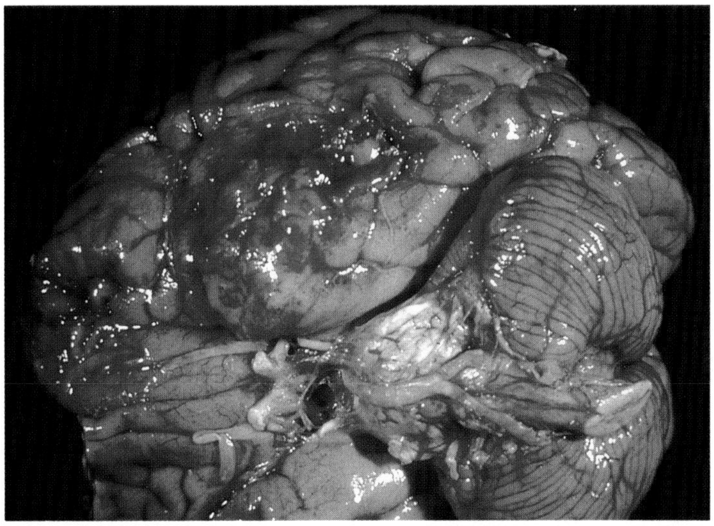

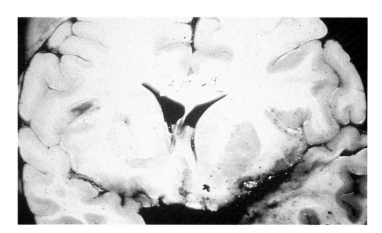

Fig. 3.42 Herpes simplex encephaltiis. Coronal section of brain showing haemorrhagic necrosis of the left anterior medial aspect of the left temporal lobe and the orbital surface of the left frontal. This is a characteristic location for the lesion of herpes encephalitis.

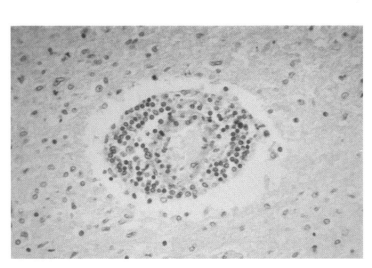

Fig. 3.41 Herpes simplex encephalitis. Gross specimen showing necrosis, haemorrhage and oedema involving the orbital surface of the left frontal lobe and the anterior, medial and lateral surface of the left temporal lobe.

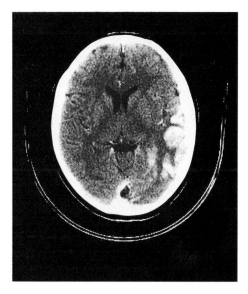

Fig. 3.44 Herpes simplex encephalitis. CT scan done late in the course of the illness, showing enhancement of gyral structures in the left temporal area and adjacent cerebral oedema. By courtesy of Dr J. Curé.

Fig. 3.43 Herpes simplex encephalitis. Perivascular monuclear inflammatory exduate associated with slight gliosis and inflammation in grey matter of the temporal lobe. H & E stain.

3.45 & 3.46) often reveal evidence of localized lesions. HSV-1 can rarely be isolated from the CSF, and culture and immunofluorescent staining of brain biopsy specimens (Figs 3.47 & 3.48) is the most reliable way to make a specific aetiological diagnosis. Recently, HSV DNA was detected in the CSF in 42 of 43 proven cases of herpes simplex encephalitis by means of a polymerase chain reaction assay, and this approach may provide a way to obtain a specific aetiological diagnosis without resort to brain biopsy. Empirical antiviral therapy is indicated in patients who develop presumed viral encephalitis in a non-epidemic setting. Without specific antiviral therapy approximately 70% of patients with herpes simplex encephalitis will die, and nearly all of the survivors will have permanent neurological sequelae. Acyclovir, given intravenously at a dosage of 10mg/kg every 8 hours, is the most effective therapeutic agent currently available. Prognosis for survival and recovery of neurological function is much better in patients treated early in the course of the illness; if therapy with acyclovir is instituted before the 5th day of illness the survival rate is approximately 90%.

Encephalitis due to varicella-zoster virus

Encephalitis is a rare complication of herpes zoster. It is seen most frequently in the elderly, in association with disseminated or cranial herpes zoster (Fig. 3.49) and in immunocompromised patients, especially those with lymphoproliferative malignancies. Whether the encephalitis is due to direct viral invasion of the CNS or results from an immunological reaction is unknown.

Common clinical features include fever, headache, confusion, memory deficit, disorientation and depressed level of consciousness, sometimes progressing to coma. CNS manifestations usually develop about a week after the appearance of skin lesions, and 1–2 days after evidence of dissemination. Untreated, the illness usually lasts approximately 14 days. Most patients recover completely without significant neurological sequelae. Diagnosis is usually made on clinical grounds. Diagnostic criteria include clinical evidence of herpes zoster, encephalopathic state, diffusely abnormal EEG and CSF abnormalities compatible with encephalitis. Most patients with herpes zoster encephalitis have a mononuclear pleocytosis and increased protein concentration in the CSF, but up to 40% of patients with herpes zoster without encephalitis have abnormalities in the CSF. Varicella-zoster virus (VZV) is rarely isolated from the CSF, but a rise in titre of serum antibody to VZV may be demonstrated. Antibody to VZV may be demonstrated in the CSF in some, but not all patients.

Treatment with high doses of acyclovir (10mg/kg every 8 hours) given intravenously usually results in rapid and dramatic clinical response, with defervescence and resolution of encephalopathy and EEG abnormalities within 72

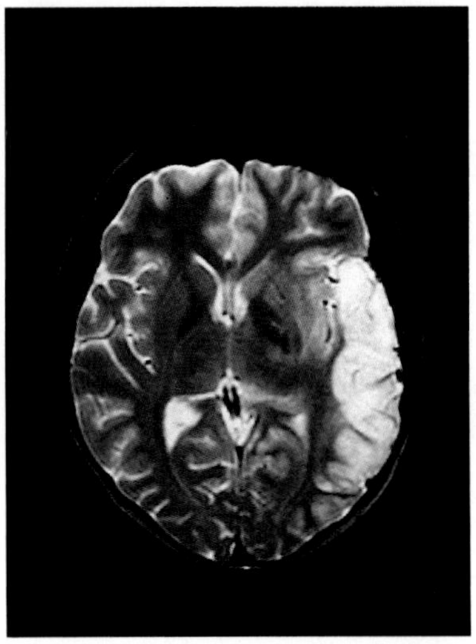

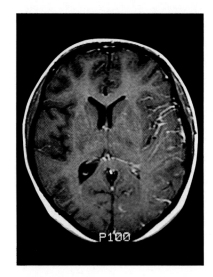

Fig. 3.45 Herpes simplex encephalitis. MRI scan showing extensive involvement of the left temporal area. By courtesy of Dr J. Curé.

Fig. 3.46 Herpes simplex encephalitis. MRI scan showing enhancement by gadolinium of gyral structures in the left temporal area. By courtesy of Dr J. Curé.

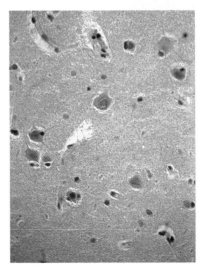

Fig. 3.47 Herpes simplex encephalitis. Intranuclear inclusion in nerve cell. × 250. H & E stain.

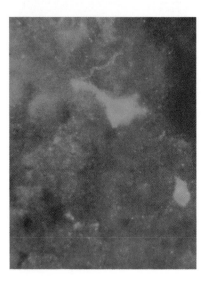

Fig. 3.48 Herpes simplex encephalitis: brain biopsy. The neurons staining bright green are heavily infected with herpes simplex virus. Immunofluorescent preparation. By courtesy of Dr S. Fisher-Hoch.

hours. Treatment should be continued for approximately 1 week.

A well-recognized but uncommon complication of chickenpox is cerebellar ataxia. This is more common in children, and usually appears within a week after the onset of the rash. In addition to ataxia, fever, vertigo, tremor, vomiting and abnormalities of speech may occur. CSF examination usually reveals lymphocytic pleocytosis and elevated concentration of protein. Resolution usually occurs within a few weeks. A more severe generalized encephalitis may also complicate chickenpox, especially in adults. These patients exhibit fever, severe headache, vomiting, disorientation, depression in the level of consciousness and frequently seizures. This type of severe encephalitis typically lasts for several weeks. The case-fatality rate may be as high as 20%, and prominent neurological sequelae occur in a significant proportion of survivors.

Other viral encephalitides

In addition to the agents already discussed, a large number of other viruses may cause encephalitis. Many of these are transmitted to man by arthropods, either mosquitoes or ticks. Some of the more important arthropod-borne encephalitides are listed in Fig. 3.50.

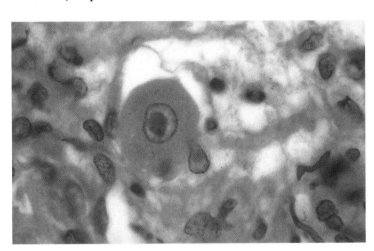

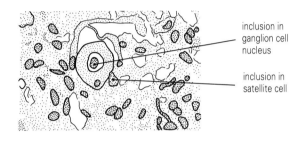

Fig. 3.49 Trigeminal herpes zoster. Cowdry type A inclusions in the nucleus of a ganglion cell and a satellite cell in a patient with Hodgkin's disease. H & E stain.

Fig. 3.50 Some important arthropod-borne encephalitides.

Some Important Arthropod-borne Encephalitides	
Disease	**Geographic Distribution**
Mosquito-borne	
Eastern equine encephalitis	Eastern, Gulf coast and southern USA
Western equine encephalitis	Western and midwestern USA; western Canada
Venezuelan equine encephalitis	South and Central America; southern USA
St. Louis encephalitis	Central, western and southern USA
Japanese B encephalitis	Japan, Korea, south east Asia, China, India
California encephalitis (La Crosse virus)	Northern USA
Murray Valley encephalitis	Australia
Rift Valley fever	Eastern and southern Africa
Tick-borne	
Colarado tick fever	Mountains of western USA.
Tick-borne encephalitis	USSR, central Europe, Scandanavia
Kyasanur Forest disease	India
Omsk haemorrhagic fever	Siberia

Sporadic cases of encephalitis occur occasionally as complications of other viral diseases, including mumps, measles, rubella, influenza, enteroviral infections and infectious mononucleosis. A distinct clinical syndrome of chronic meningo-encephalitis due to enteroviruses (primarily echoviruses) has been described in immunocompromised individuals, most commonly in those with X-linked agammaglobulonaemia.

Clinically, acute viral encephalitis is characterized by acute onset of fever, headache, stiff neck, depression of consciousness, CSF pleocytosis (predominantly mononuclear) and frequently seizures. Focal neurological deficits often develop during the course of the illness. Severity of illness and case-fatality rate vary considerably among the different arthropod-borne viral encephalitides. For example, in eastern equine encephalitis the case fatality rate in man is 50–70%, and up to 70% of survivors may have serious neurological sequelae. Severe illness is also observed commonly in Japanese B encephalitis. In contrast, fatal cases of California encephalitis (La Crosse virus) are extremely rare.

In fatal cases of viral encephalitis there is usually a prominent perivascular inflammatory reaction composed predominantly of mononuclear cells, although polymorphonuclear leucocytes may also be present. Evidence of meningitis is also present. Neurons may exhibit degenerative changes, with phagocytosis of neurons by macrophages and microglial cells (neuronophagia) (Fig. 3.51). Inflammatory cells in perivascular areas (and in CSF) are predominantly T helper cells, with smaller numbers of T suppressor/cytotoxic cells, B cells and macrophages also present. The distribution of lesions within the nervous system varies among different viral encephalitides. In Japanese B encephalitis there is often extensive infection of brain stem nuclei and structures of the basal ganglia and thalamus; this may explain the frequent occurrence of acute respiratory failure and death in patients with this infection, and the high incidence of dystonic and Parkinsonian sequelae seen in survivors.

Mycoplasma encephalitis

Encephalitis or meningoencephalitis, and occasionally other neurological complications, may occur in association with pneumonia due to *Mycoplasma pneumoniae* in up to 10% of cases (see Chapter 2).

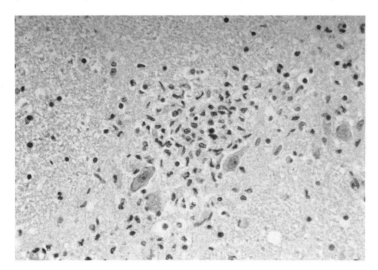

Fig. 3.51 Viral encephalitis. Mononuclear inflammatory cellular response around neurons typical of the so-called 'Babès nodule' associated with viral encephalitis. H & E stain.

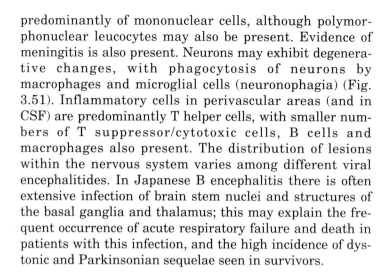

Fig. 3.52 Post-vaccinal encephalomyelitis. Perivascular demyelination and mononuclear inflammation in patient with post-vaccinal encephalomyelitis. Luxol-fast blue stain. By courtesy of Dr P. Garen.

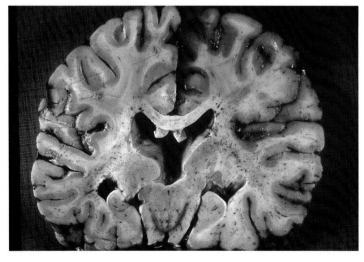

Fig. 3.53 Post-infectious encephalitis. Gross specimen of brain showing multiple punctate haemorrhages and rounded outline of the brain due to cerebral oedema.

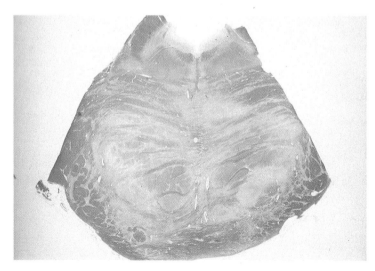

Fig. 3.54 Post-infectious encephalitis. Section of pons showing confluent areas of demyelination. Luxol-fast blue stain.

Postinfectious and postvaccinal encephalitis

Postinfectious and postvaccinal encephalomyelitis resemble, clinically and pathologically, experimental allergic encephalomyelitis produced by sensitization to central myelin, and they may be human counterparts of that condition. Postinfectious encephalomyelitis may occur following a wide variety of acute viral infections, including measles, varicella, rubella, mumps and various respiratory infections. Postvaccinal encephalomyelitis may occur following various immunizations, most commonly following administration of the older neural tissue-derived rabies vaccines. The interval between onset of the viral infection or immunization and appearance of symptoms or signs referable to the nervous system is usually between 2–12 days. The clinical picture may include evidence of encephalitis or myelitis or both. Onset of the neurological illness may be relatively abrupt, and seizures and alteration of consciousness are common. The pathological picture is characterized by perivascular infiltration of mononuclear inflammatory cells and perivenous demyelination (Fig. 3.52). In severe cases there may be pronounced cerebral oedema, multiple punctate haemorrhages and extensive demyelination and necrosis (Figs 3.53 & 3.54). Examination of the spinal fluid usually reveals elevation in protein concentration and moderate mononuclear pleocytosis. Myelin basic protein may also be present. Prognosis is uncertain, but some patients have made excellent recoveries following long periods of unconsciousness, so vigorous supportive therapy is indicated. Cerebral oedema, seizures, hypoglycaemia and inappropriate secretion of antidiuretic hormone may occur and require specific treatment.

Reye's syndrome

Reye's syndrome is a disease of unknown aetiology, affecting the liver and central nervous system, which follows a variety of viral infections, most frequently influenza B and varicella. It is seen almost entirely in children. Typically, nausea and vomiting occur a few days after onset of a viral infection, followed by a change in mental status. Neurological manifestations may include lethargy, delirium,

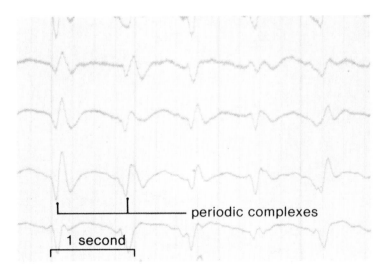

Fig. 3.55 Creutzfeldt–Jakob disease. EEG (position 8) showing periodic complexes at approximately 1.25 Hz.

seizures, stupor, coma and respiratory arrest. Hepatomegaly is present, with abnormalities in liver function tests including elevated blood ammonia and prolonged prothrombin time. Jaundice is usually absent. Examination of the CSF reveals normal protein concentration and absence of cells. Histopathological findings in the brain include cerebral oedema and anoxic degeneration of neurons, but little or no inflammation. The lesion in the liver is described in Chapter 5. A large recent study revealed an increased incidence of Reye's syndrome in children who have received aspirin for fever resulting from influenza. There is no specific therapy but intensive supportive care including administration of glucose intravenously to correct hypoglycaemia, haemodynamic monitoring, assisted ventilation and mannitol to lower increased intracranial pressure may be required. Case fatality rate ranges from 10–40%, and is highest in children who present in coma.

'Slow' viral infections

These are progressive neurological diseases caused by transmissible agents, which become manifest only after a very long incubation period of months or years. The transmissible spongiform encephalopathies (Creutzfeldt–Jakob disease, kuru and the Gerstmann-Straussler syndrome) are caused by transmissible agents called prions which differ markedly from conventional viruses; progressive multifocal leukoencephalopathy and subacute sclerosing panencephalitis are due to more typical viral agents.

The aetiological agents of the transmissible spongiform encephalopathies appear to be very small particles which contain little or no nucleic acid and are highly resistant to a number of physical and chemical agents which inactivate conventional viruses, including various types of radiation, formaldehyde, β-propiolactone, heat and nuclease enzymes. The best studied of these organisms is the agent of scrapie, a progressive neurological disease of sheep. Fibrillar or rod-shaped particles which may be proteins or glycoproteins and are closely associated with cell membranes have been visualized in the brains of affected animals and humans, and the infectious agent of scrapie has been partially purified. A 'prion protein' (PrP) of 27 000–30 000 Da molecular weight is present in normal brain tissue, and molecular studies have demonstrated altered forms of PrP in patients with spongiform encephalopathies.

Creutzfeldt-Jakob disease and other spongiform encephalopathies

Creutzfeldt–Jakob disease is an uncommon progressive cerebral disease characterized by dementia, ataxia and diffuse myoclonic jerking. In most patients dementia becomes profound within 6 months and death usually occurs within a year after onset of symptoms. The diagnosis is primarily clinical but relatively characteristic EEG findings occur at some stage of the illness in more than half of the patients (Fig. 3.55). The CSF is usually normal, although a slight elevation in protein concentration is observed occasionally. Computed tomographic (CT) scanning and magnetic resonance imaging (MRI) are usually normal. Typical neuropathological findings include diffuse loss of neurons, intense astrocytic proliferation with fibrous gliosis and intracytoplasmic vacuolation and swelling of both neuronal and astroglial processes which result in the 'spongy' state (Figs 3.56 & 3.57). In a few patients PAS-positive, amyloid-like plaques are found. In most cases the changes are most severe in the frontal lobes. Creutzfeldt–Jakob disease is worldwide in distribution, with an overall incidence of approximately one case per million population annually. A strikingly increased incidence has been observed in Libyan Jews living in Israel, possibly associated with the eating of animal brains or sheep eyeballs. Sporadic cases have apparently been acquired via person-to-person transmission following neurosurgical procedures, and via administration of growth hormone made from bovine pituitary glands. Approximately 15% of cases are familial, in a pattern which suggests autosomal dominant transmission.

Kuru is a similar disease seen only in the highlands of eastern New Guinea, primarily among tribes of the *Fore* linguistic group. It is characterized by insidious onset of cerebellar ataxia of gait and limbs, with shivering, dysarthria, pyramidal and extrapyramidal signs, involuntary movements and mood changes with eventual development of dementia, dysphagia and ventilatory failure. Neuropathological changes are similar to those of Creutzfeldt–Jakob disease, but are most severe in the cerebellum, and most patients exhibit PAS-positive, amyloid-like plaques. Transmission of kuru apparently occurs

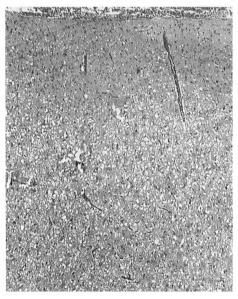

Fig. 3.56 Creutzfeldt–Jakob disease. Histological section of cerebral cortex at low magnification showing multiple vacuoles . By courtesy of Dr H. Whitwell.

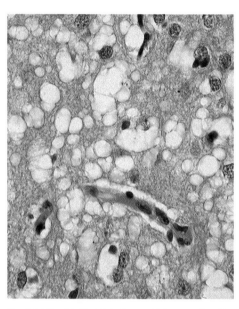

Fig. 3.57 Creutzfeldt–Jakob disease. High power view. By courtesy of Dr H. Whitwell.

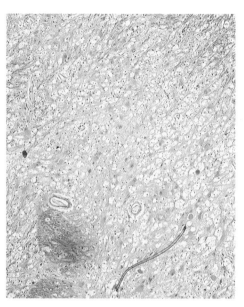

Fig. 3.58 Progressive multifocal leucoencephalopathy. Histological section showing a focus of demyelination, reactive astrocytosis and lipid-laden macrophages. Luxol-fast blue stain.

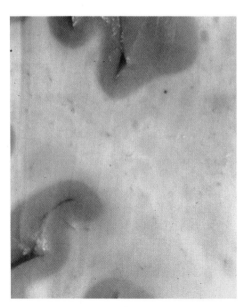

Fig. 3.59 Progressive multifocal leucoencephalopathy. Diffuse white matter loss with focal granular necrosis. By courtesy of Dr P. Garen.

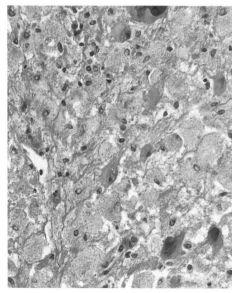

Fig. 3.60 Progressive multifocal leucoencephalopathy. Affected region of white matter displaying numerous background foamy macrophages and bizarre astrocytes with enlarged, hyperchromatic and lobulated nuclei. H & E stain. By courtesy of Dr P. Garen.

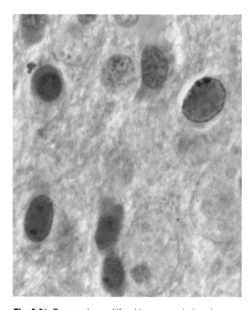

Fig. 3.61 Progressive multifocal leucoencephalopathy. Enlarged oligodendroglial nuclei with homogenous basophilic intranuclear viral inclusions. H & E stain. By courtesy of Dr P. Garen.

during ritual cannibalism of dead kinsmen, probably via cuts on the hands sustained during removal of the brains. Cessation of the practice of ritualistic cannibalism has apparently eliminated transmission of kuru.

Gertsmann–Straussler syndrome is an adult-onset, chronic cerebellar ataxia, which is usually familial. Dementia often develops late in the course of the disease. Recent investigations of families with the Gerstmann–Straussler syndrome and other dementing and ataxic illnesses have demonstrated that dementia associated with the abnormal prion protein (PrP) gene may be present in individuals who lack the characteristic neuropathological changes. Neurological disease associated with transmissible prion proteins may be more diverse and more frequent than previously suspected.

Progressive multifocal leucoencephalopathy

Progressive multifocal leucoencephalopathy is a rare, sub-acute, progressive demyelinating disease of the central nervous system which occurs almost exclusively in immunocompromised patients. The most common underlying conditions are Hodgkin's disease, chronic lymphocytic leukaemia and AIDS, although a few cases have occurred following renal transplantation. The distribution of PML is worldwide. The causative agent is the JC virus, a member of the polyoma group of papovaviruses. Approximately 75% of adults have antibody to this virus, so PML probably represents reactivation of a pre-existing latent infection. The characteristic neuropathological finding is focal destruction of myelin (Fig. 3.58), with relative preservation of axons. As the disease progresses the foci of demyelination become confluent, producing large plaques (Fig. 3.59). There is little or no inflammatory response. Giant astrocytes, with pleomorphic, hyperchromatic nuclei, sometimes with mitotic figures, indistinguishable from the malignant astrocytes seen in glioblastomas, are often present (Fig. 3.60); these cells may reflect the oncogenic potential of the polyoma virus. Viral particles, 28–40nm in diameter, may sometimes be seen in the nuclei of oligodendrocytes within the lesions (Figs 3.61, 3.62 & 3.63).

The illness usually develops rapidly, with death occurring within a few months after appearance of the first neurological symptoms. The clinical findings are diverse, depending on the location of foci of demyelination. Monoparesis, hemiparesis, ataxia, dysarthria, dysphagia, cortical blindness, personality change and mental impairment occur frequently; in the late stage of the disease extensive paralysis, severe dementia and coma may appear. CT scanning and MRI may be useful in localizing the lesions (Figs 3.64 & 3.65); the lesions of PML do not exhibit enhancement on CT scanning, which may help distinguish them from the lesions of toxoplasmosis. The cerebrospinal fluid is usually normal. At present there is no effective treatment.

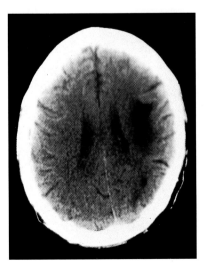

Fig. 3.62 Progressive multifocal leucoencephalopathy. Electron micrograph showing oligodendrocyte nucleus containing diffuse intranuclear viral particles of JC virus. By courtesy of Dr P. Garen.

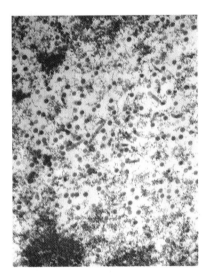

Fig. 3.63 Progressive multifocal leucoencephalopathy. Higher power demonstrating round and filamentous papovavirus particles. By courtesy of Dr P. Garen.

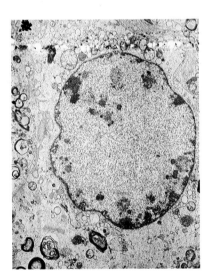

Fig. 3.64 Progressive multifocal leucoencephalopathy. CT scan showing a large hypodense lesion in the left parietal region. By courtesy of Dr J. Curé.

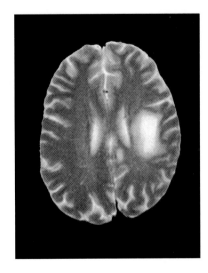

Fig. 3.65 Progressive multifocal leucoencephalopathy. MRI scan of same patient showing a large lesion in the left parietal region and a smaller lesion close to the midline. By courtesy of Dr J. Curé.

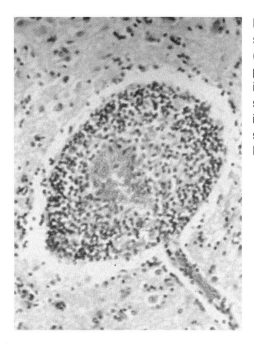

Fig. 3.66 Subacute sclerosing panencephalitis (SSPE). Very intense perivascular mononuclear inflammatory exudate, with subtle migration of inflammatory cells into the surrounding cerebral cortex. H & E stain.

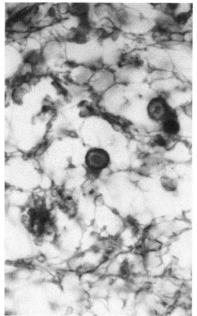

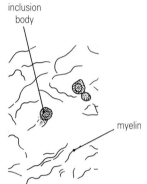

Fig. 3.67 Subacute sclerosing panencephalitis (SSPE). Eosinphilic intranuclear inclusion bodies composed of RNA and ribonuclear protein. Luxol fast blue, H & E stain.

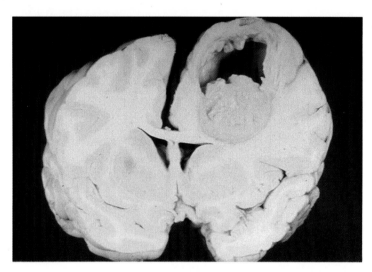

Fig. 3.68 Brain abscess: coronal section revealing chronic brain abscess due to *Staphylococcus aureus* in the left frontal lobe in a 16-year-old girl. The border of the abscess cavity reveals a linear region of brownish discolouration which represents the capsule of the abscess.

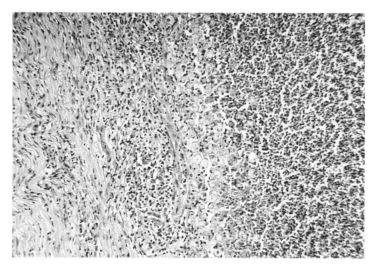

Fig. 3.69 Brain abscess. Histological section of a chronic brain abscess due to *S. aureus*. At the centre is an acute inflammatory exudate bordered by zones of macrophages, lymphocytes and plasma cells. Outside this is the layer of fibrosis in the collagenous capsule. H & E stain.

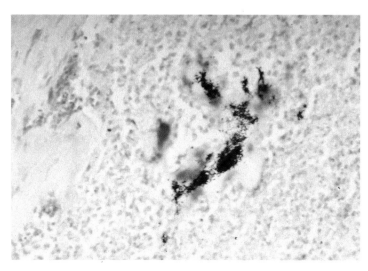

Fig. 3.70 Brain abscess. Histological section of necrotic brain tissue. Clumps of gram-positive bacteria can be seen within the necrotic material. Brown and Brenn stain. By courtesy of Dr J. R. Cantey.

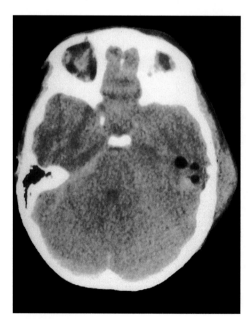

Fig. 3.71 Brain abscess due to *Clostridium perfringens*. CT scan showing gas formation in the lesion in the right parietal area and oedema of extracranial tissue.

Subacute sclerosing panencephalitis

Subacute sclerosing panencephalitis (SSPE) is a progressive inflammatory neurological disease of children and adolescents which is related to infection with measles virus. Patients with SSPE have in their brains large amounts of a defective form of measles virus, which can be cultivated only with difficulty in certain susceptible cell lines. The SSPE virus may represent a variant of measles virus resulting from mutation, or the result of recombination between measles virus and some other viral agent. It has been suggested that the host immune response may be more important in the causation of SSPE than the viral infection itself. High levels of measles antibody might damage virus-infected cells, or sensitized lymphocytes might be cytotoxic to infected target cells.

SSPE is a subacute encephalitis involving grey and white matter of both cerebral hemispheres and brain stem, with perivascular and diffuse infiltrates of lymphocytes and plasma cells (Fig. 3.66). As the disease progresses there is destruction of neurons, diffuse proliferation of glial cells and degeneration of myelin. Eosinophilic intranuclear inclusion bodies with surrounding halos (Cowdry type A inclusions) are seen in glial cells and neurons (Fig. 3.67). By electron microscopy the inclusions are seen to contain tubular paramyxovirus-like nuclear capsids, 17–19nm in diameter; these inclusion bodies stain specifically with anti-measles virus antibody. SSPE usually appears approximately 7 years after clinical measles; the disease very rarely follows measles immunization. Widespread immunization against measles in the USA and other countries has resulted in a dramatic fall in the incidence of SSPE. The average age of onset is between 7 and 8 years. The first stage of the illness is characterized by poor school performance, intellectual decline and abnormal behaviour, often diagnosed as a psychological problem. Weeks or months later, more severe intellectual deterioration, seizures, myoclonic jerks and apraxia may appear. Eventually rigidity, hyperactive reflexes, extensor plantar responses and a decorticate state ensue. Death usually occurs after a few months or years; progression is more rapid in children. A characteristic finding in the cerebrospinal fluid is increased IgG with oligoclonal bands exhibiting measles antibody activity;

these are not found in patients with measles. Titres of measles antibody in serum and CSF may continue to rise throughout the course of the illness. Radionuclide brain scan and (CT) scans may show the location and extent of the lesions, and relatively characteristic EEG abnormalities have been described. There is no effective treatment for SSPE at the present time.

OTHER INFECTIONS INVOLVING THE NERVOUS SYSTEM

Brain abscess and other intracranial bacterial infections

Bacterial abscess of the brain may arise by direct extension from a contiguous focus of infection, by the haematogenous route, following trauma, or may be unassociated with any overt underlying cause (cryptogenic abscess). The most common mechanism of spread is from a contiguous focus, usually sinusitis or otitis media, and the frontal and temporal lobes are the most common sites of brain abscess. Haematogenous spread can occur from any site of primary infection, but is most commonly associated with infections within the chest, including lung abscess, bronchiectasis and empyema. Head trauma associated with brain abscess includes skull fracture, neurosurgical procedures, pencil tip injuries to the eye in children and lawn dart injuries to the head. Many cryptogenic brain abscesses probably originate as dental infections. Two other conditions associated with a very high incidence of brain abscess are hereditary haemorrhagic telangiectasia with pulmonary arteriovenous malformations, and cyanotic congenital heart disease. In both conditions the normal pulmonary capillary filter is bypassed, and in cyanotic congenital heart disease the polycythaemia and reduced brain capillary blood flow may lead to reduced tissue oxygenation and microinfarction. In the early or 'cerebritis' stage of brain abscess there is no definite capsule around the area of necrosis but after about 10 days a capsule forms around the abscess cavity (Figs 3.68 & 3.69). Anaerobic and microaerophilic bacteria are commonly isolated from brain abscesses (Figs 3.70 & 3.71). The most common organisms encountered are microaerophilic streptococci of the *S. milleri* group, *Bacteroides* species, members of the Enterobacteriaceae and *Staphylococcus aureus*. *Actinomyces israelii* is isolated occasionally (Figs 3.72 & 3.73). Fungi, including candida (Fig. 3.74), aspergillus

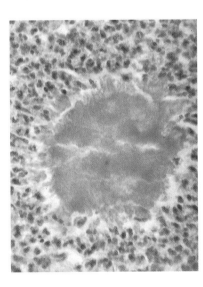

Fig. 3.72 Brain abscess. 'Sulphur granules' in necrotic inflammatory exudate in a cerebellar abscess due to *Actinomyces israelii*. H & E stain.

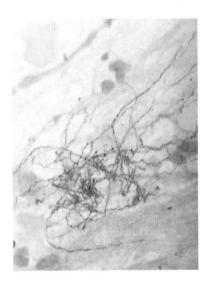

Fig. 3.73 Brain abscess. *Actinomyces israelii*, filamentous gram-positive bacilli, within inflammatory exudate. Gram's stain. By courtesy of Dr J. F. John, Jr.

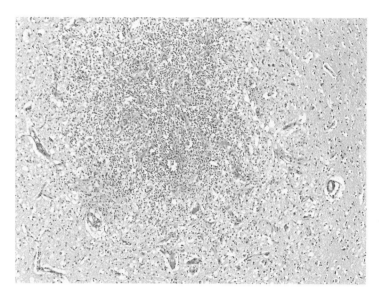

Fig. 3.74 Candida brain abscess. Focal acute cerebritis with acute inflammation caused by candida. H & E stain. By courtesy of Dr P. Garen.

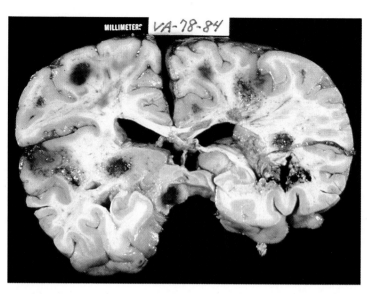

Fig. 3.75 Aspergillosis. Multiple haemorrhagic areas of acute necrosis present in both cerebral hemispheres. By courtesy of Dr P. Garen.

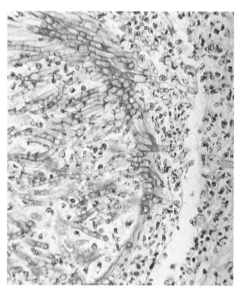

Fig. 3.76 Cerebral aspergillosis. Numerous septate hyphae invading a blood vessel wall associated with acute and chronic inflammatory reaction. Periodic acid–Schiff stain.

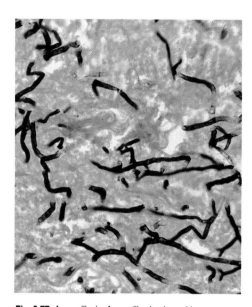

Fig. 3.77 Aspergillosis. Aspergillus hyphae with dichotomous branching and septae. Gomori methenamine silver stain. By courtesy of Dr P. Garen.

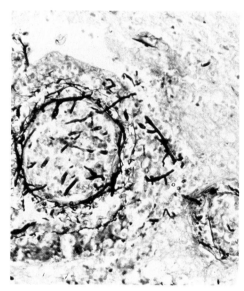

Fig. 3.78 Aspergillosis. Aspergillus hyphae ensnared in vascular thrombi. Hyphae permeate adjacent vascular wall and invade brain parenchyma. Gomori methenamine silver stain. By courtesy of Dr P. Garen.

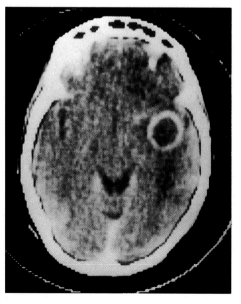

Fig. 3.79 Brain abscess due to aspergillus. CT scan showing a large abscess cavity surrounded by a thick rim in the left temporal area, and a smaller lesion in the right parietal area.

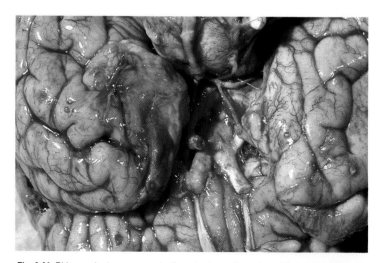

Fig. 3.80 Rhinocerebral mucormycosis. Gross brain specimen viewed from base with acute superficial necrosis of temporal lobe and thrombosis of left internal carotid artery. By courtesy of Dr P. Garen.

(Figs 3.75, 3.76, 3.77, 3.78 & 3.79), and zygomycetes (Figs 3.80, 3.81, 3.82, 3.83 & 3.84) such as rhizopus and mucor are found mainly in immunocompromised patients. Other causes of brain abscess in immunocompromised patients are *Listeria monocytogenes* (Fig. 3.85) and *Nocardia asteroides* (Figs 3.86, 3.87 & 3.88), the latter usually in associa-

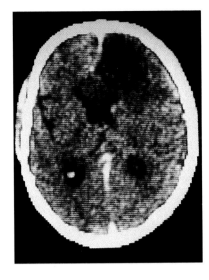

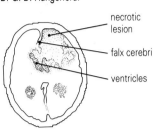

Fig. 3.81 Rhinocerebral mucormycosis. CT scan showing a large necrotic mass lesion in the left frontal lobe displacing the falx cerebri and inferior sagittal sinus. The ventricular system in the area is also distorted and displaced. By courtesy of Dr G. D. Hungerford.

necrotic lesion
falx cerebri
ventricles

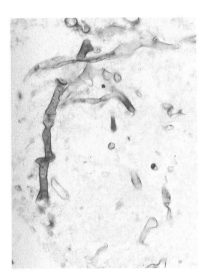

Fig. 3.82 Rhinocerebral mucormycosis. Brain biopsy from a diabetic patient showing the large nonseptate hyphae. Periodic acid–Schiff stain.

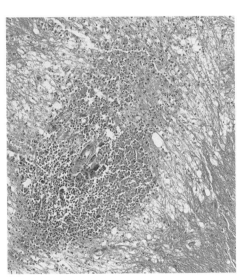

Fig. 3.83 Rhinocerebral mucormycosis. Vessel obstruction by mucor resulting in focal perivascular acute necrosis. H & E stain. By courtesy of Dr P. Garen.

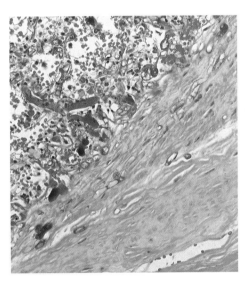

Fig. 3.84 Rhinocerebral mucormycosis. Wall of thrombosed internal carotid artery with hyphae of mucor present in thrombus and arterial wall. H & E stain. By courtesy of Dr P. Garen.

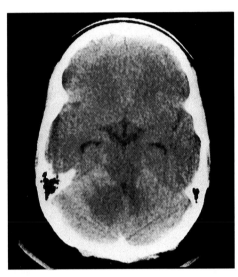

Fig. 3.85 *Listeria monocytogenes* rhombencephalitis. CT scan. Oedema (extensive hypodense lesion) involving brain stem structures with obliteration of perimesencephalic cisterns and effacement of the aqueduct of Sylvius, producing early dilatation of the temporal horns of the lateral ventricles.

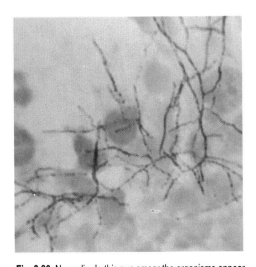

Fig. 3.86 Nocardia. In this pus smear the organisms appear mainly as irregularly staining filaments, but a variety of forms is often seen, including rods, cocci and even spiral forms. By courtesy of A. E. Prevost.

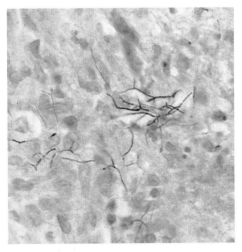

Fig. 3.87 Nocardiosis. Brain abscess revealing filamentous gram-positive bacilli of *Nocardia asteroides*. Brown and Brenn stain. By courtesy of Dr P. Garen.

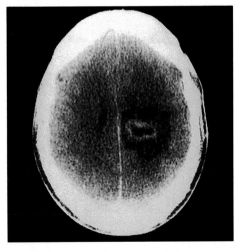

Fig. 3.88 Brain abscess due to nocardia. CT scan showing a single hypodense lesion surrounded by a thin rim and an extensive area of oedema in the left parietal region.

tion with pulmonary infection. Patients with AIDS also have an increased incidence of brain abscess due to *Toxoplasma gondii*, *Cryptococcus neoformans*, *Mycobacterium* species, and *Salmonella* group B. In certain areas of the world parasites such as *Entamoeba histolytica*, *Schistosoma japonicum* (Fig. 3.89), *Paragonimus westermani*, *Echinococcus granulosus* (Figs 3.90, 3.91, 3.92 & 3.93) and *Cysticercus cellulosae* are relatively common causes of brain abscess. Focal lesions of the brain may also be seen occasionally in Whipples disease (Fig. 3.94).

The clinical picture is highly variable. The illness usually develops more gradually than that associated with pyogenic meningitis, but 75% of patients seek medical attention within 2 weeks of the onset of symptoms. The classic triad of fever, headache and focal neurological deficits is seen in less than 50% of patients. Severe progressive headache is the most common presenting symptom. Nausea and vomiting, seizures and altered mental status are relatively common.

Lumbar puncture is contraindicated; findings in the CSF are not often helpful in the diagnosis of brain abscess and the procedure is dangerous because of the risk of herniation. CT scanning has revolutionized the diagnosis, therapy and prognosis of brain abscess. The CT scan yields evidence of brain abscess in approximately 95% of patients beyond the stage of cerebritis, and provides more accurate localization of the lesion(s) than studies available before the advent of this technique. The characteristic appearance is a hypodense centre bounded by a uniform ring of

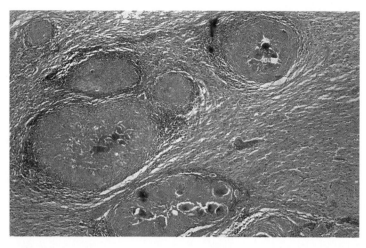

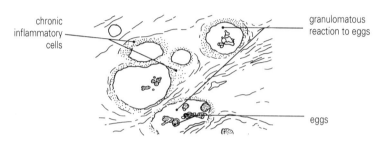

Fig. 3.89 Schistosomiasis. Eggs of *S. haematobium* in bladder wall with surrounding chronic inflammatory reaction and fibrosis. H & E stain.

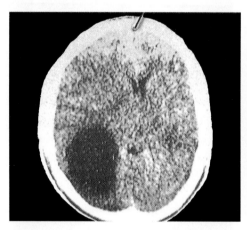
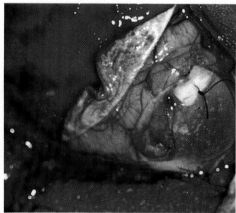

Fig. 3.90 Hydatid disease. Cyst revealed on CT scan (left) and at craniotomy (right).

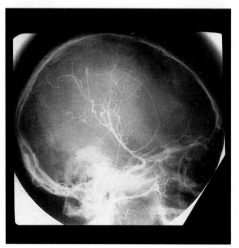

Fig. 3.91 Echinococcosis. Cerebral angiography showing displacement of vessels by a large mass in the frontal region. By courtesy of Dr H. Whitwell.

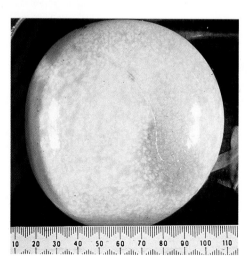

Fig. 3.92 Echinococcosis. Cyst removed from patient in Fig 3.91. By courtesy of Dr H. Whitwell.

enhancement which is surrounded by a variable hypodense region of oedema (Figs 3.95 & 3.96). Technetium 99 brain scanning and MRI may be slightly more sensitive than CT scanning during the cerebritis stage of infection. Occasionally it may be difficult to differentiate between brain abscess and a necrotic tumor; addition of the Indium–111 radionuclide scan to the CT scan may help distinguish inflammatory from neoplastic lesions.

There are relatively few direct measurements of the penetration of various antimicrobial agents into brain tissue or the interior of abscess cavities; most therapeutic recommendations are based upon studies of penetration into CSF. Penicillin G in large doses (24 million units per day intravenously) is recommended because of the frequency with which streptococci are isolated from brain abscesses, even though this agent does not cross the blood–brain barrier very well. Metronidazole and chloramphenicol (active against anaerobes), third generation cephalosporins (active against many facultative gram-negative bacilli) and trimethoprim-sulfamethoxazole (active against nocardia and many gram-negative bacilli) are appropriate choices for combination with penicillin G in various clinical and epidemiologic settings. Amphotericin B, 5-fluorocytosine and the new triazoles fluconazole and itraconazole are the agents most active against fungal causes of brain abscess. In most cases drainage of the abscess should be carried out in conjunction with antimicrobial therapy. In posterior fossa lesions or fungal infections total excision of the abscess is probably indicated. In other situations aspiration of the abscess, especially in conjunction with stereotaxic CT guidance, may be very effective. In most cases instillation of antibiotics into the abscess cavity is probably not indicated, since with a number of agents there is a risk of provoking seizures, but when highly resistant species such as *Pseudomonas aeruginosa* are implicated this may be the only way to obtain adequate local concentrations of the antimicrobial agent.

Subdural empyema is bacterial infection in the potential space between the dura and arachnoid meninges (Fig. 3.97). It most commonly arises by direct extension from infection in the frontal or ethmoid sinuses, with spread from the middle ear and mastoid being less common.

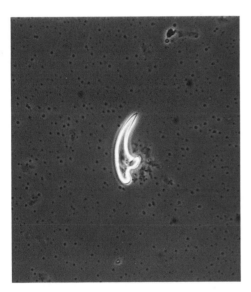

Fig. 3.93 Echinococcosis. Fluid from cyst viewed under polarized light showing hook of hydatid. By courtesy of Dr H. Whitwell.

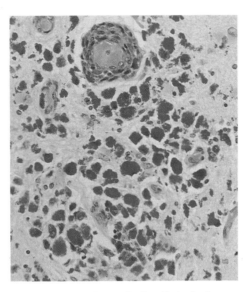

Fig. 3.94 Whipple's disease. Section of brain showing a focal lesion with many PAS-positive macrophages surrounding a small blood vessel. PAS stain. By courtesy of Dr P. Garen.

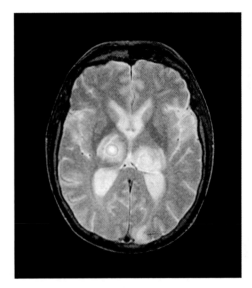

Fig. 3.95 Brain abscess. MRI scan showing bilateral abscess cavities in the region of the basal ganglia. By courtesy of Dr J. Curé.

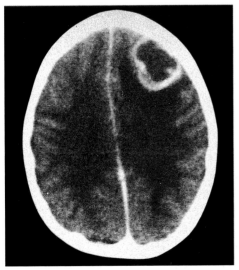

Fig. 3.96 Brain abscess. CT scan showing the typical appearance of a brain abscess in the left frontal lobe with enhancement of the capsule. The uniform thin wall is characteristic of abscess rather than tumour. By courtesy of Dr G. D. Hungerford.

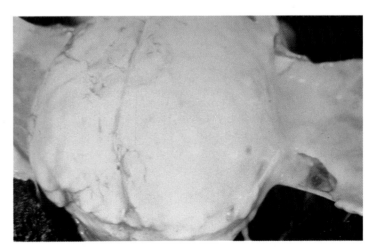

Fig. 3.97 Subdural empyema. Autopsy specimen showing bilateral subdural empyemas over the cerebral hemispheres of a child.

Streptococci and staphylococci have been isolated most frequently, but gram-negative bacteria are found in a significant number of cases, and *Haemophilus influenzae* is relatively common in children under 5 years of age. When careful attention is paid to microbiological methods, anaerobic bacteria are often found, and polymicrobial infections are common. Most infections involve the cerebral hemispheres (see Fig. 3.97). Contiguous osteomyelitis, epidural abscess and septic venous thrombosis with haemorrhagic infarction are relatively common complications. The clinical picture resembles that of meningitis or brain abscess, with fever, severe headache, vomiting and nuchal rigidity with rapid progression to focal neurological deficits, especially hemiparesis. Unless surgical treatment is undertaken promptly, the neurological picture progresses and herniation of the brain may occur.

Because of the rapidly increasing intracranial pressure, lumbar puncture is contraindicated. CT scanning and MRI are the most valuable diagnostic tests for this disease; MRI is significantly more sensitive than CT scanning for demonstration of subdural empyema. Skull films may reveal evidence of associated sinusitis or osteomyelitis. Choice of antibiotics should be based upon the principles described above for brain abscess. Mannitol or dexamethasone may be needed for treatment of cerebral oedema. Immediate surgical drainage by craniotomy or burr holes is essential to prevent rapid progression of neurological deterioration.

Spinal subdural empyema is rare and usually arises from haematogenous spread from a focus of infection outside the nervous system. *Staphylococcus aureus* is the most common aetiological agent. The clinical picture is one of cord compression and/or radicular pain. MRI is the most sensitive diagnostic procedure available; myelography is the procedure of choice if MRI is not available. Therapy should consist of prompt surgical drainage and high dose treatment with a penicillinase-resistant antistaphylococcal penicillin.

When infection occurs between the dura and the overlying bone of the skull or vertebral column, the result is an epidural abscess (Fig. 3.98). There is almost always associated osteomyelitis (Figs 3.99 & 3.100), and the infection may extend through the dura into the subdural space with formation of a concomitant subdural empyema. *Staphylococcus aureus* is the infecting organism in approximately 75% of cases. The clinical picture and diagnostic and therapeutic considerations are similar to those which apply to subdural empyema.

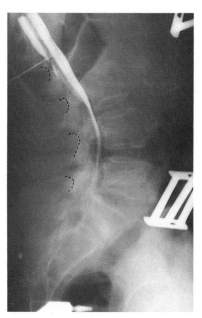

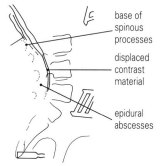

Fig. 3.98 Spinal epidural abscess. Lumbar myelogram showing anterior displacement of the column of contrast material by a posterior epidural abscess. By courtesy of Dr G. D. Hungerford.

base of spinous processes

displaced contrast material

epidural abscesses

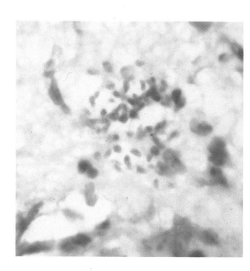

Fig. 3.99 Cryptococcosis. CT scan of vertebral body showing destructive osteomyelitis and paravertebral and epidural abscesses caused by *Cryptococcus neoformans*. By courtesy of Dr J. Curé.

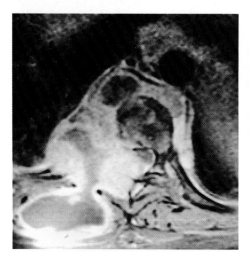

Fig. 3.100 Cryptococcosis. MRI scan of same patient showing paravertebral and epidural abscesses, destructive osteomyelitis and involvement of the spinal cord. By courtesy of Dr J. Curé.

Fig. 3.101 Toxoplasma encephalitis. Histological section of brain biopsy showing numerous tachyzoites of *T. gondii*, necrosis and inflammatory reaction. Giemsa stain.

Infection of the face, pharynx, perinasal sinuses or middle ear may spread to intracranial veins and venous sinuses by way of the emissary veins, or these structures may be involved during the course of purulent meningitis, subdural empyema or epidural abscess. The most common causative organism is *S. aureus*. The end result is venous thrombosis and suppuration, sometimes complicated by septic embolization to the lungs or other organs. Cortical vein thrombosis may produce focal neurological deficits including hemiplegia. Cavernous sinus thrombosis produces a rapidly progressive syndrome of diplopia, orbital oedema, exophthalmos, ophthalmoplegia and loss of vision. Thrombosis of the superior sagittal sinus results in bilateral leg weakness and sometimes causes communicating hydrocephalus. Thrombosis of the lateral sinus produces pain over the ear and mastoid and may also result in facial pain and sixth nerve palsy. The diagnosis may be suspected when one of the syndromes described above is present in association with an extracranial focus of infection. MRI allows the most accurate visualization and localization of the thrombosed venous structures. Culture of blood and CSF may allow specific identification of the aetiological agent. Antibiotic therapy should be based upon results of culture whenever possible; if the infecting organism has not been isolated a regimen against *S. aureus*, streptococci and anaerobic bacteria should be used. Surgical drainage and treatment of increased intracranial pressure may be required. If the disease progresses in spite of these therapeutic measures anticoagulation or surgical thrombectomy should be considered.

Toxoplasmosis

The protozoan parasite *Toxoplasma gondii* is a common cause of latent infection of the central nervous system throughout the world. Domestic cats and other felines are the definitive hosts, but humans (and many other mammals) acquire the infection incidentally by ingestion of oocysts in cat faeces, ingestion of tissue cysts in infected meat or by transmission *in utero*. Clinically apparent infection of the nervous system is seen almost exclusively in immunocompromised individuals. Although some cases of toxoplasma encephalitis have occurred in patients receiving immunosuppressing drugs, especially recipients of transplants of heart or bone marrow, this disease is the most important opportunistic infection of the CNS in patients with AIDS. In western Europe approximately 25% of patients with AIDS develop toxoplasma encephalitis, and in many developing countries the incidence is even higher. In industrialized countries most cases occur in patients already diagnosed as having AIDS, and represent recrudescence of latent CNS infection. In developing countries with a high prevalence of toxoplasmosis, encephalitis may develop early in the course of HIV infection and may represent recently acquired infection.

Toxoplasma encephalitis consists of multiple focal mass lesions, which may be granulomatous or necrotizing in nature, occurring in any part of the central nervous system but most commonly in the basal ganglia or corticomedullary junction of the cerebrum. Clinically patients usually present with altered mental status, which may progress to coma, headache and focal neurological deficits. Seizures occur in approximately a third of the patients. The syndrome of inappropriate secretion of antidiuretic hormone may be present. Examination of the CSF may reveal no abnormalities or there may be a mononuclear pleocytosis with increased protein and normal glucose.

Definitive aetiological diagnosis of toxoplasma encephalitis usually requires brain biopsy. Histopathological examination may reveal a granulomatous reaction or severe, necrotizing, focal or diffuse encephalitis. Tachyzoites (Fig. 3.101) or bradycysts (Fig. 3.102) may be seen either in haematoxylin and eosin sections of brain or in touch preparations stained with Wright–Giemsa stain. A more sensitive technique is specific immunohistological staining by the immunoperoxidase method (Fig. 3.103). Isolation of *T. gondii* from other tissue specimens or body fluids outside the CNS indicates active infection, and provides supportive evidence for the diagnosis. Approximately 97% of patients with AIDS who

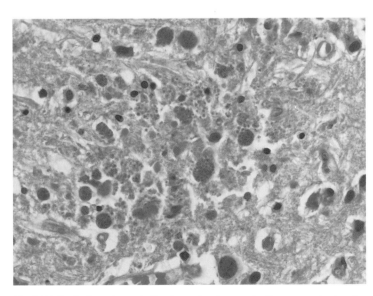

Fig. 3.102 Cerebral toxoplasmosis. Focal area of acute necrosis with numerous bradycysts and tachyzoites of *Toxoplasma gondii*. H & E stain. By courtesy of Dr P. Garen.

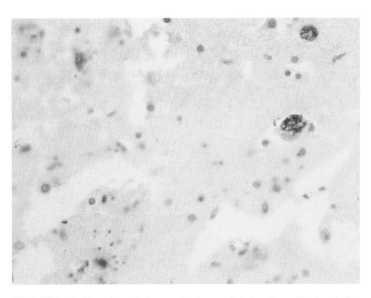

Fig. 3.103 Cerebral toxoplasmosis. Immunostaining reveals tachyzoites and bradycysts. By courtesy of Dr P. Garen.

have toxoplasma encephalitis are seropositive when first seen, so a negative IgG antibody test in serum virtually rules out this diagnosis. An IgG antibody titre in CSF which exceeds that in the serum indicates local production of antibody in the CNS and also strongly suggests the diagnosis of toxoplasmosa encephalitis. *T. gondii* can now be grown *in vitro* in tissue culture, and methods for detection of antigen in serum and CSF are being developed.

Imaging studies of the brain, especially CT scanning and MRI, may provide strong presumptive evidence of toxoplasmic encephalitis. The typical finding on CT scanning is of multiple, bilateral, hypodense, enhancing mass lesions, especially in the basal ganglia and at the corticomedullary junctions of the cerebrum (Fig. 3.104). Single lesions are occasionally seen (Fig. 3.105). 'Double-dose' enhanced CT scanning may provide increased sensitivity. MRI appears to be even more sensitive than CT scanning, and nearly always reveals multiple lesions. The finding of a single lesion on MRI suggests another diagnosis, such as intracerebral lymphoma.

Toxoplasma encephalitis in AIDS patients is invariably fatal if untreated, so patients with multiple focal lesions on imaging studies should receive immediate empirical treatment while additional diagnostic studies are being done. Standard therapy consists of pyrimethamine plus sulfadiazine, with folinic acid to reduce the toxicity of pyrimethamine to the bone marrow. Up to 40% of patients will develop leukopenia or rash during therapy with this regimen, often necessitating its discontinuation. Many adverse effects are due to the sulfadiazine, and pyrimethamine plus clindamycin may be used as an alternative regimen. Patients usually show clinical improvement within 2 weeks, and improvement in the appearance of the imaging studies in 3–4 weeks. The primary course of therapy should be continued for at least 6 weeks. Since these agents do not eradicate toxoplasma cysts, the patient remains susceptible to relapse of the infection for life, and should receive suppressive treatment with either pyrimethamine/sulfadiazine or clindamycin indefinitely.

Cysticercosis

Cysticercus cellulosae is the name applied to the intermediate stage of the pork tapeworm, *Taenia solium* (see Fig. 4.127). Humans may become intermediate hosts for the organism by ingestion of food or water contaminated with

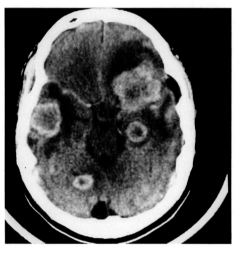

Fig. 3.104 Cerebral toxoplasmosis. CT scan showing multiple ring-enhancing, hypodense lesions, in the left fronto-temporal, right temporal, right occipital and left uncal regions, with surrounding cerebral oedema.

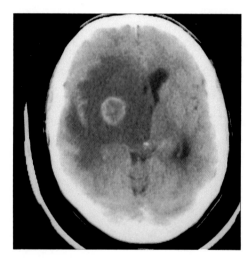

Fig. 3.105 Cerebral toxoplasmosis. CT scan showing a single ring-enhancing, hypodense lesion deep in the basal ganglia, surrounded by an extensive area of oedema.

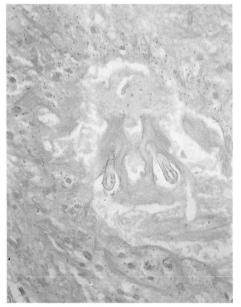

Fig. 3.106 Cysticercosis. High power histology showing hooklets. By courtesy of Dr H. Whitwell.

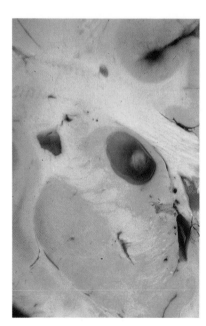

Fig. 3.107 Cerebral cysticercosis. Gross specimen of brain showing a simple cyst in the caudate nucleus. Within it can be seen the scolex of the developing tapeworm. By courtesy of Prof. H. Spencer.

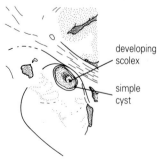

developing scolex

simple cyst

human faeces, by self-infection from anus to mouth in a person infected with the adult tapeworm, or by internal infection due to reverse peristalsis. The oncosphere penetrates the intestinal wall and rapidly develops into a fluid-filled cyst which contains the invaginated head of the larva (see Figs 4.128 & 3.106). The organism lives for several years and then dies and degenerates, and may eventually calcify (see Figs 4.129 & 4.130). The most common clinically significant site of infection is the central nervous system. Lesions may be focal and discrete when the cysts occur in the brain substance (Figs 3.107 & 3.108). If the infection occurs in the subarachnoid space at the base of the brain or in the ventricles, involvement is more diffuse, and this so-called racemose form may invade the surrounding tissue (Fig. 3.109). Clinically, patients may present with headache, papilloedema, decreased vision and focal neurological signs including hemiparesis and seizures. The most useful diagnostic tests are CT scanning (Fig. 3.110) and MRI (Figs 3.111 & 3.112), which reveal the multiple space-occupying cystic lesions and hydrocephalus. Serological tests on serum and spinal fluid are usually positive and confirm the aetiological diagnosis. Recently the drug praziquantel has proved effective in killing the larval stage of the organism. Patients who have active infection with living organisms usually exhibit marked and rapid improvement with treatment. If the organisms are already dead, treatment does not influence the clinical manifestations. Concurrent treatment with corticosteroids may also be beneficial.

Neurosyphilis

During the early stages of syphilis up to 40% of patients will have invasion of the central nervous system. A significant proportion of these will develop persistent active infection of the CNS (neurosyphilis). Patients with asymptomatic neurosyphilis have no clinical manifestations of the disease but have one or more abnormalities in the CSF, including pleocytosis, elevated protein concentration, decreased glucose concentration or positive VDRL test in the CSF. Symptomatic neurosyphilis includes meningovascular and parenchymatous forms. Meningovascular

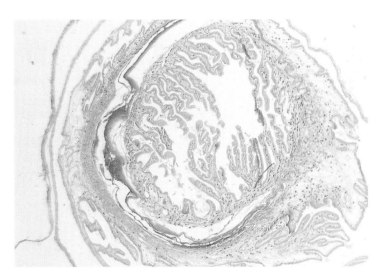

Fig. 3.108 Cysticercosis. Scolex present in lesion of brain. H & E stain. By courtesy of Dr P. Garen.

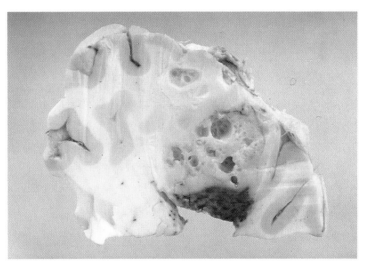

Fig. 3.109 Cerebral cysticercosis. Post mortem specimen of brain showing racemose form with diffuse involvement of surrounding tissues. By courtesy of Prof. H Spencer.

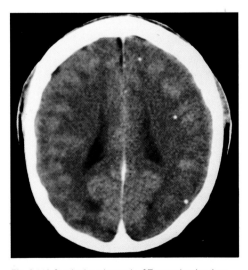

Fig. 3.110 Cerebral cysticercosis. CT scan showing three small round calcified lesions in the right cerebral hemisphere. By courtesy of Dr J. Curé.

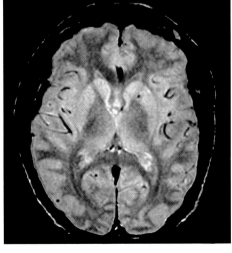

Fig. 3.111 Cerebral cysticercosis. MRI scan of same patient showing multiple small round lesions in the brain. By courtesy of Dr J. Curé.

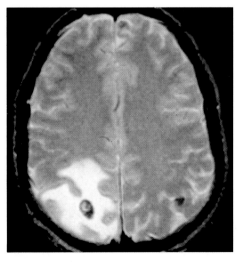

Fig. 3.112 Cerebral cysticercosis. MRI scan showing a cyst containing a developing larva, surrounded by an area of oedema. By courtesy of Dr J. Curé.

syphilis is characterized by an obliterative endarteritis affecting the small blood vessels of the meninges, brain and spinal cord (Fig. 3.113) resulting in multiple small areas of infarction. The most common clinical manifestations are focal neurological deficits including hemiparesis and aphasia, and focal or generalized seizures. Parenchymatous neurosyphilis includes general paresis and tabes dorsalis. In general paresis there is invasion of the brain substance by spirochaetes with destruction of nerve cells, principally in the cerebral cortex (Figs 3.114, 3.115 & 3.116). Common manifestations are changes in personality, intellect, affect and judgment, with hyperactive reflexes, Argyll Robertson pupil and optic atrophy (Fig. 3.117). Tabes dorsalis is characterized by demyelination of the posterior column of the spinal cord, dorsal root ganglia and dorsal roots (Fig. 3.118), resulting in eventual development of a broad-based ataxic gait, foot slap, paraesthesias, lightning pains, positive Romberg's sign, hyporeflexia, degenerative joint disease (Charcot's joint), impotence, disturbance of bowel and bladder function and sensory losses. Other forms of syphilitic involvement of

the central nervous system include localized gummata of the brain or spinal cord (Fig. 3.119), syphilitic otitis, with sensorineural hearing loss or vestibular dysfunction, and syphilitic disease of the eye, which may manifest as uveitis, chorioretinitis or episcleritis. Asymptomatic or symptomatic neurosyphilis is a relatively common late manifestation of congenital syphilis.   Definitive aetiological diagnosis of syphilitic infection of the nervous system depends upon serological studies. A positive VDRL test in the CSF indicates active neurosyphilis. A titre of specific anti-treponemal IgG antibody in the spinal fluid which is at least three times higher than that in the serum, with correction for leakage of serum proteins across the blood–brain barrier, also provides strong evidence of active infection in the CNS.

Every patient with syphilis should have examination of the CSF, and if there are any abnormalities, with or without clinical manifestations of neurosyphilis, the patient should be treated for neurosyphilis. Recommended treatment is high-dose penicillin G given intravenously for 10 days. Acceptable alternative agents are ceftriaxone, doxy-

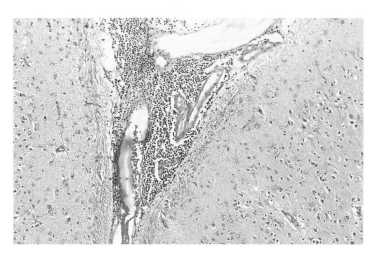

Fig. 3.113 Neurosyphilis. Meningovascular involvement in tertiary syphilis demonstrating lymphoplasmacytic meningeal infiltrate in sulcus. There is neuronal loss and marked gliosis in the underlying cortex. H & E stain. By courtesy of Dr P. Garen.

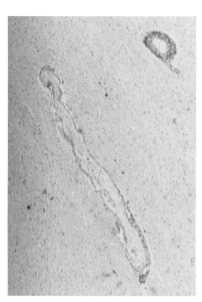

Fig. 3.114 Parenchymatous syphilis. Primarily degenerative lesion within the cerebral cortex. H & E stain.

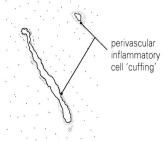

perivascular inflammatory cell 'cuffing'

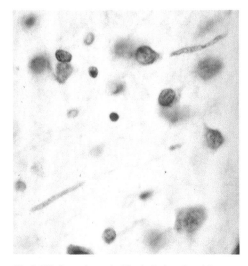

Fig. 3.115 General paresis. Histological section of the frontal cortex revealing elongate nuclei of microglial rod cells. Nissl stain.

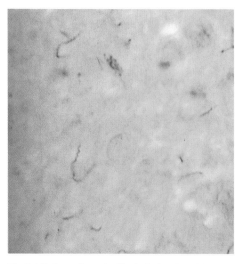

Fig. 3.116 General paresis. Histological section of the frontal cortex showing the 'corkscrew' appearance of spirochaetes. Levaditi silver stain.

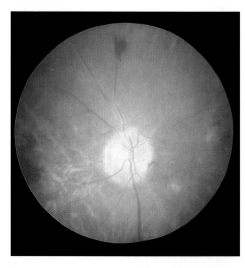

Fig. 3.117 Neurosyphilis. Fundus photograph showing optic atrophy.

cycline and the combination of oral amoxycillin and probenecid. Patients with HIV infection, including those who have not progressed to AIDS, are significantly more susceptible to infection of the nervous system by *Treponema pallidum*. Many authorities recommend that all patients infected with both HIV and *T. pallidum* receive treatment for neurosyphilis, preferably with a bactericidal agent such as penicillin G or ceftriaxone.

Tetanus

Tetanus is caused by an extremely potent neurotoxin, tetanospasmin, produced by the anaerobic spore-forming bacterium *Clostridium tetani*. Tetanospasmin is produced by vegetative cells of *C. tetani*, and enters the nervous system at the myoneural junctions. From there it travels centripetally along the axon to the spinal cord and then migrates transsynaptically to other neurons. Its most important action is the prevention of neurotransmitter release in synapses of inhibitory cells; this allows motor neurons to increase muscle tone unopposed and results in

muscular rigidity and spasm. Loss of inhibition within the autonomic nervous system may result in markedly elevated levels of plasma catecholamines.

Clostridium tetani is a motile, gram-positive, anaerobic rod which forms terminal spores (Fig. 3.120), which are highly resistant to heat and chemical disinfectants. The organism is a normal inhabitant of the gastrointestinal tract of humans and many other mammals, and the spores may remain viable for many years in soil that has been contaminated with faeces. When spores of *C. tetani* enter the body via trauma, whether or not tetanus develops depends primarily upon the immunization status of the individual and upon whether or not local conditions in the wound are favourable for germination of the spores and subsequent release of toxin. Wounds contaminated with dirt, faeces or saliva, puncture wounds and wounds associated with extensive damage to tissues, especially if other facultative microorganisms are also present, are most likely to result in development of tetanus.

The disease is most common in developing countries where the proportion of individuals who have received effective immunization is small. In such countries most cases occur in children secondary to wounds or chronic ear infections, in neonates in which the umbilical stump has been contaminated, after parturition or abortion, and following various surgical procedures performed with nonsterile instruments. In industrialized countries most cases occur in unimmunized or inadequately immunized individuals over the age of 50, in association with acute or chronic wounds, skin ulcers, abscesses, gangrene or parenteral drug abuse. In a small proportion of cases no portal of entry is evident.

The incubation period (time between injury and occurrence of the first symptom) is usually less than 2 weeks, but may range from a few days to up to 2 months. An incubation period of less than a week, or occurrence of generalized spasms within 48 hours of the first symptoms, is associated with severe disease. An early and characteristic sign is trismus or 'lockjaw', due to an increase in muscle tone and spasm in the masseter muscle. Muscular rigidity and reflex spasms increase in extent and finally

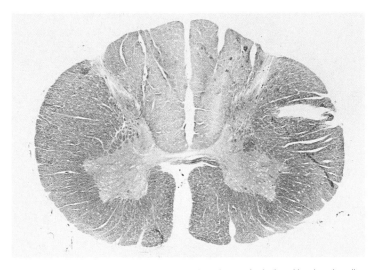

Fig. 3.118 Neurosyphilis. Degeneration of posterior columns of spinal cord in tabes dorsalis. Myelin stain. By courtesy of Dr H. Whitwell.

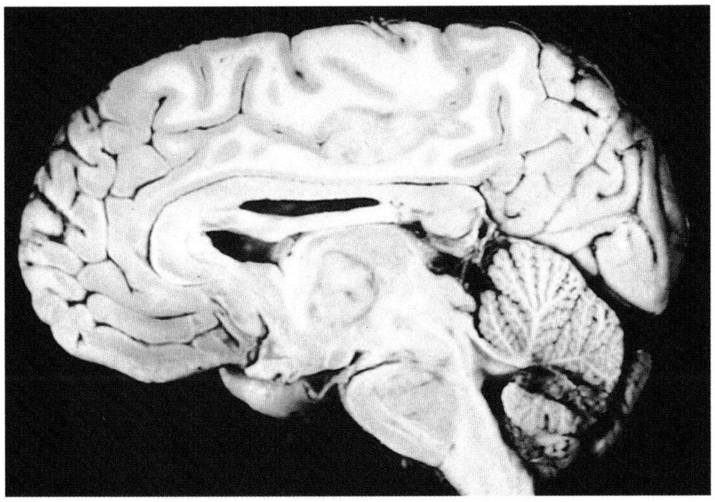

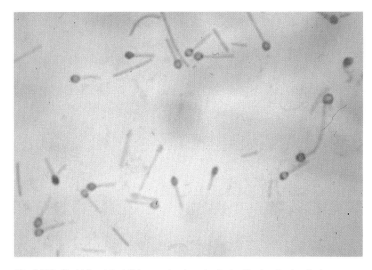

Fig. 3.119 Gumma of brain. Well-circumscribed solid mass in the thalamus of a patient with tertiary sphilis.

Fig. 3.120 *Clostridium tetani*. This organism is a slender bacillus forming terminal spores giving a 'drumstick' appearance. Spore formation occurs in tissues. Gram's stain.

become generalized to produce painful opisthotonos (Fig. 3.121), abdominal rigidity and the characteristic facial expression of 'risus sardonicus' (Figs 3.122, 3.123 & 3.124). Spasm of respiratory muscles may result in inadequate ventilation and hypoxaemia. The reflex spasms may be precipitated by stimuli such as touch or changes in the level of noise or light. Autonomic dysfunction may produce labile hypertension, tachycardia, arrhythmias, profuse sweating, fever and eventually hypotension. In uncommon cases of local tetanus the rigidity and spasms may be limited to a single extremity or to the head.

The diagnosis of tetanus depends primarily upon the characteristic clinical signs of muscle spasm and rigidity and to a lesser extent upon the history and presence of a wound. Increased tone and rigidity of the paraspinal muscles is a very helpful sign. In most cases *C. tetani* will not be isolated from cultures of the wound, and conversely the organism is sometimes isolated from wounds in patients who do not have tetanus.

Optimal treatment of tetanus requires meticulous attention to a number of important factors. Stimulation of the patient should be kept to a minimum. The constant hum of an electric fan may reduce sudden changes in the noise level, and lighting in the room should be maintained at a low but adequate level so that it will not be necessary to switch lights on and off. Benzodiazepines should as diazepam are extremely effective in inducing muscle relaxation and anxiety and producing sedation. They should be given intravenously in small frequent doses titrated to the patient's responses. In very severe cases it may be necessary to induce neuromuscular blockade with an agent such as pancuronium bromide, but this greatly complicates the maintenance of respiration and handling of secretions. If ventilatory assistance and frequent tracheal suctioning are required, tracheostomy should be performed, since this will reduce the stimulation associated with these procedures. Tetanus-immune globulin (TIG) should be administered intramuscularly at a dosage of 500 unitsimmediately to neutralize any toxin which has not already entered the nervous system. TIG (250 units) injected intrathecally has been reported to be even more effective than TIG given intramuscularly. After tetanus-

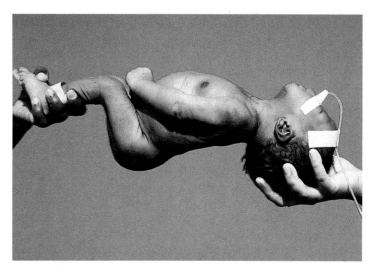

Fig. 3.121 Tetanus. Opisthotonus in an infant due to intense contraction of the paravertebral muscles. By courtesy of Dr T. F. Sellers, Jr.

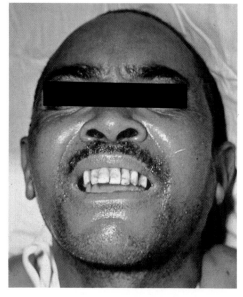

Fig. 3.122 Tetanus. *Risus sardonicus*, due to spasm of the facial muscles. By courtesy of Dr T .F. Sellers, Jr.

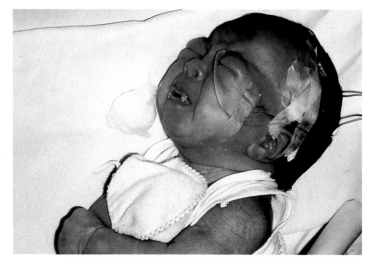

Fig. 3.123 Tetanus. *Risus sardonicus* in a newborn infant.

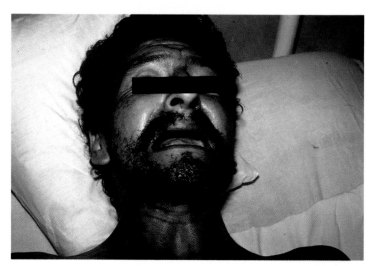

Fig. 3.124 Tetanus. Risus sardonicus in an adult.

immune globulin has been given, appropriate wound debridement or excision should be carried out, and treatment with either penicillin or metronidazole should be instituted. Since the amount of toxin released during clinical tetanus is insufficient to provide effective immunity, active immunization with tetanus toxoid should be initiated during hospitalization. Severe autonomic reactions may require use of adrenergic blocking agents or morphine.

There is essentially no natural immunity to tetanus, but the disease is entirely preventable by adequate immunization. Primary immunization consists of a series of injections of tetanus toxoid, either as a single agent or combined with full-dose diphtheria toxoid and/or pertussis vaccine in children or with reduced dose diphtheria toxoid in adults. A booster injection every 10 years will ensure maintenance of a protective level of antitoxin.

Appropriate prophylaxis against tetanus following a wound depends upon the individual's immune status and the nature of the wound. If the individual has had adequate primary immunization and has received a booster injection within the preceding 5 years, no immunoprophylaxis is indicated for any type of wound. (A booster should be given if the primary immunization series may have been with fluid toxoid.) In the immunized patient whose last booster injection was 5–10 years previously, no immunoprophylaxis need be given if the wound is clean, but those with a tetanus-prone wound should receive a booster. Immunized patients whose last booster injection was more than ten years previously should be given a booster with any type of wound. Individuals who have not been previously immunized should receive human tetanus-immune globulin, 250–500 units, depending on the nature and severity of the wound, and active immunization should be initiated.

Botulism

Botulism is a life-threatening disease characterized by descending flaccid paralysis, caused by toxins produced by the gram-positive, anaerobic spore-forming bacterium *Clostridium botulinum*. These toxins, of which there are eight distinct types, are the most potent toxins known. All are polypeptides with molecular weights of approximately 150 000 daltons. Types A, B and E are the most common causes of botulism in man. Botulism occurs in 3 forms:

• food poisoning, which results from eating food that contains the toxin;

• wound botulism, which occurs when toxin is produced by organisms contaminating a wound;

• and infant botulism, due to toxin production by organisms within the gastrointestinal tract of infants.

Botulism food poisoning was formerly associated primarily with ingestion of sausage, but at the present time more cases are related to home-canned foods. Type E botulism is usually associated with fish products such as *gefilte* fish. These toxins interfere with neurotransmission at peripheral cholineigic synapses by binding tightly to the presynaptic membrane and preventing the release of acetylcholine.

The main clinical manifestation of botulism is a symmetrical, descending flaccid paralysis which begins within hours to a few days after ingestion of food containing the toxin. Commonly associated findings which should strengthen the suspicion of botulism are postural hypotension, dilated unreactive pupils (Fig. 3.125), ophthalmoplegia, dry mucous membranes (Fig. 3.126) and absence of fever.

The diagnosis must be suspected on clinical grounds, and special studies are required to confirm it. Electromyography may reveal suggestive features such as decreased amplitude of the evoked muscle action potential to a single supramaximal nerve stimulus, as well as enhanced post-tetanic facilitation, muscle fibrillation and small-amplitude polyphasic motor unit potentials of increased number and brief duration. The diagnosis may be confirmed by demonstration of toxin in the blood, toxin and/or *C. botulinum* organisms in stool or gastric contents or toxin and/or organisms in the suspect food item. Toxin is detected by bioassay in mice. Special anaerobic culture techniques are required to isolate *C. botulinum*.

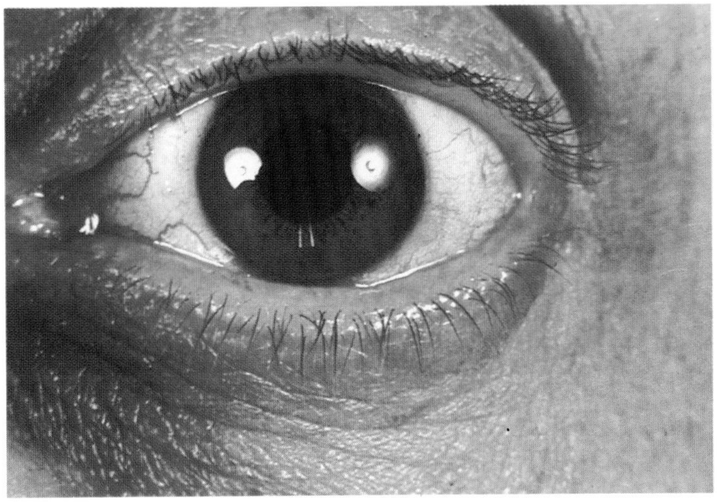

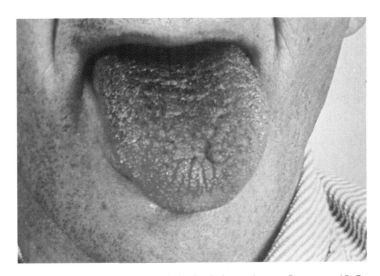

Fig. 3.125 Botulism. Clinical photograph showing dilated fixed pupil. By courtesy of Dr Z. McGee.

Fig. 3.126 Botulism. Clinical photograph showing dry furrowed tongue. By courtesy of Dr Z. McGee.

Treatment consists of maintenance of airway and ventilation, general supportive care and administration of specific antitoxin. When the toxin type is unknown a trivalent ABE antitoxin should be used (available in the USA from the Centers for Disease Control, and in the UK from the Central Public Health Laboratory at Colindale). Guanidine hydrochloride has appeared to produce clinical benefit in approximately half the patients who have received it.

Wound botulism is a rare condition in which botulinum toxin is produced by organisms within a wound. The clinical picture resembles that of botulism food poisoning. Toxin may be demonstrated in the serum and occasionally *C. botulinum* can be isolated from the wound. Treatment consists of the measures described above plus surgical debridement or excision of the wound.

Infant botulism, now recognized as the most common form of botulism in the USA, is due to release of toxin by microorganisms present within the infant's gut. The clinical picture includes constipation, generalized hypotonia, a weak and altered cry, muscle weakness and areflexia. Ingestion of honey containing spores of *C. botulinum* appears to be a common source of infection. Treatment consists of support of respiration; most infants recover without treatment with antitoxin.

Poliomyelitis

Poliomyelitis is due to infection with the polioviruses, members of the enterovirus group (Fig. 3.127). There are 3 serotypes of polioviruses; in unimmunized populations most paralytic poliomyelitis is caused by type 1. Infection is initiated by replication of virus in the gut and associated lymphoid tissues, followed by viraemic spread to reticuloendothelial tissues throughout the body. In most patients the infection is contained at this point and no symptoms result. In a few individuals replication in the reticuloendothelial system results in a major viraemia which corresponds with the non-specific febrile illness known as abortive poliomyelitis. Viraemia may also result in seeding of the leptomeninges causing an aseptic meningitis (non-paralytic poliomyelitis). In a small proportion of individuals spread of the virus to the nervous system may result in extensive necrosis of neurons in the grey matter of the spinal cord and brain with production of paralytic poliomyelitis. Destruction of neurones is accompanied by an inflammatory infiltrate of polymorphonuclear leucocytes, lymphocytes and macrophages (Fig. 3.128). The major sites of attack are the anterior horn of the spinal cord and the motor nuclei of the pons and medulla.

Up to 99% of infections are asymptomatic. Paralytic disease occurs in only approximately 0.1% of infections. The most common form of paralytic poliomyelitis involves the spinal cord with production of an asymmetrical flaccid paralysis, which affects some muscle groups while sparing others. Proximal muscles of the extremities are most commonly involved and legs are involved more commonly than arms. Bulbar poliomyelitis may involve the nuclei of cranial nerves, especially nerves IX–XII, and the respiratory and vasomotor centers. Involvement of cranial nerves may result in difficulty in swallowing and handling of secretions, and involvement of medullary centres may cause hypertension, hyperthermia, tachycardia, Cheyne–Stokes respiration and potentially fatal cardiac arrhythmias.

In developing countries in which few individuals are immunized against poliomyelitis, most cases occur in children under the age of 5 years. In industrialized countries where most individuals have been immunized, infection with wild-type virus is extremely rare and most of the few cases which occur are due to vaccine strains, especially types 3 and 2.

Paralytic disease occurs in approximately 1 out of every 2.6 million recipients of the oral, live-virus vaccine. Specific aetiological diagnosis of poliovirus infection can be made by isolation of virus from throat washings in the first week of illness, or from faeces for several weeks thereafter. Rarely the organism may be isolated from the CSF. In the absence of virus isolation the diagnosis can be established by demonstrating a significant rise in antibody titre during convalescence from the illness.

Since there are no specific antiviral agents which are effective in the treatment of poliovirus infections, management consists of supportive care and maintenance of adequate ventilation and an adequate airway. Both inactivated-virus vaccines and live attenuated oral vaccines are extremely effective in prevention of paralytic poliomyelitis.

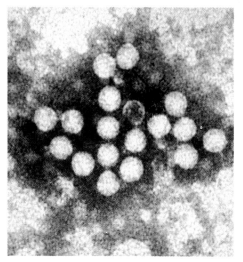

Fig. 3.127 Poliomyelitis. Electron micrograph showing spherical poliovirus particles, approximately 25nm in diameter.

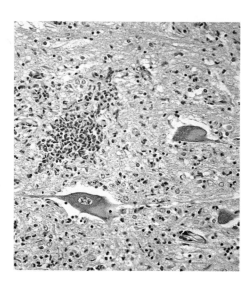

Fig. 3.128 Poliomyelitis. Histological section of spinal cord showing microglial nodules. H & E stain.

Neurological disease associated with human T-cell leukaemia virus I (HTLV-I)

HTLV-I is a human retrovirus of the oncovirus group. Infection is most common in southern Japan and the Caribbean Basin, and among Blacks in the southeast USA. Transmission occurs from mother to child (probably via breast milk), during sexual contact (via semen) and through blood transfusion or use of contaminated needles. Infection persists for life and virus can be consistently isolated from seropositive individuals.

The most important human disease related to infection with HTLV-I is adult T-cell leukaemia-lymphoma, but in endemic areas cases of a progressive neurological disease (sometimes known as tropical spastic paraplegia) have also been linked with this virus. Most of the patients have progressive bilateral spastic paraparesis, often with mild sensory involvement. Peripheral numbness or dysaesthesia, back pain and urinary frequency, urgency and incontinence are sometimes seen. Neurological examination reveals spastic paraparesis with hyperactive deep tendon reflexes. Examination of the cerebrospinal fluid may be normal or may show slight elevation in protein concentration and mild mononuclear pleocytosis. Abnormal lymphocytes similar to those seen in adult T-cell leukaemia-lymphoma may be found in the peripheral blood or CSF, and oligoclonal protein bands, viral DNA or complete virus may be found in the CSF. A favourable response to treatment with steroids has been described in some patients.

Lyme disease

Neurological abnormalities may be prominent during the course of Lyme disease (See Chapter 1). The causative organism, *Borrelia burgdorferi*, like the spirochaetes of syphilis and leptospirosis, frequently reaches the cerebrospinal fluid and tissues of the central nervous system early in the course of the infection. The microbiological diagnosis of neuroborreliosis may be made by finding a high titre of antibody against *B. burgdorferi* in the CSF, or by demonstration of *B. burgdorferi*-specific oligoclonal bands in the CSF. Early in the infection there is often a flu-like syndrome with fever, headache, myalgias and stiff neck. At this stage the cerebrospinal fluid findings are usually normal. Later, a lymphocytic meningitis with

involvement of various cranial nerves (especially Bell's palsy) and a radiculoneuritis may occur. These manifestations usually respond to antibiotic therapy. Ceftriaxone appears to be more effective than penicillins or tetracyclines. Months or years later the patient may develop a chronic progressive encephalomyelitis, distal paraesthesias or radicular pain. Serious late neurological abnormalities appear to be more common in Europe than in the USA. For treatment of the late neurological complications of Lyme disease, ceftriaxone, continued for at least 2 weeks, appears to be more effective than penicillins or other agents. Antimicrobial therapy is clearly more effective if given early in the course of the disease.

Guillain–Barré syndrome

Guillain–Barré syndrome is an inflammatory demyelinating process of peripheral nerves, predominantly involving anterior roots, which results in an ascending flaccid paralysis with paraesthesias, loss of deep tendon reflexes and muscle wasting (Fig. 3.129). Most but not all cases are preceded by an acute infection or immunization. A number of viruses, including influenza A virus, Epstein–Barr virus, human immunodeficiency virus (HIV) and various enteroviruses, as well as *Mycoplasma pneumoniae*, have been associated with this syndrome. The disease closely resembles experimental allergic neuritis, a disease induced in animals by immunization with peripheral nerve myelin, and may represent sensitization to this substance. A characteristic finding is an increased protein concentration in the cerebrospinal fluid, with few or no cells (albumino-cytological dissociation). Involvement of ventilatory muscles may necessitate respiratory assistance. Involvement of the autonomic nervous system may result in labile blood pressure which is difficult to control. Many patients benefit from plasmaphaeresis, particularly if the treatment is instituted early in the disease. Long-term prognosis is good, but improvement may occur gradually over a period of a year or more.

African trypanosomiasis

African trypanosomiasis is caused by a flagellated protozoan, *Trypanosoma brucei* (Fig. 3.130), which is transmitted

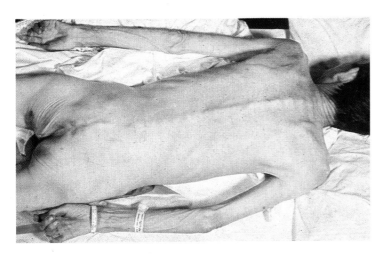

Fig. 3.129 Guillain-Barré syndrome. Limb wasting.

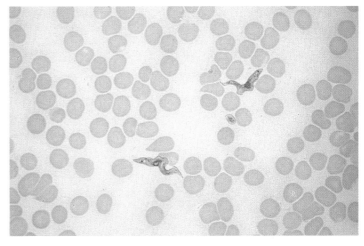

Fig. 3.130 African trypanosomiasis. Trypanosomes in a thin blood smear.

from wild and domestic animals to man by tsetse flies of the genus *Glossina* (Fig. 3.131). The range of the vectors (and the disease) includes the region of Africa between latitudes 15° north and 15° south. Both the West African form, due to *T. brucei gambiense* and the east African form, due to *T. b. rhodesiense*, cause a meningoencephalitis which is responsible for much of the morbidity and mortality of this disease. The West African form is usually a chronic disease lasting for many months, whereas the East African type is much more acute and stormy, with death from toxaemia often occurring within a few weeks after the onset of symptoms, before invasion of the central nervous system becomes apparent.

Following the bite of an infected tsetse fly, a small nodule (trypanosomal chancre) forms at the site of inoculation. Weeks or months later invasion of the bloodstream occurs with fever, general malaise, myalgias, headache, generalized lymphadenopathy (often including enlargement of the posterior cervical nodes, Winterbottom's sign (Fig. 3.132) splenomegaly, hepatomegaly and parasitaemia. During this stage of the disease (the systemic or haemolymphatic phase) the fever is usually episodic and the level of parasitaemia fluctuates due to variation in the surface antigens of the parasite which circumvents the antibody response of the host. The final, meningoencephalitic stage is characterized by increasing and persistent headache,

disturbance of sleep pattern, ataxia and other movement disorders, abnormal behaviour and depression of consciousness with stupor and progression to irreversible coma (Fig. 3.133). The patient eventually succumbs to an intercurrent respiratory or other infection. Pathologically, the brain reveals perivascular infiltration with mononuclear cells, lymphocytes, plasma cells and so-called morular or Mott cells (Fig. 3.134). The Mott cell is a distinctive form of plasma cell with large eosinophilic inclusions.

Diagnosis of African trypanosomiasis is usually made by demonstration of trypanosomes in blood during the febrile stage (see Fig. 3.130). Organisms may also be found in aspirates of lymph nodes or chancres. Serological methods of diagnosis have not proved very satisfactory, but newer tests utilizing DNA hybridization and the polymerase chain reaction are being developed. In the meningoencephalitic stage examination of the CSF reveals pleocytosis, predominantly lymphocytic, and elevated protein concentration, including elevation of IgM antibody. Morular cells (Mott cells) or motile trypanosomes may also be found (Fig. 3.135).

In early stage disease, suramin is effective in eradicating infection with *T. b. rhodesiense* or *T. b. gambiense*; pentamidime is effective only in early *T. b. gambiense* infection. In late stage disease, only melarsoprol and nifurtimox have proved effective. All of the antitrypanoso-

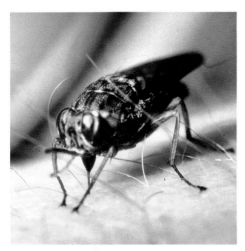

Fig. 3.131 African trypanosomiasis. Tsetse fly feeding.

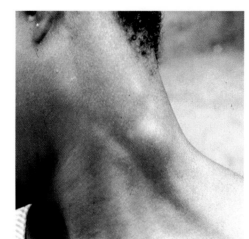

Fig. 3.132 African trypanosomiasis. Enlargement of lymph nodes in posterior cervical triangle (Winterbottom's sign). By courtesy of Prof. P. G. Janssens.

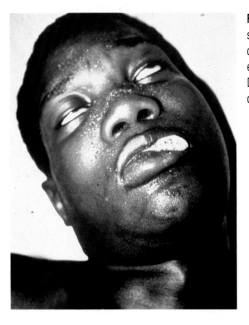

Fig. 3.133 West African sleeping sickness. Terminal coma due to generalized encephalitis. By courtesy of Dr M. E. Krampitz and Dr P. de Raadt.

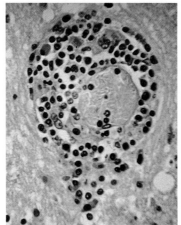
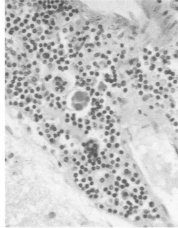

Fig. 3.134 West African sleeping sickness. Histological section of brain. Left: Prominent perivascular infiltration ('cuffing') by mononuclear cells, lymphocytes and plasma cells. Right: A prominent Mott cell. H & E stains. By courtesy of Prof. M.S.R. Hutt (left) and Prof. W. Peters (right).

mal drugs are associated with serious toxic side effects. Follow-up should be continued for at least 2 years to detect relapse, which is relatively common in these infections.

Rocky mountain spotted fever

Significant neurological involvement is common in Rocky Mountain spotted fever. Most patients complain of severe headache and photophobia, and focal neurological deficits, transient deafness, stiff neck, stupor and papilloedema without increased CSF pressure are also seen. CSF pleocytosis (usually lymphocytic) and increased protein concentration occur in approximately a third of patients. EEG may show evidence of diffuse cortical dysfunction. Prominent neurological involvement is associated with an increased case-fatality rate and a high incidence of residual neurological sequelae, especially if appropriate antimicrobial therapy is not initiated promptly. If the characteristic rash develops late in the course of the illness or is absent (10–15% of patients) it may be very difficult to distinguish this disease from other forms of encephalitis. The charac-teristic lesion is a vasculitis and perivasculitis due to direct invasion of vascular endothelial cells by the rickettsiae (Fig. 3.136), with secondary microinfarction of brain tissue (Fig. 3.137). Encephalitis has also been observed in cases of infection due to *Rickettsia conorii* (*fièvre bouttonneuse*).

Cerebral malaria

Headache, irritability, confusion and, in children, febrile convulsions occur commonly in malaria due to *Plasmodium falciparum*, but alteration in the level of consciousness, ranging from mild stupor to unarousable coma, may indicate the presence of a diffuse encephalopathy (cerebral malaria). Stiff neck, retinal haemorrhages, dysconjugate gaze and signs of upper motor neuron dysfunction (hypertonia, increased tendon reflexes with ankle clonus, extensor plantar response and absent abdominal reflexes) may also occur. Pathologically there is sequestration of parasitized erythrocytes in the microvasculature of the brain (Figs 3.138 & 139), shown by electron microscopy to be due to cytoadherence of knob-like protu-

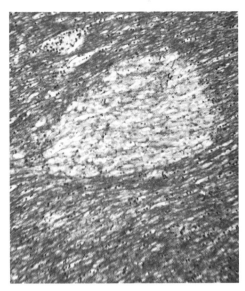

Fig. 3.135 West African sleeping sickness. Giemsa stain preparation of cerebrospinal fluid showing a typical trypanosome (no Mott cells are seen in this particular preparation). By courtesy of the Wellcome Museum of Medical Science

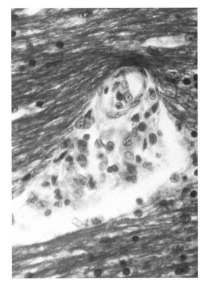

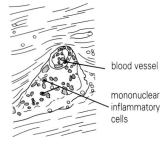

Fig. 3.136 Rocky Mountain spotted fever. Vasculitis in a small blood vessel with prominent perivascular clustering of mononuclear inflammatory cells to form a 'typhus nodule'. Luxol fast blue H & E stain.

blood vessel

mononuclear inflammatory cells

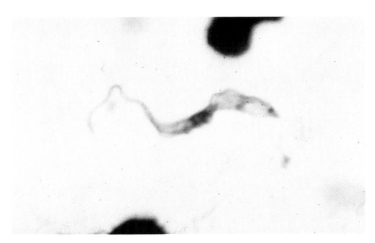

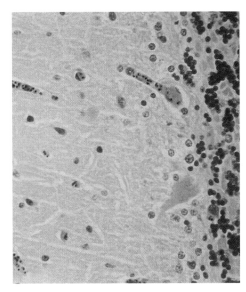

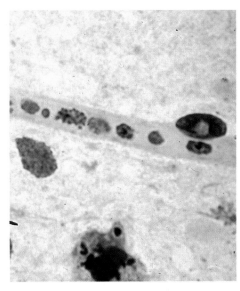

Fig. 3.137 Rocky Mountain spotted fever: microinfarct in the white matter of the brain of a child. The small infarcts are caused by the vasculitis characteristic of this disease. Luxol fast blue, H & E stain.

Fig. 3.138 Cerebral malaria. Histological section of cerebellum showing capillaries filled with parasitized red blood cells. H & E stain.

Fig. 3.139 Cerebral malaria. Histological section of cerebrum showing a capillary filled with parasitized red cells and infarction of brain tissue. H & E stain.

berances on the erythrocyte surface to vascular endothelium, resulting in obstruction of cerebral capillaries and venules, with development of ring haemorrhages around some of the obstructed vessels. Decreased deformability of infected erythrocytes may also contribute to sluggish blood flow. Metabolic abnormalities, including anaerobic glycolysis in the brain and reduced cerebral oxygen transport, have also been demonstrated. Cerebral malaria should be treated with intravenous quinine. Chloroquine, which is less toxic than quinine, may be used in areas in which only chloroquine-sensitive strains of *P. falciparum* are present. If parenteral quinine is not available quinidine gluconate may be used; the electrocardiogram and blood pressure should be monitored closely throughout the infusion period. Seizures should be managed with parenteral phenobarbital. Use of corticosteroids such as dexamethasone is contraindicated.

Leprosy

Peripheral nerve involvement in leprosy is manifested by thickened superficial nerves (Fig. 3.140) and, especially in tuberculoid leprosy, anaesthesia of the cutaneous lesions. In tuberculoid leprosy the nerve bundles are infiltrated with mononuclear inflammatory cells but few bacilli are present (Fig. 3.141). In the lepromatous form acid-fast bacilli are abundant (see Chapter 10).

CONGENITAL INFECTIONS OF THE NERVOUS SYSTEM

Three important congenital infections which may affect the nervous system are toxoplasmosis, rubella and cytomegalovirus infection.

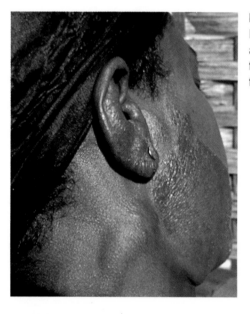

Fig. 3.140 Leprosy. Enlargement of the great auricular nerve in relationship to inflamed boderline tuberculoid lesions.

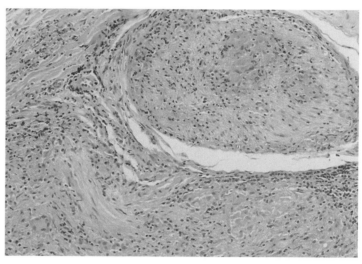

Fig. 3.141 Tuberculoid leprosy. Peripheral nerve expanded by granulomatous inflammation. Giant cells are present in nerve bundle. H & E stain. By courtesy of Dr P. Garen.

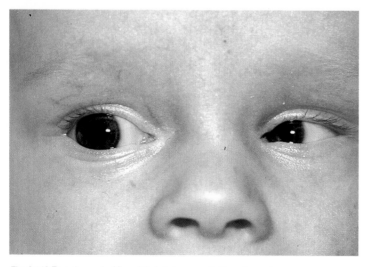

Fig. 3.142 Toxoplasmosis. Microphthalmia in congenital toxoplasmosis.

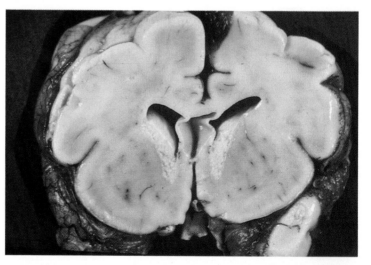

Fig. 3.143 Congenital toxoplasmosis. Brain of a premature infant revealing subependymal necrosis and calcification appearing as bilaterally symmetrical areas of whitish discolouration. The subependymal change is in the region of the caudate nucelus; the vascular congestion seen below this is probably unrelated to the primary pathological process.

Congenital toxoplasmosis

Congenital toxoplasmosis usually results from transmission of infection to the fetus following acquisition of acute toxoplasmosis by a pregnant woman. Transmission *in utero* occasionally occurs following reactivation of chronic infection in an immunocompromised pregnant woman. If the mother develops toxoplasmosis during the first trimester the rate of transmission to the fetus is approximately 25%, and the result is usually severe disease in the newborn, spontaneous abortion or stillbirth. After the first trimester the risk of infection in the fetus is much higher, but most of the affected infants will be asymptomatic at birth. Appropriate antimicrobial treatment of the mother substantially reduces the risk of transmission of infection to the fetus. Chorioretinitis (see Figs 12.66 & 12.67) is the most common manifestation of congenital toxoplasmosis, but mental and psychomotor retardation, seizure disorder, encephalitis, microcephaly, microphthalmia (Fig. 3.142),

intracranial calcification (Fig. 3.143), hydrocephalus (Figs 3.144 & 3.145) and sensorineural hearing loss are also common. Most infected infants will eventually develop signs of toxoplasmosis, but these may not appear until several months after delivery. Congenital toxoplasmosis must be differentiated from rubella, cytomegalovirus infection, HSV infection, syphilis and listeriosis. A markedly elevated concentration of protein in the CSF is typical of congenital toxoplasmosis. IgG antibody may be transferred passively from the mother to the fetus across the placenta, but a persistent or rising titre of IgG antibody or a positive test for IgM antibody provides evidence of infection in the infant. If toxoplasmosis is suspected in an apparently healthy newborn baby, therapy with pyrimethamine plus sulfadiazine should be administered for 3 weeks, followed by sulfadiazine alone until the diagnosis is confirmed or discarded. If the diagnosis is confirmed, treatment should be continued for a minimum of 6 months in infants who are asymptomatic at birth, and for a year if signs of infection are present.

Congenital rubella

Infants with congenital rubella shed large quantities of virus in body secretions for many months in spite of high titres of neutralizing antibody in the serum. How this persistent infection leads to the development of the specific manifestations of the congenital rubella syndrome is not completely understood. The effects of rubella virus on the fetus are closely related to the age of the fetus at the time infection occurs: the younger the fetus when infected the more severe the illness. The most common manifestations affecting the CNS and eye are meningoencephalitis, nerve deafness, cataract, chorioretinitis (Fig. 3.143), mental retardation, microcephaly and disorders of behaviour and language. Diagnosis of congenital rubella is made by demonstration of rubella virus or antigen with monoclonal antibody or detection of a persistent or rising titre of IgG antibody or presence of IgM antibody. Congenital rubella can be largely prevented by immunization of the popula-

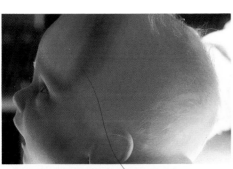

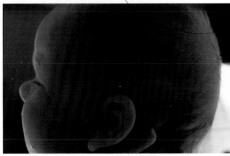

Fig. 3.144 Toxoplasmosis. Transillumination of skull with severe hydrocephalus secondary to congenital toxoplasmosis.

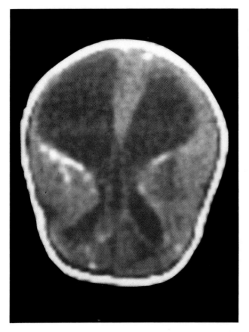

Fig. 3.145 Toxoplasmosis. CT scan of above showing severe hydrocephalus and periventricular calcification.

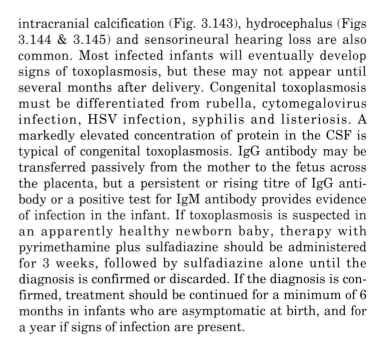

Fig. 3.146 Rubella retinopathy. Fundus photograph showing characteristic clumping of pigment and areas of retinal degeneration in the region of the macula. By courtesy of Mr G. Catford.

tion during childhood with live attenuated rubella vaccine. Women are advised not to become pregnant for at least 3 months after receiving rubella vaccine, but no cases of the congenital rubella syndrome have been attributed to the vaccine.

Congenital cytomegalovirus infection

Most cases of clinically apparent cytomegalovirus infection occur in infants of primiparous mothers who had a primary infection during pregnancy. In this situation the risk of infection in the infant is approximately 50%. The risk of infection in infants born to mothers who were seropositive at the beginning of pregnancy is much lower; immunity in the mother evidently protects the baby from infection.

Infection of the uterine cervix during pregnancy may result in transmission of infection to a neonate during passage through the birth canal. Such perinatal infections are usually asymptomatic but can be recognized when a neonate begins to secrete virus in the urine several weeks after birth. In classical fulminant congenital cytomegalovirus infection, jaundice, hepatosplenomegaly, petechial rash and evidence of multiple organ system involvement appear shortly after birth. Microcephaly, motor disability, intracerebral calcifications and chorioretinitis are often present. Infants who survive may exhibit nerve deafness, chronic seizure disorder and spastic quadriplegia. At the present time there are no established effective measures for prevention or treatment of congenital cytomegalovirus infection.

THE GASTROINTESTINAL TRACT

4

INFECTIOUS OESOPHAGITIS

The two most important aetiological agents in infectious oesophagitis are *Candida* species and the herpes simplex virus. Both of these infections are rare in immunocompetent individuals; they are encountered most frequently in patients with haematologic or lymphatic malignancies or AIDS.

Candidal oesophagitis is often seen in association with extensive oral candidiasis (thrush), but approximately one-third of patients do not have thrush. The most common symptoms are pain on swallowing, a sensation of obstruction on swallowing and substernal chest pain. Endoscopic visualization of white plaques resembling thrush (Figs 4.1, 4.2 & 4.3), hyphal elements in cytological preparations made from scrapings (Fig. 4.4) and irregularity of the oesophageal mucosa resulting from ulceration (Figs 4.5 & 4.6) are also commonly found. Definitive diagnosis is best made by endoscopic biopsy, which reveals invasion of the mucosa by hyphal elements (Fig. 4.7). The stomach, small bowel and large bowel may also be involved, and in severely immunocompromised patients concomitant infection with herpes simplex virus may be present. Oral nystatin often provides rapid relief of symptoms, but patients who fail to respond to this and those with severe infections should be treated with oral fluconazole or ketoconazole. Rarely therapy with amphotericin B given intravenously may be required. It may be impossible to completely eradicate oesophageal candidiasis in patients with AIDS; long-term suppression with fluconazole may be the best that can be achieved.

Oesophagitis due to herpes simplex virus (HSV) is seen primarily in patients with AIDS, or those with haematological or lymphoreticular malignancies, or following organ transplantation. Pain and difficulty on swallowing are common features, and significant bleeding may occur. Endoscopy reveals ulceration and frequently vesicles similar to those seen in other infections of mucous membranes due to this virus (Figs 4.8 & 4.9). Unsuspected herpetic oesophagitis is often found at autopsy, especially in patients who have had nasogastric tubes in place shortly before death. Prophylactic administration of acyclovir intravenously may prevent the development of progressive mucocutaneous and visceral herpes simplex infections in

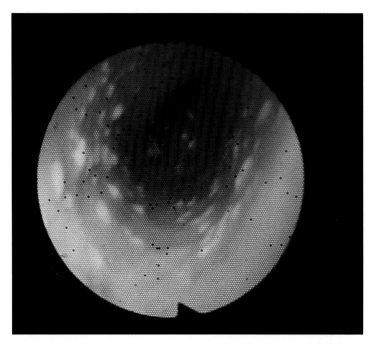

Fig. 4.1 Candida oesophagitis. Endoscopic view showing multiple cotton-wool plaques on the mucosa. This is a mild case, in which barium swallow might be normal. By courtesy of Dr J. Cunningham.

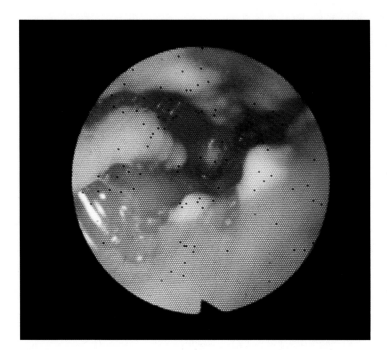

Fig. 4.2 Candida oesophagitis. A more advanced stage of severe oesophagitis with ulceration, showing discrete ulcers and thrush-like plaques on the mucosa. By courtesy of Dr J. Cunningham.

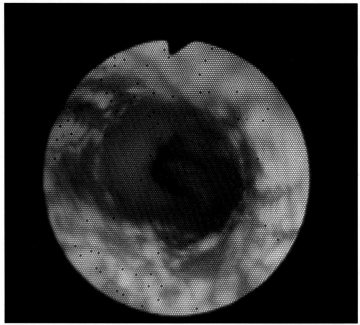

Fig. 4.3 Candida oesophagitis. Endoscopic view showing extensive areas of whitish exudate resembling the lesions of oral thrush. By courtesy of Dr I. Chesner.

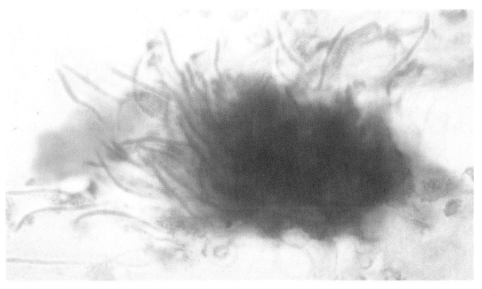

Fig. 4.4 A cytological preparation showing candidal hyphae growing outwards from a central fungal ball. ×900. Papanicolaou's stain. By courtesy of Dr E. Hudson.

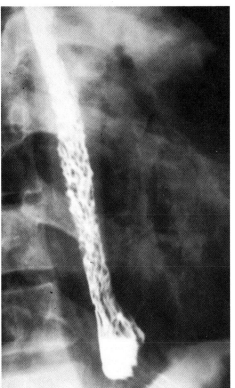

Fig. 4.5 Candida oesophagitis. Barium swallow showing multiple small ulcers, many of which contain barium, and narrowing of the oesophagus.

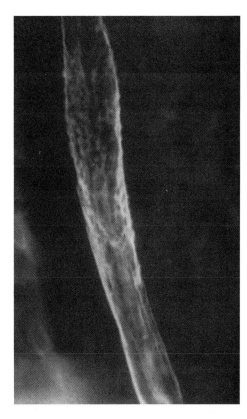

Fig. 4.6 Candida oesophagitis. Barium swallow showing multiple pinpoint ulcers. Note saw-tooth pattern along lateral sides of oesophagus produced by barium remaining in the ulcers. Herpes simplex oesophagitis can exhibit a similar picture on barium swallow. By courtesy of Dr J. Cunningham.

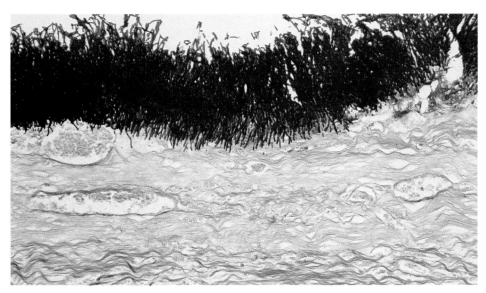

Fig. 4.7 Candida oesophagitis. Silver stain showing heavy infection of the mucosal surface by mycelial elements of *Candida albicans*, with disappearance of the epithelium. By courtesy of Dr M. J. Leyland.

certain high risk individuals, such as HSV-seropositive recipients of bone marrow transplants. Acyclovir given intravenously is also highly effective in treatment of these infections.

Ulcerative oesophageal lesions, possibly due to direct infection with the HIV virus, have been observed in patients recently infected with this virus. In rare cases the oesophagus may be involved in disseminated infection with *Mycobacterium avium–intracellulare* in patients with AIDS (Fig. 4.10).

INFECTIOUS GASTRITIS

Two important causes of gastritis are *Helicobacter pylori* (formerly *Campylobacter pylori*) and cytomegalovirus.

Helicobacter pylori

During the last few years a large body of evidence has accumulated which implicates *H. pylori* as an aetiological

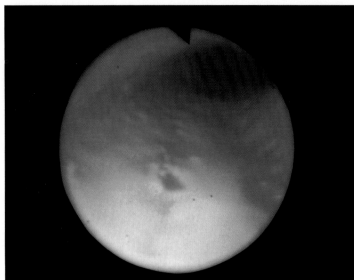

Fig. 4.8 Herpes simplex oesophagitis. Endoscopic view showing multiple pinpoint ulcers with haemorrhagic bases in a patient with severe odynophagia. By courtesy of Dr J. Cunningham.

agent in idiopathic or type B gastritis (Fig. 4.11), non-ulcer dyspepsia and duodenal ulcer. This organism is a microaerophilic, curved or spiral, gram-negative rod which produces a potent urease, an enzyme which catalyzes the hydrolysis of urea to carbon dioxide and ammonia. The bacteria live in the mucous layer overlying the gastric epithelium and apparently do not invade the tissues (Fig. 4.12). The ability of these acid-susceptible organisms to survive in the stomach may depend upon the protective effect of the mucous layer and upon local neutralization of gastric acid by ammonia (produced by the action of urease). At the present time, diagnosis of *H. pylori* infection is made by isolation of the organism from biopsy specimens, visualization of the characteristic bacteria in histological sections stained with Gram's, silver, Giemsa or acridine orange stains or demonstration of urease activity either in biopsy specimens (using the commercially available CLO test) or by means of the ^{14}C-urea breath test, which measures radiolabelled CO_2 released from urea by the action of urease, or by determination of serum antibodies to *H. pylori*. Sensitive immunofluorescent methods, using monoclonal antibodies for demonstration of the organisms in gastric biopsy material, are being developed.

H. pylori organisms are susceptible to a number of different antimicrobial agents including amoxicillin, nitrofurans, metronidazole and bismuth salts. An effective regimen has been a combination of bismuth with either tetracycline or ampicillin, administered orally for 4 weeks, with metronidazole for the first 2 weeks. When the organism is successfully eradicated by treatment, symptoms remit and the histopathological abnormalities improve. Reappearance of the organisms is followed by clinical and histopathological relapse.

Cytomegalovirus

Infection of the gastrointestinal tract by cytomegalovirus (CMV) occurs commonly in patients who are severely immunocompromised. Gastritis is the most common type of gastrointestinal infection with the virus but any level of the gastrointestinal tract may be involved. The most common symptoms are epigastric pain, anorexia, fever, nausea and vomiting, diarrhoea and gastrointestinal bleeding.

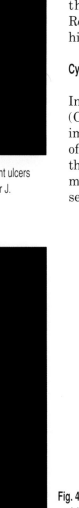

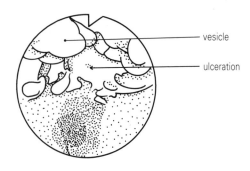

Fig. 4.9 Endoscopic view of oesophagitis due to herpes simplex virus showing herpetic vesicles and multiple ulcers.

Diagnosis is made by upper endoscopy, which reveals nodular and/or erosive gastritis, and biopsy. The tissue specimens should be examined for inclusion bodies, CMV antigen-specific immunofluorescence and culture for CMV. Ganciclovir administered intravenously (5mg/kg twice daily for a minimum of 2 weeks) is effective in the treatment of CMV infection of the gastrointestinal tract.

BACTERIAL ENTERIC INFECTIONS

Bacteria may produce diarrhoea by production of toxins, by invasion of the intestinal mucosa, or by certain other mechanisms which involve close adherence of the bacteria to the intestinal mucosal cell (see below – Diarrhoea due to *Escherichia coli*).

Toxins may include classic enterotoxins, which cause fluid secretion into the gut by stimulating adenylate cyclase or guanylate cyclase activity, as well as more general cytotoxins. Enterotoxins may be detected by their ability to produce fluid secretion in the isolated intestinal loop of the rabbit (Fig. 4.13) and by the Chinese hamster

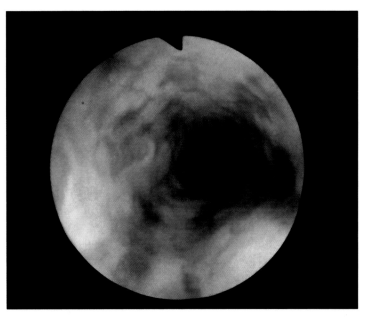

Fig. 4.10 Oesophagitis due to *Mycobacterium avium–intracellulare*. Chronic ulcerations and patches of yellow exudate with a few islands of intact mucosa. By courtesy of Dr J. Cunningham.

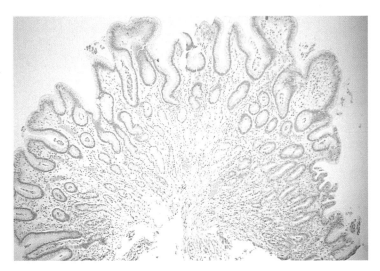

Fig. 4.11 *Helicobacter pylori* gastritis. Non-specific inflammatory changes in gastric mucosa associated with infection with *H. pylori*. By courtesy of Dr J. Newman.

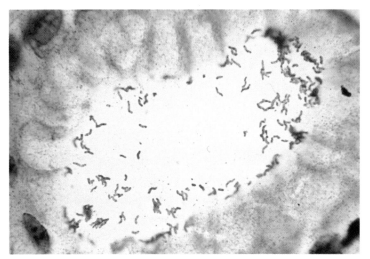

Fig. 4.12 *Helicobacter pylori* gastritis. Silver stain showing numerous comma-shaped organisms adhering to the mucosal surface. By courtesy of Dr A. M. Geddes.

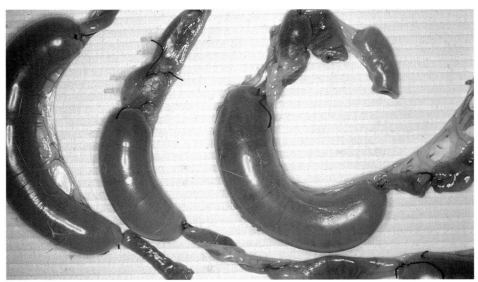

Fig. 4.13 *Escherichia coli* diarrhoea. Rabbit loop assay showing massive secretion of fluid into ligated intestinal loops which have been injected with *E. coli* enterotoxin. By courtesy of Dr H. L. DuPont.

ovary cell and Y-1 adrenal cell assays (Fig. 4.14). Classic enterotoxins such as cholera toxin produce an essentially pure biochemical lesion, with virtually no histopathological effects on the intestinal mucosa. Some important enterotoxin-producing organisms are *Vibrio cholerae, E. coli,* and *Clostridium perfringens* type A. Cytotoxins are produced by *Shigella dysenteriae* type 1, *Clostridium difficile* and certain *E. coli* serotypes (e.g. 0:157), among others.

Invasive organisms penetrate through the epithelium of the bowel into the lamina propria, and sometimes beyond, where they stimulate an intense acute inflammatory reaction with accumulation of large numbers of polymorphonuclear leucocytes (Fig. 4.15). This direct damage to the intestinal mucosa and the accompanying inflammatory reaction results in the presence of blood, mucus and inflammatory cells (polymorphonuclear leucocytes) in the stool (dysentery) (Fig. 4.16). The invasiveness of these organisms is not limited to the gut; invasiveness may be detected in cell cultures (Fig. 4.17) or by putting a drop of a culture of the organism into the eye of a rabbit, where

an intense keratoconjunctivitis is produced (the Sereny test – Fig. 4.18).

Virulence of both toxin-producing and invasive pathogens also depends upon the presence of adherence factors , which cause the bacteria to closely adhere to the mucosal cells (Fig. 4.19). Important invasive bacteria include *Shigella, Salmonella,* and *Campylobacter* species and certain strains of *E. coli.*

The clinical diseases produced by enterotoxigenic and invasive organisms differ in several respects; these are summarized in Figure 4.20.

Cholera

Cholera is the prototype of a diarrhoeal disease caused by an enterotoxin-producing microorganism. Although it has been known in India and other parts of Asia since ancient times, pandemic spread to Europe and other parts of the world first occurred early in the 19th century. Since that time the geographic distribution of cholera has expanded

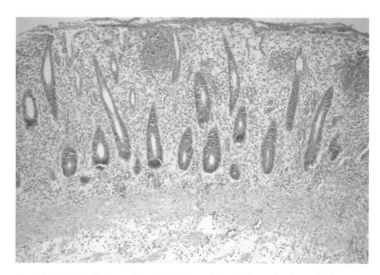

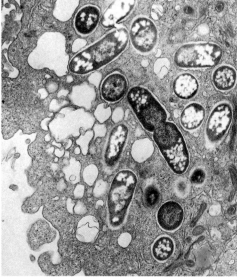

Fig. 4.14 Bacterial diarrhoea. Y1 adrenal cell assay for *E. coli* LT enterotoxin, showing normal cells (left) and cells after exposure to LT toxin (right). Note disruption of monolayer and rounding up of cells. By courtesy of Dr H. L. DuPont.

Fig. 4.15 Bacterial diarrhoea *(Campylobacter spp.).* Rectal biopsy showing marked mucosal oedema with polymorphonuclear leucocyte infiltration. Crypt degeneration has led to an attenuated appearance. H & E stain. By courtesy of Dr A. B. Price.

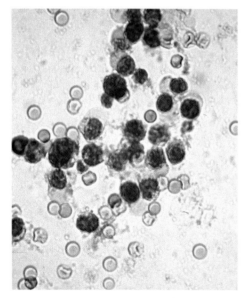

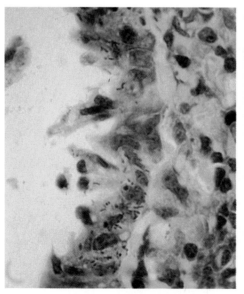

Fig. 4.16 Shigellosis. Polymorphonuclear and mononuclear leucocytes and red blood cells in the stool of a patient with shigellosis. Methylene blue wet mount under cover slip. By courtesy of Dr H. L. DuPont.

Fig. 4.17 Enteroinvasive *E. coli* infection. Invasion of mucosal layer of the intestine by *E. coli* organisms. There is necrosis of the mucosal layer at the site of invasion (left). Transmission electron micrograph showing enteroinvasive *E. coli* organisms within HEp-2 cell(right). By courtesy of Dr S. Knutton.

and contracted periodically for reasons which are poorly understood; at the time of writing (1991) the seventh recorded pandemic is in progress. The disease is most prevalent in southern Asia but small endemic foci exist in other areas, including the Coast of the Gulf of Mexico in the USA.

Vibrio cholerae is a comma-shaped gram-negative rod, closely related to the other members of the Enterobacteriaceae. It exhibits rapid motility by means of a single polar flagellum. Classical cholera vibrios (01 serotype) agglutinate with Ogawa or Inaba antisera, but similar diarrhoeal disease may be due to non-01 (non-agglutinating) organisms. Man is the only known natural host for *V. cholerae*. As John Snow elegantly demonstrated in London in the 1840s and 1850s, during epidemics the disease spreads through contamination of the water supply. Direct faecal–oral transmission within households and contamination of food are also important.

Cholera toxin is a protein which has distinct binding and active subunits. The binding subunit binds to a specific

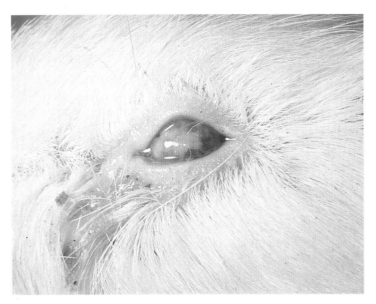

Fig. 4.18 Positive Sereny test. Keratoconjunctivitis in the rabbit produced by the instillation of shigella organisms. By courtesy of Dr H. L. DuPont.

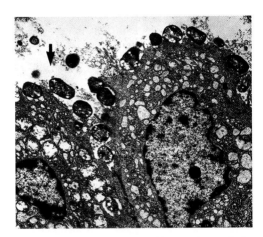

Fig.4.19 *Escherichia coli* diarrhoea. Electron micrograph of enteropathogenic *E. coli* (arrowed) attached to mucosal epithelial cells of ileum. The microvillus border of the epithelial cells has been largely destroyed by bacteria and the cells show signs of degeneration. × 3000. By courtesy of Dr J. R. Cantey.

Clinical Disease Caused by Enterotoxigenic and Invasive Organisms	
Enterotoxigenic	**Invasive**
Severe watery diarrhoea, no dysentery	Dysentery (blood, mucus, PMN)
No fever	Fever
No systemic toxicity	Severe systemic toxicity
Minimal abdominal pain and cramping	Severe abdominal pain and cramping, tenesmus
Bacteria multiply in small bowel	Bacteria multiply in colon
No PMN leucocytes in stool	PMN leucocytes in stool
Response to non–absorbable antimicrobial agents	Response to absorbable and parenteral antibiotics

Fig. 4.20 Clinical disease caused by enterotoxigenic and invasive organisms.

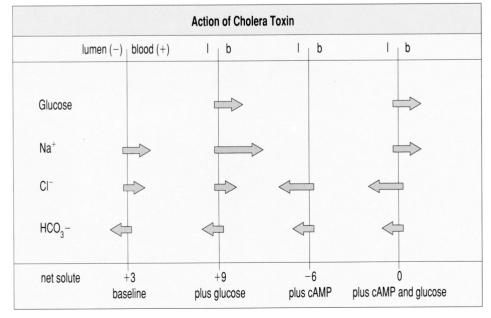

Action of Cholera Toxin

	lumen (−) blood (+)	l b	l b	l b
Glucose				
Na$^+$				
Cl$^-$				
HCO$_3$$^-$				
net solute	+3	+9	−6	0
	baseline	plus glucose	plus cAMP	plus cAMP and glucose

Fig. 4.21 Diagram showing action of cholera toxin on intestinal mucosa. The toxin stimulates the activity of cyclic AMP in the small intestinal mucosa, resulting in active secretion of chloride, with secondary loss of sodium and water. Glucose partially reverses the inhibition of sodium absorption. By courtesy of Dr M. Field.

receptor on the intestinal mucosal cell. The toxin stimulates the activity of cyclic AMP in the small intestinal mucosa, resulting in active secretion of chloride (see Fig. 4.21) with secondary loss of sodium and water.

The clinical picture of cholera consists of profound watery diarrhoea, with rapid depletion of water and electrolytes. At the height of the illness the voluminous watery stool is nearly colourless and contains flecks of mucus (the rice water stool – Fig. 4.22). If water and electrolyte losses are replaced promptly the only other symptoms may be abdominal fullness and hyperperistalsis. If replacement is inadequate, hypovolemia with shock, altered consciousness, renal failure, hypokalemia and acidosis may develop. Patients with severe cholera may lose up to 20 litres of stool per day, a total of 100 litres during the 4–7 day course of the illness.

The most important aspect of treatment is rapid replacement of the lost water and electrolytes. In most patients this can be accomplished via the oral route, but in those who are severely ill or vomiting, the intravenous route should be used. Glucose (or sucrose) must be added to oral replacement solutions since one phase of sodium absorption is glucose-dependent. Reasonably accurate estimates of the volume of fluid being lost can be made using the 'cholera cot' with a bucket and calibrated measuring stick (Fig. 4.23). Oral administration of an effective antibiotic such as tetracycline significantly shortens the duration of diarrhoea and reduces the total loss of fluid and electrolyte.

Bacteriological confirmation of the diagnosis of cholera may be made by culture of the stool or a rectal swab. Treatment must not be delayed until the bacteriological diagnosis is secured, but should be initiated immediately based upon the clinical picture.

Diarrhoeal disease due to other vibrios

In recent years it has become apparent that non-01

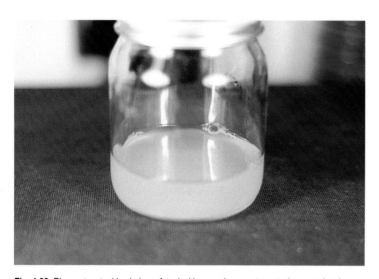

Fig. 4.22 Rice water stool in cholera. A typical large-volume watery stool excreted at the height of the illness. By courtesy of Dr A. M. Geddes.

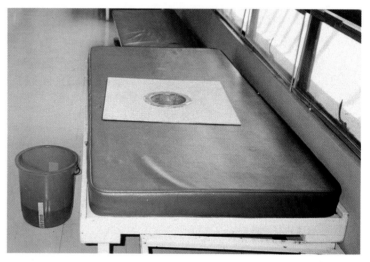

Fig. 4.23 A 'cholera cot' and bucket used for estimation of volume lost in stool. By courtesy of Dr S. Mehtar.

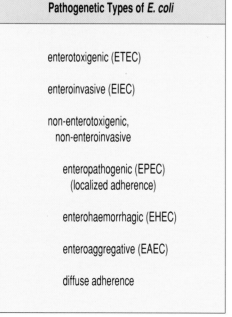

Pathogenetic Types of *E. coli*
enterotoxigenic (ETEC)
enteroinvasive (EIEC)
non-enterotoxigenic, non-enteroinvasive
enteropathogenic (EPEC) (localized adherence)
enterohaemorrhagic (EHEC)
enteroaggregative (EAEC)
diffuse adherence

Fig. 4.24 Pathogenetic types of *E. coli*.

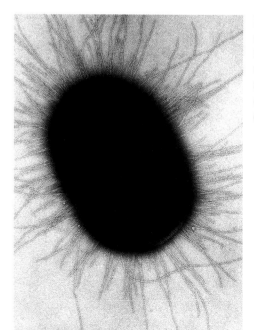

Fig. 4.25 Enterotoxigenic *E. coli* infection. Electron micrograph of the organism showing pili required for adherence to mucosal epithelial cells. By courtesy of Dr S. Knutton.

cholera vibrios, sometimes known as non-agglutinable (NAG) vibrios, which are distributed worldwide in water sources, are capable of causing diarrhoeal disease. A few patients develop severe watery diarrhoea indistinguishable from classical cholera, but in most patients the diarrhoea is less severe and resembles the traveller's diarrhoea caused by enterotoxigenic strains of *E. coli*. These organisms are isolated on thiosulphate–citrate–bile salt–sucrose (TCBS) agar. Patients with mild diarrhoea need no treatment; in more severe illness replacement of lost fluid and electrolytes by oral or intravenous routes may be required. Whether or not antimicrobial agents shorten the course of illness in severe cases has not been established.

Of the true halophilic (salt-requiring) vibrios, the most important species is *Vibrio parahaemolyticus*. This organism is an extremely important cause of diarrhoeal disease in Japan and has recently been implicated in outbreaks of disease along the Atlantic and Gulf coasts of the USA and on Caribbean cruise ships. It occurs in coastal waters around the world and is probably a common cause of diarrhoea wherever inadequately cooked seafood is eaten. Nearly all cases are related to ingestion of seafood which has either been inadequately cooked or recontaminated with sea water containing the organism. *V. parahaemolyticus* produces an enterotoxin and also invades the bowel wall, stimulating an inflammatory reaction in the tissues. The incubation period is short, usually less than 24 hours, and the onset is abrupt with explosive watery diarrhoea and cramping abdominal pain. Fever, chills and headache may also be present. Halophilic vibrios grow poorly on standard culture media and isolation is best accomplished by inoculation onto TCBS agar.

Usually no treatment is required in *V. parahaemolyticus* infections, but occasionally replacement of fluid and electrolyte losses is indicated. The infection can be prevented by adequate cooking of seafood and avoidance of recontamination of cooked seafood by sea water containing the organism. Cooked seafood which is not eaten immediately should be refrigerated promptly.

Two other important halophilic vibrios, *V. vulnificus and V. alginolyticus*, are associated primarily with wound infections and sepsis rather than diarrhoeal disease, and are discussed in Chapter 10.

Diarrhoea due to *Escherichia coli*

Worldwide, diarrhoea-producing strains of *E. coli* are a major cause of diarrhoeal disease and, in young children, of mortality. As described below, several different pathogenetic mechanisms are involved (Fig. 4.24). In general the various pathogenic types may be distinguished by serotyping of the O antigen (a lipopolysaccharide). Clinical features of the illnesses produced by the different types are also dissimilar.

Enterotoxigenic *E. coli* (ETEC) adhere to microvilli of the small intestinal mucosa by means of pili or colonization factor antigens (Figs 4.25 & 4.26) and produce two distinct enterotoxins. The heat-labile toxin (LT) is a large protein of approximately 90 000 Da and is very similar to cholera toxin. Heat-stable toxins (ST) are small proteins of approximately 2000 Da which stimulate the guanylate cyclase of the mucosal cell, resulting in an increase in cyclic guanosine monophosphate (cGMP). ETEC strains are abundant in developing countries and are responsible for at least 50% of the cases of traveller's diarrhoea; they are rarely isolated from patients with diarrhoea in industrialized countries. Transmission is primarily via faecally contaminated food or water. The incubation period varies from 12 hours to 3 days. ETEC strains produce nausea, abdominal cramps and watery diarrhoea; fever and leucocytosis are usually absent. The illness is usually mild or only moderately severe, and lasts about 5 days on average.

Enteropathogenic *E. coli* (EPEC) adhere closely to intestinal cells (Fig. 4.27) but apparently do not produce adherence pili or LT or ST. There is loss of microvilli and

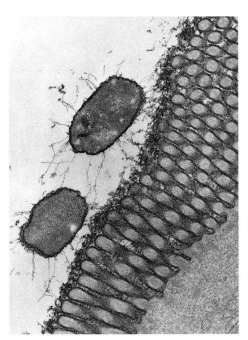

Fig. 4.26 Enterotoxigenic *E. coli* infection. Transmission electron micrograph showing bacteria adhering to the brush border of human intestinal mucosal cells. By courtesy of Dr S. Knutton.

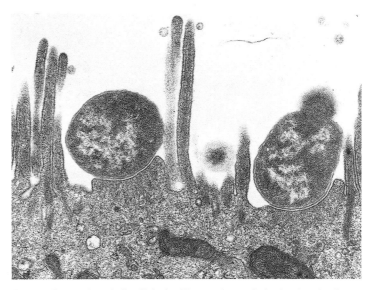

Fig. 4.27 Enteropathogenic *E. coli* infection. Electron micrograph showing close, localized adherence of bacteria to human intestinal mucosal cells and localized destruction of microvilli. By courtesy of Dr S. Knutton.

aggregation of actin adjacent to sites of adherence (Fig. 4.28). The mechanism by which they produce diarrhoea is not completely understood. EPEC occur worldwide and have produced many epidemics, mainly involving young children. Diarrhoea often lasts for 10 days or longer, sometimes a month or more. In young children this may be associated with severe depletion of water and electrolytes.

Enterohaemorrhagic *E. coli* (EHEC) adhere closely to the mucosa of the distal ileum and proximal colon, but do not invade. They produce large amounts of a Shiga-like toxins (Verotoxins), cytotoxic enterotoxins similar to the Shiga toxin originally found in strains of *Shigella dysenteriae* type 1, the Shiga bacillus (Fig. 4.29). These toxins may be responsible for the grossly bloody diarrhoea exhibited by these patients, and perhaps for the associated haemolytic uraemic syndrome. Shiga-like toxin can often be detected in the diarrhoeal stool of these patients. EHECs were originally described in the USA in 1982 asso-

ciated with ingestion of inadequately cooked hamburgers in fast-food restaurants. Most subsequent outbreaks have been associated with ingestion of contaminated food or milk, but person-to-person transmission can also occur. These organisms produce a distinctive clinical syndrome, ranging from non-bloody diarrhoea to full-blown haemorrhagic colitis, complicated in about 10% of cases by development of the haemolytic uraemic syndrome. The incubation period is longer than 8 days. Severe abdominal pain, marked abdominal distention and tenderness, especially in the right lower quadrant, are seen in most patients. X-rays show gas distending the small bowel, caecum and ascending colon and barium enema may show 'thumbprinting' of the caecum and ascending and transverse colon due to oedema and submucosal haemorrhage. On sigmoidoscopy and colonoscopy the mucosa may appear oedematous, friable and erythematous with haemorrhages and ulcerations, a picture which resembles

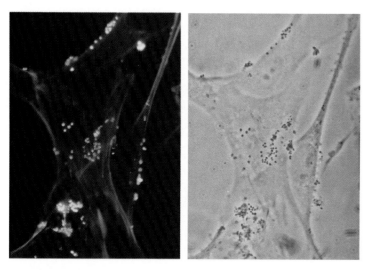

Fig. 4.28 Enteropathogenic *E. coli* infection. Fluorescent actin test specific for EPEC organisms. Left: Fluorescence microscopy showing aggregated actin. Right: Phase contrast microscopy showing location of bacteria. By courtesy of Dr S. Knutton.

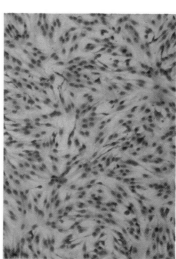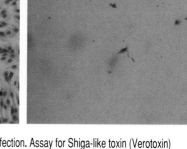

Fig. 4.29 Enterohaemorrhagic *E. coli* infection. Assay for Shiga-like toxin (Verotoxin) produced by EHEC (serotype 0:157). Left: Normal monolayer of Vero cells. Right: Destruction of Vero cells by the toxin. By courtesy of Dr S. Knutton.

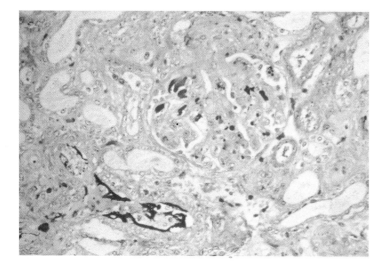

Fig. 4.30 Enterohaemorrhagic *E. coli* infection. Weigert stain showing fibrin 'thrombi' in glomerular capillaries in haemolytic uraemic syndrome. By courtesy of Dr H. R. Powell.

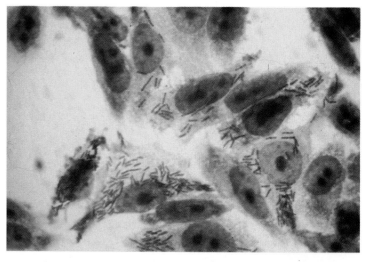

Fig. 4.31 Enteroinvasive *E. coli* infection. EIEC organisms invading HeLa cells *in vitro*. By courtesy of Dr S. Knutton.

ischaemic colitis. Patients with haemolytic uraemic syndrome exhibit deteriorating renal function, microangiopathic haemolytic anaemia and fibrin thrombi in glomerular capillaries (Fig. 4.30).

Enteroinvasive *E. coli* (EIEC) produce diarrhoea by invading and destroying the mucosal epithelium of the distal ileum and colon (Fig. 4.31). This is a rare cause of diarrhoea, although it is occasionally responsible for large foodborne outbreaks, especially in tropical countries. The clinical picture of fever, systemic toxicity, cramping abdominal pain and dysentery is one that closely resembles shigellosis.

Specific microbiological diagnosis of diarrhoea due to *E. coli* is difficult and expensive. A small number of research or public health laboratories may be able to serotype *E. coli* isolates and identify EPEC strains; only a few research laboratories can carry out the specialized procedures required to identify the other types. DNA probes and assays to identify LT, ST, Shiga-like toxins and various adherence factors are being developed.

Most cases of diarrhoea due to *E. coli* are mild and adequate oral intake of fluids is the only treatment required. In more seriously ill patients intravenous administration of fluids and electrolytes may be necessary. Bismuth subsalicylate (Pepto-bismol) and antimotility agents (loperamide or diphenoxylate) are effective in reducing diarrhoea in patients without fever or dysentery. Presence of dysentery indicates invasive infection and these patients, as well as those with severe traveller's diarrhoea, should receive antibiotic therapy. Tetracycline, doxycycline, trimethoprim–sulphamethoxazole, furazolidone, and the quinolones (nalidixic acid and the fluoroquinolones) are all effective agents. A quinolone or furazolidone would be the best choice in areas where resistance to other antibiotics is prevalent.

Shigellosis (Dysentery)

Hippocrates provided the first description of dysentery; epidemics of bacillary dysentery are known to have occurred during military campaigns at least as long ago as the Peloponnesian Wars in the 5th century BC. Shigella organisms are highly adapted to man, the only natural host, and the minimum infectious dose is only about 200 organisms. Person-to-person transmission therefore occurs readily in crowded conditions, for example in military barracks, prisons, asylums, institutions for the mentally retarded and day-care centres. Shigella infections occur most frequently in infants and young children, but secondary spread within the household to other children and adults is common. The disease is most prevalent in tropical countries, and unsatisfactory conditions of hygiene and poor nutrition increase the incidence and severity. The peak incidence is during summer. Although most spread is person-to-person via contamination of the hands with infected faeces, outbreaks due to contamination of food or water supplies have occurred (e.g. on cruise ships) and there is good evidence that the organisms can be transmitted by flies.

The geographic distribution of each of the four species of shigella (*S. dysenteriae*, *S. flexneri*, *S. sonnei* and *S. boydii*) differs significantly. In general, *S. dysenteriae* is common only in impoverished tropical countries. In many less developed countries infection with *S. flexneri* predominates. In the most highly industrialized countries of northern Europe and North America, the majority of infections are caused by *S. sonnei*.

Following ingestion, shigella organisms multiply in the distal small bowel and elicit symptoms of watery diarrhoea, cramping abdominal pain, fever, headache and other signs of systemic toxicity. In infants and young children hyperpyrexia and seizures may occur. Seizures and other neurological abnormalities may be due to Shiga or Shiga-like toxins. When the organism reaches the colon and invades the epithelium it multiplies primarily in the lamina propria, destroying the overlying mucosa (Fig. 4.32). Shigellas rarely penetrate beyond the mucosa, and bacteraemia is extremely rare. Sigmoidoscopy may reveal hyperaemia and a whitish exudate, and in severe cases an extensive pseudomembranous colitis may be present (Figs

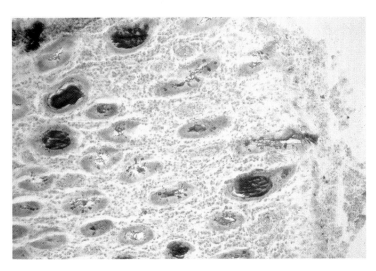

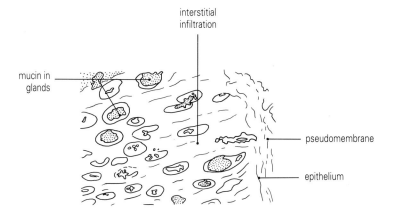

Fig. 4.32 Severe shigellosis. Histology of colon showing disrupted epithelium covered by pseudomembrane and interstitial infiltration. Mucin glands have uniformly discharged and goblet cells are empty. Colloidal iron stain. By courtesy of Dr R. H. Gilman.

4.33 & 4.34). On histopathological examination microabscesses are seen which sometimes coalesce and cause sloughing, resulting in mucosal ulceration. At this stage the signs and symptoms reflect the invasion of the colonic wall; the patient experiences cramping abdominal pain, especially in the left lower quadrant, tenesmus and dysentery (blood, mucus and pus in the stool). If a fleck of mucus is mixed with a drop of saline and methylene blue stain and examined under a cover slip, large numbers of polymorphonuclear leucocytes are usually found (see Fig. 4.16). Many patients with shigellosis exhibit large numbers of band forms in the differential leucocyte count, up to 50% of the total number of leucocytes. Most patients recover within a few days to a week. Organisms may be excreted in the faeces from 1–4 weeks after recovery; long-term intestinal carriage rarely occurs.

Microbiological diagnosis of shigellosis depends upon isolation of the lactose-positive, gram-negative rods from a stool specimen or rectal swab. Organisms are most abundant and therefore easiest to isolate early in the course of the illness. The specimen should be inoculated into culture media as soon as it is obtained. The ideal method is to plate a rectal swab directly (at the bedside) onto mildly inhibitory media and also onto more inhibitory media.

Antibiotic treatment shortens the clinical course of the illness and reduces the duration of faecal excretion of shigellas. Antibiotics that are well absorbed following oral administration are best, since the organisms are located within the tissues of the intestinal mucosa. Ampicillin, tetracyclines, trimethoprim–sulphamethoxazole, furazolidone, nalidixic acid and the fluoroquinolones are all effective against susceptible shigella strains, but resistance to the first three agents is now widespread in many tropical countries. Administration of antimotility agents is contraindicated in shigellosis, as they may interfere with elimination of the organisms by peristalsis.

Salmonellosis

Salmonella organisms are serologically extremely diverse, but at present are grouped into only three species:

• *S. typhi* – the cause of typhoid fever, an 'enteric fever';

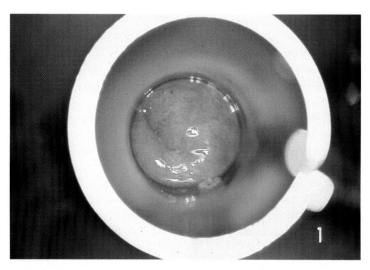

Fig. 4.33 Shigellosis. Sigmoidoscopic view of colonic mucosa in a mild case of infection due to *Shigella flexneri*. Note the thin whitish exudate, which is made up of fibrin and polymorphonuclear leucocytes. By courtesy of Dr R. H. Gilman.

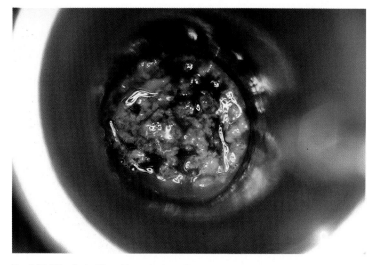

Fig. 4.34 Shigellosis. Sigmoidoscopic view of colonic mucosa in a fatal case of infection with *Shigella dysenteriae* type 1 showing extensive pseudomembranous colitis. By courtesy of Dr R. H. Gilman and Dr F. Koster.

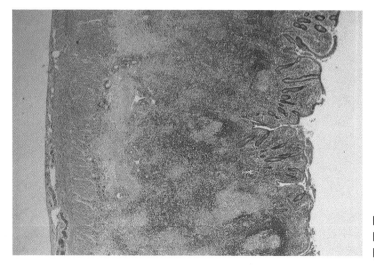

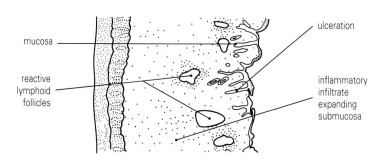

Fig. 4.35 Histological appearance of the ileum in typhoid fever showing prominent lymphoid hyperplasia and small slit-like ulcers. At this magnification the initial impression is one of lymphoma. ×10. H & E stain.

•*S. choleraesuis* – often causes a septic, bacteraemic illness with focal metastatic infection;

•*S. enteritidis* (more than 1700 serotypes) – usually causes a self-limited enterocolitis, but certain serotypes may also cause enteric fever and other syndromes.

Salmonella typhi

S. typhi is exclusively a human pathogen, and is highly adapted to man. It causes typhoid fever, an enteric fever syndrome in which diarrhoea is rarely a prominent manifestation. Most infections with *S. typhi* are acquired by ingestion of contaminated water, food or milk. Since man is the only source of *S. typhi*, it is possible to control typhoid fever by eliminating human faecal contamination from water supplies and foods. In industrialized countries most cases of typhoid fever occur either in immigrants from endemic areas or in people returning from holidays in areas where the disease is common. It is also occasionally seen in young children who have acquired the disease from an older member of the household who is a chronic carrier of *S. typhi* and prepares food for the family. This has led to the aphorism 'to culture the grandmother'.

The organism invades the intestinal epithelium, with prominent involvement of Peyer's patches (Fig. 4.35) and production of ulceration (Figs 4.36 & 4.37). The inflammatory infiltrate in the mucosa is composed primarily of mononuclear cells (Fig. 4.38) and large numbers of mononuclear cells may be present in the faeces (Fig. 4.39).

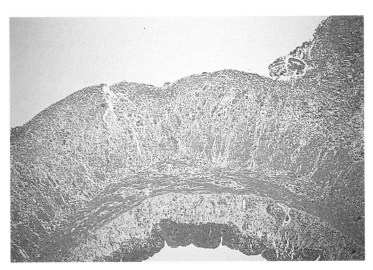

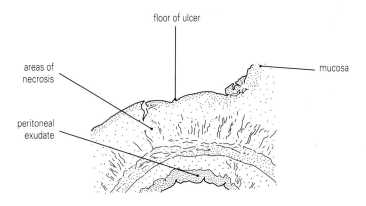

Fig. 4.36 Typhoid fever. Section of ileum showing a typhoid ulcer. There is a transmural inflammatory reaction, focal areas of necrosis and a fibrinous exudate on the serosal surface. H & E stain. By courtesy of Prof. M. S. R. Hutt.

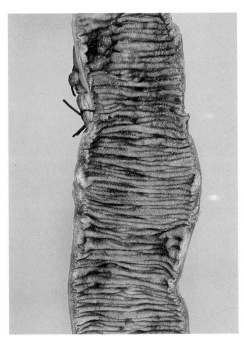

Fig. 4.37 Typhoid fever. Numerous ulcers of the small intestine overlying hyperplastic lymphoid follicles (Peyer's patches). By courtesy of Dr J. Newman.

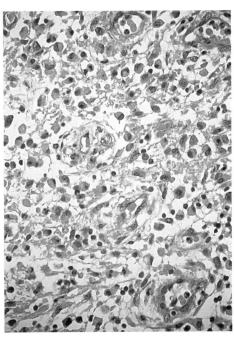

Fig. 4.38 Typhoid fever. Fig. 4.36 at higher magnification showing the typical mononuclear inflammatory cell response in the base of a typhoid ulcer. Most of the cells are macrophages. Note the absence of neutrophils. H & E stain. By courtesy of Prof. M. S. R. Hutt.

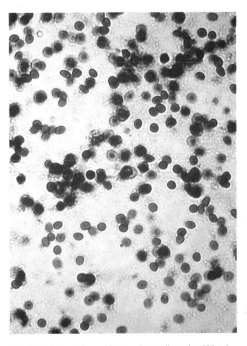

Fig. 4.39 Typhoid fever. Mononuclear cells and red blood cells in the stool. Trichrome stain. By courtesy of Dr H. L. DuPont.

Following an incubation period of 10–14 days, fever, malaise, anorexia, headache and myalgias develop. Remittent fever increases to a level of approximately 40°C by the end of the first week of illness (Fig. 4.40). Cough, sore throat, abdominal pain, chills, nausea and vomiting, diarrhoea or constipation, epistaxis, confusion, lethargy and delirium may also occur. The patient usually appears acutely ill. Rose spots, erythematous maculopapular lesions 2–4mm in diameter that blanch on pressure, often appear on the abdomen (Figs 4.41 & 4.42). Usually less than 12 lesions are present, and they disappear within a few days. Enlargement of the liver and/or spleen is observed in approximately 50% of patients. Untreated, typhoid fever usually resolves 3–4 weeks after onset of illness. Effective antibiotic therapy shortens the duration of illness and fever usually resolves 3–5 days after the insti-

tution of therapy. Serious complications, including perforation, haemorrhage and toxic megacolon (Fig. 4.43) are rare in patients receiving appropriate therapy. Clinical relapse occurs in approximately 10% of patients, treated or untreated; the relapse rate may be significantly increased in patients treated with chloramphenicol.

Excretion of the organism in the faeces for several weeks after recovery is common, but a chronic carrier state (excretion of the organism for more than one year) develops in up to 3% of patients with typhoid fever. Older age, female sex and presence of disease of the biliary tract, especially cholelithiasis (hence the 'fat female over 40') are all factors associated with increased incidence of chronic biliary carriage of *S. typhi*. Stones in the urinary tract and infection of the bladder with *Schistosoma haematobium* are associated with chronic urinary carriage of *S. typhi*.

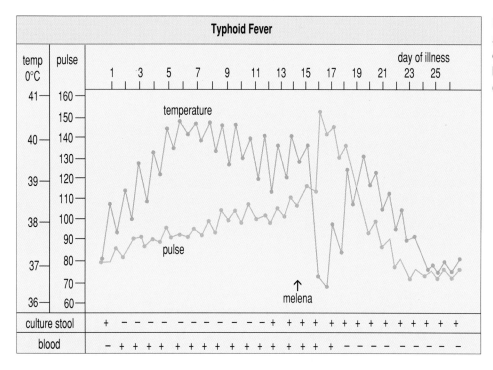

Fig. 4.40 Typhoid fever. Chart showing temperature, pulse rate and bacteriological findings in a patient whose course was complicated by a massive haemorrhage. Note the initial bradycardia with stepwise increase in the pulse rate. By courtesy of Dr H. L. DuPont.

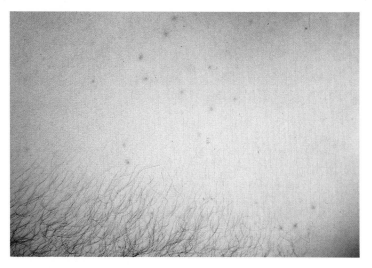

Fig. 4.41 Typhoid fever. Rose spots, small maculopapular erythematous lesions usually seen on the abdomen. By courtesy of Dr A. M. Geddes.

Fig. 4.42 Typhoid fever. Close-up view of rose spots.

Chloramphenicol, ampicillin, amoxicillin, trimethoprim-sulphamethoxazole and ciprofloxacin, given in full dosage for at least 2 weeks, have all been effective in the treatment of typhoid fever. Many other antimicrobial agents, effective against *S. typhi in vitro*, have not proved to be effective clinically. For treatment of the chronic carrier state in a patient who has a normally functioning gall bladder without evidence of cholelithiasis, ampicillin (4–6g per day) combined with probenecid (2g per day), given as four oral doses per day for six weeks is the treatment of choice. If gallbladder disease is present, and if there is no contraindication to surgery, cholecystectomy should be performed. Even without cholecystectomy about 25% of chronic *S. typhi* carriers with biliary tract disease can be cured with ampicillin. Trimethoprim–sulphamethoxazole plus rifampin and ciprofloxacin given as a single agent have also been effective in the treatment of chronic carriers of *S. typhi*.

The other species of salmonella are pathogens of lower animals which are transmitted incidentally to man. Poultry and egg products account for about 50% of human cases; meats, dairy products, pet turtles and person-to-person spread within hospitals account for most of the remainder. Many cases of salmonellosis are sporadic, but large and small outbreaks traceable to a common source also occur frequently. In a typical instance, a food handler becomes infected through the handling of infected chicken carcasses. His hands then become contaminated from his faeces and small numbers of organisms are inoculated into food which he prepares. If this food is held at a temperature favorable for growth of salmonellas, the small inoculum of organisms may grow to a large population capable of producing infection in most individuals who eat the food. Similarly, batches of powdered egg products containing thousands of eggs may become contaminated through inclusion of a single heavily infected egg. The large animal reservoir of salmonella species other than *S. typhi* has made it impossible to prevent a steady increase in the incidence of human salmonellosis during the past several decades.

Asymptomatic infection is extremely common. This is especially important in food handlers, who are both at high risk due to occupational exposure and responsible for transmission to others.

Infection with salmonella species other than *S. typhi* can cause several different clinical syndromes:

• Enterocolitis – fever, nausea and vomiting, myalgia and headache followed by diarrhoea. Usually a self-limiting disease lasting 2–3 days.

• Enteric fever – similar to typhoid fever (fever, muscle aches and headache without diarrhoea) but usually milder and of shorter duration. Severe intestinal infection may produce histopathological changes similar to those seen in typhoid fever (Fig. 4.44).

• Localized infection – metastatic infection of vascular structures, bone and a wide variety of other tissues secondary to bacteraemia . This type of disease is especially common in infection due to *S. choleraesuis*.

• Bacteraemia with recurrences following antibiotic therapy in patients with AIDS.

Faecal excretion of the organism for a few weeks following infection is very common, but persistent faecal excretion for more than a year after symptomatic or asymptomatic infection is rare (less than 1%) with organisms other than *S. typhi*.

Antimicrobial therapy is not indicated in the usual case of salmonella enterocolitis, which lasts only 2–3 days without treatment. Administration of bacteriostatic agents such as chloramphenicol may prolong the duration of faecal excretion of the organism or even exacerbate the diarrhoea. Enteric fever, localized infections and bacteraemia should be treated with antimicrobial agents. Chloramphenicol, ampicillin, amoxicillin, trimethoprim–sulphamethoxazole and ciprofloxacin have all been effective in the treatment of these more serious infections.

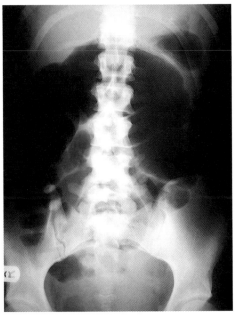

Fig. 4.43 Salmonellosis. Plain abdominal x-ray film showing distended, gas-filled colon in a patient with toxic megacolon.

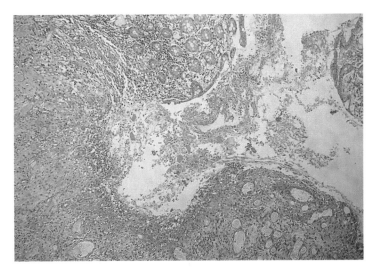

Fig. 4.44 Salmonellosis. Flask-shaped undermining ulcer with necrosis of the epithelium and extrusion of necrotic tissue, fibrin and mucus. By courtesy of Dr J. Newman.

Antibiotic resistance, including multiple resistance, is common in salmonellas and varies in different parts of the world, so therapy should be based upon determination of *in vitro* susceptibility of the infecting strain.

Bacteriological diagnosis of typhoid fever can be made by isolation of the organism from the blood during the first weeks of the illness in more than 80% of patients. Stool cultures are usually positive during the second, third and fourth weeks of the illness. In infections due to other species of *Salmonella*, the organism may be isolated from the stools in patients with enterocolitis or from the blood in patients with enteric fever or other types of bacteraemia. The organisms are lactose-negative and colonies may be differentiated from those of *E. coli* and other lactose-fermenting organisms on MacConkey agar and other selective media (Fig. 4.45). In metastatic abscesses or other types of localized infections the organisms can usually be readily isolated from specimens taken from the lesion.

Campylobacter Infection

Campylobacters are motile, non-spore-forming, comma-shaped, gram-negative rods formerly included in the genus *Vibrio* (Fig. 4.46). The half-dozen species are mainly pathogens or commensals of a wide variety of mammals and birds. The most important human pathogen is *C. jejuni*.

Campylobacter infection is a worldwide zoonosis. These organisms inhabit the gastrointestinal tracts of many wild and domestic mammals and fowl. Intestinal carriage following initial infection in these animals may be lifelong; this vast animal reservoir is the source of most human infections. Humans acquire the organism by ingesting contaminated food (especially undercooked meat), water or unpasteurized milk. Less common routes of infection are through direct contact with infected pets, occupational exposure to farm animals or person-to-person transmission. Asymptomatic infection in food handlers is uncommon, in contrast to the situation with salmonellosis. In industrialized countries this infection is probably more common than salmonellosis or shigellosis. The prevalence of asymptomatic infection is very low. In developing countries up to 40% of children under 2 years may be infected and the organism is an important cause of diarrhoea in travellers to these countries.

The infective dose for campylobacters is similar to that for salmonellas, significantly higher than the minimum infective dose for shigellas. There may be a prodrome of fever, malaise, headache and myalgias for up to a day, prior to onset of abdominal pain and diarrhoea, which may be mild or severe. Unless the proper microbiological studies are done the disease may be misdiagnosed as ulcerative colitis or Crohn's disease. *C. jejuni*, like the *Yersinia* species, may produce a pseudo-appendicitis syndrome of terminal ileitis and mesenteric adenitis. Untreated patients usually excrete the organisms for 2–3 weeks after recovery. Antibiotic treatment results in rapid elimination of campylobacter organisms from the faeces, unlike the case in salmonellosis.

Histopathological examination reveals a diffuse, haemorrhagic, oedematous and exudative enteritis often accompanied by a non-specific colitis (Fig. 4.47). Although the organisms invade the intestinal mucosa in both man and lower animals, bacteraemia is rare (less than 1%) in human infections. Both enterotoxins and cytotoxins are produced by *C. jejuni*, but their significance in the pathogenesis of the infection is unknown.

C. fetus is also an important cause of human infections.

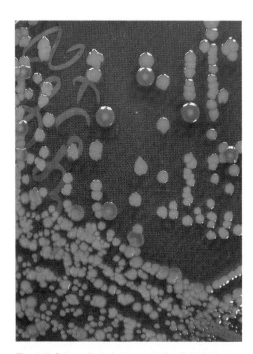

Fig. 4.45 Salmonellosis. Lactose-negative (light pink) colonies of salmonella growing on MacConkey agar, with a few lactose-positive (deep pink) colonies of *E.coli*. By courtesy of Dr J. .Hutchison.

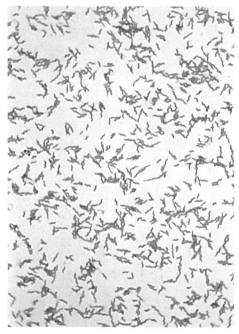

Fig. 4.46 *Campylobacter jejuni* infection. Gram stain showing gram-negative, comma-shaped bacilli of *C. jejuni*. By courtesy of Dr I. Farrell.

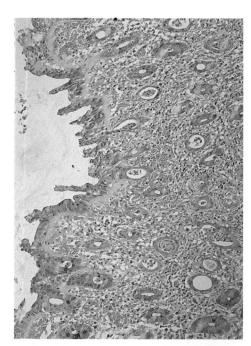

Fig. 4.47 *Campylobacter jejuni* infection. Inflammatory enteritis involving the entire mucosa with flattened, atrophic villi, necrotic debris in the lumina of the crypts and thickening of the basement membrane. Cresyl-fast violet stain. By courtesy of Dr J. Newman.

Diarrhoeal disease is less common with this species, which more often produces systemic infection with bacteraemia and a wide variety of localized infections, especially in patients in whom the immune system is impaired. The organism seems to have a special ability to produce vascular infections such as endocarditis, mycotic aneurysm and thrombophlebitis.

A diagnosis of campylobacter infection is suspected on finding the comma-shaped, S-shaped or spiral organisms in a stool specimen stained with Gram or carbol-fuchsin stains (Fig. 4.48). Microbiological diagnosis is confirmed by isolating the organism from either stools or blood, depending upon the type of infection. These organisms are microaerophilic, growing best in an atmosphere of 5–10% oxygen. Incubation at 42°C, the addition of cephalothin to the medium or passage of the specimen through a 0.65µm filter may facilitate isolation of campylobacter from faecal specimens.

Most patients with diarrhoeal disease due to campylobacters can be treated effectively with replacement of fluid and electrolyte losses, without antibiotic therapy. As with salmonellosis, no clinical benefit can be demonstrated in the treatment of mild cases of diarrhoeal disease. Antimicrobial therapy should be used in the patient who has high fever, bloody diarrhoea or more than 8 stools per day, in the patient who is getting worse or has not begun to improve by the time the diagnosis is made, and in the patient who remains symptomatic for longer than a week. Erythromycin appears to be beneficial in the treatment of severe illness. Campylobacters are extremely susceptible to the newer fluoroquinolone agents *in vitro,* and limited experience indicates that these agents are effective in the treatment of campylobacter infections. Campylobacters are resistant to the penicillins and to trimethoprim–sulphamethoxazole.

Infections due to *Yersinia enterocolitica* and *Y. pseudotuberculosis*

Yersinia enterocolitica is a widely distributed pathogen of animals which causes diarrhoea in humans primarily in cooler climates. In some northern European countries, Canada and Australia, *Y. enterocolitica* is more common than *Shigella* and rivals *Salmonella* and *Campylobacter* as a cause of enteric disease. It has been isolated from a wide variety of mammals, birds, fish and invertebrates, and also from lakes, streams, well water and vegetables. Most human infections follow ingestion of contaminated food (especially raw pork), water or milk. Person-to-person transmission is uncommon, but nosocomial spread has occurred. Serotypes 0:3, 0:8 and 0:9 are the most virulent and cause most cases of bacteraemic infection. Isolates from the inanimate environment usually belong to other, non-virulent serotypes. Virulence is associated with plasmids which code for certain specific outer membrane proteins.

The incubation period is 1–10 days. The illness usually lasts 1–2 weeks, but the organism may be found in the stool for several weeks after clinical recovery. In children under the age of 5 years, the most common type of illness is enterocolitis, characterized by diarrhoea, low-grade fever and abdominal pain. White and red blood cells are found in the stools, which are sometimes grossly bloody. Most of these infections are self-limited and serious complications are uncommon.

In older children terminal ileitis (Figs 4.49, 4.50 & 4.51) and mesenteric adenitis (Figs 4.52 & 4.53) are most common. Most patients exhibit fever, leucocytosis, abdominal pain and tenderness in the right lower quadrant. Nausea, vomiting and diarrhoea are present in a minority. The

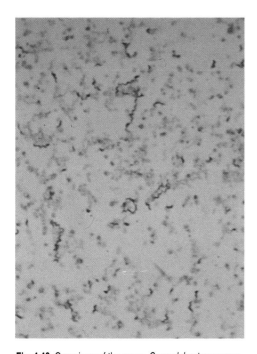

Fig. 4.48 Organisms of the genus *Campylobacter* are now recognized as an important cause of gastroenteritis. They are gram-negative rods; many are curved or show a 'seagull' configuration.

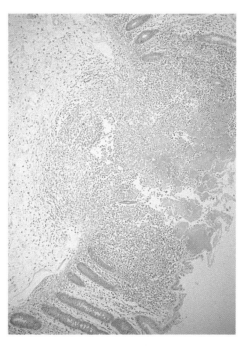

Fig. 4.49 Yersinia infection. Necrosis and ulceration of intestinal mucosa overlying a hyperplastic lymphoid follicle. The inflammatory infiltrate is composed primarily of mononuclear cells. By courtesy of Dr J. Newman.

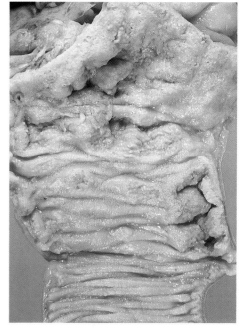

Fig. 4.50 Yersinia infection. Gross specimen of ileum, showing superficial necrosis of the intestinal mucosa with several well-defined deep and superficial ulcers. By courtesy of Dr J. Newman.

clinical picture may be indistinguishable from acute appendicitis and appendectomy has been performed in many patients. Physical examination may reveal a tender, sausage-shaped mass in the right lower quadrant. Ultrasonography is valuable in distinguishing between the terminal ileitis/mesenteric adenitis syndrome and appendicitis. In these patients the appendix is normal or only slightly inflamed, but the wall of the terminal ileum is grossly thickened with mucosal ulcerations and involvement of Peyer's patches and, on microscopic examination, exhibits inflammation and oedema (see Figs 4.49 & 4.50). *Y. enterocolitica* can be cultured from the tissue of the terminal ileum and from involved lymph nodes.

Bacteraemia and focal extraintestinal infections are seen primarily in older adults. Focal infections include pharyngitis, cellulitis and localized abscesses in various organs. Cirrhosis and haemochromatosis are associated with an increased incidence of bacteraemia due to this organism. Reactive polyarthritis and erythema nodosum also occur most commonly in older patients.

Diagnosis is best made by isolating the organisms, which are lactose-negative, on MacConkey agar. Since *Y. enterocolitica* multiplies at cold temperatures, isolation from stool specimens can be facilitated by cold-enrichment techniques. Agglutinating antibodies appear during the first week and reach a peak in the second week of illness. Cross-reactions occur between antigens of *Y. enterocolitica* and those of *Brucella abortus*, rickettsias, salmonellas and thyroid tissue.

The organism is sensitive to trimethoprim–sulphamethoxazole, aminoglycosides, tetracyclines, third-generation cephalosporins and fluoroquinolones. It is resistant to most penicillins and first-generation cephalosporins. Treatment with antibiotics is not required in cases of enterocolitis or the terminal ileitis/mesenteric adenitis syndrome, but more invasive types of infection such as bacteraemia and focal abscesses should be treated.

Yersinia pseudotuberculosis is primarily a pathogen of wild and domestic mammals and birds around the world. Human infection is uncommon and occurs primarily in individuals who have contact with infected domestic animals. The illness produced in man by *Y. pseudotuberculo-*

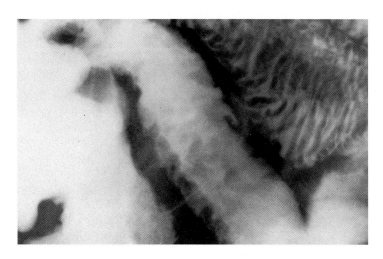

Fig. 4.51 Barium study in a patient with yersinia ileitis showing nodularity and shallow ulceration in the distal ileum.

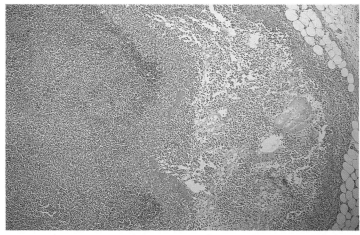

Fig. 4.52 Yersinia infection. Hyperplasia and inflammatory infiltration of a mesenteric lymph node. By courtesy of Dr C. Edwards.

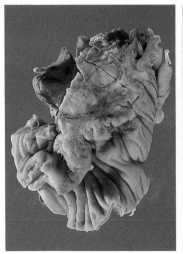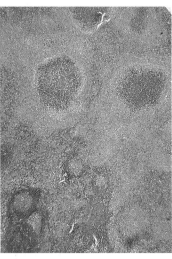

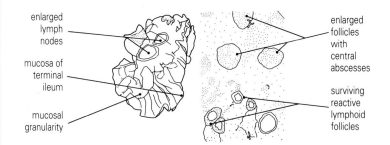

Fig. 4.53 Yersiniosis. Left: Resected ileum showing two enlarged fleshy nodes in the mesentery and some overlying mucosal granularity. The nodes contained the classical necrotic inflammatory foci. Right: The basic nodal architecture is preserved in yersiniosis but many of the follicular germinal centers are replaced with polymorphs with some necrosis from tiny micro-abscesses. ×10. H & E stain.

sis resembles that resulting from *Y. enterocolitica*. Most patients have an appendicitis-like syndrome with fever and pain in the right lower quadrant of the abdomen, caused by terminal ileitis and mesenteric adenitis. A few patients with sepsis and bacteraemia have been reported. *Y. pseudotuberculosis* is more antibiotic-sensitive than *Y. enterocolitica*; otherwise the recommended treatment for the two types of infection is the same.

Clostridium perfringens

Clostridium perfringens type A is a very common cause of food poisoning, and *C. perfringens* type C causes a much more serious necrotizing enteritis in various parts of the world. *C. perfringens* food poisoning is due to a heat-labile enterotoxin released during germination of spores in the food or in the gastrointestinal tract after ingestion. The clinical picture consists of diarrhoea and abdominal cramps, usually without fever or vomiting. Outbreaks usually follow ingestion of meats and gravies. The classic vehicle is a meat pie with a crust: the vegetative cells but not the spores are killed during cooking; the crust maintains anaerobic conditions while the spores germinate; and the bacteria release toxin as the pie cools. Necrotizing enteritis is most often associated with invasion of the bowel wall by *C. perfringens* type C and may be due to the action of the β-toxin, which is a potent lecithinase that causes cell lysis (Fig. 4.54). Sporadic cases are seen around the world, in adults and especially in children. Epidemics have been described in northern Germany (in Darmbrand) in the mid-1940s, and in the highlands of New Guinea during ritual orgiastic feasting on inadequately cooked pork (*pig-bel*). The illness begins suddenly with severe abdominal pain, vomiting, bloody diarrhoea, prostration and shock. Pathological findings include acute patchy necrotizing lesions (Fig. 4.55), which may progress rapidly to segmental gangrene with gas in the mucosa,

mesentery or regional lymph nodes. Gas may be seen radiographically in the wall of the small bowel. Treatment includes supportive care with replacement of food and electrolyte losses and decompression of the bowel. Penicillin G should be given intravenously in large doses and *C. perfringens* type C antiserum containing β-antitoxin should be administered if available. Complications of paralytic ileus, strangulation and perforation of the bowel may necessitate abdominal exploration and resection of involved segments of the intestine.

Antibiotic-associated colitis

Many patients develop mild, transient diarrhoea during or following antibiotic therapy, probably due to alterations in the normal flora of the intestine. A more serious antibiotic-associated colitis (AAC), which may progress to full-blown pseudomembranous colitis, is associated with the presence of *Clostridium difficile* and its cytotoxins. This organism is present in the intestinal tract in approximately 3% of normal adults. The prevalence may be much higher in some populations, especially in hospitalized patients who are elderly or debilitated or who have recently undergone abdominal surgery. AAC may follow treatment with a wide variety of antimicrobial agents, most commonly ampicillin, clindamycin and cephalosporins, but also including tetracyclines, erythromycin, trimethoprim–sulphamethoxazole and even metronidazole, which is used in the treatment of this disease. The incidence varies widely from one geographical area to the next; the presence of clusters of cases strongly suggests person-to-person spread of the organism. The spores are resistant to many environmental influences and can persist for long periods on the hands of hospital personnel. Most strains of *C. difficile* isolated from patients with AAC produce toxins A and B; the colitis apparently results from production of toxin in the intestinal lumen. Approximately 90% of adult

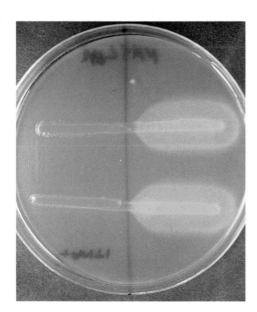

Fig. 4.54 *Clostridium welchii (perfringens)*. Nagler's reaction detects the lecithinase produced by *C. welchii* which gives a precipitate in egg yolk media. There are two parallel streams of growth. Zones of opacity are seen on the right half but not on the left, on which antitoxin was placed before inoculation.

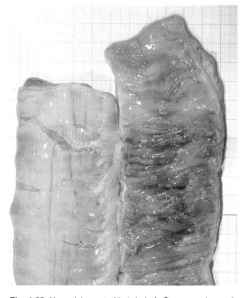

Fig. 4.55 Necrotizing enteritis (*pig-bel*). Gross specimen of small bowel from a case seen in Uganda. The lower piece of opened jejunum shows the greyish-black areas of necrosis, particularly involving the superficial part of the transverse mucosal folds. By courtesy of Professor M. S. R. Hutt.

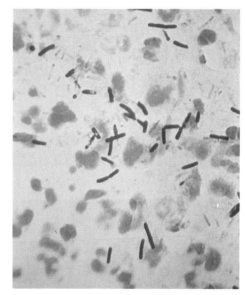

Fig. 4.56 Antibiotic-associated colitis. Gram stain of faeces showing large gram-positive spore-forming rod-shaped cells of *C. difficile*, along with small numbers of gram-negative organisms and many inflammatory cells. By courtesy of Dr R. Fekety.

patients with antibiotic-associated diarrhoea who have either *C. difficile* or its toxins demonstrated in the faeces have either gross or microscopic evidence of colitis. On the other hand, up to 50% of newborn infants may be colonized at least transiently with *C. difficile*; these infants remain well in spite of the presence of large amounts of toxin in the bowel.

The role of antibiotic therapy in precipitating AAC is not fully understood. These agents may suppress the normal bacterial flora, allowing overgrowth of *C. difficile* (Fig. 4.56), or they may stimulate production of toxins by this organism. A similar if not identical disease was observed in the pre-antibiotic era, and not all patients who develop pseudomembranous colitis at the present time have received antibiotics.

The disease usually begins 4–10 days after initiation of antibiotic therapy with the explosive onset of profuse, watery or mucoid, green, foul smelling diarrhoea. In about one-third of patients diarrhoea begins after discontinuation of antibiotics, usually within a few days but occasionally up to 6 weeks after therapy has been stopped. Crampy abdominal pain, abdominal tenderness, fever up to 41°C and leucocytosis are commonly present. Approximately half have leucocytes present in the diarrhoeal stools. Signs of acute surgical abdomen, toxic megacolon, perforation of the colon and peritonitis occur in a few patients. The case fatality rate is 10–20% in untreated cases.

The diagnosis is made by demonstrating colitis in association with *C. difficile* and/or its toxins. The characteristic plaques of pseudomembranous colitis are yellowish white, 1–5mm in diameter, with an erythematous border or base (Figs 4.57 & 4.58). They may occur anywhere in the colon, but are most common in the rectosigmoid region where they are readily seen on sigmoidoscopy (Figs 4.59, 4.60 & 4.61). Irregularity of the mucosal outline may be seen on plain x-ray films of the abdomen or on barium enema examination (Fig. 4.62). In a few cases plaques occur only in the proximal colon and colonoscopy is required to visualize them. On microscopic examination they are found to be composed of fibrin, mucus, necrotic epithelial cells and leucocytes (Fig. 4.63). In less severe cases only a diffuse microscopic colitis without plaque formation is present. *C. difficile* is readily isolated from most cases of AAC by culturing stool specimens anaerobically at 35–37°C on selective media. *C. difficile* toxin B may be detected with assays employing monolayers of fibroblasts or other cell lines (Fig. 4.64). Most patients with AAC due to C. *difficile* have large amounts of toxin in their stool filtrates. Neutralization of the cytopathic effects by appropriate antiserum establishes the identity of the toxin.

If the patient has only mild diarrhoea, treatment should consist only of discontinuation of the antibiotic and replacement of fluid and electrolyte losses. If the diarrhoea is severe and/or systemic illness is present, or if the

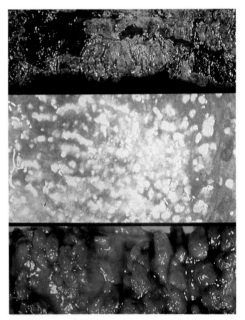
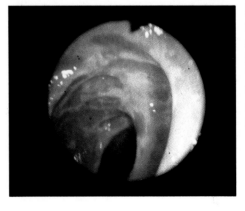

Fig. 4.57 Gross specimens of colons from fatal cases of antibiotic-associated colitis. Top: Extensive inflammatory pseudomembrane. Middle: numerous small plaques, some almost confluent. Bottom: Confluent pseudomembrane covering most of the epithelial surface. By courtesy of Dr F. Pittman (top) and Dr R. Fekety (middle and bottom).

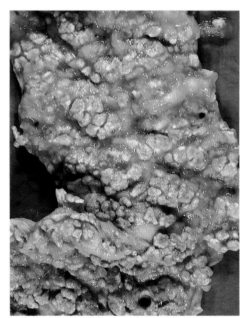

Fig. 4.58 Macroscopic appearance of typical pseudomembranous colitis showing the discrete yellow plaques.

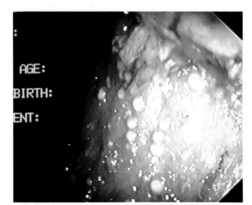

Fig. 4.59 Sigmoidoscopic view of pseudomembranous colitis due to antibiotic treatment. The yellow-white 'membrane' contrasts with the reddened colonic mucosa. By courtesy of Prof. R. Hunt.

Fig. 4.60 Antibiotic-associated colitis. Sigmoidoscopic view demonstrating multiple pseudomembranous lesions in a patient with antibiotic-associated colitis due to *Clostridium difficile*. By courtesy of Dr J. Cunningham.

patient fails to improve within 48 hours on supportive therapy, antimicrobial therapy should be initiated. The most effective agent is vancomycin, given orally. Treatment should be continued for 5–7 days, or until toxin disappears from the stools. In less severe cases, metronidazole may be given. This drug is much less expensive than vancomycin. Limited experience indicates that bacitracin is also effective in the treatment of this disease. Recurrences develop in 10–20% of patients. These should be treated with vancomycin, regardless of which drug was used for initial treatment. Use of opiates and other antimotility agents should be avoided.

Rectal spirochaetosis

Rectal spirochaetosis is a poorly understood condition seen in approximately 36% of homosexual men and less commonly in heterosexual individuals. It is sometimes associated with chronic diarrhoea. The numerous organisms often form a superficial haematoxyphilic layer covering the epithelium (Figs 4.65 & 4.66).

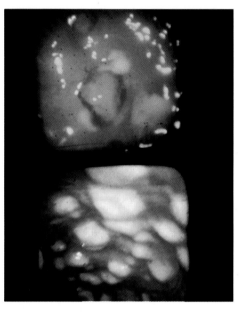

Fig. 4.61 Colonoscopic views of antibiotic-associated colitis. Top: Several whitish or yellowish plaques surrounded by haemorrhagic borders. Bottom: Numerous characteristic whitish plaques. By courtesy of Dr F. Pittman (top) and Dr R. Fekety (bottom).

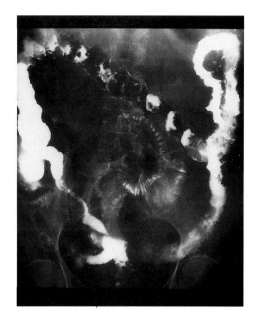

Fig. 4.62 Antibiotic-associated colitis. Barium follow-through showing narrowing of the lumen of the colon, thickened haustral folds ('thumbprinting') and numerous small mucosal ulcerations. By courtesy of Dr R. Noble.

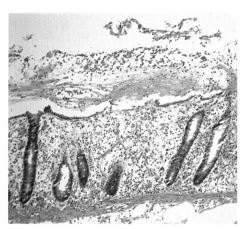

Fig. 4.63 Antibiotic-associated colitis. A section of colon showing intense inflammatory response with the characteristic 'plaque'. H & E stain.

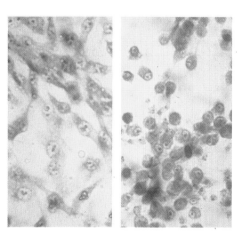

Fig. 4.64 Antibiotic-associated colitis. Assay for *Clostridium difficile* toxin showing normal baby hamster kidney cells (left) and cells after exposure to toxin (right). Note the rounding up of cells following exposure to toxin. By courtesy of Dr R. Fekety.

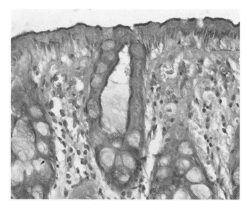

Fig. 4.65 Rectal spirochaetosis. The numerous organisms form a superficial PAS-positive layer over the epithelium. There is also superficial oedema between the basal cell layer and the distorted basement membrane and lymphocytic infiltration of the lamina propria. By courtesy of Dr J. Newman.

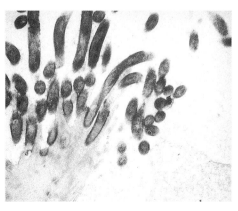

Fig. 4.66 Rectal spirochaetosis. Electron micrograph showing numerous organisms attached to the epithelial surface of the intestinal mucosa. By courtesy of Dr J. Newman.

Tuberculous enteritis

Infection of the gastrointestinal tract by the tubercle bacillus may be either primary or secondary to pulmonary or miliary tuberculosis. Prior to widespread pasteurization of milk, intestinal tuberculosis was often caused by *Mycobacterium bovis*; now in industrialized countries nearly all cases are caused by *M. tuberculosis*. The ileocaecal area is involved most often (Figs 4.67 & 4.68), although extensive involvement of the small bowel and colon may also be seen (Figs 4.69 & 4.70). The most common clinical features are fever, abdominal pain, weight loss and diarrhoea, sometimes with a fixed palpable mass in the ileocaecal area. Obstruction, haemorrhage and malabsorption are occasional complications. On barium studies and even at surgery the hypertrophic or ulcerative lesions may be difficult to distinguish from carcinoma or Crohn's disease (Figs 4.71). Other diseases which may resemble intestinal tuberculosis are sarcoidosis, actinomycosis, amoeboma

and periappendiceal abscess. Definitive diagnosis often requires demonstration of acid-fast bacilli in the tissue by stain or culture (Fig. 4.72). Caseation necrosis is often absent from the intestinal lesion but may be seen in the mesenteric nodes (Figs 4.73 & 4.74). Treatment is the same as for other forms of extrapulmonary tuberculosis.

Mycobacterium avium–intracellulare

Approximately 50% of AIDS patients who have disseminated infection with *Mycobacterium avium–intracellulare* (MAI) have involvement of the intestine. These patients have, in addition to the fever, malaise and weight loss exhibited by all patients with disseminated MAI infection, have chronic diarrhoea and abdominal pain. Like other patients with disseminated MAI infection, they have persistent bacteraemia, but also have positive stool cultures for this organism. Histopathological studies of the gut typically show absent or poorly formed granulomas and acid-

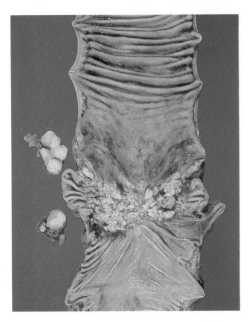

Fig. 4.67 Tuberculous enteritis. Transverse ulceration and caseous necrosis involving the intestinal wall and adjacent lymph nodes. By courtesy of Dr J. Newman.

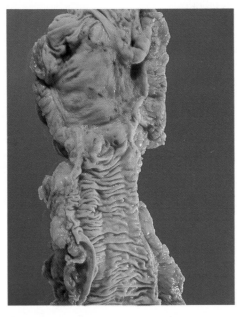

Fig. 4.68 Macroscopic appearance of the ileocaecal region in intestinal tuberculosis, showing the thickened, flattened, featureless caecal mucosa and small haemorrhagic ulcers.

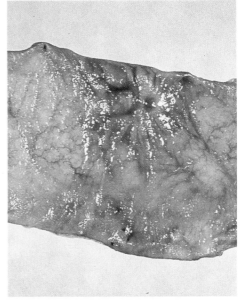

Fig. 4.69 Tuberculosis enteritis. Autopsy specimen of colon showing an oval ulcer. The bowel wall is generally somewhat thickened.

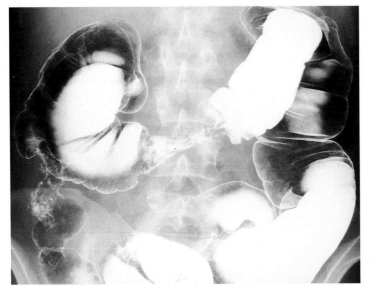

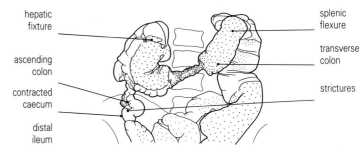

Fig. 4.70 Barium enema showing tuberculous stricturing in the transverse colon and ascending colon.

fast bacilli within macrophages (Fig. 4.75). There are two clinical syndromes, which may overlap: chronic diarrhoea and abdominal pain in patients with invasion of the colon; and chronic malabsorption and steatorrhoea with Whipple's disease-like histopathological changes in the small bowel (Fig. 4.76). The latter patients have large numbers of mycobacteria within macrophages in the lamina propria of the small intestine and enlarged mesenteric lymph nodes infiltrated with acid-fast bacteria (Fig. 4.77).

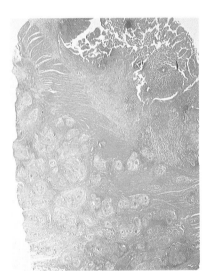

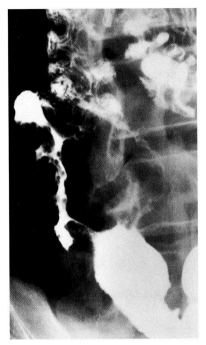

Fig. 4.71 Barium enema in hypertrophic TB, mainly affecting the ascending colon in a 32-year-old Indian presenting with a large mass in the right iliac fossa.

transverse colon
ascending colon
hypertrophic mass
appendix
ileocaecal sphincter
contracted caecum
distal ileum

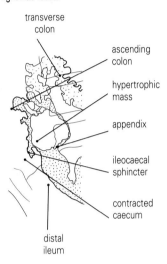

Fig. 4.72 An acid-fast mycobacterium (M). ×1200. Ziehl-Neelsen stain.

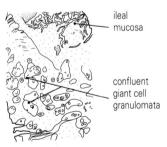

Fig. 4.73 Confluent giant cell granulomata penetrating the full thickness of the intestinal wall in tuberculosis. By contrast, in Crohn's disease the granulomata are smaller and usually solitary. ×10. H & E stain.

ileal mucosa
confluent giant cell granulomata

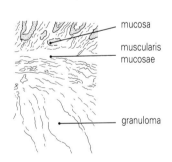

Fig. 4.74 Tuberculous enteritis. Histological section of colon showing a granuloma with lymphocytes, epithelioid cells and giant cells, but without caseation, in the submucosa. H & E stain.

mucosa
muscularis mucosae
granuloma

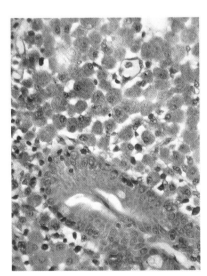

Fig. 4.75 Enteritis due to *Mycobacterium avium–intracellulare*. FITE stain showing acid-fast organisms (red) and intense chronic inflammatory response without granuloma formation in a patient with AIDS. By courtesy of Dr M. B. Cohen.

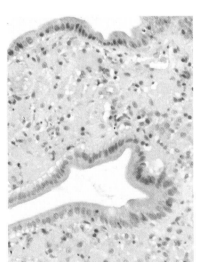

Fig. 4.76 Enteritis due to *Mycobacterium avium–intracellulare*. Section of small intestine from a patient with AIDS with a Whipple's disease-like syndrome, showing many foam-filled microphages in the lamina propria. By courtesy of Dr R. S. Markin.

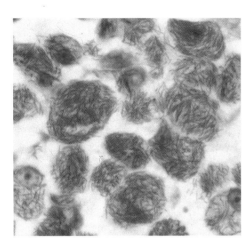

Fig. 4.77 Enteritis due to *Mycobacterium avium–intracellulare*. Acid-fast stain of a section of small intestine in a patient with AIDS, showing abundant acid-fast bacilli in macrophages. By courtesy of Dr R. S. Markin.

Most isolates of MAI are susceptible to ansamycin (rifabutine), clofazimine, cycloserine, ethambutol and ethionamide, but are resistant to isoniazid and rifampin. However, treatment with even the most active agents has been ineffective. In most patients bacteraemia, diarrhoea and abdominal pain continue unabated until death, which usually occurs within 6 months of onset of the clinical syndrome. Whether or not it is worthwhile even to attempt antimicrobial treatment of these patients is an undecided question.

Tropical sprue

Tropical sprue is an inflammatory disease of the small

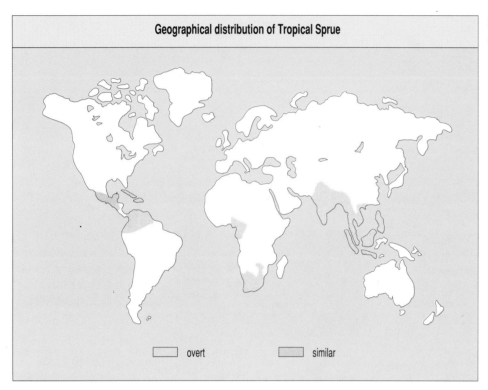

Geographical distribution of Tropical Sprue

☐ overt   ☐ similar

Fig. 4.78 Map showing the distribution of tropical sprue and disorders resembling sprue.

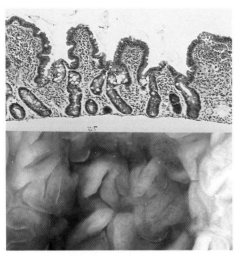

Fig. 4.79 Partial villous atrophy in tropical sprue. Top: Jejunal biopsy showing moderate partial villous atrophy. The villi are squat and the ratio of villus height to crypt depth approaches unity. ×10. H & E stain. Bottom: The dissecting microscope view shows the pattern of convolutions or ridges representing severe partial villous atrophy.

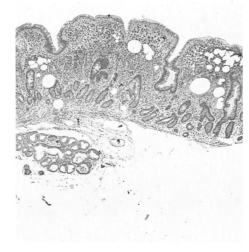

Fig. 4.80 Whipple's disease. Small intestinal biopsy. Subtotal villous atrophy with marked blunting of villi. By courtesy of Dr J. Cunningham

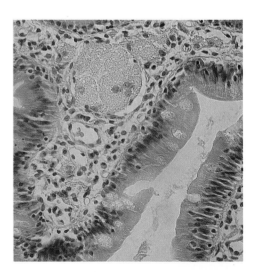

Fig. 4.81 Whipple's disease. Focus of large lipid-containing macrophages in the lamina propria of the intestine. PAS stain. By courtesy of Dr C. Edwards.

bowel mucosa with many features which suggest that it is an infectious disease. The geographic distribution includes the Caribbean area, northern South America, tropical and southern Africa, India and southeast Asia (Fig. 4.78). It occurs in both natives and expatriates from temperate regions, usually after one or two years residence in the tropics. Both sporadic and epidemic cases are seen.

Onset, at least in expatriates, is often acute with explosive diarrhoea accompanied by fever, malaise, weakness and nausea; this is followed by chronic diarrhoea, abdominal distention and crampy abdominal pain. Examination of fluid from the upper small intestine reveals contamination by coliform bacteria, most commonly *Klebsiella pneumoniae*, with *E. coli* or *Enterobacter cloacae* found less frequently. Most bacterial strains isolated from patients produce heat-labile and heat-stable enterotoxins which differ from the LT and ST toxins of *E. coli*. Many of the strains also produce ethanol, which may damage the intestinal mucosa. Tropical sprue may be a consequence of chronic contamination of the small intestine by toxigenic coliform bacteria following an initial episode of acute bacterial enteritis.

Eventually symptoms of folate deficiency develop, including glossitis, anaemia and weight loss. There is net secretion of water and electrolytes in the small bowel and malabsorption of carbohydrate, amino acids, fats and vitamins.

Definitive diagnosis is made by examination of the stools to exclude giardia and other parasites and intestinal biopsy to exclude gluten enteropathy, Whipple's disease and lymphoma. Histopathological findings include broadening and shortening of the villi, with infiltration of the mucosa by chronic inflammatory cells (Fig. 4.79).

Treatment with folate alone often relieves the symptoms but usually does not restore intestinal morphology and function to normal. Addition of tetracycline and a vitamin B_{12} regimen usually results in prompt clinical improvement and eventual healing of the inflammatory lesion.

Whipple's disease

Whipple's disease is a chronic multisystem disease in which the small intestine and associated lymph nodes are prominently involved. Diarrhoea is present in nearly all cases. Microscopic examination of the small intestine shows villous atrophy (Fig. 4.80), dilated lacteals containing fat droplets (Fig. 4.81), and large numbers of macrophages with foamy cytoplasm which contains many periodic acid–Schiff (PAS) positive 'sickle-form' particles (Fig. 4.82 & 4.83). Similar findings may be present in the draining lymph nodes (Fig. 4.84). Electron microscopy

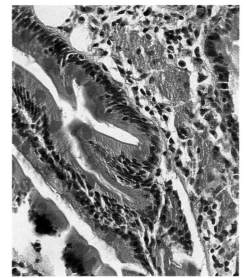

Fig. 4.82 Whipple's disease. High power view showing the diagnostic diastase-resistant PAS-positive material in submucosal macrophages. By courtesy of Dr J. Cunningham.

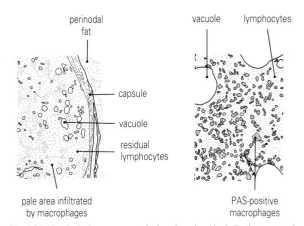

Fig. 4.83 Whipple's disease. Intestinal mucosa stained by the PAS reagent method showing typical PAS-positive material within large macrophages in the lamina propria. By courtesy of Dr C. Edwards.

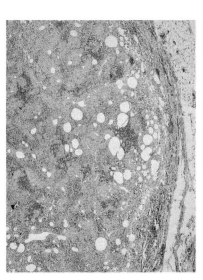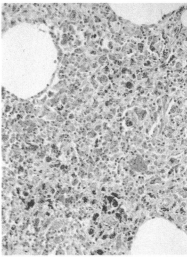

perinodal fat

capsule

vacuole

residual lymphocytes

pale area infiltrated by macrophages

vacuole

lymphocytes

PAS-positive macrophages

Fig. 4.84 Histological appearance of a lymph node with similar features to those in the small bowel. The architecture is distorted by the macrophage infiltrate and large vacuoles. Left: ×30. H & E stain. Right: ×180. PAS stain.

reveals the presence in many tissues of small rod-shaped microorganisms, approximately $0.2 \times 2.0\mu m$ in size, with a homogenous cell wall (Fig. 4.85). These organisms are most abundant in the extracellular spaces of the lamina propria of the small intestine, but have been found in many other tissues of the body. Thus far it has not been possible to grow these organisms in culture or to transmit them to experimental animals. In addition to diarrhoea, a wide variety of other manifestations including fever, weight loss, anaemia, intermittent arthralgias, malabsorption, abdominal pain, lymphadenopathy, skin pigmentation, polyserositis, nonbacterial endocarditis, dementia and various neurological abnormalities may be present. Barium enema may reveal dilated jejunal loops with thickened, nodular folds (Fig. 4.86).

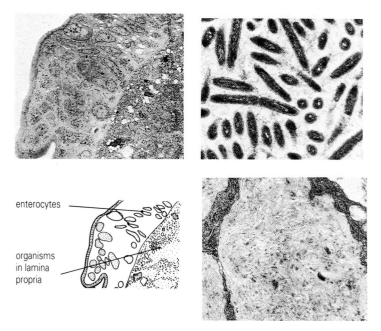

enterocytes

organisms in lamina propria

Fig. 4.85 Electron micrographs of Whipple's disease in the small intestine. Top left: Large numbers of rod-shaped organisms lying free in the lamina propria. ×700. Top right: Individual organisms under high power. ×14 000. Bottom right: Macrophage containing the empty shells of bacteria. Such cells persist long after the active disease state. ×14 000.

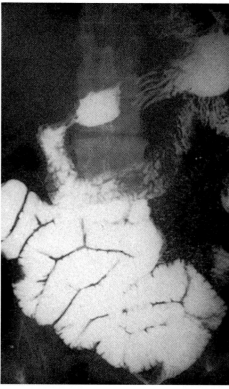

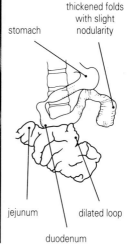

Fig. 4.86 Barium examination of the small intestine in Whipple's disease showing dilated jejunal loops with some thickened, slightly nodular folds proximally.

thickened folds with slight nodularity

stomach

jejunum

dilated loop

duodenum

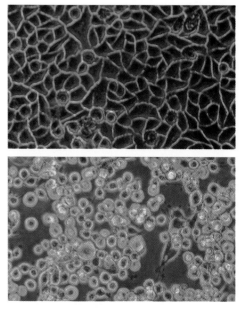

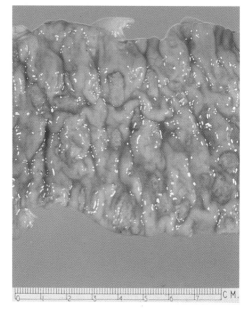

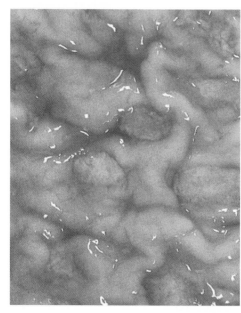

Fig. 4.87 Amoebic colitis. HeLa cell assay for *Entamoeba histolytica* cytotoxin showing normal cell monolayer (top) and cells after exposure to the toxin (bottom). Note the disruption of the monolayer and the rounding up of cells. By courtesy of Dr F. Pittman.

Fig. 4.88 Amoebic colitis. Colon showing discrete ulcerations with surrounding oedema and hyperaemia. (Compare with shigellosis where the entire mucosa is inflamed.) By courtesy of Prof. M. S. R. Hutt.

Fig. 4.89 Macroscopic appearance of the colonic surface showing amoebic ulcers. By courtesy of Dr S. Lucas.

Many patients with Whipple's disease experience prompt remission of symptoms after treatment with antibiotics. In these patients the bacilli disappear from jejunal biopsy specimens and there is improvement in mucosal anatomy. A recommended regimen is penicillin plus streptomycin for two weeks, followed by oral tetracycline administration for approximately one year. About one-third of patients eventually relapse, but the average remission lasts for about 4 years. Treatment with tetracycline alone is less effective. Shorter courses of therapy are usually followed by early relapse. Many relapses after antimicrobial therapy involve the nervous system. This finding has led to the recommendation that patients receive an antibiotic that crosses the blood–brain barrier in the absence of meningeal inflammation, such as trimethoprim–sulphamethoxazole.

The underlying defect which allows the development of Whipple's disease is unknown. A good possibility is that the monocytes and macrophages of these individuals, although able to engulf the bacilli seen in this disease, are unable to destroy and digest them.

As noted above, involvement of the gut by MAI in patients with AIDS may mimic the clinical, histopathological and radiological findings of Whipple's disease.

PROTOZOAL ENTERIC INFECTIONS

Amoebiasis

Entamoeba histolytica is a protozoan parasite which inhabits the wall and lumen of the human colon. It moves by means of pseudopodia and feeds by phagocytosis. There is still debate about whether or not a non-invasive form,

which inhabits only the lumen of the gut and is incapable of damaging the tissues, also exists. The life cycle of this organism is relatively simple. The motile trophozoites invade the bowel wall and also inhabit the lumen. Under certain conditions the trophozoite undergoes encystment within the lumen of the bowel. The cyst passes out of the host in the faeces and, if ingested, passes through the stomach unharmed to reach the small intestine. There it undergoes cell division and conversion into a trophozoite. The cyst form is responsible for transmission via contaminated water or vegetables or by direct faecal–oral spread.

Approximately 10% of the world's population is infected with *E. histolytica*, and more than 10 million cases of invasive amoebiasis occur each year. The prevalence depends upon factors which determine the opportunities for transmission; these factors include sanitation, degree of crowding, socioeconomic status and cultural habits. In some countries 40–50% of individuals may be infected. In the USA the overall prevalence of infection is approximately 4%; however, it is as high as 70% in institutions for the mentally retarded and is about 30% among male homosexuals in New York City. Incidence is also high among migrant workers, immigrants and travellers from endemic areas.

E. histolytica adheres to intestinal mucosal cells by means of specific receptors and produces cytotoxic factors (Fig. 4.87) which enable it to invade the colon with lysis of the mucosal cells. The lesions in the colon range from a non-specific colitis to flask-shaped ulcers which may extend through the mucosa and muscularis mucosae into the submucosa (Figs 4.88 & 4.89). Microscopic examination reveals trophozoites of *E. histolytica* and inflammatory cells in the lamina propria (Figs 4.90, 4.91 & 4.92) and

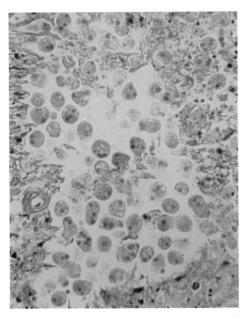

Fig. 4.90 Amoebic colitis. Histological section of bowel wall showing trophozoites of *Entamoeba histolytica*, many containing ingested red blood cells. Due to the shrinkage artifact, the amoebae appear to be lying within a space. H & E stain. By courtesy of Dr K. Juniper.

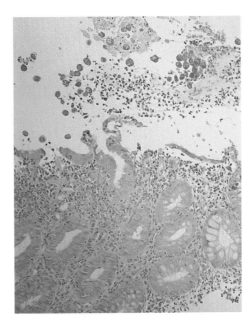

Fig. 4.91 Amoebic colitis. Section of colon showing trophozoites of *Entamoeba histolytica* (stained magenta with the PAS reagent method) embedded in purulent material in the lumen, and an inflammatory infiltrate composed primarily of polymorphonuclear leucocytes in the lamina propria. The lysosomes of the PMN leucocytes also stain magenta with the PAS reagent method. By courtesy of Dr C. Edwards.

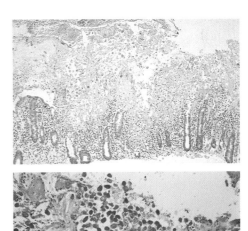

Fig. 4.92 Rectal biopsy in amoebiasis. Top: Invasion of the mucosa can be seen as well as many organisms in the surface debris. ×75. H & E stain. Bottom: Surface debris should be examined carefully, as it may be the only site at which organisms are found. Periodic acid–Schiff reagent stains amoebae magenta; it is the best way of detecting small numbers of organisms. ×180. PAS stain.

on the epithelial surface (Figs 4.93 & 4.94). In the tissue the rounded amoebae are surrounded by a halo which is a result of fixation artifact; the organisms may be distinguished from the host cells by the nuclear morphology, PAS staining and the presence of intracellular erythrocytes (Fig. 4.95). Cell-mediated immunity appears to be more important than humoral immunity in prevention of recurrence of invasive colonic or hepatic disease.

Asymptomatic infection is the most common form of infection with *E. histolytica*. The spectrum of illness pro-

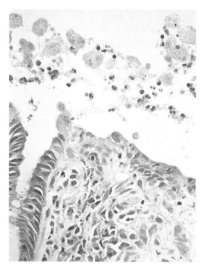
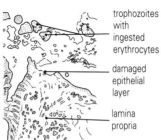

Fig. 4.93 Amoebic colitis. Intestinal biopsy showing loss of mucosal lining cells and sparse infiltrate of inflammatory cells in the lamina propria. Trophozoites and polymorphs are present in the lumen. H & E stain.

trophozoites with ingested erythrocytes

damaged epithelial layer

lamina propria

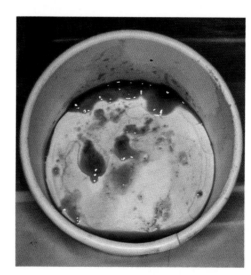

Fig. 4.94 Amoebic colitis. Biopsy of colon showing numerous organisms embedded in fibrin and necrotic material in the lumen, with an acute inflammatory infiltrate composed predominantly of polymorphonuclear leucocytes. By courtesy of Dr C. Edwards.

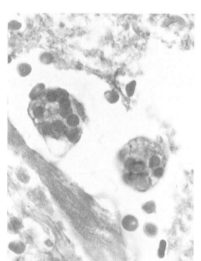

Fig. 4.95 Amoebae with ingested erythrocytes. ×660. H&E stain. By courtesy of Dr S. Lucas.

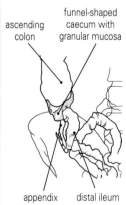

Fig. 4.96 Amoebic colitis. Typical dysentery stool (small volume, blood and mucus) from a patient with acute amoebiasis. By courtesy of Dr H. L. DuPont.

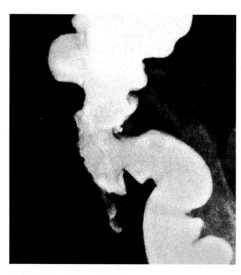

constricted caecum

ileocaecal junction

appendix

Fig. 4.97 Amoebic colitis. Barium study showing amoeboma of caecum. Note constriction and distortion of the caecal region. By courtesy of Dr F. Pittman.

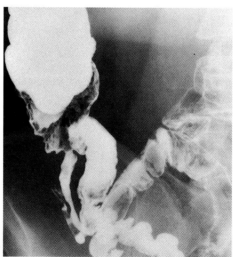

ascending colon

funnel-shaped caecum with granular mucosa

appendix

distal ileum

Fig. 4.98 Barium enema radiograph in chronic amoebic colitis showing a funnel-shaped caecum with granular deformity.

duced by this organism is very broad. The most common type is chronic, mild, intermittent diarrhoea with colicky abdominal pain. More severe diarrhoeal disease may also occur with fever, dysentery (blood, mucus and pus in the stool – Fig. 4.96) and severe abdominal pain and tenderness. Massive infection may be complicated by development of an acute surgical abdomen with severe abdominal pain and distention, vomiting and absent bowel sounds due to perforation of the bowel and combined amoebic and bacterial peritonitis. Toxic megacolon occurs occasionally, especially in patients who have been receiving corticosteroid therapy. Amoeboma, usually occurring in the caecum and ascending colon, may manifest as an annular lesion mimicking carcinoma of the colon or as a palpable mass which resembles a pyogenic abscess (Figs 4.97, 4.98 & 4.99). Chronic intermittent diarrhoea lasting for more than a year may follow an episode of acute amoebic colitis and may resemble non-infectious inflammatory bowel disease.

Extraintestinal infection most often involves the liver (see Chapter 5). From the liver, infection may extend into the pleural space with production of empyema and lung abscess, or into the pericardium. Rarely, brain abscess may occur. In extraintestinal infection there may be no evidence of active amoebic colitis, and the stools may be negative for amoebae.

In intestinal infection, the diagnosis is made by identifying either cysts (Fig. 4.100) or trophozoites (Fig. 4.101) of *E. histolytica* in the stool. Fresh material from a lesion seen at sigmoidoscopy may be suspended in saline and examined on a warm microscope stage for trophozoites. Trophozoites may also be identified in smears stained with iron–hematoxylin or Wheatley's trichrome stains. A stool specimen may be suspended in a formalin–ether solution and the cysts concentrated at the formalin–ether interface by centrifugation and identified after staining with diluted iodine solution. A few laboratories are able to culture *E. histolytica* from clinical specimens. At least three stool specimens should be examined; administration of a saline purge can increase the yield of positive examinations.

Sigmoidoscopy usually reveals a hyperaemic, oedematous mucosa with punctate haemorrhages and small ulcers (Fig. 4.102). The large confluent ulcers described in

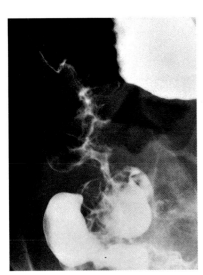
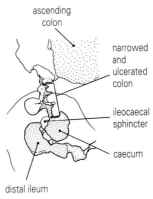

Fig. 4.99 Barium enema showing an amoeboma in the ascending colon.

ascending colon

narrowed and ulcerated colon

ileocaecal sphincter

caecum

distal ileum

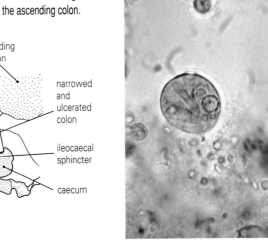

Fig. 4.100 Amoebic colitis. Cyst of *Entamoeba histolytica* showing round shape, refractile wall and multiple nuclei. Iodine stain.

Fig. 4.101 Amoebic colitis. Trophozoites of *Entamoeba histolytica* showing amoeboid form and internal organelles. Eosin stain.

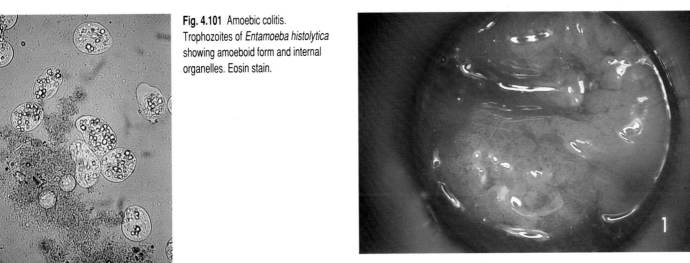

Fig. 4.102 Amoebic colitis. Sigmoidoscopic view of colonic mucosa in a typical case of amoebic dysentery showing the non-ulcerated diffuse colitis which is the predominant form of the disease. By courtesy of Dr R. H. Gilman.

textbooks are seen less commonly (Figs 4.103 & 4.104). In early infections the mucosa may appear normal.

The indirect fluorescent antibody test is usually negative in asymptomatic cyst passers, but is positive in approximately 85% of cases of invasive amoebic colitis and is nearly always positive in amoebic liver abscess.

The optimum treatment regimen varies with the type of disease being treated. Asymptomatic intraluminal infection can be treated with tetracycline in combination with either diiodohydroxyquin or diloxanide furoate. Invasive intestinal disease should be treated with metronidazole followed by treatment with either diiodohydroxyquin or diloxanide furoate. Extraintestinal infection may be treated with the same regimens used in the treatment of invasive intestinal disease. Since a few liver abscesses are not cured with metronidazole plus diiodohydroxyquin or diloxanide furoate, some authorities would add treatment with chloroquine.

Giardiasis

Giardia lamblia is a flagellated protozoan which is a major cause of diarrhoeal disease throughout the world. The organism exists as a free-living trophozoite and as a thin-walled cyst form. Infection is acquired by ingesting the cysts, usually in faecally contaminated water. The disease is a common cause of chronic debilitating diarrhoea in travellers. Well-publicized outbreaks have occurred in visitors to Leningrad and among campers and hikers in western states of the USA. *G. lamblia* infects many animal species including beavers, which may contaminate the water of mountain streams. Up to 50% of children in day-care centres may be infected and the organism is readily spread to family members. Infection is also common among homosexual men and in crowded custodial institutions.

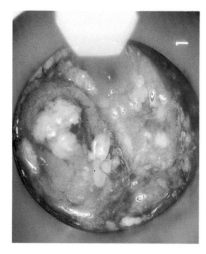

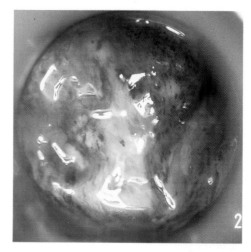

Fig. 4.103 Amoebic colitis. Sigmoidoscopic view of colonic mucosa showing the 'textbook', but less common form of amoebic dysentery, with deep ulcers and overlying purulent exudate. By courtesy of Dr R.H. Gilman.

Fig. 4.104 Amoebic colitis. Sigmoidoscopic view of colonic mucosa showing extensive ulceration with a 'Dyak hair ulcer'. By courtesy of Dr R.H. Gilman.

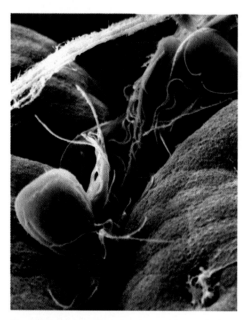

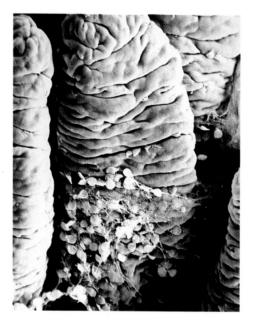

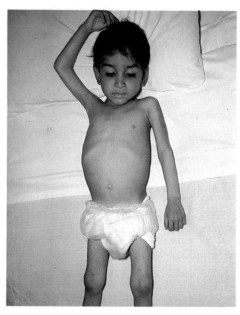

Fig. 4.105 Giardiasis. Scanning electron micrograph of *Giardia lamblia* trophozoites in a crevice of a human jejunal villus. The slightly concave ventral adhesive disc and ventral flagella are seen in the organism upper left; the irregular dorsal surface can be seen in the giardia lower right. ×1550. By courtesy of Dr R.L. Owen.

Fig. 4.106 Electron micrograph showing villi of the mouse jejunum with *Giardia lamblia* trophozoites adhering to the surface near the bases of the villi, wedged into furrows and lying in mucus. By courtesy of Dr R. L. Owen.

Fig. 4.107 Giardiasis. Child with chronic severe infection with *Giardia lamblia*, showing abdominal distention and evidence of malnutrition.

The organism adheres by means of its disc to the brush border of the small intestine (Figs 4.105 & 4.106), sometimes disrupting the integrity of the brush border. *G. lamblia* apparently does not produce an enterotoxin and the mechanism by which it causes diarrhoea is not fully understood. Both cell-mediated and humoral mechanisms appear to be important in recovery from disease and in resistance to infection with *G. lamblia*. Patients with common variable immunodeficiency and X-linked agammaglobulinemia are predisposed to infection with this organism, and selective IgA deficiency may also increase susceptibility to infection.

Infection with *G. lamblia* may result in asymptomatic cyst passage, an acute self-limited episode of diarrhoea, or chronic diarrhoea with malabsorption and weight loss (Fig. 4.107). Symptomatic patients usually have diarrhoea, with stools that are greasy, foul smelling and may float, as well as abdominal cramps, bloating and flatulence, anorexia, malaise and nausea.

Diagnosis is made by finding the organism in the stools or in duodenal aspirate or biopsy material. Liquid stool may be examined directly in a wet mount for the motile trophozoites or cysts (Fig. 4.108). Fresh stool or stool preserved in polyvinyl alcohol may be stained with iron–haematoxylin or trichrome stains. Organisms are found in only about 50% of cases when a single stool specimen is examined. If three stools are examined the detection rate approaches 90%. If stools are negative, duodenal material may be sampled by the Enterotest technique. In this test a nylon string is contained in a gelatin capsule; the free end of the string is secured at the mouth and the capsule is swallowed. After 4–6 hours, or overnight, the string is removed and examined fresh under a wet mount or stained (Fig. 4.109). Examination of aspirated duodenal fluid, duodenal brushings or biopsy specimens may also provide the diagnosis.

Both quinacrine and metronidazole are highly effective in the treatment of giardiasis. Provision of a safe water supply and maintenance of good personal hygiene will prevent transmission of this infection. Travellers in endemic areas should boil water for one minute before drinking, or add halazone (5 tablets per litre) and allow to stand for 30 minutes before drinking.

Cryptosporidiosis

Until recently, *Cryptosporidium* species were thought to be an uncommon cause of mild diarrhoeal disease, occurring primarily in children. Improved techniques for detecting the organism in stool specimens have shown that this infection is relatively common and, in some localities, that it is the most common enteric protozoan infection. In immunocompetent individuals this organism usually causes asymptomatic infection or a transient watery diarrhoea lasting up to ten days, accompanied by abdominal cramps and nausea. Both the symptoms and faecal excretion of organisms subside without antimicrobial treatment. More recently, infection by *Cryptosporidium* species has been found to be a major opportunistic infection in patients with AIDS. Infection in these patients usually results in a relentless, progressive, watery diarrhoea which persists until death. Occasional patients have appeared to respond to therapy, especially with spiramycin, but no treatment has been consistently effective. Involvement of the biliary tract sometimes occurs in patients with AIDS, resulting in a picture of acute biliary colic.

Diagnosis of cryptosporidiosis is made by finding the oocysts in the faeces, using either modified acid fast stains (Fig. 4.110) or iodine stains. The cryptosporidia are acid-fast, but iodine negative. These minute organisms (2–4μm) may also sometimes be seen lining intestinal

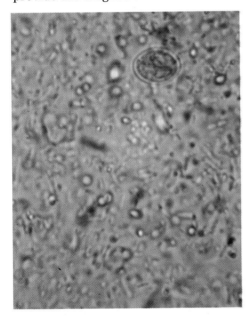

Fig. 4.108 Giardiasis. Cyst of *Giardia lamblia* showing ovoid shape, prominent cyst wall, granular cytoplasm and at least two nuclei. By courtesy of Dr H. L. DuPont.

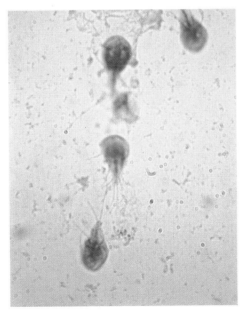

Fig. 4.109 Giardiasis. Trophozoites of *Giardia lamblia* obtained from mucus stripped from an Enterotest string pulled from the duodenum after overnight passage. Note the characteristic shape, paired nuclei and multiple flagella. The patient also had adult acquired hypogammaglobulinaemia. Three stool examinations for *Giardia* had been negative. Trichrome stain. By courtesy of Dr F. Pittman.

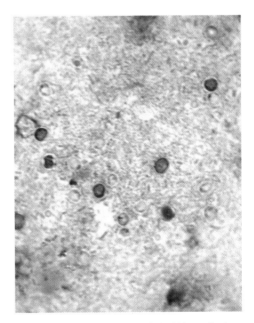

Fig. 4.110 Cryptosporidiosis. Modified acid-fast stain of stool specimen showing characteristic acid-fast *Cryptosporidium* organisms.

epithelial cells in small bowel biopsy specimens (Figs 4.111, 4.112 & 4.113).

Isospora belli

Like organisms of the genus *Cryptosporidium*, *Isospora belli* is a coccidian protozoan parasite which usually produces a mild self-limited diarrhoeal disease in immuno-competent patients, but can produce a severe progressive disease in patients with AIDS (Fig. 4.114). The infection is diagnosed by finding the large (20–30mm) ellipsoidal acid-fast oocysts in the faeces (Fig. 4.115). However, *Isospora belli* infection is not a zoonosis. It usually responds promptly to treatment with either oral trimethoprim–sulphamethoxazole or pyrimethamine–sulphadoxine.

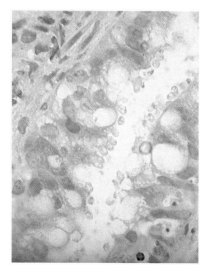

Fig. 4.111 Cryptosporidiosis. Numerous organisms in the brush border of the intestine. By courtesy of Dr J. Newman.

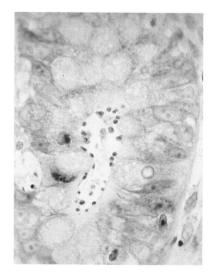

Fig. 4.112 Cryptosporidiosis, with numerous organisms in the brush border of the intestine. Giemsa stain. By courtesy of Dr J. Newman.

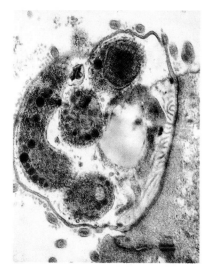

Fig. 4.113 Cryptosporidiosis. Electron micrograph showing mature schizont with several merozoites attached to the intestinal epithelium.

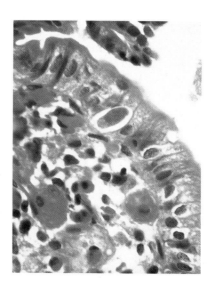

Fig. 4.114 Human coccidiosis. Enteric infection in a patient with AIDS. A single *Isospora belli* organism is seen within an epithelial cell, and there is a chronic inflammatory reaction in the lamina propria. By courtesy of Dr G. N. Griffin.

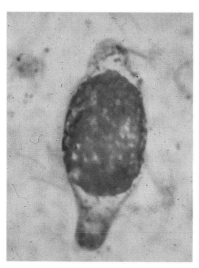

Fig. 4.115 *Isospora belli.* Oocyst in faeces. Modified acid-fast stain. By courtesy of Dr G. N. Griffin.

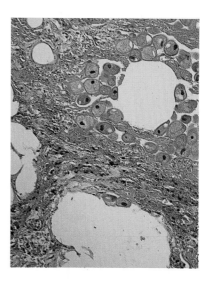

Fig. 4.116 Balantidiasis. Numerous large trophozoites in the wall of the intestine in a patient with AIDS.

Balantidium coli

Balantidium coli is a very large (100μm) oval-shaped ciliated protozoan that causes disease in a number of different mammalian species. Human disease usually occurs in individuals who have close contact with swine. The organism penetrates the mucosa of the colon and multiplies in the submucosa, producing a colitis with blood and mucus in the stool (dysentery). The diagnosis is made by finding the very large cysts or trophozoites in the stool or in biopsy specimens of the bowel (Figs 4.116 & 4.117). The infection can be treated with tetracycline, metronidazole or paromomycin.

Blastocystis hominis

This organism, originally identified as a trichomonad, then long considered a yeast, has finally been identified as a sporozoan protozoa. It is commonly found in intestinal contents of healthy individuals. Its status as a human pathogen is controversial, and many patients who have diarrhoeal disease ascribed to *B. hominis* also have other, better-established enteric pathogens present concomitantly. However, recent reports have associated it with diarrhoea in severely immunocompromised patients, including several patients with AIDS. In a few cases the diarrhoea has responded to treatment with diiodohydroxyquin.

HELMINTHIC ENTERIC INFECTIONS

Schistosomiasis

The schistosomes or blood flukes are parasitic flatworms. Three species are important causes of human infection: *Schistosoma mansoni*, *S. japonicum* and *S. haematobium*. Together they infect more than 200 million people worldwide and the incidence of human infection is increasing. The adult forms of *S. mansoni* and *S. japonicum* inhabit the portal and mesenteric veins; *S. haematobium* inhabits the vesical plexus of the bladder and is discussed in Chapter 6. Man is the principal definitive host for these three species of schistosomes. The worm lives in the venous system of the intestines (Fig. 4.118). The female worm inhabits a groove in the lateral edge of the body of the male (Fig. 4.119) and produces approximately 300 (*S. mansoni*) or 3000 (*S. japonicum*) eggs every day. These find their way into the lumen of the bowel and are excreted in the faeces (Fig. 4.120). In fresh water the eggs hatch and release motile ciliated miracidia which penetrate the body of the intermediate host, usually a snail of the genus

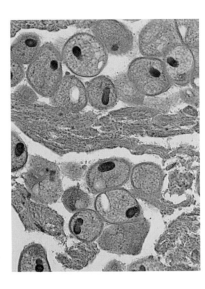

Fig. 4.117 Balantidiasis. Higher magnification showing typical foamy cytoplasm and bean-shaped macronucleus of *B. coli*. By courtesy of Dr J. Newman.

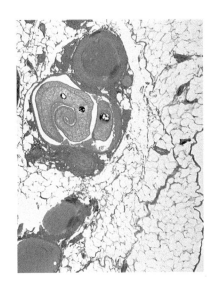

Fig. 4.118 Schistosomiasis. Section of mesentery showing adult *Schistosoma mansoni* worm lodged in the mesenteric vein. H & E stain.

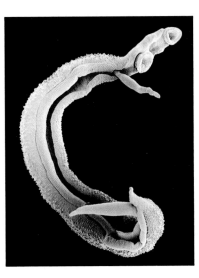

Fig. 4.119 Schistosomiasis. The slender female worm lies in a groove (the gynecophoral canal) in the lateral edge of the body of the male. Scanning electron micrograph. By courtesy of Dr V. Southgate and the publishers of *Systematic Parasitology*.

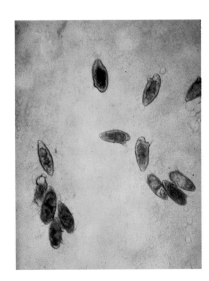

Fig. 4.120 Schistosomiasis. Eggs of *S. mansoni* in faeces showing characteristic lateral spine.

Biomphalaria (*S. mansoni*) or *Oncomelania* (*S. japonicum*). The miracidia multiply asexually inside the snail; within a few weeks, hundreds of motile fork-tailed cercariae emerge. When the cercariae encounter human skin they penetrate it, lose their tails and change into schistosomula forms which migrate to the lungs and liver. In approximately 6 weeks they mature into adult worms which mate and pass through the venous system to their final habitat, where they may live for up to 10 years.

The geographic range of each species of schistosome is determined primarily by two factors: the presence of the specific snail that is the intermediate host; and the method of disposal of human excreta. *S. mansoni* occurs in Arabia, Africa, South America and many Caribbean islands. *S. japonicum* is found in China, Japan, and the Philippines. *S. haematobium* occurs in Africa and the Middle East.

Three major disease syndromes occur in schistosomiasis. They are:

• Schistosome dermatitis;

• Katayama fever;

• Chronic schistosomiasis

Schistosome dermatitis is a pruritic papular skin eruption also known as swimmer's itch. It occurs only in individuals who have been previously exposed to schistosome antigens and represents a sensitization reaction. It may occur up to 24 hours after swimming in contaminated water. It is usually caused by infection with avian rather than human schistosomes and thus is common in temperate regions where human schistosomes are not endemic.

Katayama fever is a serum sickness-like syndrome which occurs in heavy infections at the onset of egg deposition. The clinical picture includes fever, chills, sweating, headache, cough, hepatomegaly, splenomegaly, generalized lymphadenopathy and eosinophilia. The symptoms and signs usually disappear within a few weeks but in massive infection due to *S. japonicum* death may occur.

In chronic schistosomiasis there is a progressive increase in the worm burden which affects primarily the intestines (Figs. 4.121 & 4.122) and liver (Fig. 4.123). Chronic granulomatous lesions occur in these organs and may result in portal hypertension, massive splenomegaly and gastrointestinal bleeding from oesophageal varices (Fig. 4.124). The patient experiences fatigue, abdominal pain and diarrhoea, and in the most severe cases jaundice

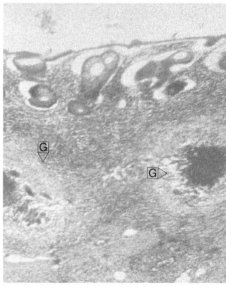

Fig. 4.121 Schistosomiasis. Eggs of *S. mansoni* in mucosa of colon with surrounding granulomatous reaction(G). H & E stain.

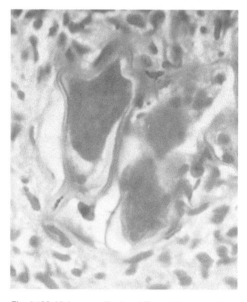

Fig. 4.122 Higher magnification of Fig. 4.121 showing the characteristic lateral spine on one of the eggs. H & E stain.

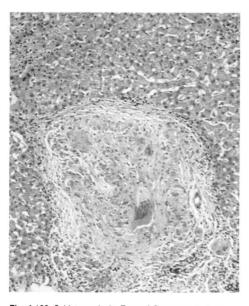

Fig. 4.123 Schistosomiasis. Eggs of *S. mansoni* in liver with surrounding granulomatous reaction. H & E stain.

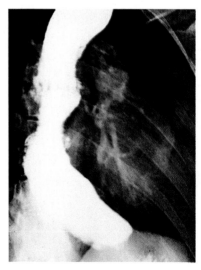

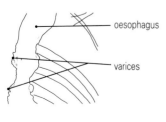

Fig. 4.124 Schistosomiasis. Barium study of oesophagus showing oesophageal varices secondary to portal hypertension in *S. mansoni* infection. By courtesy of Dr I. G. Kagan.

— oesophagus

— varices

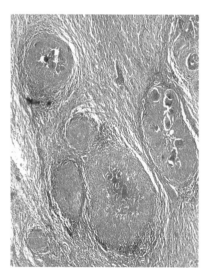

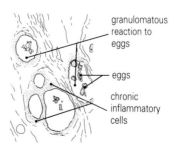

Fig. 4.125 Schistosomiasis. Eggs of *S. japonicum* in gliotic brain with surrounding macrophage and chronic inflammatory cell response. H & E stain.

granulomatous reaction to eggs

eggs

chronic inflammatory cells

and liver failure. Occasionally eggs may bypass the liver via the portalsystemic collateral circulation and give rise to granulomas in the lung with pulmonary hypertension and cor pulmonale, or lesions in the brain (4.125) or spinal cord which may produce the picture of a space-occupying lesion, generalized encephalopathy or transverse myelitis.

Schistosomiasis is diagnosed by finding the characteristic schistosome eggs in the faeces, in the urine or in a biopsy specimen, usually of the rectal mucosa (see Fig. 4.121). Serological tests have been developed but are not of much practical help in most cases. Development of praziquantel has dramatically improved the effectiveness of drug therapy of schistosomiasis. Administration of this drug either cures or drastically reduces the worm burden in nearly all cases. The dosage for *S. mansoni* and *S. haematobium* infection is 40mg/kg, given as a single oral dose; for *S. japonicum* infection the dose is 60mg/kg given as three doses of 20mg/kg on one day. Adverse effects are usually mild and include headache, fever and abdominal discomfort.

Taeniasis

Man is the only definitive host for the beef tapeworm, *Taenia saginata* (Fig. 4.126). Infection occurs when inadequately cooked meat of infected cattle is eaten. The encysted larva (cysticercus) in the meat passes through the stomach; in the presence of bile acids in the intestine the larva is released. It attaches to the wall of the intestine and develops into an adult worm, releasing eggs into the lumen of the gut. When these eggs are ingested by cat-

tle the oncospheres penetrate the intestinal wall and the larval forms develop in the muscle tissue. Human tissue does not support growth of the cysticerci, so man is unable to serve as an intermediate host for this organism, although it can serve as an intermediate host for the pork tapeworm, *T. solium* (see below). Infection with *T. saginata* occurs throughout the world. It is most prevalent in Yugoslavia, Moslem countries, Ethiopia and Kenya. It also occurs, albeit less frequently, in Central and South America. Symptoms are usually minimal and consist only of mild abdominal cramps. Rarely a large mass of proglottids causes intestinal or appendiceal obstruction. Segments of worm up to several feet in length may be passed per rectum. The only systemic reaction to the worm is mild eosinophilia.

Eggs of *T. saginata* are indistinguishable from those of *T. solium* (Fig. 4.127) but presence of taenia eggs in the faeces should stimulate a search for proglottids (tapeworm segments) by which the two species can be distinguished. Niclosamide (4 tablets chewed thoroughly following a light meal) causes expulsion of the adult worm from the intestine. Paromomycin and praziquantel are also effective. Infection with *T. saginata* can be prevented either by thorough cooking of meat or prevention of human faecal contamination of ground upon which cattle are grazing.

Man can serve as both definitive and intermediate host of the pork tapeworm, *T. solium*. The pathogenesis, symptomatology, diagnosis and treatment of intestinal infection with the adult tapeworm are the same as described for *T. saginata*. Man may become the intermediate host for this organism by ingestion of food or water contaminated with

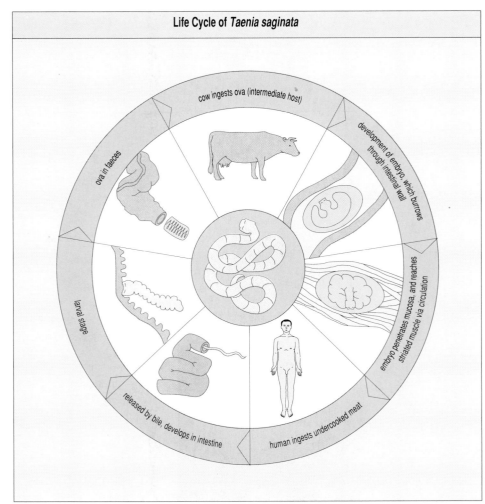

Life Cycle of *Taenia saginata*

cow ingests ova (intermediate host)

development of embryo, which burrows through intestinal wall

ova in faeces

embryo penetrates mucosa, and reaches striated muscle via circulation

larval stage

released by bile, develops in intestine

human ingests undercooked meat

Fig. 4.126 Life cycle of the tapeworm, *Taenia saginata*. A human becomes infected by eating undercooked infected beef. The parasite, released by bile, enters the small intestine where it matures in 2–3 months into a long segmented worm attached to the wall of the intestine by the suckers on its scolex. As segments of the tail mature they are shed into the bowel lumen and escape through the anus. These segments release thousands of eggs, which find their way onto pastures grazed by cattle, especially when sewage is used as fertilizer. If the egg is swallowed by a cow, it develops into an oncosphere, which penetrates the gut wall and enters the circulation. Upon reaching striated muscle it develops into the cysticercus, the infective stage for man. By courtesy of Dr J. Taverne.

infected human faeces, by autoinfection from anus to mouth in an individual already infected with the adult tapeworm and by reverse peristalsis and internal infection. After penetrating the host's intestinal wall the oncosphere develops rapidly and after 10 weeks there is a fully infective larva within the cyst wall (Fig. 4.128). The cysts can develop in almost any part of the body and may produce small mass lesions in the eye, heart, skeletal muscle (Fig. 4.129), skin (Fig. 4.130), or peritoneal cavity. The most important form of cysticercosis is infection of the central nervous system (described in Chapter 3). Both praziquantel and mebendazole are effective in killing the larval stage of the organism, although in many cases the larva has already died and is degenerating at the time symptoms appear.

Diphyllobothrium latum

The adult form of the fish tapeworm *Diphyllobothrium latum* is the largest tapeworm of man, reaching up to 15 metres in length. The eggs released from the gravid proglottids pass out of the body in the faeces and after reaching fresh water, develop into a ciliated oncosphere, the coracidium. This free-swimming form must be eaten within a few days by a copepod (a crustacean), in which it develops into a mature larva called a procercoid. When the copepod is ingested by a fish the procercoid develops into a plerocercoid, or sparganum. If the fish is eaten raw by a mammal the plerocercoid develops after a few weeks into the adult form of *D. latum*.

This infection occurs wherever ingestion of raw fish is common, such as in Scandinavian and Baltic countries, Japan and among Eskimos in Canada and Alaska. In the USA, Israel and elsewhere it is seen among Jewish cooks who sample *gefilte* fish during its preparation.

The symptoms of infection are usually mild but occasionally large masses of the adult worm produce intestinal obstruction. The worm competes with the host for vitamins including vitamin B_{12}; diminished absorption of this vitamin may lead to megaloblastic anaemia or even neurological manifestations of pernicious anaemia, including numbness, paraesthesias, unsteady gait and weakness.

Diagnosis of *D. latum* infection is made by finding the characteristic operculated eggs and proglottids in the faeces. The adult worm may be visualized during barium studies of the upper gastrointestinal tract. Niclosamide, paromomycin and praziquantel are all effective in treatment. Infection with this tapeworm can be prevented by thorough cooking of freshwater fish.

Hymenolepis nana

Man can serve as both intermediate and definitive host for the dwarf tapeworm, *Hymenolepis nana*. The cycle of internal autoinfection can thus be maintained in a single individual and the infection spread to other humans by faecal contamination of the environment. *H. nana* infection is found throughout the world, but is particularly common in Africa, South America and Eastern Europe. In industrialized countries it is seen most often in children living in crowded institutions. The adult worm is only 25–50mm in length. Eggs produced by gravid proglottids may either pass out of the body in the faeces or develop into oncospheres which penetrate the villi of the mucosa of the original host. The oncospheres rupture from the villi after approximately 4 days and mature into adult worms in 10–12 days, completing the life cycle. The cycle of internal autoinfection may result in gradually increasing numbers of adult worms in an infected individual. Symptoms of abdominal cramps and diarrhoea may be due to mucosal

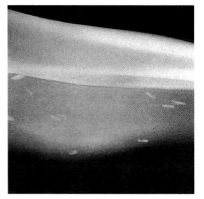

Fig. 4.127 Taeniasis (tapeworm infection). An egg of either *T. solium* or *T. saginata* in faeces containing hexacanth larvae. By courtesy of Dr T.W. Holbrook.

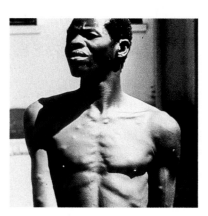

Fig. 4.128 Taeniasis. Scolex of immature *T. solium* in cystic lesion of cysticercosis. H & E stain.

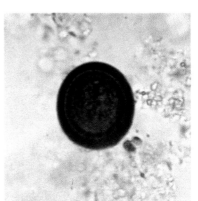

Fig. 4.129 Taeniasis. Radiograph of leg showing characteristic elongated calcified cysts of *T. solium*. At this site they produce no symptoms.

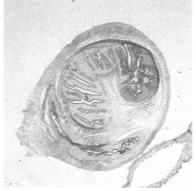

Fig. 4.130 Taeniasis. Infection with the larval form of *T. solium* (cysticercosis) showing multiple subcutaneous cystic lesions containing the larvae, which are known as *Cysticercus cellulosae*. By courtesy of Dr M. G. Schultz.

irritation by adult worms or to rupture of the larvae from the villi. Neurological symptoms of dizziness or seizures may be due to a poorly understood toxin produced by the worms. Diagnosis is made by finding the eggs with their characteristic double membrane in the stools (Fig. 4.131). Treatment with niclosamide should be continued for 5–7 days to eradicate all of the drug-sensitive adult worms as they mature from the drug resistant cysticercoid stage. Paromomycin and praziquantel are also effective in treatment of this infection.

Trichuriasis

Worldwide approximately 500 million people are infected with the whipworm, *Trichuris trichiura*. The infection is most common in tropical areas with poor sanitation facilities. The adult worm inhabits the human caecum and ascending colon. The anterior whiplike portion of the worm is embedded in the wall of the gut while the more robust posterior portion extends into the lumen (Figs 4.132 & 4.133). Eggs are released into the lumen. After excretion in the faeces the embryo develops on moist soil for 2–4 weeks. When the embryonated egg is ingested the larva escapes from the shell and eventually develops into an adult in the caecum or ascending colon.

Most infections are asymptomatic but in a few individuals mild anaemia, bloody diarrhoea and rectal prolapse may develop. Diagnosis is made by finding the characteristic lemon-shaped ova in the faeces (Fig. 4.134). Mebendazole cures or at least drastically reduces the worm burden in nearly all patients.

Enterobiasis

Infection with the pinworm *Enterobius vermicularis* is prevalent throughout the world, especially among school children in temperate regions. It is common at all socio-economic levels, but the highest rates of infection are in crowded populations and among close family of an infected child. The small (10mm) adult worm inhabits the caecal area and the gravid females migrate at night to the perianal region to release their eggs. The embryonated eggs are transmitted via the hands, night clothes, bedding, air and dust. The lifespan of the adult worm is brief, only about a month, but in highly endemic areas reinfection is common.

Many infections are asymptomatic and in most other infected individuals symptoms are limited to pruritus of the perianal region and perineum, which may interfere with sleep. Rarely migration of the parasite may result in appendicitis (Fig. 4.135), chronic salpingitis or ulcerative lesions of the bowel. Diagnosis is made by examination of

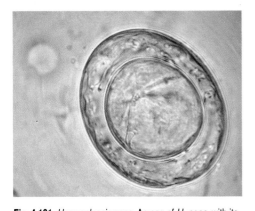

Fig. 4.131 *Hymenolepsis nana*. An egg of *H. nana*, with its characteristic double membrane. By courtesy of Dr I. Farrel.

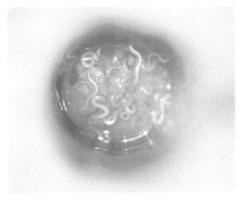

Fig. 4.132 Trichuriasis. Numerous adult *T.trichiura* seen on proctoscopic examination in a healthy infected child. The thin anterior 'whip' end of the worm is secured within the intestinal mucosa, and the thicker posterior end is seen within the lumen. By courtesy of Dr R. H. Gilman.

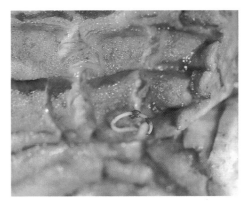

Fig. 4.133 Trichuriasis. A whipworm with its head buried in the ileal mucosa.

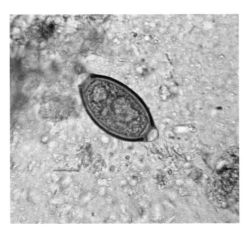

Fig. 4.134 Trichuriasis. Egg of *Trichuris trichiura* in faeces. Note the barrel shape, thick shell and translucent polar prominences.

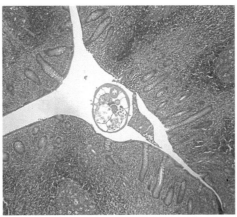

Fig. 4.135 Enterobiasis (pinworm or threadworm infection). Left: Section showing adult pinworm *(Enterobius vermicularis)* in lumen of appendix. Right: Showing numerous eggs within the coiled uteri. H & E stain.

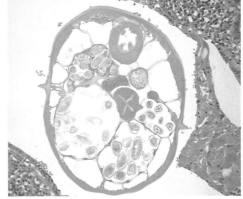

a transparent adhesive tape pressed against the perianal region early in the morning (Fig. 4.136). If 5 examinations are done, 99% of infections will be detected. Since the infection rate within families is so high, all members of a family in which a member is found to be infected should be examined. All infected members of the family should receive mebendazole, which has cure rates of 90–100%.

Ascariasis

Approximately a billion people around the world are infected with the roundworm *Ascaris lumbricoides* (Fig. 4.137). Although this organism is worldwide in distribution, infection is most prevalent in tropical countries. The

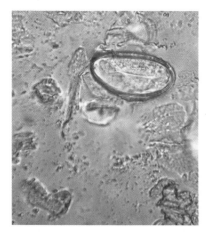

Fig. 4.136 Enterobiasis (pinworm or threadworm infection). A characteristic egg of *E. vermicularis*, collected by adhesive cellophane tape pressed against the perianal area.

adult worm, 15–35cm in length (Figs 4.138 & 4.139), normally inhabits the lumen of the jejunum and middle ileum. Each female worm produces an enormous number of eggs, approximately 200 000 per day. These are passed from the body in the faeces and, under warm moist conditions, develop into mature infective embryos within 10 days. After ingestion they hatch in the small intestine; the embryos penetrate the wall of the gut and migrate through the venous system to the heart and lungs (Figs 4.140 & 4.141) where they break out into the alveoli, pass up through the bronchial system and are swallowed, finally reaching the intestine to develop into mature worms. Most infections are asymptomatic, but heavy infection can interfere with intestinal absorption and lead to malnutrition. Rarely a mass of worms (Fig. 4.142) may obstruct the lumen of the small bowel and produce an acute illness with vomiting, abdominal distention and cramping pain. During such an attack worms may be passed in vomitus or in stools. A worm may invade the common bile duct, producing obstruction with colicky abdominal pain, nausea and vomiting (Figs 4.143 & 4.144). When large numbers of larvae migrate through the lungs in an individual who is sensitized to ascaris antigens, an allergic pneumonitis resembling Löffler's syndrome may result, with respiratory symptoms and eosinophilia in the peripheral blood.

The diagnosis can be made by finding the unfertilized or embryonated eggs on direct examination of a stool specimen (Figs 4.145, 4.146 & 4.147). Occasionally an adult

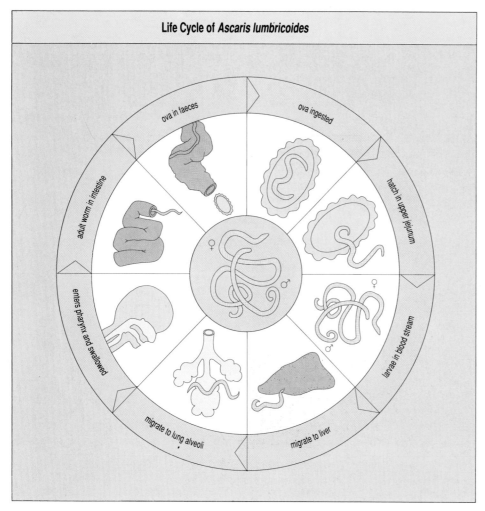

Life Cycle of *Ascaris lumbricoides*

ova in faeces

ova ingested

adult worm in intestine

hatch in upper jejunum

enters pharynx and swallowed

larvae in blood stream

migrate to lung alveoli

migrate to liver

Fig. 4.137 Life cycle of *Ascaris lumbricoides*. *A. lumbricoides* is transmitted to man directly from the soil, without the mediation of a vector. Following ingestion of the ova, the larvae hatch in the small intestine and are carried in the bloodsteam to the liver, from where they migrate to the lungs. They then pass through the trachea, throat and oesophagus, and return to the intestine where they mature in 2–3 months into adult worms. The adult worms live in the intestinal lumen for 12–18 months, so that infection does not persist in the absence of re-exposure. Eggs pass out in the faeces at the single cell stage. The eggs may survive in the soil for months or even years. If the temperature and humidity are suitable, they develop into active embryos and can become fully infective within 2–3 weeks. By courtesy of Dr J. Taverne.

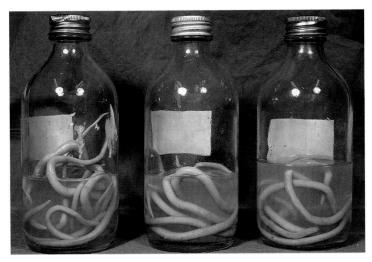

Fig. 4.138 Ascariasis. Large adult worms of *Ascaris lumbricoides*.

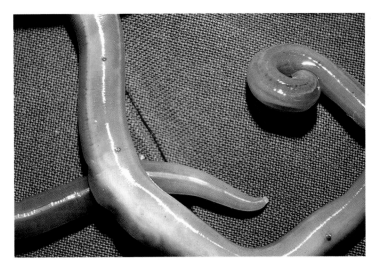

Fig. 4.139 Ascariasis. Large adult worms of *Ascaris lumbricoides*.

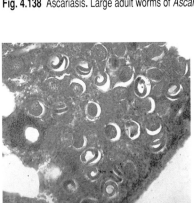

Fig. 4.140 Ascariasis. Section of lung showing very heavy infection with larvae of *A. lumbricoides*. H & E stain.

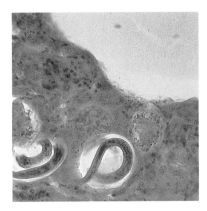

Fig. 4.141 Ascariasis. Higher magnification of Fig. 4.140 showing detail of larva and surrounding inflammatory reaction. H & E stain.

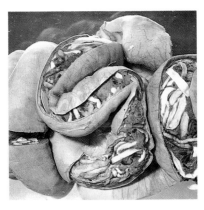

Fig. 4.142 Bolus of ascaris worms in the gut causing intestinal obstruction. By courtesy of Dr D. R. Davies.

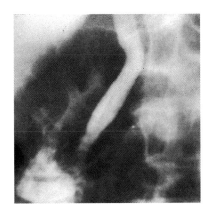

Fig. 4.143 Ascariasis. A single *A. lumbricoides* is visible within the common bile duct. Contrast material can also be seen in the alimentary tract of the worm, which was subsequently removed by sphincterotomy. By courtesy of Dr J. Cunningham.

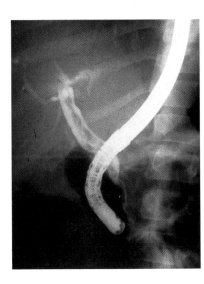

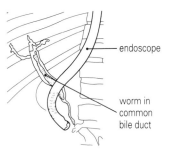

endoscope

worm in common bile duct

Fig. 4.144 ERCP showing an ascaris worm in the common bile duct of a young African patient presenting with acute pancreatitis and cholangitis. By courtesy of Dr A. Hatfield.

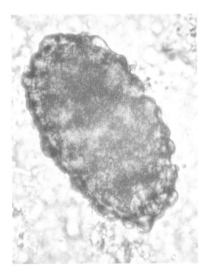

Fig. 4.145 Ascariasis. Unfertilized egg of *A. lumbricoides* in faeces showing pronounced ellipsoidal shape and indistinct internal structure. This type of egg may be seen in patients harbouring only female worms and they are occasionally mistaken for vegetable cells.

worm is seen during barium examination of the small intestine (Figs 4.148 & 4.149). The most effective treatment for intestinal infection with *A. lumbricoides* is mebendazole. If intestinal or biliary obstruction is suspected, piperazine citrate should be used, as this drug narcotizes the worms and prevents further aggravation of the obstruction.

Hookworm Infection

Infection with one of the two species of hookworm, *Necator americanus* and *Ancylostoma duodenale*, affects approximately one billion individuals, mainly in tropical and subtropical regions. The adults are small (10mm), cylindrical worms which live attached to the mucosa of the upper

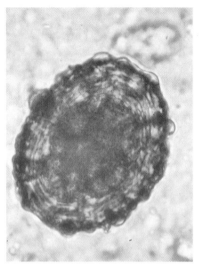

Fig. 4.146 Ascariasis. Fertilized egg of *A. lumbricoides* in faeces showing more rounded shape and corticated outer shell.

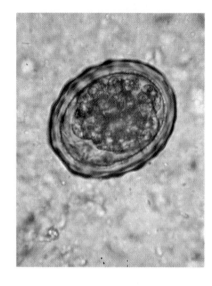

Fig. 4.147 Ascariasis. Embryonated egg of *A. lumbricoides* containing more mature embryo and showing less pronounced cortication of outer shell.

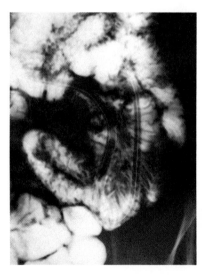

Fig. 4.148 Ascariasis. Barium study of small bowel in a patient with ascariasis. The intestinal tract of one of the adult worms is also well-outlined with barium which it has ingested.

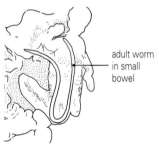

adult worm in small bowel

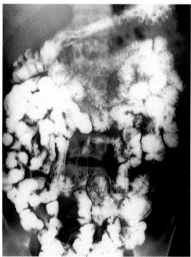

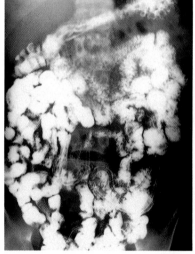

Fig. 4.149 Barium study showing ascaris in the small intestine.

ascaris

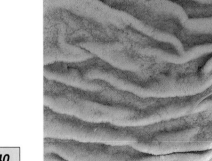

Fig. 4.150 Hookworm infection. A short section of infected intestine. By courtesy of Dr D. R. Davies.

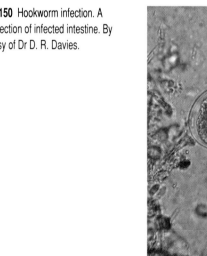

Fig. 4.151 Hookworm infection. Nonembryonated egg of *Necator americanus* in a freshly-passed stool specimen. (Eggs of *N. americanus* and *Ancylostoma duodenale* are difficult to distinguish from one another, although adults can be differentiated easily.)

small intestine by means of their buccal capsules (Fig. 4.150). The eggs pass out of the body with the stools and under suitable conditions of temperature and humidity hatch into larvae which can penetrate intact human skin. They are carried through the venous system to the lungs where they penetrate the alveolar walls, make their way up the trachea and are swallowed, to reach their final habitat in the small intestine. Efficient transmission thus depends on two factors: the disposal of human faecal waste on the ground, and the habit of walking barefoot.

Iron deficiency anaemia and hypoalbuminaemia due to intestinal blood loss are the major clinical manifestations of hookworm infection. 'Ground itch', (an intense pruritus, erythema and papulovesicular rash) may result from the penetration of larvae through the skin. As the larvae migrate through the lungs, a Löffler–like syndrome may occur with cough, wheezing and sputum production, with infiltrates on the chest x-ray and eosinophilia in the sputum and peripheral blood. In heavy infections abdominal pain, diarrhoea and weight loss may be occur.

The diagnosis is made by finding the eggs in the faeces.

The two species cannot be distinguished by the appearance of the eggs. In freshly passed stool specimens the eggs seen are non-embryonated (Fig. 4.151), but if the specimen has been at room temperature for several hours, embryos of various stages may be seen within the eggs (Figs 4.152 & 4.153). Because of the potential for production of significant clinical illness, heavy hookworm infection should be treated with mebendazole. The anaemia should be treated with iron.

Strongyloidiasis

Infection with the nematode *Strongyloides stercoralis* is uncommon in comparison with the nematode infections discussed above, but is nontheless widely distributed in tropical countries. The prevalence of infection may be as high as 4% in some southern states of the USA. The adult worms inhabit the upper small intestine where the females burrow through the mucosa, depositing ova in the tissues (Figs 4.154 & 4.155). The larvae hatch in the mucosa and bore through the epithelium into the lumen,

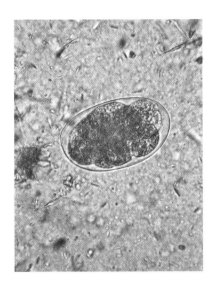

Fig. 4.152 Hookworm infection. Embryonated egg of *N. americanus* in which cell division has begun.

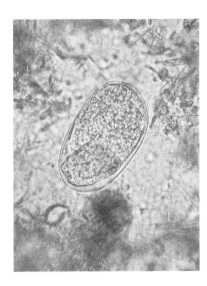

Fig. 4.153 Hookworm infection. Egg of *N. americanus* in faeces containing a relatively mature embryo.

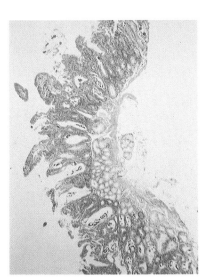

Fig. 4.154 Strongyloidiasis. Section of duodenal mucosa showing the very small adult worms of *Strongyloides stercoralis* in the crypts of the mucosa. H & E stain.

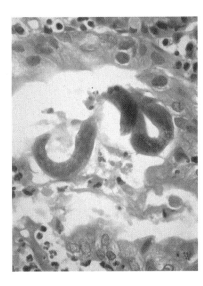

Fig. 4.155 Strongylyoidiasis. Higher magnification showing adult *S. stercoralis* in crypt in jejunal mucosa. H & E stain.

where they are normally passed in the faeces (Fig. 4.156). After leaving the body they may develop into either free-living adults or infective filariform larvae. If the latter come into contact with human skin, they may penetrate it, pass by way of the venous system to the lungs, ascend to the glottis where they are swallowed and finally reach the small intestine. Some larvae may develop into filariform worms in the lumen of the gut and penetrate the intestinal mucosa of the individual in which they originated.

A pruritic skin rash may be produced at the site of penetration of the larvae through the skin. A pneumonitis resembling Löffler's syndrome can occur as the larvae migrate through the lungs. Invasion of the intestinal mucosa by the organisms may produce colicky abdominal pain, diarrhoea, nausea, vomiting and weight loss. Eosinophilia is usually present. Autoinfection may result in massive larval invasion of the lungs and other organs, particularly in immunocompromised hosts (Fig. 4.157).

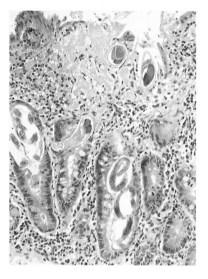

Fig. 4.156 Stronglyloides. Ulcerated jejunal mucosa showing adult and larval forms of *Strongyloides stercoralis*. No eggs are visible here. ×120. H & E stain.

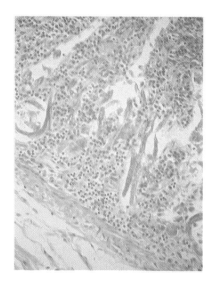

Fig. 4.157 Strongyloidiasis. Massive invasion of a lymph node by larvae of *S. stercoralis* in disseminated infection in an immunocompromised patient. H & E stain.

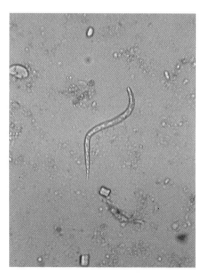

Fig. 4.158 Strongyloidiasis. Rhabditiform larva of *S. stercoralis* in faeces. At this magnification it is very difficult to distinguish from the larvae of hookworms.×100.

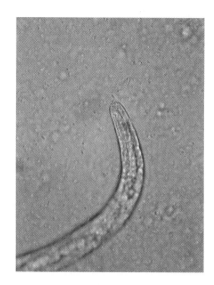

Fig. 4.159 Strongyloidiasis. Higher magnification of rhabditiform larva of *S. stercoralis* showing the short buccal capsule. Larvae of hookworms have a much longer buccal capsule.×400.

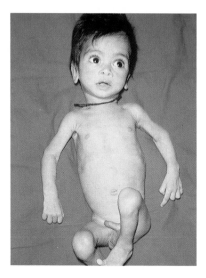

Fig. 4.160 Viral gastroenteritis. Note the alert expression, flaccid posture and general appearance of dehydration and malnutrition.

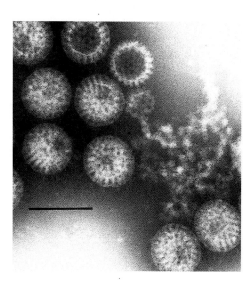

Fig. 4.161 Rotavirus. Electron micrograph showing negatively-stained particles approximately 75nm in diameter in faeces. The 'spoked-wheel' appearance is characteristic. Bar = 100nm. By courtesy of Regional Virus Laboratory, East Birmingham Hospital, Birmingham, England.

This type of disseminated infection has been described following chemotherapy for lymphomas and leukaemias, in patients with lepromatous leprosy and in individuals treated with corticosteroids. Treatment with corticosteroids may suppress the eosinophilia which is usually observed in these patients. Patients with overwhelming autoinfection may exhibit severe generalized abdominal pain, diffuse pulmonary infiltrates, ileus, shock and meningitis or sepsis from gram-negative bacilli. Recurrent meningitis due to intestinal bacteria has been reported in a few cases.

The diagnosis is made by demonstrating the larvae of *S. stercoralis* in the faeces or duodenal fluid (Fig. 4.158 & 4.159). Concentration of the specimen by the zinc sulphate method may be necessary. Duodenal contents may be sampled by the Enterotest technique used in the diagnosis of *Giardia lamblia* infection. The only drug effective in the treatment of *S. stercoralis* infection is thiabendazole. In the hyperinfection syndrome treatment should be continued for 2–3 weeks.

VIRAL ENTERIC INFECTIONS

Acute viral gastroenteritis is a major global cause of serious morbidity, especially in infants and young children, in whom diarrhoea and vomiting may rapidly lead to malnutrition, dehydration and serious electrolyte imbalance (Fig. 4.160). Acute gastroenteritis affects approximately 500 million children per year worldwide. In less developed countries it is the leading cause of death in children under the age of 4 years. In developed countries viral gastroenteritis is second in prevalence only to viral upper respiratory tract illness. During the last 20 years a number of viruses associated with acute gastroenteritis have been identified. These include the rotaviruses, fastidious faecal adenoviruses, Norwalk virus and Norwalk-like agents, caliciviruses, astroviruses and coronaviruses.

Rotaviruses

Rotaviruses are members of the family *Reoviridae*. They possess a double layer of icosahedral shells approximately 70nm in diameter, and have a core of double-stranded RNA (Fig. 4.161). They have been classified into a number of different types based on the electrophoretic mobility of the 11 different segments of the RNA genome. Segments which exhibit similar electrophoretic mobility do not necessarily exhibit RNA homology, but the electrophoretic patterns are useful in epidemiological studies. At least 4 and possibly as many as 6 serotypes of human rotaviruses have also been identified.

Diarrhoeal disease due to rotaviruses most commonly affects young children. Infected neonates are often asymptomatic and the parents of infected children may exhibit only a rise in serum antibody titres. Rotaviruses are prevalent in day-care centres, where they are readily transmitted by the faecal–oral route to other children and to family contacts. The illness may be relatively severe in the elderly, and fatal infections have occurred in individuals living in nursing homes. Rotaviruses are responsible for approximately 50% of all cases of paediatric gastroenteritis requiring hospitalization in the world's temperate zones. The two most common features of rotavirus disease are diarrhoea and vomiting. The vomiting often precedes the diarrhoea. It is not known for certain whether rotaviruses cause respiratory symptoms. The diarrhoea often lasts 5–8 days and, in small children, often results in dehydration and electrolyte imbalance.

Rotaviruses primarily effect the small intestine; virus replication takes place in epithelial cells at the tips of the villi. The patchy mucosal changes include shortening and blunting of the villi and increased infiltration of the lamina propria with mononuclear cells. The epithelial cells become more cuboidal and less regular than normal. Reovirus-like particles may be seen by electron microscopy in the epithelial cells of the duodenal mucosa (Fig. 4.162). Functionally, low levels of activity of maltase, sucrase and lactase occur; these abnormalities return to normal after 4–8 weeks. Most children exhibit malabsorption of lactose and lactose intolerance; an increase in the diarrhoea may occur after ingestion of lactose.

Large amounts of rotavirus are excreted in the stool during acute gastroenteritis and the virus can be seen upon direct examination of the stool by electron microscopy (EM) (see Fig. 4.161). Immune electron microscopy (IEM), in which the faecal suspension is mixed with specific antiserum, is even more sensitive than direct examination. However, electron microscopic procedures are time con-

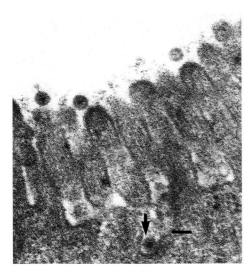

Fig. 4.162 Rotavirus. Electron micrograph showing thin section of enterocyte with heavy infective load of rotaviruses. One has penetrated the brush border. Bar = 100 nm. By courtesy of Dr K. Coehlo.

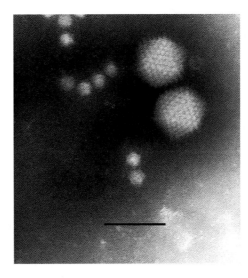

Fig. 4.163 Adenovirus. Electron micrograph showing negatively-stained particles of approximately 80nm diameter , isolated from faeces. Note the typical hexagonal outline produced by the icosahedral structure. The very small particles are adeno-associated (satellite) viruses. Bar = 100nm. By courtesy of Regional Virus Laboratory, East Birmingham Hospital Birmingham, England.

suming and expensive, so most laboratories employ the enzyme-linked immunosorbent assay (ELISA) or latex agglutination (LA) tests, for which several commercial kits are available.

The mechanisms involved in protection and recovery from rotavirus infection are complex and appear to involve both local and systemic humoral and cell-mediated responses and also possibly other non-specific factors. Vaccine development has concentrated on oral vaccines which stimulate production of local intestinal IgA antibody. Vaccines utilizing attenuated strains of both bovine and monkey rotaviruses, as well as reassortant vaccines, are under investigation.

Treatment of rotavirus infections (and of other diarrhoeal diseases due to viruses) is based on the replacement of water and electrolytes in dehydrated patients. Although a few patients require initial therapy with intravenous fluids, by far the great majority of patients can be treated with oral replacement solutions. These solutions contain both electrolytes and glucose; the latter is required for glucose-coupled sodium transport in the small intestine. After dehydration and electrolyte imbalance are corrected, feedings begin with breast milk or dilute formula and progress to full-strength formula over two or three days. Bland carbohydrate solid foods which do not contain lactose, such as rice, cereal and potatoes, are reintroduced as soon as tolerated.

Adenoviruses

Adenoviruses are probably second only to rotaviruses in importance as viral causes of diarrhoeal disease (Fig. 4.163). These are 70–75nm, non-enveloped, icosahedral, double stranded DNA viruses which infect many species of mammals and lower animals. Of the 41 serotypes which infect man, types 40 and 41 are designated 'fastidious' adenoviruses, as they cannot be isolated in routine cell cultures and exhibit DNA restriction patterns which differ from those of the other serotypes. Although non-fastidious respiratory adenoviruses may cause diarrhoeal disease in humans, the fastidious adenoviruses appear to be more important causes of viral gastroenteritis. Whether or not these agents can also cause respiratory disease is unknown. Fastidious adenoviruses cause infection and disease primarily in children under the age of 2 years.

Diarrhoea with or without vomiting is the predominant symptom. Severity may range from a mild afebrile illness to a severe or even fatal disease with profound dehydration. Most patients infected with adenoviruses have milder disease with less pronounced vomiting, less fever and less diarrhoea than patients infected with rotaviruses. Respiratory symptoms are more common in patients infected with adenoviruses.

Type-specific ELISA using monoclonal antibodies to the fastidious types 40 and 41 have been developed, but these tests are not in routine clinical use at the present time.

Norwalk virus and Norwalk-like agents

Norwalk virus is a small round virus, 25–30nm in diameter, which cannot be cultivated *in vitro*. A number of other Norwalk-like viruses, some of which are antigenically similar to Norwalk virus, have also been found in association with outbreaks of acute non-bacterial gastroenteritis (Fig. 4.164). Transmission apparently occurs via ingestion of contaminated water or food or by person-to-person spread. In industrialized countries Norwalk and similar viruses tend to infect older children and adults, suggesting that exposure to these viruses is uncommon during early childhood. In the USA and Canada, antibody to Norwalk virus is found in only 5% of children up to the age of 12 years, but prevalence of antibody increases rapidly during adolescence and young adulthood. In less developed countries antibody usually appears during childhood.

The incubation period is usually 24–48 hours. Onset of illness is sudden with nausea and vomiting, which is often

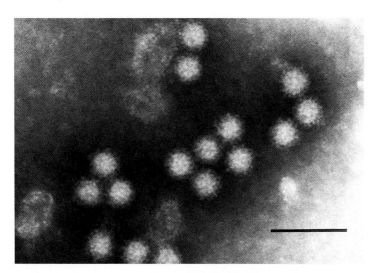

Fig. 4.164 Small round structured virus (similar morphology to Norwalk agent). Electron micrograph showing negatively-stained particles of 33–38nm diameter. These particles show little organized surface structure, but the appearance is consistent. Bar = 100 nm. By courtesy of Regional Virus Laboratory, East Birmingham Hospital Birmingham, England.

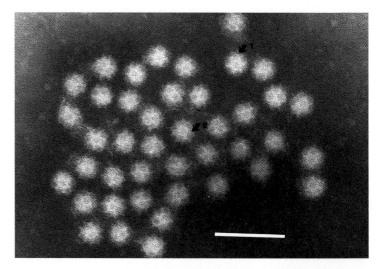

Fig. 4.165 Calicivirus. Electron micrograph showing negatively-stained particles of 33–38nm diameter in faeces. A characteristic appearance is the 6-pointed star of David with a central hole (1). Also shown is a 10-pointed sphere (2). Bar = 100 nm. By courtesy of Regional Virus Laboratory, East Birmingham Hospital Birmingham, England.

severe, low-grade fever and diarrhoea, which may be mild. Other symptoms include mild abdominal pain or cramps, headache and malaise. The attack rate in outbreaks may be as high as 50%. Respiratory symptoms apparently do not occur as a result of infection with Norwalk or similar viruses. In children vomiting is usually the predominant symptom, whereas adults are more likely to experience diarrhoea. Hospitalization is rarely required, but a few cases of serious illness have been reported. Intestinal mucosal biopsy has revealed mild changes similar to those seen in gastroenteritis due to other viruses, and transient deficiency in intestinal enzyme activity may occur.

Only small numbers of Norwalk and similar viruses are present in the faeces in infected individuals, so the agent can rarely be detected by direct EM. Clumps of viral particles can often be visualized by the more sensitive technique of IEM. Radioimmunoassays and ELISAs have been developed and utilized in epidemiological studies, but are rarely available in clinical microbiology laboratories.

Immunity to Norwalk virus appears to be complex. Most volunteers given Norwalk virus who become ill have pre-existing Norwalk antibody, whereas the majority of volunteers who do not become ill have little or no pre-existing antibody in the serum. Protective mechanisms other than serum antibody must be important.

Other viral causes of acute gastroenteritis

Three other groups of viruses, the caliciviruses, astroviruses and coronaviruses, have been implicated in acute gastroenteritis in humans.

Caliciviruses are small RNA viruses, approximately 30nm in diameter. There are 32 cup-shaped depressions on ,the surface of the virion, which gives the particle a spiky appearance and a six-pointed Star of David configuration at certain orientations. These viruses cause gastroenteritis primarily in infants and young children. In most areas of the world a majority of individuals exhibit

antibody to caliciviruses by the age of 5 years. The symptoms of calicivirus infection are similar to those of rotavirus infection. Diarrhoea is usually the predominant feature, but in some studies vomiting has also been common. Upper respiratory tract symptoms and fever occur in a significant minority of patients. Caliciviruses may be seen in the stools by direct EM and IEM (Fig. 4.165), but cannot be isolated in routine cell cultures.

Astroviruses are 28–30nm round virus particles which have a smooth edge. The particles may have either a 5- or 6-point star-like configuration. These viruses may be detected in stool suspensions by direct EM (Fig. 4.166) and also can be propagated in HEK cells. There are at least five distinct serotypes of human astroviruses. Children from infancy up to the age of 7 years are most often affected. Symptomatic children have watery diarrhoea, vomiting or both. The illness is usually less severe than that seen with rotavirus infection.

Coronaviruses are enveloped, single-stranded RNA viruses approximately 80–150nm in diameter which are well-documented causes of upper respiratory tract illness. Projections on the surface of the rounded particles give the appearance of the corona of the sun. Coronavirus-like particles have been seen by direct EM in the stools of patients with acute non-bacterial gastroenteritis (Fig. 4.167). The evidence that these agents cause acute gastroenteritis consists of the findings that in certain areas, such as southern Arizona in the USA, coronavirus-like particles are seen much more frequently in the stools of patients with diarrhoea than in healthy individuals; convalescent sera from these patients reacts with certain coronaviruses. These enteric coronavirus-like agents cannot be propagated in routine cell types and most investigators have not been able to propagate them at all. Most cases of diarrhoea associated with these agents occur in children less than 2 years old; the illness is usually dominated by diarrhoea, with or without vomiting.

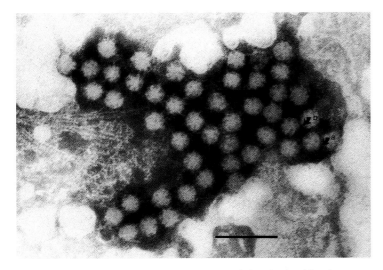

Fig. 4.166 Astrovirus. Electron micrograph showing negatively-stained particles of 28–32nm diameter in faeces. Surface morphology shows (a) 5- and (b) 6-pointed stars. Bar = 100 nm. By courtesy of Regional Virus Laboratory, East Birmingham Hospital Birmingham, England.

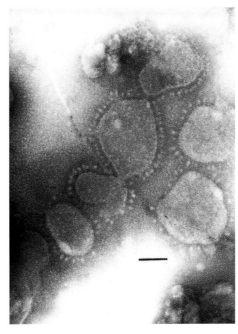

Fig. 4.167 Coronavirus. Electron micrograph showing negatively-stained pleomorphic particles which can vary in size from 80–300nm in diameter. The particles are covered by evenly spaced pin-like projections which can look like a fringe or 'crown'. Bar = 100 nm. By courtesy of Regional Virus Laboratory, East Birmingham Hospital Birmingham, England.

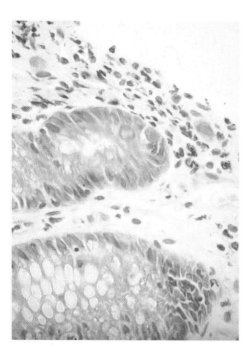

Fig. 4.168 Cytomegalovirus colitis. Section of colon showing several giant cells with eosinophilic intranuclear inclusions and infiltration of inflammatory cells in the lamina propria. By courtesy of Dr C. Edwards.

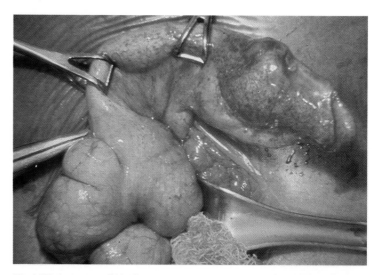

Fig. 4.169 Acute appendicitis. Operating room photograph showing a globoid tip secondary to obstruction of appendiceal lumen by a faecalith. There is a pronounced hyperaemia and oedema of the appendix wall with petechial haemorrhages on the surface and dilatation of the lumen distal to the obstruction. By courtesy of Dr M. Anderson.

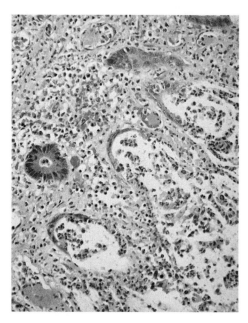

Fig. 4.170 Acute appendicitis. Histological section of the wall of the appendix showing acute inflammation, destruction of glands and intense vascular congestion with fibrin microthrombi. H & E stain.

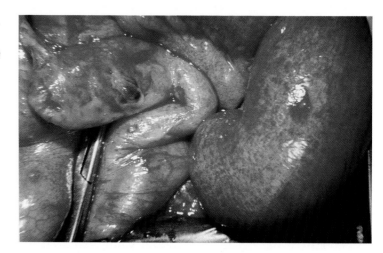

Fig. 4.171 Acute appendicitis. Operating room photograph showing an area of necrosis in the wall of the appendix with perforation at the site of obstruction by a faecalith. There is vascular congestion and fibrinous exudate on the adjacent serosal surface. By courtesy of Dr M. Anderson.

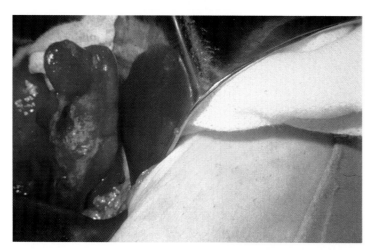

Fig. 4.172 Acute appendicitis. Operating room photograph showing acute gangrenous appendicitis with intense hyperaemia of the serosal surface of the appendix and a creamy exudate on the surface. Perforation has occurred in the middle third of the appendix, and there is a greenish gangrenous area adjacent to the perforation. By courtesy of Dr W. M. Rambo.

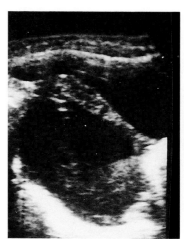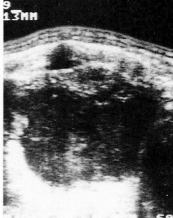

Fig. 4.173 Appendiceal abscess. Ultrasound studies showing an abscess in the pouch of Douglas secondary to a ruptured appendix. Lateral view (left) and transverse view (right). By courtesy of Dr A. E. A. Joseph.

Cytomegalovirus colitis

Colitis due to infection with cytomegalovirus (CMV) is seen almost exclusively in patients with suppression of the immune system. At least 5–10% of patients with AIDS develop CMV colitis. In about one-third of the cases CMV colitis is the initial opportunistic infection experienced by the patient. Nearly all patients have diarrhoea and abdominal pain. Colonoscopy reveals focal or diffuse areas of erythema, mucosal oedema and mucosal erosion. Haemorrhage and mucosal ulcers 5–10mm in diameter are commonly observed. Diagnosis of CMV colitis can be made only by biopsy of colonic or rectal mucosa. Typical findings are CMV inclusions in swollen endothelial cells associated with neutrophilic infiltration of blood vessels (Fig. 4.168). CMV can often be cultured from biopsy specimens. Isolation of CMV from stool cultures is not adequate to establish the diagnosis of CMV colitis.

Many patients with CMV colitis associated with AIDS have now been treated with the antiviral agent ganciclovir and a majority have had a clinical response with decrease in diarrhoea and abdominal pain. Unless maintenance therapy is continued for an indefinite period clinical and virological relapse usually occurs.

INFECTIONS OF THE PERITONEUM AND PERITONEAL CAVITY

Appendicitis

Acute appendicitis is due to acute inflammation of the wall of the appendix, usually associated with some degree of obstruction of the appendiceal lumen. Classic clinical findings are tenderness at or near McBurney's point in the right lower quadrant of the abdomen, with rebound tenderness, voluntary guarding or rigidity, low-grade fever and leucocytosis. Anatomically, there is frequently an obstructing faecalith in the lumen of the appendix with distension of the lumen, infiltration with acute inflammatory cells and oedema in the wall, and hyperaemia and petechial haemorrhages on the serosal surface (Figs 4.169 & 4.170). Persistent obstruction of the appendiceal lumen by a faecalith leads eventually to gangrene and rupture of the appendix (Figs 4.171 & 4.172). Spillage of pus from the inflamed appendix into the peritoneal cavity may result in generalized peritonitis; alternatively the infection may be walled off with formation of an appendiceal abscess (Fig. 4.173).

Peritonitis and intra-abdominal abscess

Primary peritonitis, in which no primary focus of infection is apparent, occurs most commonly in association with alcoholic cirrhosis and ascites. *E. coli* and related species are isolated most frequently. Spread of infection from an intra-abdominal organ into the peritoneal space results in secondary peritonitis (Fig. 4.174). Organisms may reach the peritoneal cavity either by transmural spread through the intact wall of a severely inflamed viscus, or by rupture of a viscus with spillage of its contents into the surrounding space. The intense inflammatory response of the peritoneum to bacterial infection includes deposition of fibrin and migration of polymorphonuclear leucocytes, both of which tend to limit the spread of bacteria to a localized area. Complete walling off of the infection without eradication of the microorganisms results in formation of an intra-abdominal abscess. In addition to appendicitis, important sources for peritonitis and intra-abdominal abscess include rupture of the gallbladder, perforation of a peptic ulcer, ruptured intestinal diverticulum, acute pancreatitis, chronic peritoneal dialysis (Fig. 4.175) and pelvic inflammatory disease. Most cases of secondary peritonitis are polymicrobial in nature, with mixtures of anaerobic

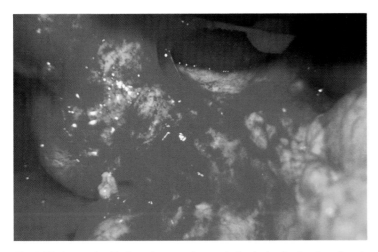

Fig. 4.174 Acute peritonitis. Operating room photograph showing localized acute peritoneal inflammation with oedema, acute inflammatory exudate, intense vascular congestion and petechial haemorrhage, associated with acute cholecystitis. By courtesy of Dr M. Anderson.

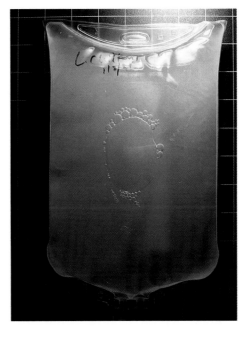

Fig. 4.175 Acute peritonitis. Cloudy, infected peritoneal dialysate removed from a patient undergoing chronic peritoneal dialysis.

and facultative enteric bacteria. New imaging methods such as computerized tomographic (CT) scanning (Fig. 4.176), radionucleide scanning (Figs 4.177 & 4.178) and ultrasound studies (Fig. 4.179) have greatly facilitated the prompt and accurate diagnosis of intra-abdominal abscess. Empirical treatment of secondary peritonitis should include an agent or agents active against both anaerobic and facultative organisms, such as imipenem or a combination of metronidazole or clindamycin with a third-generation cephalosporin. If abscess formation has occurred, catheter or surgical drainage will also be required.

Tuberculous peritonitis

Tuberculous peritonitis is usually due to rupture of a caseous abdominal lymph node. It may or may not be accompanied by active pulmonary disease. Pleural effusion is frequently present. The peritoneal disease may be manifested by abdominal masses and a doughy abdomen or by presence of ascites and signs of peritonitis. Low-grade fever, anorexia, weight loss and abdominal pain are common. The clinical picture may mimic many other intra-abdominal diseases, and the diagnosis is particularly difficult in the presence of co-existing cirrhosis with

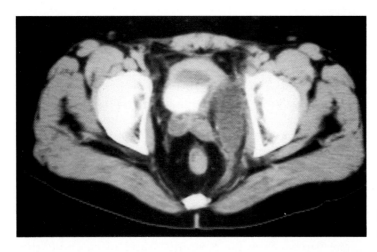

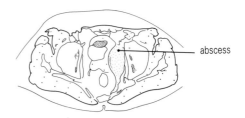

Fig. 4.176 Intra-abdominal abscess. CT scan at the level of the seminal vesicles showing an elliptical abscess to the left of the midline.

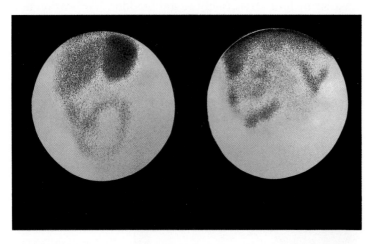

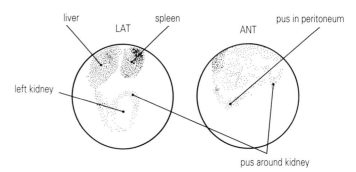

Fig. 4.177 Intra-abdominal abscess. Leucocytes labelled with indium-111 have concentrated in regions of purulent peritoneal fluid. Activity is normally seen by this technique in the liver and spleen. By courtesy of Dr D. Ackery.

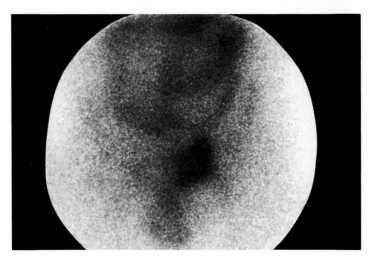

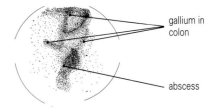

Fig. 4.178 Intra-abdominal abscess. Gallium scan showing an area of increased uptake of the radionucleide in the left lower quadrant of the abdomen. Gallium is also seen in the lumen of the colon.

ascites and in patients undergoing chronic peritoneal dialysis. The tuberculin test is often negative. The peritoneal fluid usually contains 500–2000 cells, predominantly lymphocytes. Smears of the fluid are rarely positive and culture yields *M. tuberculosis* in only 25% of cases. Surgical exploration or laparoscopy often reveals fibrous adhesions, ascites and tubercles scattered over the peritoneal surface (Figs 4.180, 4.181 & 4.182) and biopsy of these lesions yields the diagnosis in up to 85% of cases. Treatment is the same as for pulmonary tuberculosis.

Abdominal actinomycosis

Abdominal actinomycosis usually occurs following abdominal surgery, trauma or rupture of a colonic diverticulum or duodenal ulcer. The latent period between this event and subsequent development of manifestations of actinomycosis may be several years, so the connection between the two is not always immediately apparent. The ileocaecal region is most frequently involved and the lesion may be mistaken for a caecal carcinoma, tuberculosis or amoebiasis. A mass lesion is frequently produced with contiguous spread and fistula formation involving the body wall, perianal region or other internal organs (Fig. 4.183). Pus

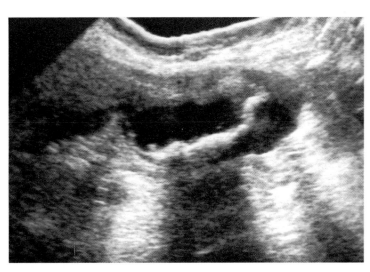

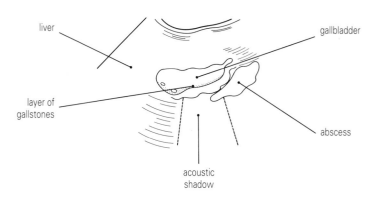

Fig. 4.179 Pericholecystic abscess. Ultrasound study showing sonolucent abscess cavity adjacent to the gallbladder in a patient with a pericholecystic abscess secondary to perforation of the gallbladder. By courtesy of Dr A. E. A. Joseph.

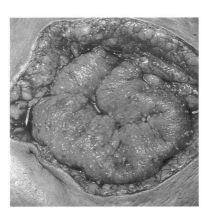

Fig. 4.180 Tuberculous peritonitis. Operating room photograph showing oedematous bowel with numerous focal white lesions on the peritoneal surface. By courtesy of Dr M. Goldman.

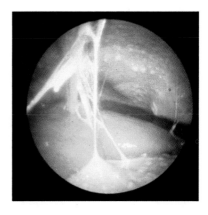

Fig. 4.181 Tuberculous peritonitis. Laparoscopic view in a patient with the chronic serous type of TB peritonitis, showing fibrous adhesions attached to the left lobe of the liver and numerous tubercles on the parietal peritoneum. By courtesy of Dr J. Cunningham.

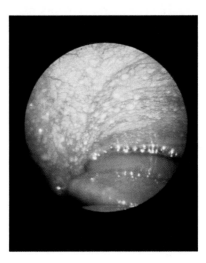

Fig. 4.182 Tuberculous peritonitis. Laparoscopic view in a patient with extensive acute exudative tuberculous peritonitis, showing vascular engorgement, multiple granulomas on the parietal peritoneum and ascites. By courtesy of Dr J. Cunningham.

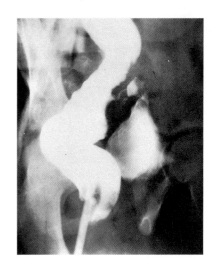

Fig. 4.183 Abdominal actinomycosis. Barium enema showing an area of mucosal abnormality in the sigmoid colon, with a fistulous tract extending from the sigmoid colon to the urinary bladder, which is filled with contrast material.

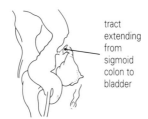

obtained by aspiration or surgical drainage may reveal sulphur granules (Fig. 4.184). Gram's stain reveals the characteristic beaded, filamentous, gram-positive organisms (Fig. 4.185) and *Actinomyces israelii* can be grown anaerobically (see Chapter 7).

Echinococcosis

Echinococcosis (hydatid disease) is caused by human infection with the tapeworm *Echinococcus granulosus*. Man becomes involved accidentally by ingesting the eggs which are present in the faeces of infected dogs. The most common location of hydatid cysts are the liver, usually the right lobe (see Chapter 5), followed by the lung. Usually a single cyst is present. Rupture of the cyst through the capsule of the liver into the peritoneal cavity results in the formation of new daughter cysts throughout the peritoneum and omentum (Fig. 4.186). Rupture through the diaphragm may lead to dissemination throughout the pleural space. The new larvae (scolices) (Fig. 4.187) develop in large numbers from the germinal layer of brood capsules within the wall of the cyst.

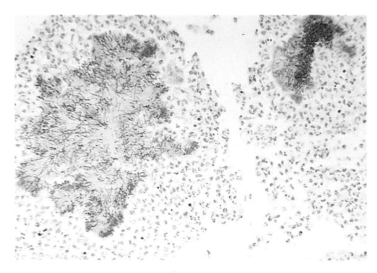

Fig. 4.184 Abdominal actinomycosis. Inflammatory exudate containing a typical sulphur granule. By courtesy of Dr C. Edwards.

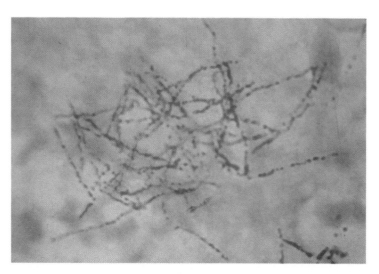

Fig. 4.185 Abdominal actinomycosis. Pus drained from an intra-abdominal abscess showing tangled, beaded, gram-positive filaments of *Actinomyces israelii*. Gram's stain. By courtesy of A. E. Prevost.

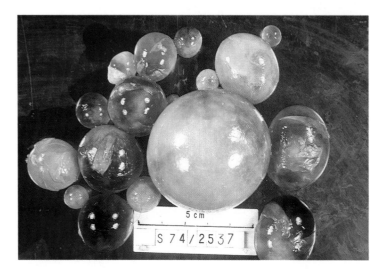

Fig. 4.186 Echinococcosis. Surgical specimen showing multiple hydatid cysts from the omentum of a patient who had infection disseminated throughout the peritoneal cavity.

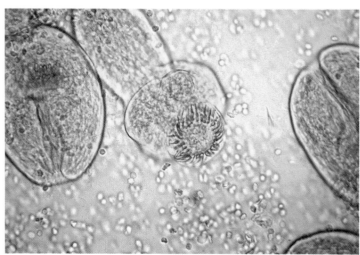

Fig. 4.187 Echinococcosis. Light microscopy of scolices from a hydatid cyst showing both invaginated and evaginated hooklets and suckers. By courtesy of Prof. W. Peters.

5

THE LIVER AND BILIARY TRACT

ACUTE HEPATITIS

Acute hepatitis may be caused by a large number of different viruses, the most important of which are the hepatitis B virus (HBV), the hepatitis A virus (HAV) and the non-A, non-B (NANB) group. Clinical and morphological features of all three types of infection are similar. Hepatitis is the predominant manifestation of yellow fever, and is a common feature of cytomegalovirus infection and infectious mononucleosis, caused by the Epstein-Barr virus. Less commonly, the liver may be involved in disseminated herpes simplex infection and in varicella (chickenpox). Nonviral forms of acute hepatitis include Q fever, bacterial hepatitis, leptospirosis and Reye's syndrome.

Pathologically, viral hepatitis is characterized by spotty necrosis scattered throughout the liver lobule with varying degrees of degeneration of liver cells, including necrosis, infiltration of the liver by mononuclear cells and variable degrees of cholestasis (Fig. 5.1). In HBV infections, 'ground-glass' hepatocytes and specific staining of HBV surface antigen may be demonstrated (Figs. 5.2 and 5.3). Hepatic cell necrosis is usually focal and limited in extent, but occasionally, especially in HBV infection, massive hepatic necrosis (acute yellow atrophy) occurs with loss of nearly all liver cells and complete collapse of the hepatic architecture (Figs. 5.4 and 5.5). As discussed below, some types of viral hepatitis may persist and produce chronic lesions in the liver, including postnecrotic cirrhosis.

Hepatitis B Virus Infection

Infection with HBV (hepatitis B), formerly known as serum hepatitis, is the most prevalent type of acute hepatitis worldwide. Persistent infection with the virus is common, and in highly endemic areas approximately 10% of the population are chronic carriers of HBV; in many individuals infection persists for life. The total number of chronic carriers worldwide exceeds 230 million. Formerly a major cause of transfusion-associated hepatitis, HBV infection is now most frequently spread by sexual contact, intravenous drug abuse and transmission from mothers to their newborn infants.

Three types of viral particles are found in the blood of infected individuals (Fig. 5.6). The complete virion (Dane particle) is 42 nm in diameter. The hepatitis B surface antigen particle (HB$_S$Ag), which may be spherical, filamentous or rod-shaped, is 22 nm in diameter. The virion core, also 22 nm in diameter, contains the core antigen (HB$_C$Ag), the viral DNA, DNA polymerase, protein kinase activity and the 'e' antigen (HB$_e$Ag), which is closely associated with infectivity. The genome of HBV is complex and unique; its replication involves the activity of reverse transcriptase which is unique among human DNA viruses. This replication mechanism, and the nucleotide sequence homology between HBV and retroviruses, suggests a possible phylogenetic relationship between these two families of viruses.

Man is the only important reservoir of HBV. Blood and blood products are the best documented sources of the virus, but it is also found in faeces, urine, bile, semen, saliva and other body fluids. The most important vehicles for infection are probably blood, semen and saliva. Transmission commonly occurs via percutaneous inoculation of virus during administration of contaminated blood or blood products, haemodialysis, tattooing, ear piercing, acupuncture, sharing of needles by intravenous drug

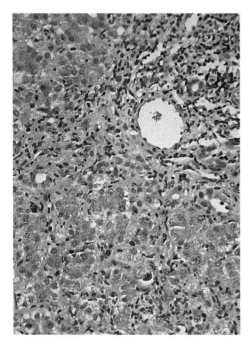 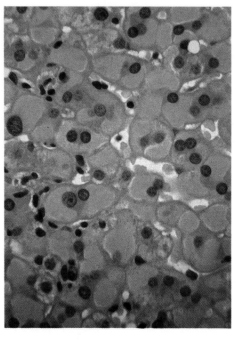 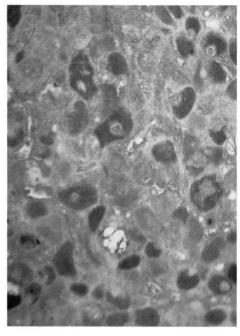

Fig. 5.1 Acute viral hepatitis: histological section of liver showing hepatocytes in degeneration, necrosis and regeneration. Haematoxylin and eosin (H&E) stain. By courtesy of Dr. R.D. Johnson.

Fig. 5.2 Viral hepatitis: histological section of liver showing 'ground-glass' hepatocytes. H&E stain.

Fig. 5.3 Viral hepatitis: histological section of liver in hepatitis B virus infection showing specific staining of hepatitis B surface antigen in hepatocytes. Shikata stain. By courtesy of Dr. R.D. Johnson.

abusers, or accidental needle stick injuries by hospital personnel, and also during heterosexual and homosexual contact. In areas of the world where the prevalence of chronic HBV infection is very high, transmission from infected mothers to infants occurs frequently during late pregnancy, parturition or during the first two months' postpartum.

The incubation period of acute hepatitis B is usually between two and six months. In patients who develop jaundice, 10-20% have a prodromal serum sickness-like illness with fever, maculopapular erythematous rash, arthralgias and urticaria for several days to several weeks before the appearance of signs of liver disease.

The severity of acute hepatitis B varies widely, and many cases are clinically inapparent. In these subclinical cases and in anicteric cases, serum transaminases are usually elevated. In icteric cases, malaise, fever, headache, anorexia and nausea, sometimes with vomiting, appear 2-7 days before the appearance of jaundice. Anorexia is often pronounced and accompanied by aversion for tobacco; the smell of food or tobacco may induce nausea. Pain and tenderness in the right upper quadrant are common. The liver is often enlarged, palpable and tender. Icterus of the sclerae and other mucous membranes and skin are usually noted when the concentration of serum bilirubin is ≥3 mg/100 ml.

Laboratory abnormalities include a striking increase in serum transaminases (SGPT > SGOT), with a peak of 1,000 U/ml or greater reached within the first week of illness. Serum bilirubin rises during the first 10-14 days and then declines over the next 2-4 weeks in most cases.

Although most cases of hepatitis B have a relatively mild and self-limited course, fulminant hepatitis with

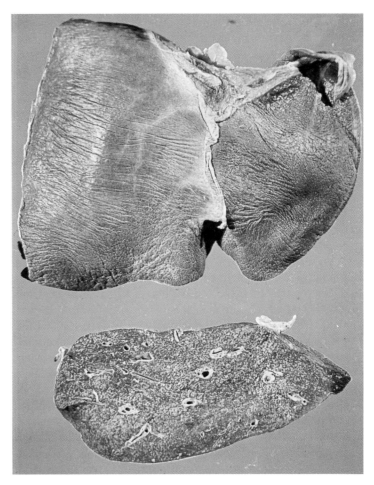

Fig. 5.4 Viral hepatitis: gross specimen of liver showing massive hepatic necrosis. The capsular surface (upper) is wrinkled. The cut surface (lower) has a 'nutmeg' appearance due to cell loss and congestion in the central lobular zones. Light foci represent remaining liver cells; areas of necrosis appear darker. The hepatic architecture has collapsed and the organ has shrunk in size. By courtesy of Dr. J. Newman.

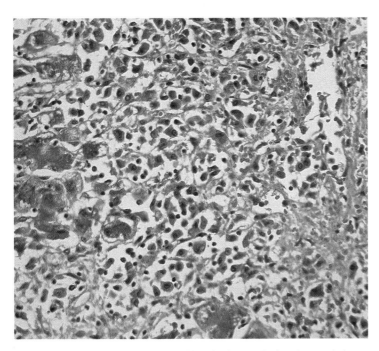

Fig. 5.5 Viral hepatitis: histological section of liver showing massive hepatic necrosis due to hepatitis A virus infection. There is a paucity of hepatocytes and large numbers of pigment-laden macrophages. H&E stain. By courtesy of Dr. R.D. Johnson.

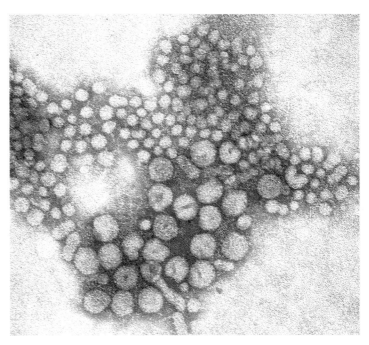

Fig. 5.6 Viral hepatitis: electron micrograph of hepatitis B virus, serum specimen. The smaller rounded structures are non-infectious particles containing HBsAg determinant on their surfaces. HBsAg can also be seen in tubular or filamentous form. The larger (40-50 nm diameter) rounded bodies are Dane particles, probably the fully assembled infectious virus. By courtesy of Professor C.R. Madely.

hepatic failure and encephalopathy may occur. The case fatality rate is very high, with death usually occurring within three weeks of onset. Concomitant infection with hepatitis delta virus (HDV) (see below) is associated with an increased risk of fulminant hepatitis.

During the active stage of self-limited hepatitis, both HBsAg and HBeAg can be detected in the blood. These antigens disappear after weeks or months, and antibodies against surface antigen (anti-HB$_s$), core antigen (anti-HB$_c$) and 'e' antigen (anti-HB$_e$) appear and persist, at gradually declining titres, for years (Fig. 5.7). In persistent infection HB$_s$Ag, with or without HBeAg, persists indefinitely. Anti-HB$_c$ and anti-HB$_e$ are also present, but not anti-HB$_s$ (Fig. 5.8).

In 5-10% of adults, and virtually 100% of newborns, persistent infection occurs. This may be associated with a histologically normal liver and normal liver function, but it often results in lesions designated 'chronic persistent' hepatitis, in which the basic hepatic architecture is preserved (Fig. 5.9), or 'chronic active' hepatitis in which there is disruption of lobular architecture and degeneration and regeneration of hepatocytes (Fig. 5.10). The presence of HBeAg in persistent infection is usually associated with chronic hepatitis. Chronic active hepatitis may eventually result in postnecrotic cirrhosis, with extensive fibrosis and distortion of the lobular architecture of the liver.

Hepatitis B infection is also closely associated with development of hepatocellular carcinoma which, after skin cancer, is the most common malignant tumour worldwide.

Hepatitis B viral DNA, often integrated into the genome of liver cells, can be demonstrated in approximately 75% of hepatocellular carcinoma cases; exactly how the virus is involved in carcinogenesis is not known. Extrahepatic manifestations of persistent HBV infection, possibly related to circulating immune complexes, include a serum sickness-like syndrome, polyarteritis nodosa and membranous glomerulonephritis.

Vaccines prepared from heat-inactivated serum containing HBsAg, or by recombinant DNA techniques, provide effective protection against HBV infection. Immunization is of no value in individuals with pre-existing antibody to HBsAg or in chronic HBsAg carriers. Administration of hepatitis B vaccine is recommended particularly for individuals with a high risk of infection, such as male homosexuals, intravenous drug abusers, household and sexual contacts of hepatitis B carriers, dialysis patients, recipients of clotting factors VIII or IX, medical and laboratory workers with frequent exposure to blood or blood products, mortuary workers, and residents and staff members of institutions for the mentally retarded. Adults should receive 1 ml vaccine intramuscularly at 0, 1 and 6 months; children under 10 years should receive 0.5 ml on the same schedule. If exposure to HBV occurs via needle stick injury or other means, such as sexual intercourse, oral exchange of saliva by kissing or sharing a toothbrush of an unimmunized individual, prompt administration of serum immunoglobulin with high titres of anti-HBs antibody (HBIG) can provide partial protection. As soon as possible

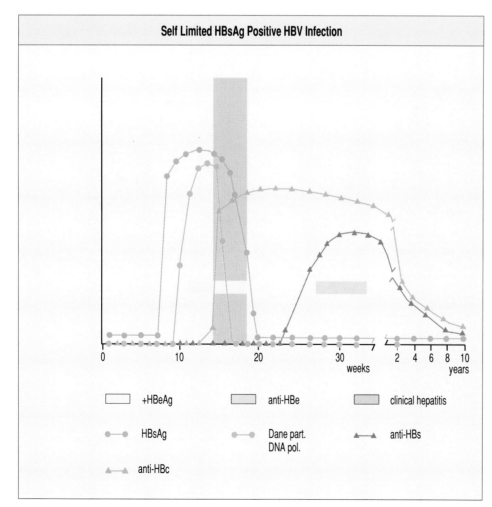

Fig. 5.7 Hepatitis B: schematic representation of viral markers in the blood throughout the course of self-limited, HBsAg-positive primary HBV infection. Adapted from Robinson WS. Hepatitis B virus and hepatitis delta virus. In: Mandell GL, Douglas RG, BennettJE, eds. *Principles and Practice of Infectious Diseases, Third Edition,* Churchill Livingstone, New York, 1990.

after exposure, 0.06 ml/kg HBIG should be given intramuscularly, followed either by immediate institution of active immunization with hepatitis B vaccine, or by a second dose of HBIG after one month.

No therapeutic measure has been shown to be beneficial in the treatment of acute viral hepatitis. Progression of chronic active hepatitis has been favourably affected by administration of corticosteroids or azathioprine. In some patients, liver function returns towards normal and cirrhosis appears to be prevented. The best results have been observed in HBsAg-negative patients, and in women treated at an early stage of disease. Unfortunately, corticosteroid therapy enhances replication of HBV, and may be associated with the appearance or rise in titre of HBsAg, HBeAg and Dane particles. Corticosteroid therapy is therefore recommended only for patients who are

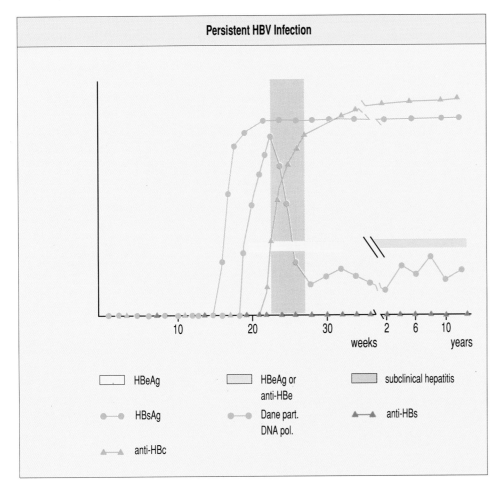

Fig. 5.8 Hepatitis B: schematic representation of viral markers in the blood throughout the course of HBV infection that becomes persistent. For source see.Fig. 5.7.

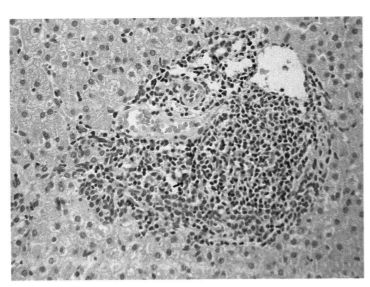

Fig. 5.9 Chronic persistent hepatitis: histological section of liver showing inflammatory nodule in a portal triad. Hepatic architecture is otherwise preserved and the limiting plate is intact. H&E stain. By courtesy of Dr. R.D. Johnson.

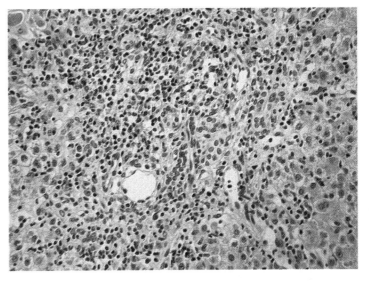

Fig. 5.10 Chronic active hepatitis: histological section of liver showing extensive infiltration by inflammatory cells with loss of the limiting plate, disruption of lobular architecture and degeneration and regeneration of hepatocytes. H&E stain. By courtesy of Dr. R.D. Johnson.

symptomatic, HBsAg negative and have severe histological lesions in liver biopsies.

Two antiviral agents, human leucocyte alpha interferon and adenine arabinoside, have also produced beneficial results in limited trials. Further studies are required to determine their place, if any, in the treatment of chronic hepatitis B infection. Serial determination of alpha-fetoprotein levels and ultrasound examination of the liver in HBsAg carriers with cirrhosis may allow detection of hepatocellular carcinoma at a stage when the tumour can be cured by surgical resection.

Hepatitis A Virus Infection

Infection with HAV, formerly known as infectious hepatitis, also occurs worldwide. The causative agent of hepatitis A is a small single-stranded RNA virus, similar to the enteroviruses, 27 nm in diameter (Fig. 5.11). Viral particles are present in hepatocytes and in faeces during the late incubation period and early stage of clinical hepatitis. Unlike HBV, with HAV there is no persistent state of infection with prolonged viraemia, so transmission by blood or blood products via parenteral routes almost never occurs. Humans represent the only significant reservoir of infection. Faeces appear to be the only important source of virus and transmission occurs most often via the faecal-oral route, or via food or water contaminated by sewage. Shellfish such as clams, oysters and mussels concentrate the virus during filter feeding and are common sources of hepatitis A infection. High risk groups include male homosexuals, children and staff members in day care centres, and other populations living in crowded settings such as prisons, military facilities and certain schools. Infection in young children is usually asymptomatic; most recognized cases occur in household contacts of children. There is little evidence for sexual transmission between heterosexual partners. The highest attack rates are found in developing countries, where housing and sanitation are inadequate. In some developing countries more than 90% of young adults have serological evidence of prior infection, as compared with approximately 20% of adults in the United States. About one-half of

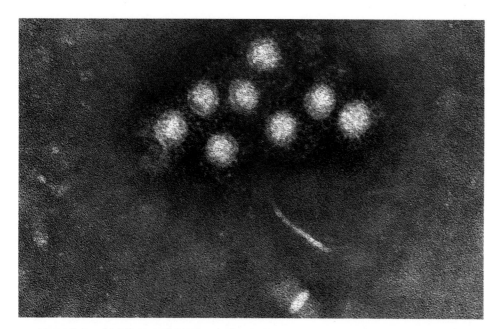

Fig. 5.11 Hepatitis A virus: electron micrograph of negatively stained particles. Small round particles of 27 nm diameter from human faeces, agglutinated with anti-MS-1 antiserum. By courtesy of Regional Virus Laboratory, East Birmingham Hospital.

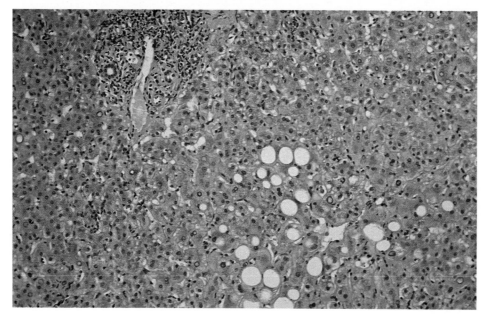

Fig. 5.12 Non-A, non-B hepatitis: acute spotty hepatitis with macrovesicular fat in the centrilobular area, diffuse microvesicular fat and infiltration of inflammatory cells in the portal triad. By courtesy of Dr. J. Newman.

acute viral hepatitis cases occurring in the United States are due to HAV.

The pattern of secondary infections in household contacts of patients with hepatitis A indicates that the patient is most infectious late in the incubation period or soon after the onset of symptoms, and this corresponds with the presence of the largest numbers of viral particles in the faeces. Faecal excretion of virus ends at about the time serum transaminases rise and jaundice appears in icteric cases. Although a transient viraemia may occur late in the incubation period, percutaneous transmission by blood or serum occurs very infrequently and is insignificant as a mode of HAV transmission.

Approximately 90% of cases of HAV infection are asymptomatic. In patients who become ill the clinical picture of the acute hepatitis is indistinguishable from that produced by HBV or by NANB viruses. The incubation period is usually from 2-6 weeks. Illness begins with fever, malaise, fatigue, headache, anorexia, nausea and vomiting, myalgias and epigastric or right upper quadrant pain. Diarrhoea, arthralgias, rash and respiratory symptoms of cough, coryza, and sore throat occur occasionally. Onset of symptoms may be more abrupt in hepatitis A than in hepatitis B, in which the illness usually develops gradually. As in hepatitis B, increased serum transaminases, dark urine and rising serum bilirubin precede the appearance of clinical jaundice. The illness usually lasts an average of two weeks, but in adults jaundice may last for one month or more. The histopathological findings are indistinguishable from those seen in acute hepatitis B. In contrast to hepatitis B, hepatitis A virus infection is not followed by chronic hepatitis.

Infection with HAV is followed by long-lasting immunity to reinfection. Serum IgG antibodies to HAV (anti-HAV)) appear during the convalescent stage and persist for years; IgM antibody is present during acute infection and disappears after 3-6 months. The best method of making a serological diagnosis of hepatitis A is by detection of anti-HAV IgM antibody during or shortly after the clinical illness; IgM antibody is not likely to be acquired passively via blood transfusion.

Careful attention to hand washing and proper disposal of infectious faeces and disposal or disinfection of contaminated objects can reduce the transmission of HAV infection. Household bleach diluted 1:32 can be used to disinfect objects or surfaces contaminated with HAV. Water can be rendered non-infectious by boiling for one minute or by adequate chlorination; the concentration of chlorine required depends upon the amount of organic matter in the water. Immunoglobulin can provide effective pre- or post-exposure passive protection against hepatitis A infection; it is recommended for household or sexual contacts, staff of day care centres, residents and staff of prisons or institutions for the mentally retarded, and for travellers to highly endemic areas. A single injection of immunoglobulin 0.02 ml/kg given intramuscularly within a few days of exposure to HAV reduces the attack rate of clinical hepatitis A by 80-90%; protection against further exposures lasts from 2-6 months. For travellers or residents in highly endemic settings, 0.06 ml/kg given intramuscularly provides protection for at least five months. The dose can be repeated every five months. A killed virus vaccine has been developed and appears to be immunogenic, but it is not yet available for general use.

Non-A, Non-B Hepatitis Virus Infection

Occurrence of cases of post-transfusion hepatitis without serological evidence of either hepatitis B or A infection led to the recognition of 'non-A, non-B' hepatitis. At least two distinct viruses are involved. In industrialized countries approximately 90% of cases of post-transfusion hepatitis are caused by the hepatitis C virus, an RNA virus which may be related to the arthropod-borne encephalitis viruses. Approximately 150,000 cases of hepatitis C infection occur in the United States every year. Only 5-10% are associated with blood transfusions; about 40% are associated with intravenous drug use, and 10% occur in heterosexual individuals with multiple sexual partners or household or sexual contacts of a patient with hepatitis. No source of infection can be identified in 40% of cases. Chronic liver disease develops in approximately 50% of individuals infected with the hepatitis C virus, and both cirrhosis and hepatocellular carcinoma are common sequelae. In recent studies approximately one-half of patients with chronic hepatitis C responded to administration of alpha interferon, but relapse was frequent after discontinuation of therapy. Corticosteroids are ineffective in the treatment of chronic hepatitis C infection.

Epidemics of water-borne hepatitis in less developed countries have been linked to an immunologically distinct virus, designated hepatitis E virus. This small RNA virus is present in the faeces of infected individuals, and has been demonstrated in the hepatocytes of experimentally-infected cynomolgus macaque monkeys. Hepatitis E virus appears to be one of the most common causes of acute hepatitis and jaundice in the Third World, but is rare in the United States.

The clinical illness produced by the hepatitis C and E viruses is usually mild, but there is a high case fatality rate in pregnant women who become infected with hepatitis E virus. Transient improvement followed by relapse is commonly seen in infection with hepatitis C virus The histopathological features are not always distinctive, but in some cases there is a disproportionate sinusoidal infiltrate and fat may be present (Fig. 5.12). Chronic hepatitis, which commonly follows infection with hepatitis C virus, is not seen in association with water-borne infections due to hepatitis E virus.

Delta Hepatitis

The hepatitis delta virus (HDV) is a defective RNA virus which is capable of replication only during concomitant infection with HBV. Thus it occurs only in patients who have HBsAg in the serum. It was discovered by immunofluorescent staining as a nuclear antigen distinct from the antigens of HBV, and is found in hepatocytes and serum of infected individuals. The hepatitis delta virus is a 35 nm particle which has an external coat of HBsAg provided by the genome of HBV (the helper virus) and an internal delta antigen (HDV-Ag) provided by the genome of HDV. The genome of HDV is smaller than that of any animal virus, and resembles that of the viroids of plants.

The virus can cause either acute or chronic hepatitis. Acute delta hepatitis resembles other forms of acute hepatitis, but is more severe, with a case fatality rate of 2-20% (compared with less than 1% in acute hepatitis B). Chronic delta hepatitis is also more severe than other forms of chronic viral hepatitis; 70-80% of patients develop cirrhosis with portal hypertension. Acute delta hepatitis occurs as either coinfection or superinfection. Coinfection is the simultaneous occurrence of acute hepatitis B and acute delta infection. Superinfection is the occurrence of acute HDV infection in a chronic HBV carrier. Acute delta coinfection is usually mild and self limited, rarely leading to chronic hepatitis. In contrast, acute delta superinfection leads to chronic hepatitis in more than 80% of patients.

Diagnosis of delta hepatitis is made by detecting antibodies to HDV in the serum of a patient who has HBsAg-positive hepatitis. Delta hepatitis should be suspected in any patient with acute or chronic hepatitis B infection, especially if the disease is severe or fulminant, or if the patient has a history of intravenous drug abuse or repeated exposure to blood or blood products. Clinical features suggesting delta infection are a biphasic illness in acute hepatitis or a history of jaundice or worsening of disease during the course of chronic hepatitis B infection.

Delta hepatitis occurs in three epidemiological settings. Endemic infection is especially common in the Mediterranean area and in the Middle East. The highest prevalence is reported from Kuwait and Saudi Arabia, where 20-40% of HBsAg carriers have antibody to HDV.

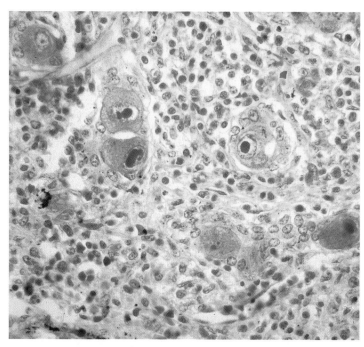

Fig. 5.13 Cytomegalovirus hepatitis: histological section of liver, portal area, showing intranuclear inclusion bodies in giant cells formed from bile duct epithelial cells, with surrounding mononuclear cell infiltrate. Phloxine-tartrazine stain.

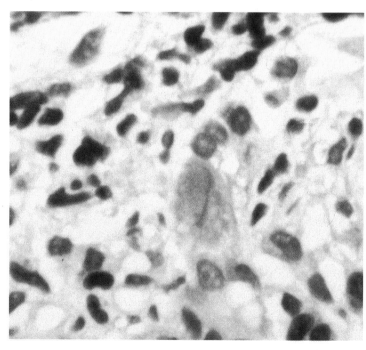

Fig. 5.14 Cytomegalovirus hepatitis: specific staining of CMV-infected giant cell using a DNA probe. By courtesy of Dr. Rodney S. Markin.

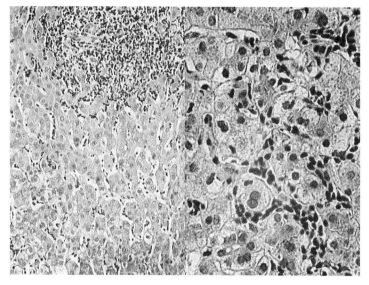

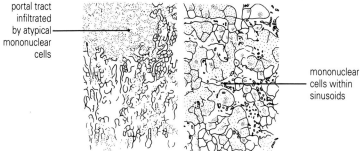

portal tract infiltrated by atypical mononuclear cells

mononuclear cells within sinusoids

Fig. 5.15 Infectious mononucleosis: histological sections of liver showing (a) a portal tract infiltrated by atypical mononuclear cells (by courtesy of Dr. I. Talbot), (b) mononuclear cells extending into the sinusoids. H&E stain.

Delta hepatitis is rare in northern Europe, the United States and most of South America, and is also uncommon in southeast Asia and China, where the prevalence of chronic HBV infection is very high. The disease occurs in epidemic form in isolated populations in certain underdeveloped areas of the world, especially in northern South America and the Amazon Basin. In these outbreaks the disease is strikingly severe, with sudden onset of fulminant hepatitis and a rapidly fatal course. The epidemic form occurs most frequently in children. In northern Europe and the United States delta hepatitis occurs primarily in certain high risk groups, including intravenous drug addicts and patients who receive multiple blood transfusions or antihaemophilic globulin. Although sexual transmission of delta hepatitis can occur, it is rare in most but not all populations of male homosexuals.

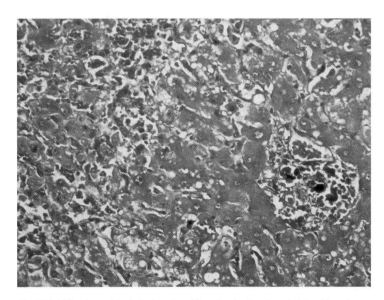

Fig. 5.16 Yellow fever: histological section of liver showing the characteristic midzonal necrosis between central vein and portal tract. Masson trichrome stain.

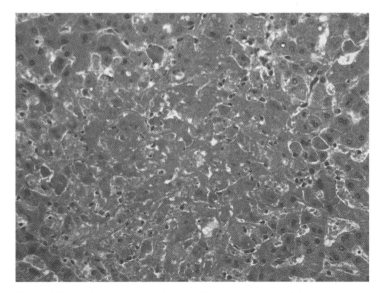

Fig. 5.17 Herpes simplex: histological section of liver showing a necrotic focus with little surrounding inflammation. H&E stain.

Immunization against HBV infection also provides immunity against delta hepatitis. Unfortunately there is no way to prevent HDV superinfection in HBsAg carriers, other than avoidance of contact. There is no established therapy for delta hepatitis. Corticosteroids are not effective in modifying the course or preventing progression of the disease. Alpha interferon inhibits replication of HDV and has produced clinical improvement in some patients, although discontinuation of therapy appears to be followed by relapse in nearly all cases. Results of liver transplantation in chronic delta hepatitis have been good, and some long-term survivors have remained both HBsAg- and HDV-negative after transplantation.

Other Forms of Acute Hepatitis

Clinical hepatitis due to cytomegalovirus occurs mainly in immunocompromised patients, in whom the disease may be severe or even fatal. It is clinically indistinguishable from HBV hepatitis, but the histopathological picture is distinctive because of the intranuclear inclusions in giant cells produced by coalescence of proliferating bile duct epithelium, and infiltration of mononuclear cells (Fig. 5.13). Virus and antigens can be identified by culture or by immunofluorescent staining in blood and liver (Fig. 5.14), and in other body fluids and tissues.

A mild, self-limited hepatitis, manifested by elevation of hepatocellular enzymes in the serum, occurs in 80-90% of patients with infectious mononucleosis due to the Epstein-Barr virus (Fig. 5.15). Occasionally severe hepatitis with jaundice is observed. Progression to chronic hepatitis or cirrhosis occurs rarely, if ever.

Yellow fever is an acute viral illness caused by a group B arbovirus transmitted by the mosquito *Aedes aegypti*. The virus is viscerotropic and produces damage in the liver, kidney, heart and gastrointestinal tract. The name 'yellow fever' refers to the jaundice which is present in severe infections. After an incubation period of a few days the illness begins abruptly with fever and chills, headache, myalgias, nausea and vomiting and leucopenia. After a few days the patient appears to improve, but the illness returns with fever, jaundice, haemorrhages, albuminuria and renal failure. Death often occurs in 7-10 days, following a terminal stage characterized by agitation, delirium, shock and coma.

The hepatic lesion consists of acute coagulative necrosis of the midzonal portion of the lobule (Fig. 5.16). Intracellular hyaline deposits (Councilman bodies) and intranuclear eosinophilic inclusions (Torres bodies) may be seen. Even in severe cases there is a conspicuous absence of infiltration by inflammatory cells. Yellow fever formerly occurred throughout much of the world (except Asia), but is now found only in tropical America and Africa. Control of yellow fever has been achieved primarily by elimination of the insect vector from much of its former range, and the live attenuated 17D vaccine provides essentially life-long protection from infection.

In immunocompromised individuals with herpes simplex infection or varicella (chickenpox), the virus may disseminate to visceral organs, including the liver. The characteristic hepatic lesion is focal coagulative necrosis with little surrounding inflammation (Figs. 5.17 and 5.18).

In Q fever, a rickettsial disease, there may be hepatic necrosis and lipogranulomatous lesions with eosinophilic material surrounding the central vacuole (Fig. 5.19).

In congenital syphilis (see Chapter 7), there is a hepatitis characterized by fibrosis around individual hepatocytes (Fig. 5.20), and there are abundant spirochaetes in the liver. In tertiary syphilis the typical lesion is the gumma, a necrotic nodule surrounded by granulation tissue (Fig. 5.21), which produces deep scars (hepar lobatum) as it heals by fibrosis.

Most infections with *Leptospira* (see Chapter 13) are either asymptomatic or result in mild anicteric infections without evidence of significant hepatic involvement. In severe cases of leptospirosis (Weil's disease), jaundice and impaired liver function are characteristically present. The jaundice is usually not associated with hepatocellular necrosis and leptospires are rarely seen in the liver (Fig. 5.22). After recovery, hepatic function returns to normal.

Jaundice is a well-recognized complication of severe bacterial infection in newborns, but this syndrome occurs rarely in adults. Occasionally in severe bacteraemic infections, especially those due to *Escherichia coli* and related members of the family *Enterobacteriaceae*, cholestatic jaundice is observed. Serum bilirubin and alkaline phos-phatase levels are elevated, but transaminases are usually normal or elevated only slightly. Histopathological examination reveals intrahepatic cholestasis with little or no hepatocellular necrosis.

Reye's syndrome is a syndrome of unknown aetiology seen primarily in children following influenza B (less commonly influenza A), varicella and a number of other viral infections. The incidence appears to be increased in children who have received aspirin. Involvement of the central nervous system is the most serious aspect of Reye's syndrome, and most deaths are due to cerebral oedema. In the liver the predominant findings are fatty infiltration of hepatocytes, with multiple small droplets of lipids uniformly distributed throughout the cells (Figs. 5.23 and 5.24). Swelling and pleomorphism of hepatic mitochondria are seen using electron microscopy. Inflammatory changes are absent, and there is little or no hepatocellular necrosis.

GRANULOMATOUS HEPATITIS

Formation of granulomas in the liver is observed in a wide variety of diseases, both infectious and non-infectious. The essential event in granuloma formation is the trans-

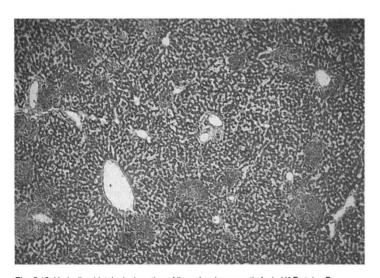

Fig. 5.18 Varicella: histological section of liver showing necrotic foci. H&E stain. By courtesy of Dr. I. Talbot.

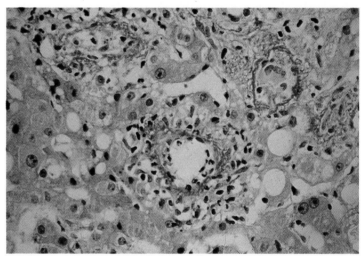

Fig. 5.19 Q fever: histological section of liver showing the characteristic lipogranulomatous-like lesion - a granuloma with a central vacuole and a red 'fibrinoid' rim. Martius scarlet blue stain.

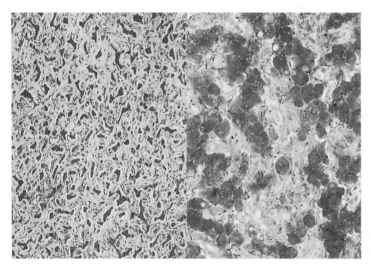

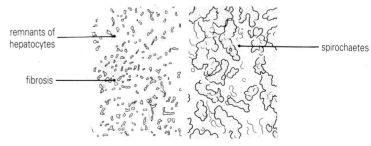

Fig. 5.20 Congenital syphilis: histological section of liver showing (a) diffuse pericellular fibrosis (H&E stain), (b) spirochaetes (Levaditi stain). By courtesy of Dr. I. Talbot.

formation of the monocyte/macrophage into an epithelioid cell. This event is stimulated by the presence of antigen, either soluble or particulate (e.g. micro-organisms and/or their products) in a sensitized cell.

The most common infectious disease associated with granuloma formation in the liver is tuberculosis. Outside the liver, tuberculous granulomas usually exhibit caseation necrosis, but hepatic granulomas due to tuberculosis are

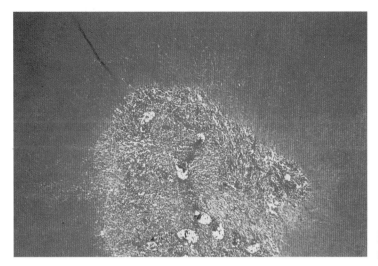

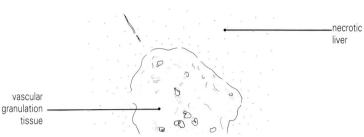

Fig. 5.21 Tertiary syphilis: histological section of liver showing a gumma. H&E stain. By courtesy of Dr. I. Talbot.

Fig. 5.22 Leptospirosis: hepatocytes contain large amounts of bilirubin. There are scattered lymphocytes and numerous irregularly-shaped nuclear fragments. By courtesy of Dr. J. Newman.

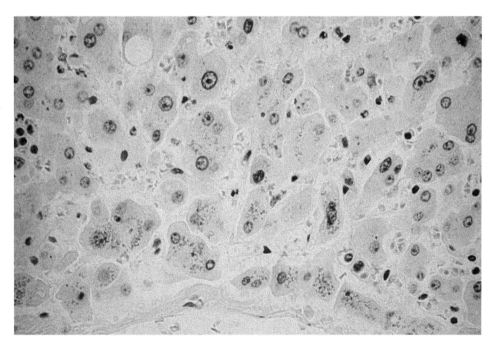

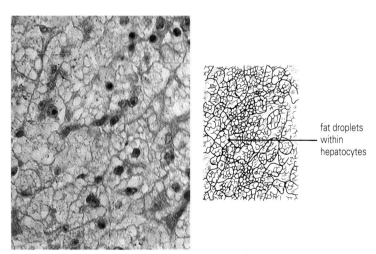

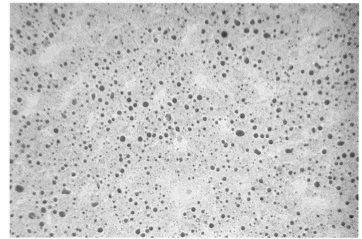

Fig. 5.23 Reye's syndrome: histological section of liver showing fat within cytoplasmic microvesicles. H&E stain. Courtesy of Dr. I. Talbot.

Fig. 5.24 Reye's syndrome: liver section with fat globules stained by oil red O. By courtesy of Dr. I. Talbot.

characteristically noncaseating (Fig. 5.25). Hepatic granulomas are present in more than 90% of patients with miliary tuberculosis, but are also extremely prevalent in pulmonary and in other extrapulmonary forms of the disease (70-80%). Tubercle bacilli can be demonstrated either by staining techniques or culture in approximately half of patients with miliary tuberculosis (Fig. 5.26), but are detected much less frequently in the granulomas associated with other forms of tuberculosis.

Infections due to *Mycobacterium tuberculosis* and *M. avium-intracellulare* are very common in patients with AIDS. Most AIDS patients with tuberculosis have disseminated or other extrapulmonary forms of the disease, and lesions are commonly found in the liver. Sometimes typical granulomas are found, but often the granulomas are poorly formed or the lesions are abscesses rather than granulomas. Infection with *M. avium-intracellulare* usually occurs late in the course of AIDS, in patients who are profoundly immunocompromised. In such patients granulomas are poorly formed or absent (Fig. 5.27).

Disseminated fungal infections are also commonly associated with granulomas in the liver. In the United States, disseminated histoplasmosis is the most common fungal infection associated with hepatic granulomas (Fig. 5.28), and liver biopsy is a valuable technique in the diagnosis of this infection (Fig. 5.29) and in the diagnosis of disseminated African histoplasmosis (Fig. 5.30). Hepatic candidiasis appears to be increasing in frequency among patients with cancer; in these patients the lesions often resemble abscesses rather than granulomas. Hepatic involvement is occasionally seen during systemic infection with a wide variety of other fungal organisms including *Cryptococcus neoformans* (Fig. 5.31).

The adult trematode worms *Schistosoma mansoni* (see Chapter 4) and *S. japonicum* reside in the portal and mesenteric veins (Fig. 5.32), and granulomas surrounding the eggs of these organisms may occur in the liver (Fig. 5.33). If infection is extensive, portal hypertension, hepatosplenomegaly and oesophageal varices may result (Fig. 5.34). Extensive liver involvement may also occur in visceral leishmaniasis (kala-azar) (see Chapter 13). In this disease there is marked proliferation of Kupffer cells,

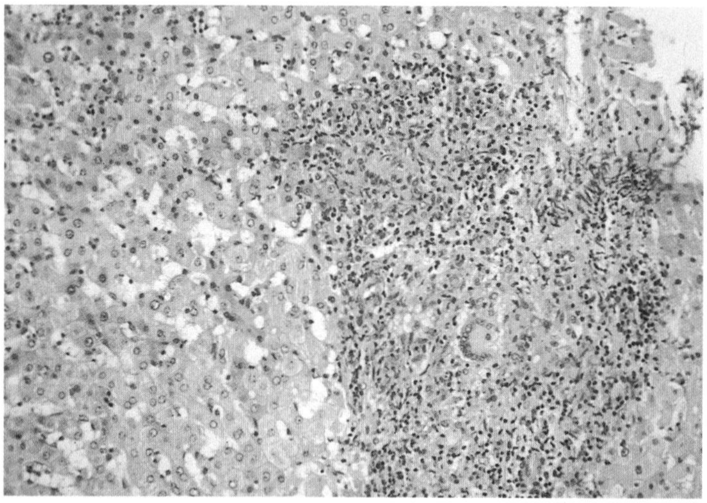

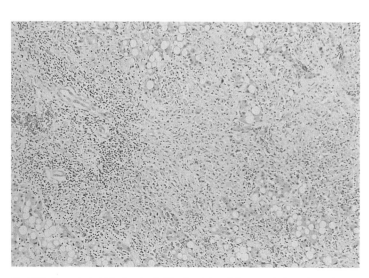

Fig. 5.25 Miliary tuberculosis: liver biopsy showing two contiguous tubercles and epithelioid cells, a few Langhans-type giant cells and lymphocytes. There is no caseation. H&E stain.

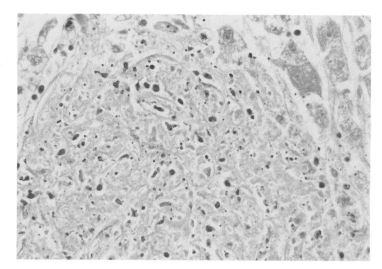

Fig. 5.26 Miliary tuberculosis: acid-fast stain of hepatic granuloma showing a few red-staining tubercle bacilli. By courtesy of Dr. Terry Gramlich.

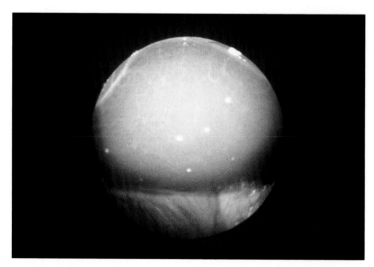

Fig. 5.27 Disseminated infection due to *M. avium-intracellulare*: poorly formed granuloma in the liver of a patient with AIDS. By courtesy of Dr. Terry Gramlich.

Fig. 5.28 Histoplasmosis: laparoscopic view of the surface of the liver showing healed granulomatous lesions in a patient with old, healed histoplasmosis. Biopsy of the lesions revealed calcification. By courtesy of Dr. John T. Cunningham.

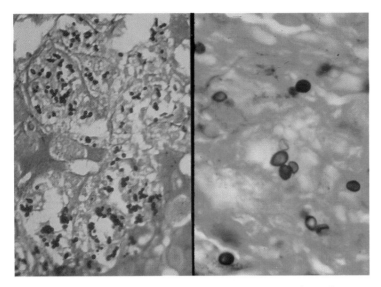

Fig. 5.29 Disseminated histoplasmosis: (a) section of liver showing yeast forms of *Histoplasma capsulatum* in hepatic sinusoids, (b) yeast forms of *H. capsulatum* from a lesion of the vocal cord. Gomori-methenamine silver stains. By courtesy of Dr. H.P. Holley, Jr.

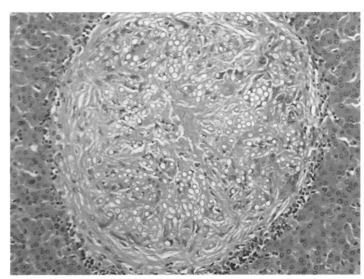

Fig. 5.30 Histoplasmosis: hepatic granuloma in African histoplasmosis, showing round vacuolated *H. duboisii* organisms. H&E stain.

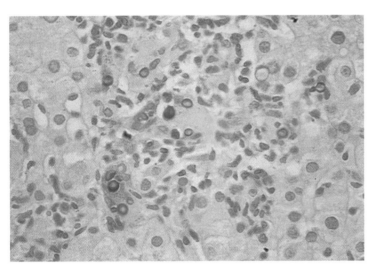

Fig. 5.31 Histological section of liver showing cryptococci staining blue with alcian blue stain.

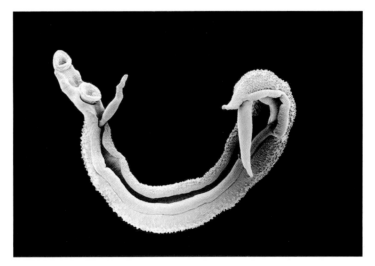

Fig. 5.32 Schistosomiasis: paired male and female adult schistosomes. The slender female lies within the gynecophoral canal of the male. By courtesy of Dr. V. Southgate and *Systemic Parasitology* (Kluwer Academic Publishers).

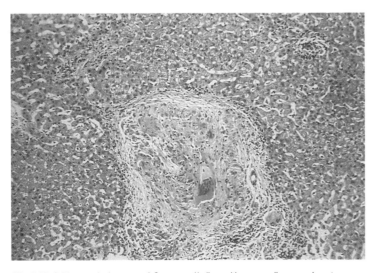

Fig. 5.33 Schistosomiasis: eggs of *S. mansoni* in liver with surrounding granulomatous reaction. H&E stain.

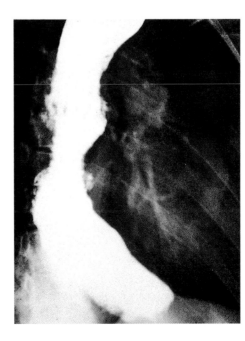

Fig. 5.34 Schistosomiasis: barium study of oesophagus showing oesophageal varices secondary to portal hypertension in *S. mansoni* infection. By courtesy of Dr. I.G. Kagan.

many of which are filled with the amastigote forms of *Leishmania donovani* (Fig. 5.35). Other infectious diseases in which liver granulomas are sometimes observed include toxoplasmosis, visceral larva migrans, Q fever (see Fig. 5.19), cat scratch disease, CMV infection, hepatitis B, and infectious mononucleosis.

Among non-infectious diseases, sarcoidosis is the disease most commonly associated with hepatic granulomas. In sarcoidosis and in other non-infectious causes of hepatic granuloma formation, the granulomas are noncaseating (Fig. 5.36). Hepatic granulomas are also seen in Hodgkin's disease and in various hypersensitivity states such as erythema nodosum. In approximately 50% of patients with granulomas in the liver, the lesions appear to be limited to the liver and no cause can be found. Presence of extensive granuloma formation in the liver is often associated with fever, and this condition is a common cause of 'fever of undetermined origin'.

HEPATIC ABSCESS

Abscesses in the liver may be due to *Entamoeba histolytica* or to various bacterial organisms. Clinical differentiation between the two types on the basis of such features as height of the temperature, leucocytosis or local pain and tenderness is notoriously unreliable. Amoebic liver abscesses are characteristically single and located in the right lobe and may be extremely large (Figs. 5.37 and 5.38). Most patients do not give a history consistent with preceding or current amoebic dysentery. An enlarged, tender liver, elevated diaphragm on chest X-ray, leucocytosis and elevated serum alkaline phosphatase levels are usually observed. Radioisotope scanning, computed tomography and ultrasonography are valuable for demonstrating the abscess. A serological test for amoebiasis is almost always positive in amoebic liver abscess. Occasionally, multiple amoebic abscesses are present (Figs. 5.39 and 5.40). The abscess cavities contain whitish, incompletely liquified, necrotic material which is

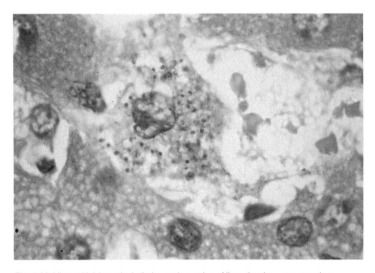

Fig. 5.35 Visceral leishmaniasis (kala-azar): section of liver showing a mononuclear phagocytic cell in a sinusoid containing many amastigote forms of *L. donovani*. H&E stain.

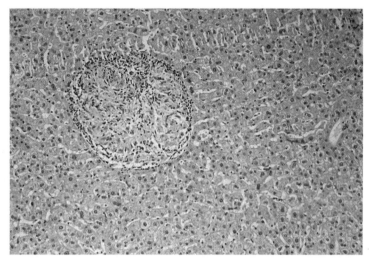

Fig. 5.36 Sarcoidosis: histological section showing a discrete noncaseating granuloma in the liver, composed primarily of epithelioid cells, surrounded by a thin rim of lymphocytes. H&E stain.

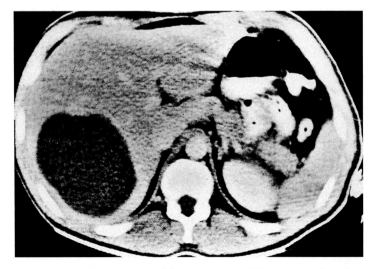

Fig. 5.37 Amoebic liver abscess: computerized tomographic (CT) scan showing large single amoebic abscess in the right lobe of the liver. Courtesy of Dr. F. Pittman.

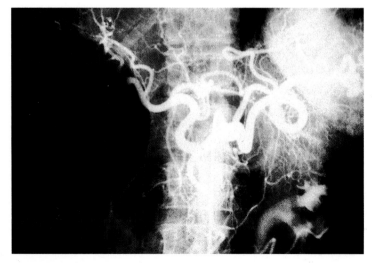

Fig. 5.38 Amoebic liver abscess: coeliac angiogram showing absence of vascular structures in a large amoebic liver abscess. The liquified necrotic material has been aspirated from the abscess and replaced by air. Courtesy of Dr. J. Cunningham.

sharply distinct from the normal liver tissue, and thick, brownish, odourless, liquified material consisting of necrotic liver tissue, inflammatory cells, and small or large numbers of amoebae (Fig.5.41). This material is regarded by some as resembling anchovy paste. Medical therapy with metronidazole or other drugs is usually effective and surgical drainage is rarely required.

Bacterial liver abscesses may occur secondary to nearby infection in the biliary tract, or the organisms may reach the liver via the portal vein (from intra-abdominal infections such as appendiceal abscess) or the systemic circulation. They are more likely than amoebic abscesses to be multiple. If the source of the abscess is infection in the biliary tract, the most common aetiological agents are *E. coli* and other members of the *Enterobacteriaceae*, including salmonella. If the infection has reached the liver via the portal vein, anaerobic bacteria, with or without aerobic species, are usually found. Streptococci of the *S. intermedius* (*S. milleri*) group are found in up to 80% of the lesions. Radionuclide scanning (Fig. 5.42), computed

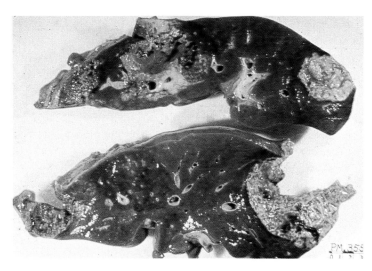

Fig. 5.39 Amoebic liver abscess: cut surface of liver showing multiple amoebic abscesses. Note the large central abscess containing 'anchovy paste' material and thick irregular lining of abscess cavities, composed of necrotic liver which has not yet liquified. Courtesy of Dr. J.T. Galambos.

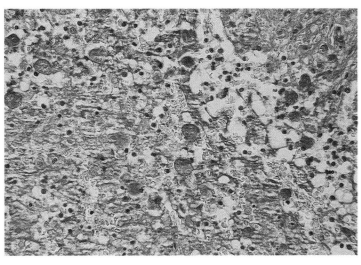

Fig. 5.40 Amoebic liver abscess: trophozoites of *Entamoeba histolytica* in necrotic liver tissue. By courtesy of Dr. C. Edwards.

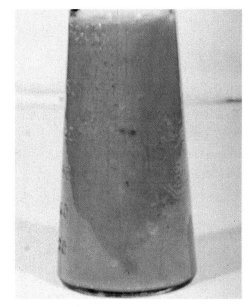

Fig. 5.41 Amoebic liver abscess: 'anchovy paste' material aspirated from an amoebic abscess of the liver. This fluid, unlike that found in pyogenic liver abscess, is odourless. Amoebae may or may not be readily found upon microscopic examination. By courtesy of Dr. K. Juniper.

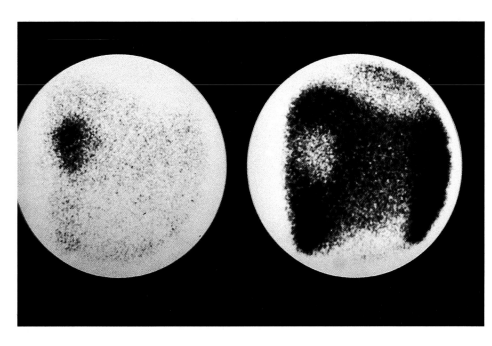

Fig. 5.42 Pyogenic liver abscess: gallium (left) and technetium (right) radionuclide scans of the liver. Gallium is picked up by inflammatory cells in the wall and cavity of the abscess, and thus outlines the abscess itself. Technetium is deposited in the Kuppfer cells of normally functioning liver, so activity is absent from the area involved by abscess. By courtesy of Dr. H. P. Holley, Jr.

tomographic scanning (Figs. 5.43 and 5.44) and ultra-sonography (Fig. 5.45) are valuable for confirming the presence of suspected liver abscesses. Percutaneous catheter drainage, using computed tomography to achieve precise placement of the catheter (Fig. 5.46), has obviated the need for surgical drainage in most cases of bacterial liver abscess. When multiple abscesses are present it may be necessary to drain several of the largest cavities. Treatment with an antibiotic effective against the infecting organisms should be administered for from one to several months. Amoebic liver abscesses are sometimes secondarily infected with bacteria; this type of combined infection may be very difficult to diagnose.

Echinococcosis (Hydatid Disease)

Adults of the dog tapeworm, *Echinococcus granulosus*, inhabit the intestinal tract of dogs. Sheep and cattle ingest the cysts in food contaminated by canine faeces. The cysts dissolve in the stomach and the liberated ova penetrate the intestinal wall. Dogs become infected by eating the viscera of dead, infected sheep and cattle, and the cycle is maintained (Fig. 5.47). Man is an accidental dead-end host, infected by contact with contaminated dog faeces, and plays no role in the cycle of infection. After penetrating the bowel wall the embryos travel via the portal blood to the liver and other organs. They may die and calcify (Fig. 5.48) or they may slowly enlarge over many years, producing disease by pressure effects or rupturing into the peritoneal cavity or pleural space with dissemination of the larvae (scolices) and production of multiple new lesions (Figs. 5.49-5.51).

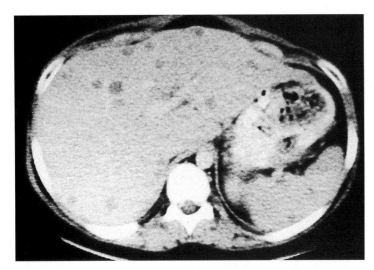

Fig. 5.43 Pyogenic liver abscess: CT scan showing multiple liver abscesses due to *Pseudomonas aeruginosa* in a severely neutropenic patient with chronic aplastic anaemia. By courtesy of Dr. N. Holland.

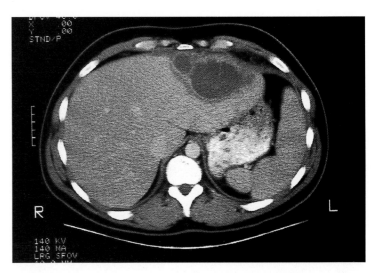

Fig. 5.44 Pyogenic liver abscess: CT scan showing a large abscess in the left lobe of the liver, with septum formation between compartments of the abscess. By courtesy of Dr. Randy Noble.

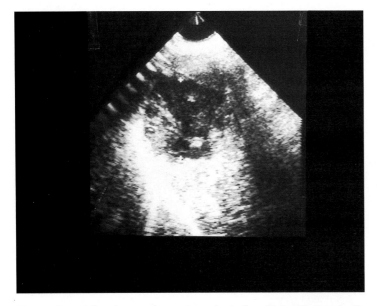

Fig. 5.45 Pyogenic liver abscess: ultrasound scan showing large intrahepatic abscess, with incomplete septum formation within the abscess cavity. By courtesy of Dr. Randy Noble.

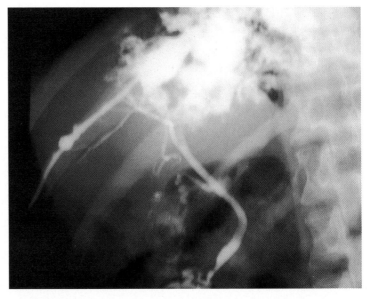

Fig. 5.46 Pyogenic liver abscess: percutaneous drainage of liver abscess. Injection of contrast material to delineate extent of abscess formation.

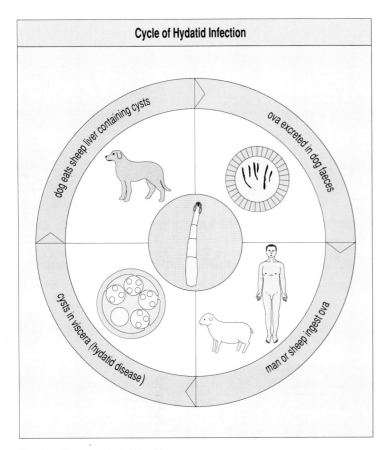

Cycle of Hydatid Infection

dog eats sheep liver containing cysts

ova excreted in dog faeces

cysts in viscera (hydatid disease)

man or sheep ingest ova

Fig. 5.47 The cycle of hydatid infection.

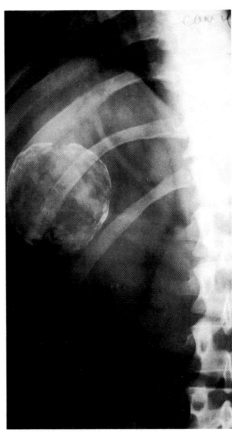

Fig, 5.48 Echinococcosis: abdominal radiograph showing a calcified hydatid cyst in the liver.

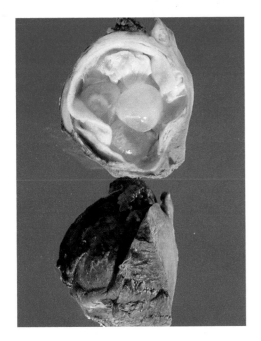

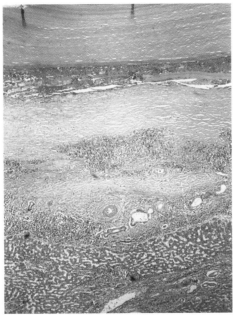

Fig. 5.49 Echinococcosis: an echinococcal cyst showing daughter cysts, resected from the liver (left), and histological section showing the layers of an hydatid cyst (right). H&E stain.

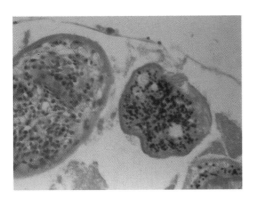

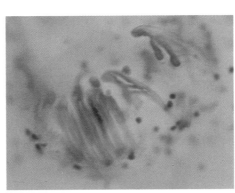

Fig. 5.50 Echinococcosis: (a) scolices of *E. granulosus* (H&E stain); (b) Hooklet at a higher magnification. Ziehl-Neelsen stain.

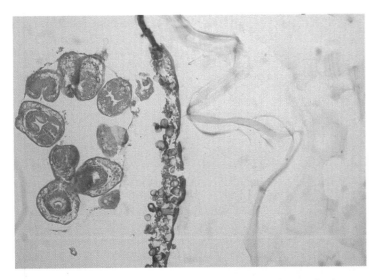

Fig. 5.51 Echinococcosis: cyst in liver showing (from right) laminated, non-nuclear layer, nucleated germinal layer with many brood capsules attached, and multiple scolices within the cyst cavity. By courtesy of Dr. C. Edwards.

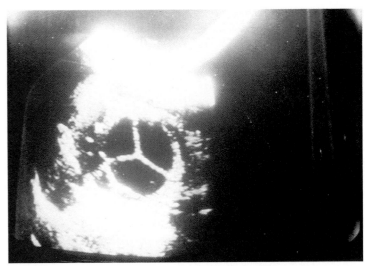

Fig. 5.52 Echinococcosis: ultrasound scan showing multiloculated cyst in liver.

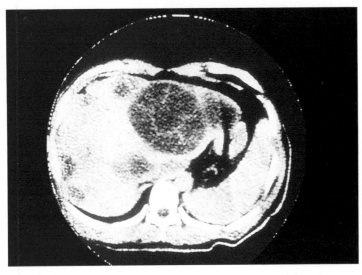

Fig. 5.53 Echinococcosis: CT scan showing large multiloculated cyst in left lobe of liver.

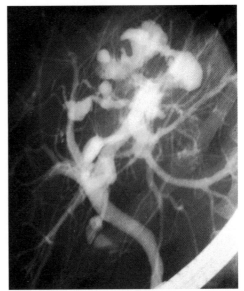

Fig. 5.54 Echinococcosis: Endoscopic retrograde cholangio-pancreatography (ERCP) showing intrahepatic hydatid cystic spaces draining into the biliary tree.

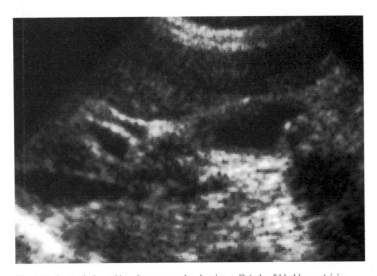

Fig. 5.55 Acute cholecystitis: ultrasonography showing a dilated gall bladder containing sludge and a single gallstone, with pericholecystic effusion. By courtesy of Dr. Randy Noble.

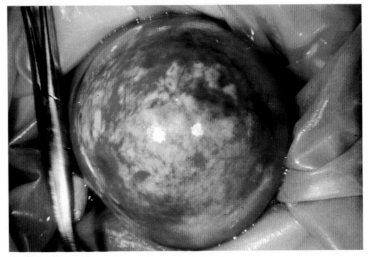

Fig. 5.56 Acute cholecystitis: operating room photograph showing multiple dark greenish areas with surrounding yellow border on surface of gallbladder, indicating transmural necrosis. There is also marked vascular engorgement of the serosal surface, indicative of the severity of the inflammatory process, and grayish areas of exudate on the serosal surface. By courtesy of Dr. M. Anderson.

The cysts can be visualized by ultrasonography (Fig. 5.52) or computed tomographic scanning (Fig. 5.53) or other imaging techniques (Fig. 5.54), and serological tests may provide a specific aetiological diagnosis. In cases where treatment is required, surgical removal, marsupialization and sterilization of cyst contents with formalin, hypertonic sodium chloride or iodine solution, or therapy with anthelminthic agents such as mebendazole, albendazole or praziquantel, may be effective. Infection in dogs can be prevented by proper disposal of sheep and cattle carcasses.

BILIARY TRACT INFECTION

Infection of the gallbladder (cholecystitis) may be acute or chronic, or the two types may coexist. In more than 90% of cases, stones are present in the cystic duct. Common clinical findings include pain in the right upper quadrant of the abdomen, fever. jaundice and a palpable gallbladder. Ultrasonography (Fig. 5.55) and hepatobiliary radionuclide scanning with an acetanilide iminodiacetic acid (IDA) derivative are both rapid and sensitive techniques for diagnosing this disease. The causative bacteria are most commonly *E. coli* and other organisms of the family *Enterobacteriaceae* and streptococci. Anaerobic bacteria are found occasionally, but seem to be involved less frequently than in most other types of intra-abdominal infection.

In acute cholecystitis (Figs. 5.56 and 5.57) there is an intense acute inflammatory reaction which may involve the full thickness of the gallbladder wall and may progress to transmural necrosis and perforation. In emphysematous cholecystitis, a severe form occurring primarily in diabetics, gas may be seen within the lumen and wall of the gallbladder (Fig. 5.58). In chronic cholecystitis, the wall of the gallbladder may be markedly thickened; multiple stones may be present inside the gallbladder, and chronic inflammatory changes and fibrosis may be apparent in the wall and on the serosal surface (Fig. 5.59).

Most cases of acute cholecystitis resolve within a few days, but elderly or seriously ill patients, or those who

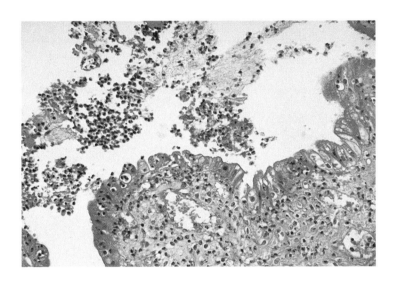

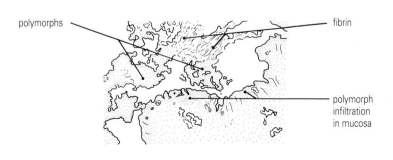

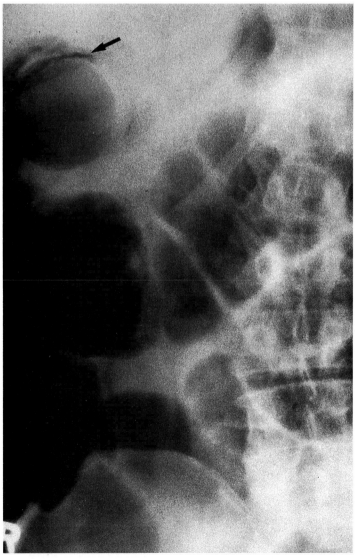

Fig. 5.57 Acute cholecystitis: histological section of gallbladder mucosa and submucosa. Note the purulent exudate in the lumen and infiltration within the epithelial lining and mucosa. H&E stain. By courtesy of Professor M.S.R. Huth.

Fig. 5.58 Emphysematous cholecystitis: plain abdominal X-ray. The gallbladder is seen as a gas-filled viscus. Gas is present in the wall of the gallbladder due to infection by *Clostridium perfringens*. By courtesy of Dr. M. Anderson.

develop complications such as perforation or gangrenous (emphysematous) cholecystitis, should be treated with antibiotics effective against Gram-negative bacilli and anaerobic bacteria, e.g. piperacillin, mezlocillin, or a combination of an aminoglycoside plus metronidazole or clindamycin. Immediate surgical intervention (cholecystectomy or cholecystectomy with drainage) is required for perforation, pericholecystic abscess or gangrenous cholecystitis. Acute cholecystitis is often associated with extension of infection into the extrahepatic and intrahepatic biliary system (ascending cholangitis) (Fig. 5.60). The cholangitis may become complicated by multiple intrahepatic abscesses (Fig. 5.61).

Ascending cholangitis usually produces severe systemic illness with high fever and chills, jaundice and severe pain and tenderness over the liver. "Charcot's triad' (fever, chills and jaundice) is present in 85% of cases. Ascending cholangitis is frequently associated with bacteraemia; the organisms isolated most commonly are *E. coli, Bacteroides fragilis* and *Clostridium perfringens*. Prompt therapy with appropriate antibiotics administered intravenously and relief of biliary obstruction is required. The technique of endoscopic retrograde cholangio-pancreatography (ERCP) has revolutionized the diagnosis and treatment of this condition by allowing direct visualization of gallstones in the common bile duct (Fig. 5.61). Either sphincterotomy with stone extraction (Fig. 5.62) or non-operative decompression of the biliary system by placement of an indwelling stent (Fig. 5. 63) may be employed to relieve the obstruction.

Clonorchiasis

Man is an incidental host for the oriental liver fluke *Clonorchis sinensis*, a parasite of fish-eating mammals of the Far East. Millions of people in China and Southeast Asia are infected with this organism. The adult worms live in the distal biliary passages (Fig. 5.64), where they

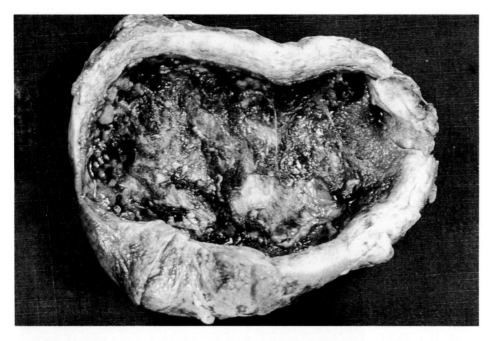

Fig. 5.59 Acute on chronic cholecystitis: macroscopic specimen showing loss of mucosa and necrosis, with haemorrhage in the submucosa (acute changes). There is also marked thickening of the gallbladder wall secondary to scarring, multiple stones lining the lumen of the gallbladder, and a shaggy nontranslucent appearance to the serosal surface (chronic changes).

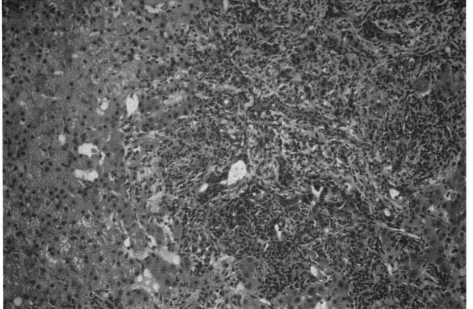

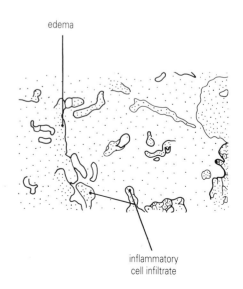

Fig. 5.60 Ascending cholangitis. The portal tract is edematous and filled with inflammatory cells.

edema

inflammatory cell infiltrate

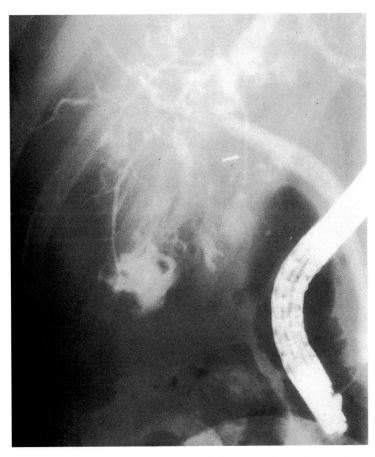

Fig. 5.61 Ascending cholangitis: multiple intrahepatic abscesses and several stones in the common bile duct demonstrated by ERCP. The endoscope is visible in the lower right hand corner. By courtesy of Dr. John T. Cunningham.

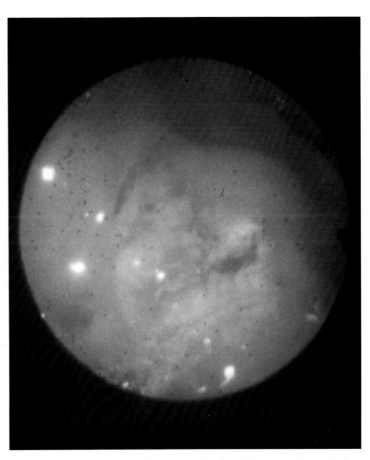

Fig. 5.62 Ascending cholangitis: endoscopic view showing sphincterotomy of ampulla of Vater in treatment of ascending cholangitis. By courtesy of Dr. John T. Cunningham.

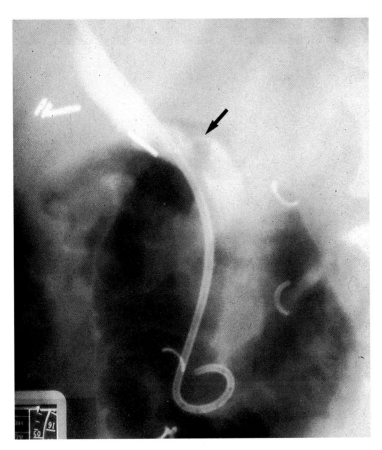

Fig. 5.63 Ascending cholangitis: a double pig-tailed endoprosthesis has been placed by ERCP to bypass the single stone in the common bile duct to prevent recurrent cholangitis. By courtesy of Dr. John T. Cunningham.

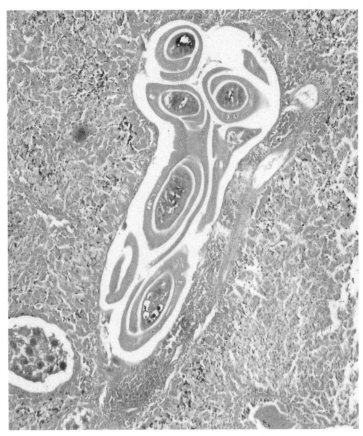

Fig. 5.64 Clonorchiasis: section of liver showing multiple adult worms of *Clonorchis sinensis* in a distal biliary duct. H&E stain.

produce eggs which pass down the biliary system and out of the body in the faeces. The eggs are ingested by snails, in which they hatch into miracidia. These multiply within the snail, producing large numbers of cercariae that emerge into the water. The cercariae penetrate under the scales of certain freshwater fish, in which they encyst as metacercariae, the forms which are infective when ingested by mammals.

Man acquires the disease by eating inadequately cooked fish. The metacercariae encyst in the duodenum and pass through the ampulla of Vater, where they mature into adult worms inside the bile ducts. Most infected individuals are asymptomatic, but heavy infection may produce cholangitis and hepatitis. Infection with this fluke is associated with an increased incidence of adenocarcinoma arising from the epithelium of the bile ducts. Diagnosis is made by finding the characteristic eggs in the faeces. No satisfactory treatment for this infection is available.

Fascioliasis

Infection with the liver fluke *Fasciola hepatica* occurs throughout the world wherever sheep are raised. The adult worms live in the biliary system of sheep, cattle and man (Fig. 5.65), where they deposit their eggs. The eggs pass into the intestines and are eliminated in the faeces. They complete their development into miracidia in freshwater and infect the intermediate snail host. Multiplication occurs within the snail and cercariae emerge and undergo encystment into metacercariae attached to aquatic plants. When these are ingested they excyst and the larvae penetrate through the intestinal wall and peritoneum, passing through the capsule of the liver and eventually reaching the biliary tract. The clinical illness is characterized by fever, eosinophilia and painful enlargement of the liver. Occasional cases have resulted in biliary obstruction or cirrhosis. Diagnosis is made by finding the eggs in faeces or bile. There is no proven effective treatment for the infection.

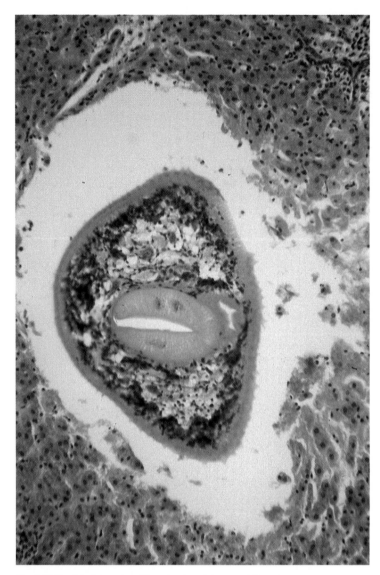

Fig. 5.65 Fasciolasis: section of liver showing adult worm of *Fasciola hepatica* lying within a bile duct. H&E stain.

6 THE URINARY TRACT

Infections of the urinary tract are among the most common of all bacterial infections. They tend to occur in four groups: schoolgirls, sexually active young women, men with prostatic hypertrophy, and the elderly. The vast majority of these infections occur in females, presumably because of the shorter urethra, which provides easier access into the bladder for microorganisms present on the perineal surface.

The term urinary tract infection (UTI) refers only to the presence of 'significant bacteriuria', and may or may not be accompanied by clinical symptoms. It is also usual to indicate whether infection involves only the bladder (cystitis) or also include the renal parenchyma (pyelonephritis).

Although the distal urethra of both sexes may be colonized by a variety of organisms, the remainder of the normal urinary tract is bacteriologically sterile. The most important route of urinary infection is the ascent of urethral organisms into the bladder and thence up the ureters to the renal pelvis and parenchyma. Haematogenous spread of infection to the renal parenchyma does occur but this usually results in abscess formation.

The major source of the bacteria that cause UTI is the faecal flora, particularly *Escherichia coli*. In women, the organisms first colonise the perineum, introitus and distal urethra and then ascend to the bladder. Factors facilitating ascent of bacteria to the bladder are urethral trauma, sexual intercourse and the turbulent urine flow in the short female urethra. Infection is much less frequent in men, probably due to the longer male urethra and the bactericidal activity of prostatic secretions. Bladder catheterization is almost invariably followed by infection within 3–4 days.

Once bacteria have gained access to the bladder, they are usually rapidly cleared by the flow of urine and complete bladder emptying. If bladder emptying is incomplete, due to obstruction or neurological disease, then high numbers of organisms may remain and produce infection.

Other local defences are phagocytic cells and local secretion of immunoglobulins (IgA and IgG).

Aetiology

Almost any bacterium can cause UTI, but some bacterial strains are particularly likely to do so: they possess a number of virulence factors. Chief amongst these are fimbrial adhesins that allow them to adhere to uroepithelium (Fig. 6.1), the quantity of K antigen, the production of haemolysins, and the ability to resist serum killing. These properties are particularly important in the pathophysiology of acute pyelonephritis but are also found more often in strains that cause lower UTIs than in control strains.

Some surveys have suggested that women with recurrent UTIs have more frequent vaginal colonization with *E. coli* than women with infrequent infections and that the vaginal and uroepithelial cells from women with recurrent attacks of cystitis have increased attachment of uropathogenic *E. coli* than cells from control women. Nonsecretor status and the use of diaphragms for contraception have also each been linked with an increased propensity for recurrent UTI, possibly by affecting the attachment of *E. coli* to uroepithelium.

In order to diagnose urinary tract infection (UTI) it is not necessary to obtain a specimen of urine from the bladder by direct aspiration. The diagnosis is usually based upon examination of voided urine specimens and therefore has to take into consideration contamination of the specimen by organisms from the anterior urethra. With regard to a clean, voided, midstream urine (MSU) specimen, the diagnosis of bacterial UTI is based upon the presence of the number of bacteria needed to meet the criterion of 'significant bacteriuria'. This depends upon the sex of the individual and whether the person has symptoms of UTI or not. A concentration of greater than 10^5/ml of bacteria of a single type in pure culture (usually expressed as colony-forming units [cfu/ml]) has a predictive accuracy of bladder bacteriuria of 80% in asymptomatic women and about 95% in women with symptoms of UTI. Two consecutive

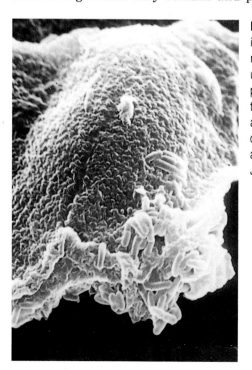

Fig. 6.1 Urinary tract infection. Scanning electron micrograph of an exfoliated urothelial cell obtained from a patient with an acute urinary tract infection, showing attached bacteria. By courtesy of Dr T. S. J. Elliott and the Editor of *British Journal of Urology*.

Prevalence of Bacteriuria in Populations	
Population	Prevalence (%)
Males	
Schoolboys	0.03
Adult men	0.1
Men over 65 years	10
Females	
Schoolgirls	1–3
Adult Women	1–3
Pregnant woman	4–7
Women over 65 years	20

Fig. 6.2 Prevalence of bacteriuria in various different populations.

positive cultures of 10^5cfu/ml increase the predictive accuracy to 95% in asymptomatic women. If there are colony counts of 10^4–10^5cfu/ml without associated signs and symptoms of UTI, then this is almost always due to contamination – in only 5% will a second specimen contain greater than 10^5cfu/ml. In symptomatic women, it is now appreciated that lesser bacterial concentrations are meaningful (see below). In the presence of symptoms, only concentrations less than 10^2cfu/ml cfu/ml should be disregarded. The same should probably be said for men, whether symptomatic or not,as the likelihood of contamination is much less than in women. The isolation of more than 10^2cfu/ml from a suprapubic aspiration of the bladder is significant. Specimens from patients with indwelling urinary catheters are best obtained by direct puncture of the catheter and aspiration with a sterile needle rather than by opening the closed drainage system or culturing the urine from the bag. If samples are taken in this way, contamination is most unlikely and a concentration of greater than 10^5cfu/ml is 95% predictive of true bladder infection.

A standard technique for urinalysis is recommended. Microscopic examination of the sediment from approximately 5ml of centrifuged urine may permit a presumptive diagnosis. The presence of more than 20 white blood cells per high power field (hpf) of the sediment is correlated with a bacterial colony count of greater than 10^5cfu/ml in most cases. The presence of bacteria in each hpf of a Gram stain of uncentrifuged urine also correlates with significant bacteriuria. Negative urine microscopy does not, however, rule out significant bacteriuria.

Differentiation between infection of the upper and the lower urinary tract has therapeutic and prognostic implications but is unreliable on the basis of clinical symptoms. Ureteral catheterization is reliable but invasive. Attempts have been made to detect antibody-coated bacteria (as evidence of invasive upper UTI) using fluorescein-conjugated antihuman IgG. A positive test is found in more than 80% of cases of acute pyelonephritis but there are false-positive and false-negative results in some groups of patients and it has not gained wide acceptance other than as an epidemiological tool.

Asymptomatic bacteriuria

Screening programmes have shown bacteriuria in a significant percentage of persons, particularly females (Fig. 6.2). In children, 1–3% of preschool or school age girls and 0.03 per cent of boys have bacteriuria. In young adults, the prevalence is 1–3% in non-pregnant women and 0.1% in men. In the elderly the prevalence increases dramatically to 10% of men and 20% of women. The majority of these asymptomatic patients have infection of the lower urinary tract only. In pregnancy there is a greater than 20% risk of asymptomatic bacteriuria leading to acute pyelonephritis, which is a risk factor for prematurity or stillbirth. Hence, asymptomatic bacteriuria in pregnancy requires therapy and regular review. Otherwise, asymptomatic bacteriuria in women only needs to be treated when there is obstruction present. There is no point in treating asymptomatic infection in the catheterized person: the urine cannot be sterilized because the catheter acts as a foreign body and the only consequence is the selection of resistant organisms in the bowel flora (which subsequently cause further UTIs).

Acute cystitis

Acute cystitis probably affects at least 20% of women at some time during their lives. It is characteristically associated with symptoms of dysuria, frequency and urgency. Sometimes there is suprapubic discomfort and occasionally there is frank haematuria. Fever is unusual and there are rarely any systemic signs. Acute cystitis is not usually associated with any anatomical or functional abnormality of the urinary tract. Predisposing factors are present in about 5% of women with cystitis. These factors are usually conditions that allow residual urine to remain in the bladder, or that disturb urinary flow.

If bacteria multiply to significant numbers in the bladder, then there are inflammatory changes in the bladder wall. In mild cases the mucosal oedema and cellular infiltrate may be largely superficial, but in severe cases this may involve the entire bladder wall (Fig. 6.3). In some cases, particularly in catheterized patients, severe mucosal

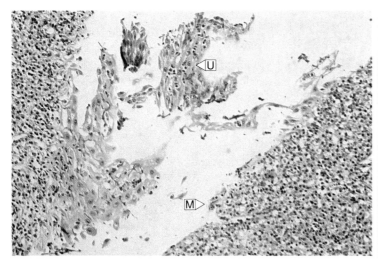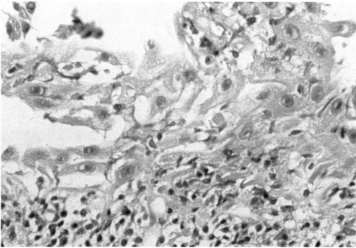

Fig. 6.3 Acute cystitis. Left: Severe cystitis causes extensive sloughing of uroepithelium (U) and may result in extensive mucosal denudation (M). Right: A higher magnification shows marked reactive changes with characteristic large nuclei in the partially detached uroepithelium.

hyperaemia and petechiae may produce haemorrhagic cystitis (Fig. 6.4).

E. coli is responsible for more than 90% of episodes of acute bacterial cystitis. *Staphylococcus saprophyticus*, a coagulase-negative staphylococcus, is the second most common cause of cystitis in young women. Other responsible pathogens are enteric bacteria, for instance strains of *Klebsiella*, *Proteus*, and *Enterobacter* species. These organisms, which are often resistant to many antibiotics, are particularly likely to cause hospital acquired UTIs. Other causes of cystitis, especially in the catheterized, diabetic or immunosuppressed person are *Pseudomonas aeruginosa*, and yeasts such as *Candida* and *Torulopsis glabrata* (Fig. 6.5). An unusual but spectacular form of cystitis is emphysematous cystitis (Fig. 6.6), caused by infection with gas-forming organisms, including some *E. coli* strains, clostridia and yeasts. This causes the diagnostic radiographic appearance of gas in the lumen of the bladder (Fig. 6.7) and may lead to passage of gas bubbles in the urine (pneumaturia).

Cystitis due to viruses can occur. Infection due to adenoviruses is particularly likely to cause haemorrhagic cystitis (see Fig. 6.4). This is much more common in schoolboys than in girls.

Patients with indwelling urinary catheters frequently develop cystitis. When prolonged catheterization is needed, prophylactic systemic antibiotics only prevent infections for about 4 days, after which there is no reduction in the infection rate as compared with controls and there is an increased risk of development of resistant organisms. Careful use of closed systems and aseptic techniques are the most important aspects of indwelling bladder catheterization.

Radiographic examination of the urinary tract is not indicated in all patients with cystitis, but should be performed in groups with a high risk of renal parenchymal damage (Fig. 6.8). In young children there is a strong possibility of renal scarring if infection is accompanied by vesicoureteric reflux: voiding cystourethrography should be performed (Fig. 6.9). Patients with recurrent attacks of cystitis may have a thickened bladder wall with irregular mucosa on intravenous urography and occasionally vesicoureteric reflux and residual urine on voiding cystourethrography. Some of these findings are transient and

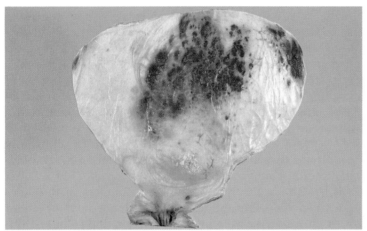
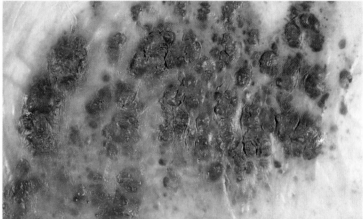

Fig. 6.4 Haemorrhagic cystitis. Left: Gross specimen showing discrete and confluent areas of haemorrhage in the bladder mucosa. Right: Close-up of same specimen. By courtesy of Dr J. Newman.

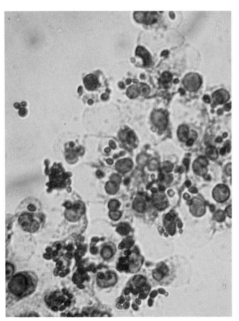

Fig. 6.5 *Torulopsis glabrata* infection. Centrifuged urine sediment showing many yeast cells and macrophages. The yeast cells are seen both inside and outside the phagocytic cells. *Sedistain* urine stain. By courtesy of A. E. Prevost.

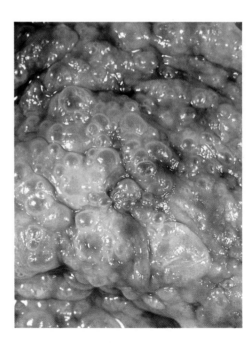

Fig. 6.6 Emphysematous cystitis. The blebs are gas bubbles in the submucosal connective tissue of the bladder. They are presumed to be caused by gas-forming bacteria. By courtesy of Dr J. Newman.

due to inflammation interfering with the normal, sphincter-like action of the ureterovesical junction: hence, where possible, radiographic studies should be delayed for at least 6 weeks after resolution of the infection.

The treatment of cystitis should take into consideration the prognosis of the infection in different individuals, the presence or absence of symptoms, and the inconvenience and adverse effects of the various antimicrobial agents. Symptomatic patients are usually treated – in asymptomatic patients, bacteriuria has been shown to have serious consequences only in preschool children and pregnant women. The usual drugs used for the treatment of acute cystitis are trimethoprim, cotrimoxazole, cephalosporins, amoxycillin/clavulanate, quinolones, and nitrofurantoin. These are all readily absorbed from the gastrointestinal tract, concentrated in the urine, of low toxicity and inex-

pensive. The choice of agent depends upon the patterns of resistance in the urinary pathogens prevalent in the locality and can be adjusted once the results of urine culture are available (at 48–72 hours). Sulphonamides and ampicillin/amoxycillin are no longer recommended owing to the high rates of resistance in *E. coli* in most places. Conventional therapy is continued for 7–14 days, but for uncomplicated cystitis a single dose or three days of antibiotic is commonly used (Fig. 6.10).

Investigations	
Investigation	**Patient groups**
IVU and/or ultrasound	All children
	Men
	Women with:
	Acute pyelonephritis
	History of childhood UTI
	Recurrent infections with same organism (relapses)
	Painless haematuria
	Calculi or obstruction
	UTI with bacteraemia
Voiding cystourethrography	All boys after first UTI
	Preschool girls after UTI

Fig. 6.8 Patients with UTI in whom radiological investigation of the urinary tract is indicated.

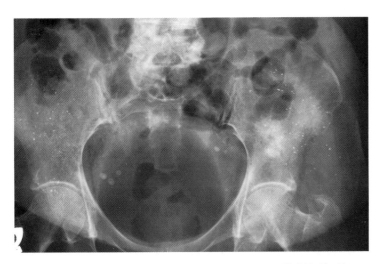

Fig. 6.7 Emphysematous cystitis. Plain abdominal x-ray showing gas-filled bladder. The multiple tiny densities in the gluteal regions are residua from intramuscular injections of bismuth given many years previously as treatment for syphilis. A few calcified phleboliths in the pelvic veins are also seen. By courtesy of Dr H. P. Holley, Jr. and the *Journal of the American Medical Association* (1981) **246**: 363–4. Copyright 1981, American Medical Association.

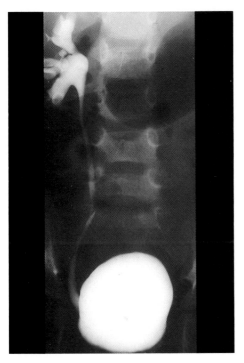

Fig. 6.9 Vesicoureteric reflux. Micturating cystoureterography in a young child showing right-sided reflux of contrast material into ureter and renal calices.

Patients Unsuitable for Single Dose Therapy
Patients with:
Symptoms of acute pyelonephritis
Antibody-coated bacteria test positive
Symptoms for more than 7 days
Anatomical abnormalities
Previous UTI with relatively resistant bacteria
Men
Children or infants
Pregnant women

Fig. 6.10 Groups of patients for whom single dose antibiotic therapy should not be given.

Causes of Urethral Syndrome			
Infection	Colony count	Pyuria	Antimicrobial therapy
Lower UTI	100–10 000	+	+
Urethritis	0–100	+	±
Vaginitis	0–100	–	+
Unknown cause	0–100	–	–

Fig. 6.11 Features of the various forms of urethral syndrome in women.

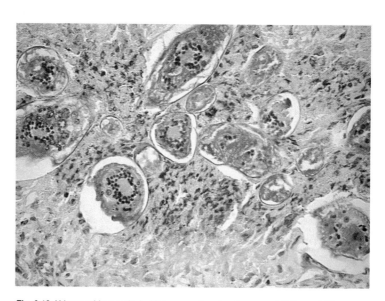

Fig. 6.12 Urinary schistosomiasis. High power view showing eggs of *S. haematobium* surrounded by granulomatous reaction within bladder wall. By courtesy of Dr J. Newman.

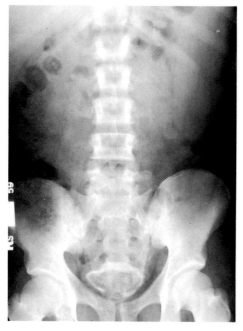

Fig. 6.13 Schistosomiasis. Plain abdominal x-ray showing calcification outlining the bladder wall, a late reaction in the chronic granulomatous reaction due to *S. haematobium* infection. By courtesy of Dr D. Tudway.

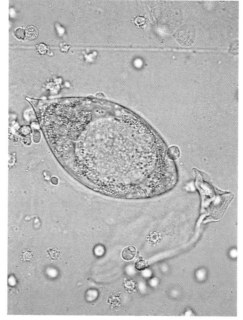

Fig. 6.14 Urinary schistosomiasis. Egg of *S. haematobium* in the urinary sediment. Note the terminal spine. By courtesy of Dr M. H. Winterborn.

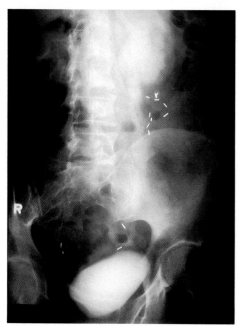

Fig. 6.15 Obstructive uropathy. Intravenous pyelogram showing markedly dilated left renal collecting system due to ureteral obstruction by tumour. There is also thinning of the renal parenchyma indicating a chronic obstructive process. By courtesy of Dr Randy Noble.

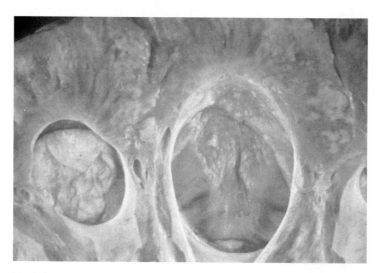

Fig. 6.16 Acute pyelonephritis. The obstructed kidney is particularly prone to infection. The dilated calices have a granular dull mucosa focally covered by a shaggy exudate. The confluent pale parenchymal nodules, which obliterate the normal corticomedullary markings, represent numerous abscesses.

Given that those with occult upper tract infection will not be cured or will relapse after such short courses, and that differentiation of upper from lower UTIs is not possible clinically, follow-up cultures should be taken 1–2 weeks after stopping therapy. In children it is prudent to continue follow-up with regular urinary cultures for at least 2 years. Those who fail should receive a conventional course of antibiotics. If infections occur repeatedly or the underlying cause for a relapsing infection can not be eradicated, then chronic suppressive therapy with daily low-dose cotrimoxazole, trimethoprim or nitrofurantoin (which have little effect on the bowel flora) can be used. Similar prophylactic antibiotics can be given to women in whom UTI frequently follows sexual intercourse.

Acute urethral syndrome

Almost 50% of women with symptoms of frequency and dysuria, but without fever and systemic symptoms, do not have 'significant bacteriuria' (greater than 10^5cfu/ml). These women are said to have the urethral syndrome (Fig. 6.11). It is now recognised that many women with these common symptoms do indeed have acute cystitis but with low counts of bacteria in the urine (10^2–10^4cfu/ml). Patients in this group usually have pyuria and are helped by antimicrobial therapy. Urethritis caused by sexually-transmitted agents such as *Chlamydia trachomatis* (which is also accompanied by pyuria and may be cured by tetracycline therapy), herpes genitalis or the various forms of vaginitis may also cause similar symptoms (see Chapter 7). Other women have frequency and dysuria but no infective cause can be determined.

Schistosomiasis

Urinary schistosomiasis is due to infection with the blood-fluke *Schistosoma haematobium*, which is endemic in Africa and the Middle East. The life cycle of the parasite is similar to that of *S. mansoni* (see Chapter 4), except that the adult worms live in the venous plexus around the urinary bladder. The adult worms constantly produce large numbers of eggs, many of which are retained in the tissues and induce a granulomatous reaction (Fig. 6.12). The inflammation leads to extensive fibrous tissue and scarring, which results in urinary obstruction or irregularity of the bladder wall. Eventually these lesions may calcify, producing a characteristic radiographic appearance (Fig. 6.13). Chronic *S. haematobium* infection is associated with both the salmonella urinary-carrier state and carcinoma of the bladder.

Persons infected with *S. haematobium* usually have terminal haematuria and dysuria, other symptoms resulting from obstruction or recurrent urinary infections. A definitive diagnosis can be made by finding schistosome eggs in the urine, best collected in the early afternoon (Fig. 6.14). The therapy for schistosomiasis is now best given with a single oral dose of praziquantel (40mg/kg body weight), which is effective against all human schistosomes and is remarkably free of serious adverse effects. Metrifonate is also active, but only against *S. haematobium* and must be given three times.

Acute pyelonephritis

Pyelonephritis refers to inflammation of the kidney parenchyma, calices and pelvis, usually due to bacterial infection. When infection reaches the kidney, it usually does so by ascending the ureters from the lower urinary tract, though blood-borne infection can also occur. Abnormalities of the urinary tract, such as vesicoureteric reflux and other causes of residual bladder urine, obstruction at various levels of the urinary tract due to stones or other pathology (Figs 6.15 & 6.16), and renal parenchymal damage are important predisposing factors to the development of pyelonephritis. Vesicoureteric reflux in the presence of infection, particularly in children under the age of 5, is associated with the development of renal scarring. Such scars often do not progress after this age and the reflux may disappear with time.

Magnesium ammonium phosphate (struvite) stones occur in association with infection due to urea-splitting organisms (*Proteus* species). They may form a virtual cast of the renal pelvis, when they are known as staghorn calculi (Fig. 6.17). Bladder stones (Figs 6.18 & 6.19) are nearly

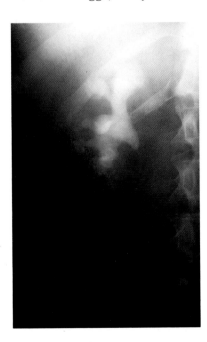

Fig. 6.17 Staghorn calculus. Detail from plain film of the abdomen demonstrating a staghorn calculus virtually filling the entire collecting system of the right kidney. By courtesy of Dr Randy Noble.

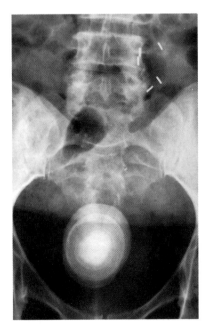

Fig. 6.18 Bladder calculus. Plain x-ray of pelvis showing a single large laminated stone in the bladder. By courtesy of Dr C. N. Griffin.

always found in males, in association with obstruction due to prostatic hypertrophy, urethral stricture or anatomical abnormality at the bladder neck.

There are several virulence factors that are important in the development of upper UTI. So-called P-fimbriae are essential for *E. coli*, *Proteus* species and *Klebsiella* species to infect renal epithelial cells. Another virulence factor in *E. coli* that favours the development of pyelonephritis is the presence of certain K antigens (polysaccharide capsular antigens that are poorly immunogenic).

The classic clinical features of acute pyelonephritis are systemic: fever, rigors and pain and tenderness in the costovertebral angle, associated with the symptoms and signs of lower UTI. Nausea, vomiting and diarrhoea may be prominent. However, it is now recognised that many patients with symptoms suggestive only of lower UTI do in fact have subclinical pyelonephritis. A useful sign is the presence of casts containing white blood cells in the urinary sediment (Fig. 6.20): these are formed in the renal tubules and collecting ducts and thus signify involvement of the kidney. Bacteraemia complicates up to 40% of cases of acute pyelonephritis. The kidney in acute pyelonephritis is usually enlarged and oedematous with many polymorphonuclear leucocytes in the tubules and interstitial areas (Fig. 6.21). Pathological changes are most prominent in the medulla, probably reflecting an ascending route of infection and increased susceptibility of the medullary tissue to infection. Multiple microabscesses are usually present in severe cases (Fig. 6.22), particularly after haematogenous spread of infection due to *S. aureus* or *Candida* species. Occasionally a large intrarenal abscess (renal carbuncle) may occur (see below). In the absence of obstruction, recurrent UTIs in adults rarely lead to progressive renal damage and infection alone probably never leads to chronic pyelonephritis (see below).

Fungal pyelonephritis is usually due to *Candida albicans* and results from systemic infection rather than ascending UTI. It is particularly likely to occur in immunosuppressed individuals. Small abscesses are seen scattered through the cortex of the kidney (Fig. 6.23) and

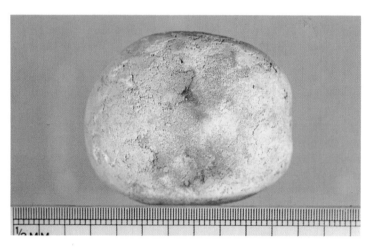

Fig. 6.19 Bladder calculus removed from patient with chronic cystitis and prostatic hypertrophy. By courtesy of Dr J. Newman.

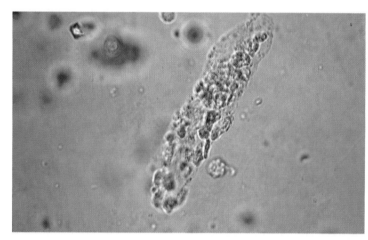

Fig. 6.20 Acute pyelonephritis. High power view of urine sediment showing a tubular cast containing many white blood cells in various stages of degeneration. By courtesy of Dr S. Rous.

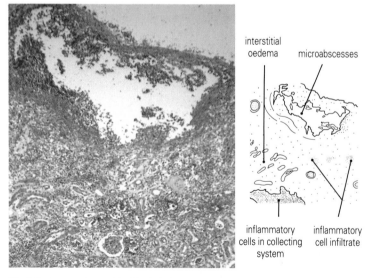

interstitial oedema   microabscesses

inflammatory cells in collecting system   inflammatory cell infiltrate

Fig. 6.21 Acute pyelonephritis. Histological section of kidney showing intense infiltration by inflammatory cells, severe interstitial oedema, many inflammatory cells in the collecting system and an intrarenal abscess. H & E stain.

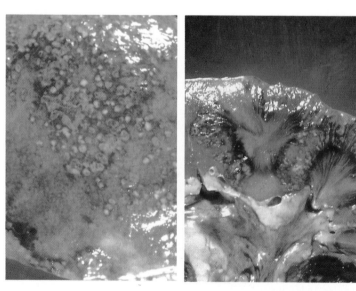

Fig. 6.22 Acute pyelonephritis. Left: Cortical abscess in pyelonephritis, which produces discrete or confluent, raised, yellow-white, rounded nodules with surrounding hyperaemia. Right: The cut surface also contains abscesses, and there are straight yellow streaks and hyperaemia in the medullae. The pelvic mucosa is congested, granular and dull.

microscopically these are seen to contain large numbers of fungi (Fig. 6.24).

Whether patients with symptomatic pyelonephritis should be treated in hospital or as outpatients depends largely upon clinical judgement. Those who are severely ill or who have bacteraemia will need parenteral antibiotics: an aminoglycoside, cephalosporin, cotrimoxazole or quinolone for those with community-acquired infections and imipenem or ceftazidime for those with possible pseudomonas or highly-resistant Enterobacteriaceae infection (nosocomial or catheter-associated infections). Those who are less unwell can be managed as outpatients with oral trimethoprim, cotrimoxazole, amoxycillin clavulanate or ciprofloxacin. Therapy should be given for 10–14 days. Relapse occurs in 10–50% of patients after 2 weeks of therapy; these should be treated again with a 4-week course of antibiotics. Radiological investigation should be undertaken. Follow-up urine cultures should be taken in children, pregnant women, and those with obstruction of the urinary tract.

Renal abscess

The pathogenesis of intrarenal abscess (Fig. 6.25) has changed over the years. In the past they arose as complications of staphylococcal infections elsewhere, occurring as a result of bacteraemic spread. Nowadays they are frequently seen as complications of acute pyelonephritis and are caused by gram-negative organisms. These patients usually present with high fever, loin pain and flank tenderness suggestive of acute pyelonephritis; those with renal abscesses secondary to haematogenous spread may sometimes present more chronically with symptoms of malaise and weight loss. Urine culture is often normal if *S. aureus* is the causative organism, but when gram-negative bacteria are responsible urine culture usually shows the same organism. The diagnosis can occasionally be suggested by the presence of gas within the renal shadow on a plain abdominal x-ray but is usually made by intravenous or retrograde urography (Fig. 6.26) and ultrasonography. When an abscess is

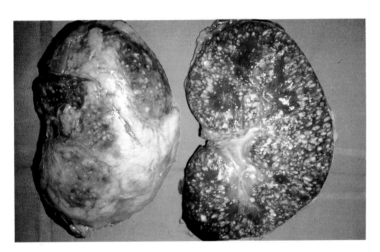

Fig. 6.23 Candida pyelonephritis. Numerous small abscesses scattered throughout the cortex in a patient who died from Candida endocarditis.

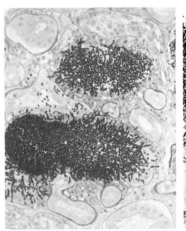
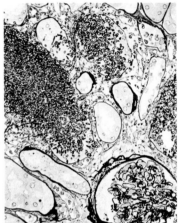

Fig. 6.24 Fungal pyelonephritis. Microscopic examination of the kidney of a renal transplant patient showing large numbers of candida organisms visible in the interstitium. Left: PAS stain. Right: Grocott stain. By courtesy of Dr J. Newman.

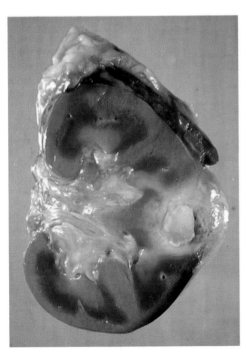

Fig 6.25 Renal abscess. Gross specimen showing large abscess in the cortical, subcapsular tissues. By courtesy of Dr J. Newman.

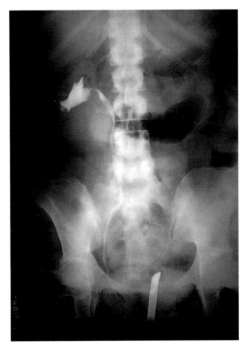

Fig. 6.26 Renal abscess. Parenchymal destruction from acute pyelonephritis may result in a large renal cortical abscess evident radiographically. This retrograde pyelogram shows deformation and displacement of the collecting system of the right kidney by a very large abscess in the lower pole. By courtesy of Dr Randy Noble.

confirmed, empirical parenteral antibiotic therapy directed against the likely pathogens should be started and ultrasound guided percutaneous aspiration attempted. This enables the pus to be cultured and usually provides a route for the introduction of a fine-bore drainage catheter to decompress the abscess. This often makes surgical drainage unnecessary.

Papillary necrosis

Renal papillary necrosis may occur in association with severe pyelonephritis, especially in diabetics and in individuals with urinary tract obstruction, sickle-cell disease or trait, or analgesic abuse. Wedge-shaped areas of necrosis, often with a congested border, develop in the pyramids and portions of the necrotic papillae may break off.

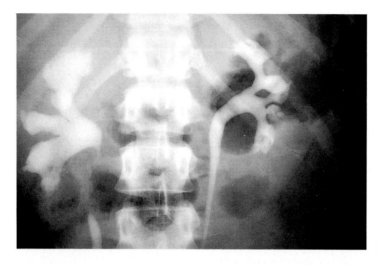

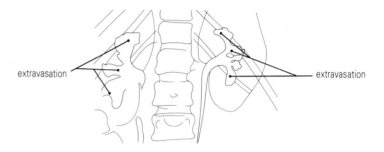

Fig. 6.27 Renal papillary necrosis. Intravenous pyelogram showing extravasation of contrast material from several calices of each kidney into the cavities created by necrosis of renal papillae, in a patient with sickle cell trait. By courtesy of Dr D. Tudway.

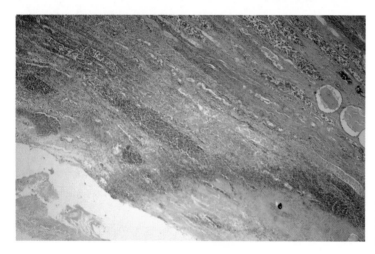

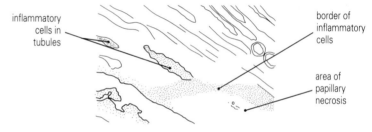

Fig. 6.28 Acute papillary necrosis. Histological section of kidney showing intense inflammatory cell infiltration in the tubules and interstitium, and a zone of acute inflammatory cells bordering the area of necrosis. H & E stain.

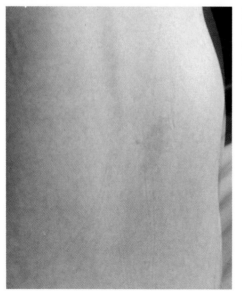

Fig. 6.29 Perinephric abscess. Clinical photograph showing prominent bulge in the right flank. By courtesy of Dr P. Hohl.

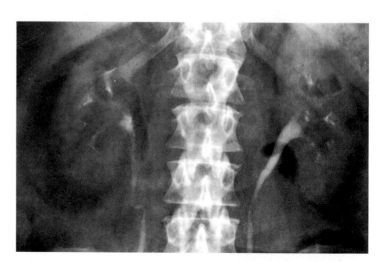

Fig. 6.30 Intravenous urogram of perinephric abscess. The nephrogram phase shows normal-sized kidneys but on the right there is a perirenal gas halo due to the abscess and obliteration of the psoas shadow on that side.

A characteristic radiographic appearance may be seen on intravenous pyelography, consisting of collections of contrast material outside the caliceal system in cavities produced by the necrosis and sloughing of the papillary tissue (Fig. 6.27).

Microscopically there is coagulation necrosis of the papillary tissue which is sharply demarcated from the surrounding medulla by a zone of inflammatory cells (Fig. 6.28).

Perinephric abscess

Renal infection may extend through the capsule of the kidney into the perinephric fat to produce an abscess, usually in patients with severe pyelonephritis associated with obstruction of the urinary tract or renal calculi or who are diabetic. Rarely it may be secondary to bacteraemia. As for intrarenal abscesses the infecting organisms are typically gram-negative bacteria or, in the case of perinephric abscess secondary to bacteraemia, *S. aureus*. The patient complains of fever and chills associated with abdominal and flank pain, often of several days duration. Examination may or may not reveal a mass in the flank (Fig. 6.29). Urine culture is generally positive.

The intravenous urogram is abnormal in most cases. If films are taken on inspiration and standing it will be seen that the local adhesions mean that the kidney does not descend as in the normal individual. A perinephric gas halo (Fig. 6.30), a gas pattern over the kidney and the loss of the psoas shadow on the affected side may also be seen. Ultrasonography, CT scanning (Fig. 6.31) and gallium scanning may establish the diagnosis. Treatment consists of drainage of the abscess after starting parenteral antibiotic therapy. Antibiotic choice may need to be empirical but is usually governed by the urine culture results). Drainage can often be undertaken percutaneously.

Chronic pyelonephritis

This is a confusing term which is used differently by different authorities. It is often applied to a group of pathological findings associated with chronic inflammation and fibrosis of the kidney, which may be due to infection but which almost certainly can result from urinary tract obstruction, analgesic nephropathy, vascular disease and urate nephropathy. Many patients with these pathological findings do not have bacteria in the urine, and the response to antimicrobial therapy is poor.

Typically there is asymmetric contraction and distortion of the kidney (Fig. 6.32) with deep cortical scars overlying dilated and blunted calices (Figs 6.33 & 6.34).

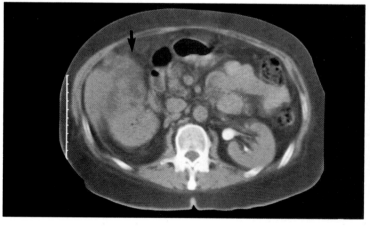

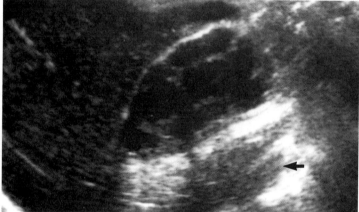

Fig. 6.31 Perinephric abscess. Left: CT scan showing a large abscess in the right perinephric space (arrowed). Right: Ultrasound study of pyonephrotic kidney displaced anteriorly by abscess (arrowed). By courtesy of Dr P. Hohl.

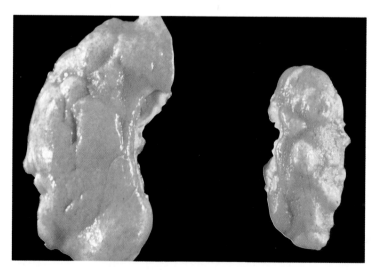

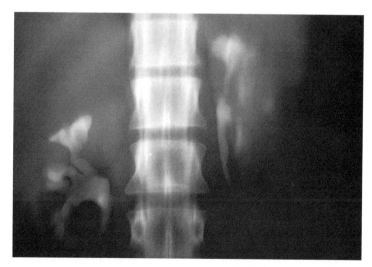

Fig. 6.32 Chronic pyelonephritis. Typical asymmetrical changes with irregular large flat scars. The finely granular appearance of the intervening cortex is secondary to hypertensive nephrosclerosis.

Fig. 6.33 Chronic pyelonephritis. Tomogram of intravenous urogram shows blunting and distortion of calices of both kidneys with marked thinning of the overlying renal cortex. By courtesy of Dr D. Tudway.

Microscopically, there is interstitial infiltration with chronic inflammatory cells progressing to interstitial fibrosis, periglomerular fibrosis, which eventually destroys and replaces the glomerulus, and plugging of tubules with inspissated hyaline proteinaceous material and atrophy of tubular epithelium ('thyroidization' – Fig. 6.35).

Xanthogranulomatous pyelonephritis

This is a rare form of chronic suppurative pyelonephritis. It is always unilateral and is characterized by the presence of yellowish nodules adjacent to areas of necrosis and suppuration (Fig. 6.36). The nodules contain granuloma-

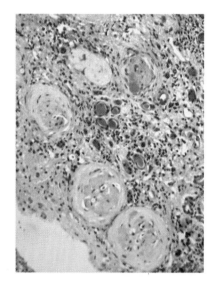

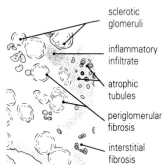

Fig. 6.35 Chronic pyelonephritis. Histological section of end-stage kidney showing sclerotic glomeruli, interstitial fibrosis, a moderate chronic inflammatory infiltrate and atrophic tubules. H & E stain.

- sclerotic glomeruli
- inflammatory infiltrate
- atrophic tubules
- periglomerular fibrosis
- interstitial fibrosis

Fig. 6.34 Chronic pyelonephritis. Intravenous urogram at 15 minutes showing deep cortical scarring of the right kidney opposite blunted calices. By courtesy of Dr C. N. Griffin.

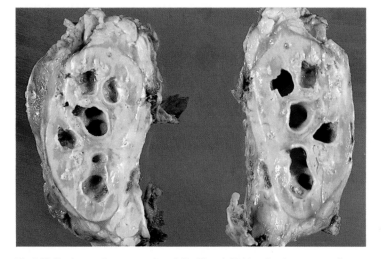

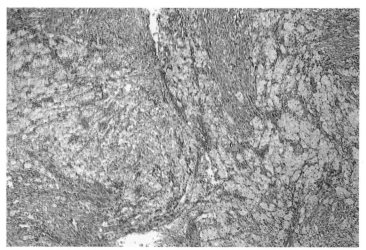

Fig. 6.36 Xanthogranulomatous pyelonephritis. There is friable yellow tissue surrounding the dilated calices. The renal capsule is markedly adherent. By courtesy of Dr J. Newman.

Fig. 6.37 Xanthogranulomatous pyelonephritis. Numerous, characteristic lipid-laden histiocytes impart the yellow colour seen macroscopically. By courtesy of Dr J. Newman.

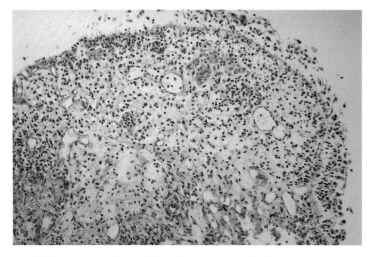

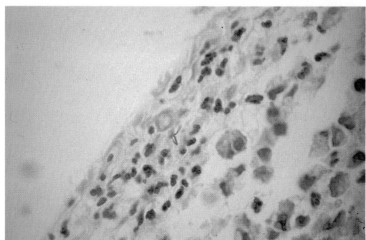

Fig. 6.38 Tuberculous cystitis. Left: Histological appearance of bladder showing chronic inflammation with giant cells. H & E stain. Right: Scanty acid-fast bacilli. Ziehl–Neelsen stain.

tous lesions with large macrophages laden with fat and cholesterol esters (Fig. 6.37). A staghorn calculus may be present and radiological diagnosis occasionally indicates an obstructed non functioning kidney. *Proteus* species and staphylococci are often isolated from the lesions but antibiotic therapy alone is rarely successful and surgery is usually required.

Urinary tract tuberculosis

Any part of the genitourinary system may be affected by tuberculosis. The first lesion is most commonly in the kidney from which infection may extend to bladder (Fig. 6.38), prostate and seminal vesicles. Ascending infection also occurs. Tuberculous epididymitis (see below) is a common feature of genitourinary tuberculosis in the male. About 50% of cases have evidence of extrarenal disease (usually inactive) and genitourinary tuberculosis often only emerges into clinical significance at a very late stage in the natural history and may be seen in elderly patients in whom tuberculosis has remained latent for many years or even decades.

Patients usually do not have constitutional symptoms and many are truly asymptomatic. There usually is pyuria or haematuria and culture of three early morning urine specimens confirms the diagnosis in almost all cases. Most patients are tuberculin positive. The IVU is frequently abnormal, usually unilaterally. At an early stage, the changes are non-specific: only poor or delayed concentration and some 'motheaten' irregularity of the calices may be seen. This can also be seen in the retrograde pyelogram (Fig. 6.39). Later, the IVU changes become more specific with caliceal abscesses extending into the cortex, 'pipe stem' changes in the ureter and focal or gross parenchymal calcification.

The gross appearance of advanced renal tuberculosis is shown in Fig. 6.40. Histologically, the early stages (Fig. 6.41) consist of typical tuberculous granulation tissue, which then caseates. In long-standing disease, the caseous areas have begun to calcify and have become more sharply demarcated by fibrous tissue. The end stage of renal disease is shown in Figs 6.42 and 6.43.

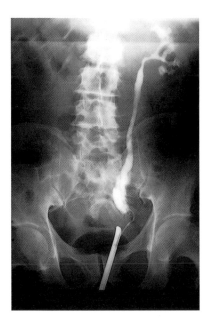

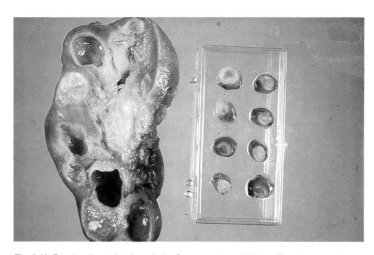

Fig. 6.39 Renal tuberculosis. Retrograde pyelogram showing 'motheaten' destructive changes of the caliceal system of the left kidney. There is also a stricture of the distal ureter with more proximal ulceration of the ureteric mucosa and extravasation of contrast material. By courtesy of Dr Randy Noble.

Fig. 6.40 Renal and ureteric tuberculosis. Gross specimen of kidney. There is hydronephrosis and most of the renal parenchyma is atrophied. The calices are thickened focally and sections of the ureter (right) show variable lumen diameter due to chronic inflammation of the wall. By courtesy of Dr J. Newman.

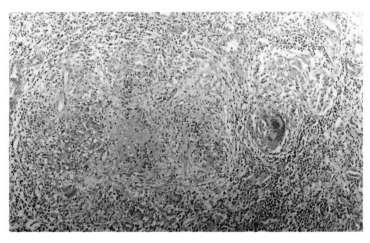

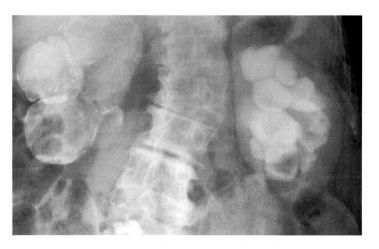

Fig. 6.41 Renal tuberculosis. Histological section of kidney showing only a few renal tubules remaining at the edges of the section. The rest consists of a typical tuberculous granuloma, poorly-defined and of recent development. H & E stain.

Fig. 6.42 Renal tuberculosis. Intravenous urogram in advanced renal tuberculosis. The right kidney is a calcified pyonephrosis and is non-functioning. The left kidney is hydronephrotic with distended pelvis and calices.

Treatment with chemotherapy regimens containing rifampicin and isoniazid is usually sufficient alone to cure urinary tract tuberculosis. The minimum necessary duration of therapy has not been determined but it seems that short courses, similar to those required for pulmonary disease, are adequate. Surgery may be needed if scarring produces obstruction.

PROSTATITIS

The term prostatitis is used as an explanation for a wide range of lower abdominal or perineal complaints in men. Often the diagnosis is based on poor evidence and it is important for therapy to distinguish several different forms of prostatic infection.

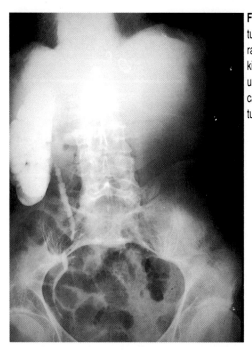

Fig. 6.43 Renal tuberculosis. Plain radiograph of a 'plaster cast' kidney. The right kidney and ureter are extensively calcified from chronic tuberculosis.

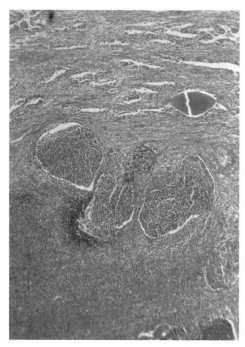

Fig. 6.44 Acute prostatitis. Histological section of prostate showing destruction of normal architecture by intense inflammation and distension of ducts by intraductal abscesses. By courtesy of Dr J. Newman.

Fig. 6.45 Localization of lower urinary tract infection using sequential urine cultures.

Localization Studies	
Specimen	**Description**
Voided bladder 1 (VB1)	The initial 10ml of urine is collected into the first container
Voided bladder 2 (VB2)	A midstream urine specimen is collected into a second container
Expressed prostatic secretions (EPS)	Digital prostatic massage is performed and the expressed secretions collected
Voided bladder 3 (VB3)	The first 10ml or urine after prostatic massage is collected

Interpretation of Results

1. If colony count in VB1 exceeds that VB3, the infection is localized to the anterior urethra

2. If colony counts in VB1 and VB2 are negative or very low and those in EPS and VB3 are high, then bacterial prostatitis is likely

3. In chronic prostatitis examination of the EPS reveals white blood cells and culture is usually positive (although only small numbers of bacteria may be present)

Acute bacterial prostatitis

Acute bacterial prostatitis presents with high fever and acute perineal pain together with symptoms of a lower UTI. Most cases are caused by Enterobacteriaceae or pseudomonads although a few are due to *Staphylococcus saprophyticus* or *Streptococcus faecalis*. The patient is usually obviously ill and rectal examination reveals an exquisitely tender, tense prostate. Prostatic localization studies (see below) should not be done as they can lead to bacteraemia. Examination of a routine urine specimen demonstrates pyuria and culture is positive. Biopsy specimens are seldom obtained (Fig. 6.44). Antibiotic therapy, even with agents that do not penetrate well into the uninflamed prostate, readily cure the infection. Suitable agents for empirical therapy are cotrimoxazole or one of the quinolones, such as ciprofloxacin or norfloxacin. Most cases recover completely but prostatic abscess or chronic prostatitis occasionally follow.

Chronic bacterial prostatitis

Chronic bacterial prostatitis is an important cause of relapsing lower UTI in the adult male. Between episodes of symptomatic urinary infection, the man is free of problems and examination of the prostate is generally entirely normal. The only means of confirming the diagnosis is by localization studies (Fig. 6.45). Antibiotic therapy is not always successful. Co-trimoxazole (TMP–SMZ), given for 6–12 weeks, is curative in about one-third of cases, suppressive (needing long term low-dose therapy after the initial course) in another third, but of no benefit in the remainder. Ciprofloxacin and several other quinolones have shown excellent results in chronic prostatitis due to *Enterobacteriaceae* but are of less value when pseudomonads or enterococci are responsible.

Nonbacterial prostatitis

This condition is very common. Patients experience a range of lower abdominal and perineal pain or discomfort, but there are no abnormal signs. There is no evidence of bacterial infection on careful localization studies (see above) but expressed prostatic secretions show an excess of white cells. The aetiology of this condition is unclear and opinion is divided over the role of *Chlamydia trachomatis* and *Ureaplasma urealyticum*. A small number of cases do improve with tetracycline or erythromycin therapy, but most are not helped.

EPIDIDYMITIS

Inflammation of the epididymis is common. It may be acute (Fig. 6.46) or chronic (Fig. 6.47) and either sexually transmitted or related to urinary tract problems. It produces a painful swelling of the scrotum, often associated with dysuria and/or a urethral discharge. Initially the inflamed epididymis is felt as a tender swelling in the posterior scrotum; later the testis often becomes inflamed and it can be difficult to determine the anatomical limitation of the inflammatory mass. A hydrocele is commonly present. In young men epididymitis is usually sexually transmitted and caused by *C. trachomatis* or *N. gonorrhoeae* (see Chapter 7). There may not be a history of urethral discharge but diagnosis depends upon appropriate cultures of urethral swabs. Therapy should be with drugs appropriate for both pathogens and treatment of sexual partners is important. In men over 35 years old, epididymitis is usually caused by coliforms, other gram-negative bacilli, or gram-positive cocci. It commonly follows urinary tract surgery or instrumentation in the presence of bacteriuria, or accompanies prostatitis. Medical management with antibiotics for both gram-negative bacilli and gram-positive cocci is usually effective.

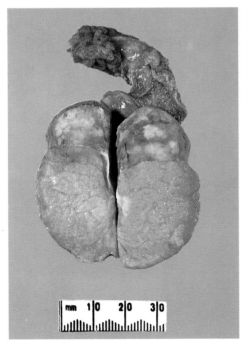

Fig. 6.46 Acute epididymitis. Gross specimen showing an enlarged epididymis with necrosis and microabscess formation. By courtesy of Dr J. Newman.

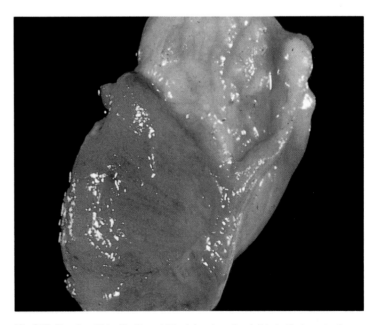

Fig. 6.47 Chronic epididymitis. The epididymis is enlarged and distorted by long standing inflammation with resultant scarring.

Tuberculous epididymo-orchitis

Male genital tuberculosis is usually present concurrently with renal tuberculosis (see above). Epididymitis (Fig. 6.48) generally follows prostatic infection and presents as a palpable painful scrotal swelling with a 'beadlike' feel to the vas deferens. Chronic infection can result in scrotal sinuses. The tuberculin skin test is usually positive and the diagnosis can be confirmed by biopsy and culture. Standard antituberculous therapy is effective.

ORCHITIS

Infection of the testis without prostatitis and epididymitis is nearly always due to viral infections, although blood-borne bacterial infections can occur.

Viral orchitis

The most common cause of orchitis is mumps (see Chapter 1). Orchitis occurs in about 20% of postpubertal males who develop mumps, but is very rare in the prepubertal. The typical clinical picture is abrupt onset of unilateral testicular swelling starting during the first week of the parotitis. This is accompanied by a variable degree of testicular pain and, in the severe cases, by high fever, vomiting and constitutional symptoms. The testis is tender and warm and the scrotum erythematous. In about one third of cases the other testis becomes involved a few days later. Resolution can take anything from a few days to several weeks. Following resolution there is testicular atrophy of variable severity but, contrary to popular belief, sterility seldom results. Bed rest and support of the affected testis make the patient more comfortable. High dose steroid therapy during the acute phase seems to reduce the symptoms of mumps orchitis but has no effect upon the subsequent testicular atrophy.

Acute orchitis has also been recorded in infections due to coxsackie viruses (particularly coxsackie B) and echovirus 6. The disease is clinically identical to mumps orchitis.

Bacterial orchitis

Epididymo-orchitis is described above. Occasionally orchitis can follow haematogenous spread. The patient is acutely ill with high fever, severe pain, marked testicular tenderness and often an acute hydrocele. The testis is swollen and large areas of necrosis and abscess may form (Fig. 6.49). Parenteral antibiotic therapy is needed and surgical drainage may be necessary if an abscess or pyocele develops.

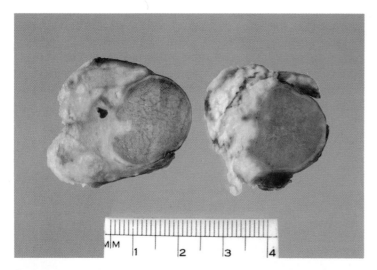

Fig. 6.48 Tuberculous epididymitis. Cheesy white caseation and chronic inflammation replacing the epididymis. By courtesy of Dr J. Newman.

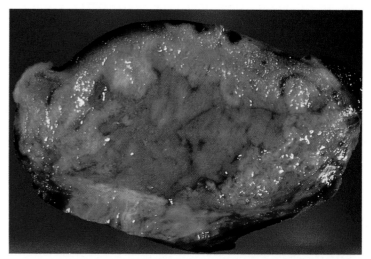

Fig. 6.49 Acute suppurative orchitis. Transected testis from patient with acute suppurative orchitis shows a large abscess cavity.

7

THE GENITAL TRACT

GONORRHOEA

A steady increase in the incidence of gonorrhoea occurred in all countries in which records are kept over the three decades prior to 1985. Although the number of new cases has declined a little since awareness of the AIDS epidemic led to a modification in sexual behaviour, gonorrhoea remains one of the major uncontrolled epidemics of infectious disease. *Neisseria gonorrhoeae* is a gram-negative diplococcus that is characteristically seen intracellularly in clinical specimens (Fig. 7.1).

Gonococcal infection in adults is almost always transmitted sexually, although gonococcal ophthalmia neonatorum (see Chapter 12) is acquired from the mother's birth canal. Subclinical infection has long been recognised in up to 50% of females and it is now clear that infection may also be asymptomatic in 5–25% of males. These asymptomatic individuals are the major source of disease transmission. The common acute manifestation is urethritis in either sex (Fig. 7.2) and cervicitis in the female (Fig. 7.3). Symptoms start 2–5 days after infection and consist of dysuria and urinary frequency followed by a purulent urethral or vaginal discharge. Anorectal infection is also seen in both sexes and is often asymptomatic although anal irritation, pain, bleeding and muco-purulent discharge may be produced (Fig. 7.4). Oropharyngeal infection also occurs but rarely causes symptoms.

Gram stains and cultures of urethral swabs or cervical exudate should be performed; intracellular gram-negative diplococci (Fig. 7.5) are highly specific for gonorrhoea. This is a very sensitive test in males; however, only 50% of symptomatic females give a positive result. In both women and homosexual men rectal swabs should also be cultured routinely. Pharyngeal swabs should also be cultured on a selective medium as the presence of non-pathogenic strains of *N. gonorrhoeae* within the pharynx makes Gram-smear microscopy useless.

Local complications of gonorrhoea are relatively uncommon. In the male the most common complication of untreated urethral gonorrhoea is epididymitis, but prostatitis, infection of the seminal vesicles and abscesses in Cowper's glands (Fig. 7.6), can also occur. Stricture formation in the bulbous urethra may follow gonococcal urethritis, with multiple fistulous tracts due either to infection or to instrumentation with the creation of false passages (Fig. 7.7). In 10–15% of females infection spreads to the fallopian tubes and then may extend to cause adnexal abscesses, peritonitis or pelvic abscesses (see below –

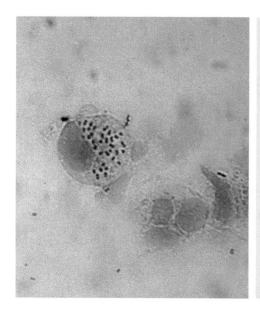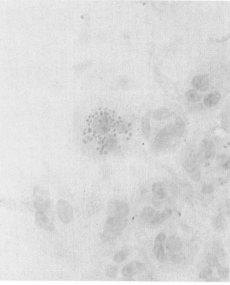

Fig. 7.1 Specimens of urethral pus showing polymorphonuclear leucocytes that have ingested *Neisseria gonorrhoeae*, seen as kidney-shaped diplococci. Left: Gram stain. By courtesy of Dr V.E. Del Bene. Right: Sandiford's stain. By courtesy of Dr I. Farrell.

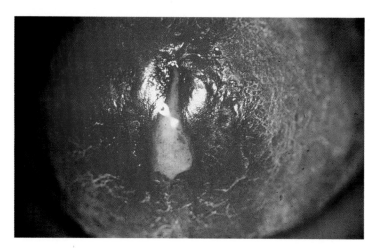

Fig. 7.2 Gonococcal urethritis. Typical purulent meatal discharge with inflammation of the glans. By courtesy of Dr J. Clay.

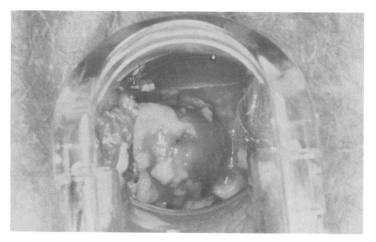

Fig. 7.3 Gonococcal endocervicitis. View through vaginal speculum showing reddened external os through which mucopurulent secretion is exuding. By courtesy of Dr S. E. Thompson.

Pelvic inflammatory disease). Rectal disease does not extend into the sigmoid colon and local abscesses are very rare. Disseminated gonococcal infection occurs in about 1% of patients infected and most frequently produces a rash, tenosynovitis and arthritis (see Chapter 8).

The treatment of gonorrhoea has been much complicated by the development of antibiotic resistance in *N. gonorrhoeae*. Resistance to sulphonamides emerged rapidly after their introduction while a slower diminution in penicillin susceptibility led to the need for increasing doses of penicillin in treatment. Since 1976 the situation has been further complicated by the emergence of highly penicillin-resistant strains. Some of these strains possess a plasmid that confers the ability to produce a penicillinase (β-lactamase) and are known as PPNG (penicillin-producing *N. gonorrhoeae*). In others the resistance is chromosomally mediated and is not due to β-lactamase production. These latter strains are also resistant to tetracyclines. The choice of therapy therefore depends upon the site of infection, any history of penicillin-allergy and the prevalence of penicillin-resistant strains in the community where the infection was acquired. PPNG strains are particularly prevalent in the Far East and in parts of Africa.

Another important concern in treating gonorrhoea is the coexistence of chlamydial infection in up to half the cases. Treatment of gonorrhoea should, therefore, be followed by a course of tetracycline therapy (see below – *Chlamydia trachomatis* infections). For uncomplicated gonococcal urethritis, cervicitis, or rectal infection, therapy is usually undertaken with a single-dose regimen. When the infection is from a source known for certain not to have penicillin-resistant gonorrhoea, either oral amoxicillin (3g) with probenecid, or intramuscular procaine penicillin (2.88g) with probenecid may be used. Otherwise the recommended therapy is intramuscular ceftriaxone (250mg) or spectinomycin (2g), either of which will deal with PPNG strains. Oral cefuroxime axetil plus probenecid or a quinolone such as ciprofloxacin also seem suitable. In pharyngeal gonorrhoea spectinomycin is unreliable – procaine penicillin, ceftriaxone, or a week of an oral tetracycline are used. The place of the oral quinolones in the treatment of these infections remains to be determined.

CHLAMYDIA TRACHOMATIS INFECTIONS

Non-specific or non-gonococcal urethritis and cervicitis,

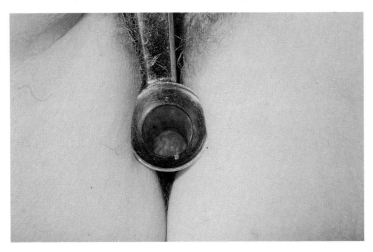

Fig. 7.4 Gonococcal proctitis. View through a proctoscope showing mucopurulent anal secretions in a woman. By courtesy of Dr J. Clay.

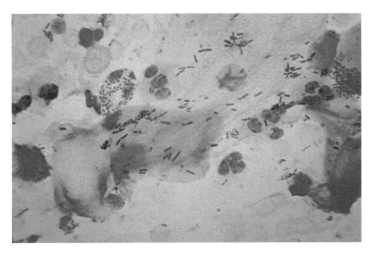

Fig. 7.5 Gonococcal endocervicitis. Gram stain of pus from cervix. This illustrates the difficulty which may be experienced in identifying *Neisseria gonorrhoeae* microscopically, since its presence is often obscured by other bacteria. By courtesy of Dr S.E. Thompson.

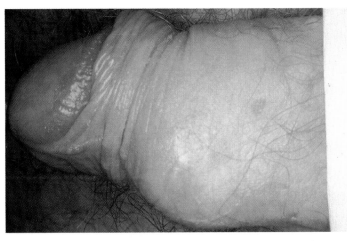

Fig. 7.6 Gonococcal urethritis. Early complication showing swelling of shaft of penis due to a periurethral abscess. By courtesy of Dr J. Clay.

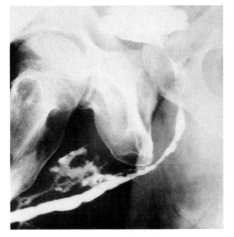
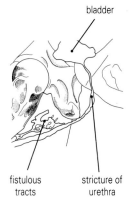

bladder

fistulous tracts

stricture of urethra

Fig. 7.7 Gonococcal urethritis. Late complications of urethral stricture. The urethrogram shows stricture of the bulbous urethra and multiple fistulous tracts. By courtesy of Dr C. N. Griffin.

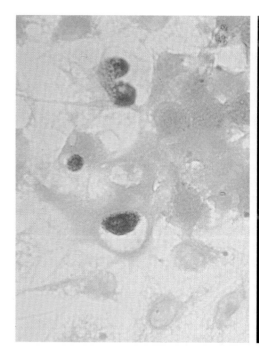
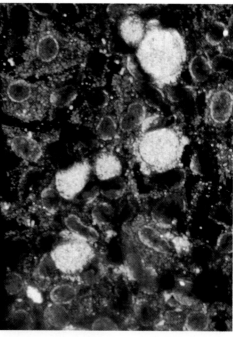

Fig. 7.8 Chlamydia. Tissue culture of *C. trachomatis* in McCoy cells of mouse. Left: Iodine stain, showing intracytoplasmic inclusions. Right: Giemsa stain with dark ground illumination – the inclusions appear as bright yellow areas. By courtesy of Dr G. L. Ridgway.

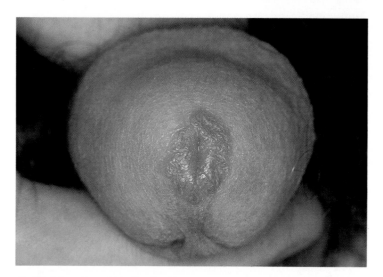

Fig. 7.9 Chlamydia urethritis. Meatitis with non-purulent urethral discharge. By courtesy of Dr J. Clay.

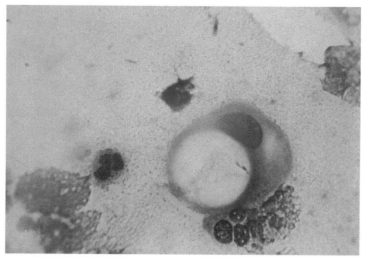

Fig. 7.10 Chlamydia urethritis. Urethral discharge showing typical large intracytoplasmic inclusion body. Wright's stain. By courtesy of Dr J. Clay.

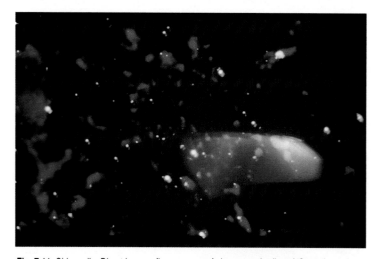

Fig. 7.11 Chlamydia. Direct immunofluorescence of elementary bodies of *C. trachomatis*, which appear as bright green dots. By courtesy of Dr G. L. Ridgway.

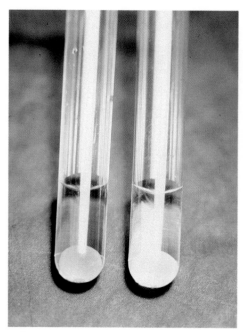

Fig. 7.12 Chlamydia. Rapid enzyme-linked immunoassay technique for diagnosis of *C. trachomatis* infection in a specimen from the urethra or cervix. A colour change (left-hand tube) indicates a positive result. By courtesy of Dr G. Ridgway.

like gonorrhoea, has increased enormously in frequency in the last two decades and *C. trachomatis* has emerged as the most important cause (Fig. 7.8). The genus *Chlamydia* is divided into three species, *C. psittaci,* the cause of psittacosis, *C. pneumoniae,* a recently recognized respiratory pathogen and *C. trachomatis,* of which different groups of serovars are found respectively in non-gonococcal urethritis (serovars D–K), in lymphogranuloma venereum (LGV) (serovar L) and in endemic trachoma (serovars A–C). Originally isolated in yolk sac culture, the cultivation of these organisms in tissue culture has enabled their place to be more fully elucidated. In addition to their role in acute genital infection, strains of *C. trachomatis* have been isolated from many female patients with chronic pelvic sepsis and constitute an important cause of infertility. Asymptomatic women are an important reservoir of infection, transmitting infection to their sexual partners and to their neonates, producing neonatal ophthalmia and pneumonia (see below and Chapters 2 and 12).

Urethritis due to chlamydia is a common problem in men attending genitourinary medicine clinics (Fig. 7.9). *C. trachomatis* can be found in about half the cases of non-gonococcal urethritis (NGU) and two-thirds of the female partners of these culture-positive cases will have chlamydial endocervicitis. NGU in men produces a mucoid urethral discharge and dysuria. Examination of the discharge reveals pus cells but no evidence of intracellular gonococci (although concurrent infections may occur). Inclusion bodies may be detected by means of Giemsa or Wright's staining (Fig. 7.10) of swab material. However, diagnosis is now chiefly undertaken by detection of chlamydial antigens by direct immunofluorescence using a monoclonal antibody test (Fig. 7.11) or an enzyme-linked immunosorbent assay (ELISA) (Fig. 7.12) and, where culture facilities are available, by isolation of *C. trachomatis* in McCoy cell culture. Serological tests are not useful for the oculogenital strains of *C. trachomatis*, unlike the serovars causing

LGV (see below). Untreated NGU in men may lead to prostatitis or epididymitis (see Chapter 6).

Symptomatic urethritis may occur in women, but *C. trachomatis* is more often a cause of endocervicitis (Fig. 7.13). Often this is asymptomatic but usually there is a mucopurulent vaginal discharge and cervicitis visible on speculum examination. In a sexual contact of a man with NGU or mothers of neonates with chlamydial infection, cervical smears and cultures should be taken. Salpingitis and the other complications of cervical infection are dealt with below.

NGU is treated with doxycycline (100mg every 12 hours) or erythromycin, for 7 days. Control cannot be expected unless sexual partners are traced and treated concurrently while refraining from sexual intercourse.

TRICHOMONIASIS

Trichomonas vaginalis is a common infection of women throughout the world and is frequently found asymptomatically in the urethra or prostate of men. It is a flagellated protozoan with optimal growth and motility at pH 5.5–6.5 (higher than normal vaginal pH). Asymptomatic infections may occur in women but the most common manifestation of infection is vaginitis with a thin, frothy, offensive discharge (Fig. 7.14). The symptoms often occur when there is a natural increase in vaginal pH with menstruation or at the menopause. The vagina often has a granular inflamed appearance. Diagnosis is most easily made by visualizing the motility of unstained organisms in a wet preparation examined rapidly on a slide or as a hanging drop (Fig. 7.15). Cervical cytology is a less specific method and direct staining of smears with monoclonal antibodies is sensitive but costly. In the male most infections are asymptomatic but may be accompanied by mild chronic urethritis.

Full treatment should be given to all sexual partners as

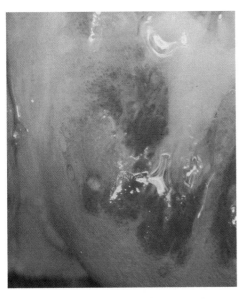

Fig. 7.13 Chlamydia endocervicitis. Colposcopic view showing mucopurulent discharge and beefy red mucosa of columnar epithelium. By courtesy of Mr D. W. Sturdee.

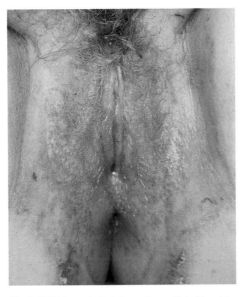

Fig. 7.14 Trichomoniasis. Inflammation and intertrigo of the vulva and perineal skin due to copious vaginal discharge from trichomoniasis. By courtesy of Dr J. Clay.

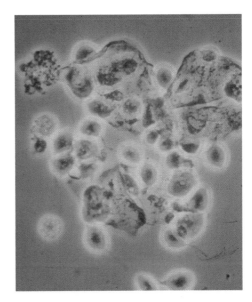

Fig. 7.15 Trichomoniasis. Wet preparation of *Trichomonas vaginalis*. Direct examination of a vaginal secretion shows pus cells interspersed with the pear-shaped nucleated and flagellated causal organisms. By courtesy of Dr S. E. Thompson.

well as to the index case in order to prevent relapses. Systemic therapy is better than local applications and the preferred treatment is with a single dose of oral metronidazole (2g). A second dose usually deals with those infections that fail to respond initially.

GENITAL CANDIDIASIS

In the female, *Candida albicans* is one of the most common causes of vaginitis. Sexual transmission only has a limited role in the condition. Many patients with candidal infection are asymptomatic and symptoms are related to factors that increase vaginal secretions such as pregnancy, antibiotic therapy, oral contraceptive use and diabetes mellitus. The chief symptoms are intense irritation of the vulva and vagina and dyspareunia, sometimes with a white, thick, cheesy discharge (Fig. 7.16). The vaginal mucosa is often red and white patches may be seen on the vagina and vulva. In the male infection may be subclinical or accompanied by the characteristic irritation and rash on the glans and prepuce (Fig. 7.17).

The diagnosis depends upon clinical findings as candida is frequently found as a vaginal commensal. The organism is usually identified in a Gram stain (Fig. 7.18) or KOH-prepared wet mount of the vaginal discharge (Fig. 7.19), or by culture. Treatment is usually given with topical antifungals: nystatin pessaries should be given for 14 days but miconazole or clotrimazole pessaries or cream are effective as shorter courses (3 or 7 days). Oral fluconazole or itraconazole is also effective in treating vaginal candidosis, but is usually not indicated. Routine treatment of male partners is unnecessary but when infection recurs, evidence of balanitis should be sought and penile swabs taken. If candida is found then the man should use an antifungal cream and wear a condom during sexual intercourse while the woman is being treated.

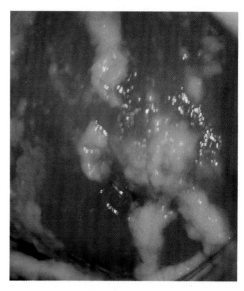

Fig. 7.16 Vulval candidiasis. Thick white cheesy discharge typical of candida infection. By courtesy of Mr. D. W. Sturdee.

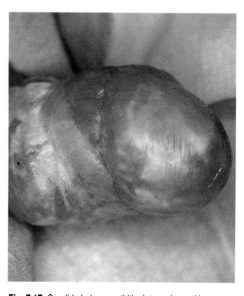

Fig. 7.17 Candida balanoposthitis. Intensely pruritic inflammation of the glans and prepuce with white cheesy exudate. By courtesy of Dr J. Clay.

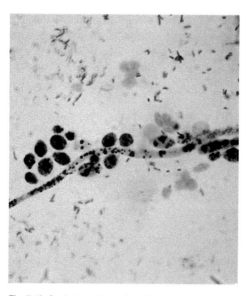

Fig. 7.18 Genital candidosis: *Candida albicans* in Gram stain of vaginal secretion showing yeast and mycelial forms. The diagnosis may be confirmed by culture of the fungus on Sabouraud's medium. By courtesy of Dr J. Clay.

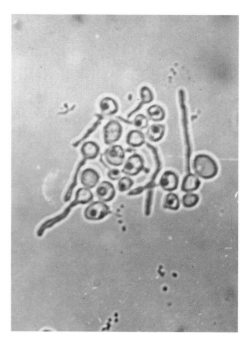

Fig. 7.19 Genital candidiasis. *Candida albicans* in a KOH preparation of vaginal secretion showing both yeast and mycelial forms of this common fungus. By courtesy of Dr S. E. Thompson.

Diagnostic Criteria for Bacterial Vaginosis
Vaginal pH ⩾ 5
Thin homogenous vaginal discharge
Release of an amine-like odour when the vaginal discharge is mixed with 10% KOH
Clue cells present in wet preparation or Gram stain

Fig. 7.20 The four criteria of bacterial vaginosis. In order for the diagnosis to be made at least three of these must be present.

BACTERIAL VAGINOSIS

Bacterial vaginosis (also called non-specific vaginitis or anaerobic vaginosis) is a clinical diagnosis based upon at least three of four criteria (Fig. 7.20). The patient complains of a mild to moderate, thin, greyish, vaginal discharge, itching and a vaginal odour, which is classically described as 'fishy'. Wet mount of the discharge reveals vaginal epithelial cells studded with small coccobacilli – the so-called 'clue cells' (Fig. 7.21). There is still controversy as to whether this is a sexually-transmitted disease. No single organism is responsible for the condition but both aerobic and anaerobic bacteria seem to play important roles. The principal organisms are *Gardnerella vaginalis*, a Gram-negative facultatively anaerobic coccobacillus, and anaerobes in the *Bacteroides*, *Peptostreptococcus*, and *Mobinculus* genera.

The treatment options are oral therapy with metronidazole, another nitroimidazole or clindamycin, or the use of metronidazole or chlorhexidine pessaries. The need to routinely treat the male partner(s) in bacterial vaginosis remains uncertain, but many physicians would treat if the condition were to recur or fail to respond to initial therapy.

HERPES GENITALIS

Genital herpes is now one of the most important sexually transmitted disease in the Western World, having increased dramatically in incidence over the 1970s and early 1980s. In some parts of the USA the disease is considered to be of epidemic proportions with reported rates of more than 200 per 100 000. Herpes simplex virus (HSV) is a DNA virus found in two serological forms – HSV-1 and HSV-2. Both types may cause genital disease, although that caused by type 2 is more common (about 80% of genital herpes infections) and recurs more frequently. Transmission is by sexual or other physical contact. Following primary infection HSV establishes latency in neurones of the sensory or autonomic ganglia. The mechanisms of latency are poorly understood.

Primary infection produces lesions a few days after exposure. Depending upon the sexual practices involved, it results in multiple clusters of painful vesicles or ulcers on the skin or mucous membranes of the penis (Fig. 7.22), labia (Fig. 7.23), introitus, anorectal area or adjacent areas; the cervix is commonly involved (Fig. 7.24). The lesions and shedding of virus last about 10 days and complete

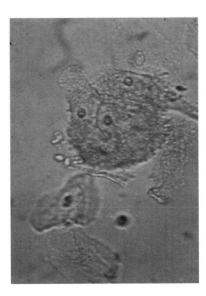
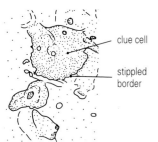

Fig. 7.21 Bacterial vaginosis. The clue cell – a vaginal epithelial cell with attached microorganisms. The attached bacteria give the clue cell a stippled appearance. By courtesy of Prof. G. P. Schmid and Dr R. J. Arko.

clue cell

stippled border

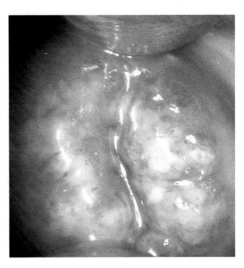

Fig. 7.22 Genital herpes. Primary infection of the penis showing groups of typical painful ulcers on the glans and shaft. By courtesy of Dr B. K. Fisher.

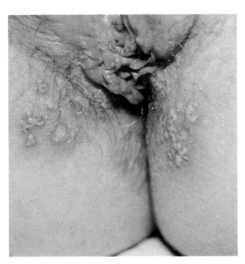

Fig. 7.23 Genital herpes. Vesicles and ulcers on the labia and surrounding skin. The virus can be visualized on electron microscopy or cultured from the vesicular fluid. By courtesy of Dr J. Clay.

Fig. 7.24 Cervical herpes. Area of superficial erosions and ulcers on the cervix in a case of primary herpes genitalis. The cervix is involved in about 90% of primary infections. By courtesy of Dr J. Clay.

healing may take a further week. Viraemia is common in primary infection and fever, headaches and myalgia result: depending upon the site involved, inguinal lymphadenopathy, discharge from the urethra, vagina, cervix or anus, urinary retention, tenesmus and constipation may also occur. Rarely there is a true meningitis or meningomyelitis.

Recurrent episodes of genital herpes are much less severe. They occur within the first year in about half of those with primary HSV-1 infection and in 80% of those with HSV-2. The frequency of recurrence in individuals is very variable but in some may be as often as once a month. The precipitating factors are poorly understood but patients offer a variety of explanations including menstruation, sexual intercourse and stress. Prodromal tingling or paraesthesiae in the area are often noted for 1–2 days before the lesions appear. Both the number and the duration of the lesions is less than in primary attacks (Fig. 7.25) and constitutional symptoms are rare. Subclinical attacks are common in both men and women

and have important bearings upon the transmission of the infection to sexual partners and to the neonate (see below). Extensive perianal herpes and HSV proctitis may be seen in patients with AIDS.

HSV infection of the neonate is usually acquired at the time of delivery. The infant may suffer generalized infections with involvement of the liver, lungs, and CNS and some will have a typical vesicular rash. Others only have involvement of one organ, usually the skin, brain or eyes. Treatment is with parenteral vidarabine or acyclovir, but the mortality and morbidity resulting from neonatal HSV remain high. Attempts to reduce the transmission from mother to baby have not been entirely successful: most cases result from asymptomatic viral shedding from the cervix at the time of delivery and there is no way of predicting this other than by viral cultures at term. Certainly, however, Caesarian section would be prudent when the mother has clear evidence of genital lesions at or near the time of delivery. The association between genital herpes and carcinoma of the cervix, whether as a cause or

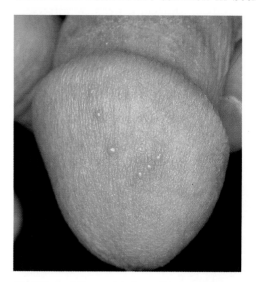

Fig. 7.25 Genital herpes. Irritating vesicles on the glans during a recurrence of genital herpes. The lesions are fewer in number and shorter-lived than in primary disease. By courtesy of Dr B. K. Fisher.

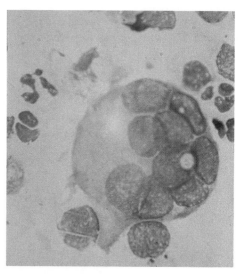

Fig. 7.26 Genital herpes. Scraping from the bottom of an unroofed vesicle showing characteristic multinucleated giant HSV-infected cell. Giemsa stain. By courtesy of Dr J. Clay.

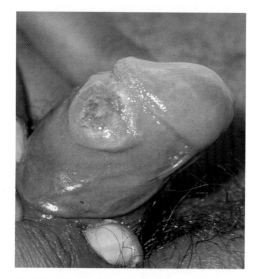

Fig. 7.27 Primary syphilis. Typical penile chancre showing rounded, raised and well-defined lesion with central ulceration. The lesion and the enlarged lymph nodes are both painless. By courtesy of Dr R. D. Catterall.

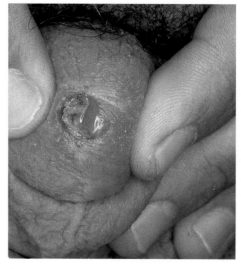

Fig. 7.28 Primary syphilis. A primary intrameatal chancre. By courtesy of Dr B. K.Fisher.

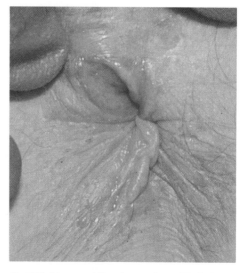

Fig. 7.29 Primary syphilis – chancre of anus. The lesion is firm and painless and the inguinal nodes are enlarged. By courtesy of Dr R. D. Catterall.

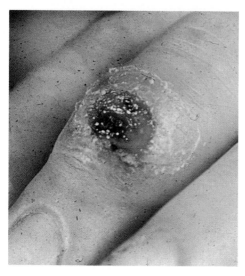

Fig. 7.30 Primary syphilis – chancre on the finger.

as a covariable with papillomaviruses (see below) is still uncertain.

The diagnosis of genital herpes may be suggested by the typical clinical appearances but can be confirmed by viral isolation. Direct immunofluoresence, Giemsa stain of scrapings (Fig. 7.26) or Tzanck preparations may also be used but are less sensitive. A patient with genital herpes is often apprehensive and in need of reassurance and explanation about the risks and consequences of the infection. General advice about the steps that will minimise the transmission of the virus and about personal hygiene during an attack is important but, although some may derive a measure of symptomatic relief from salt baths etc., only acyclovir therapy has been proven to shorten the acute attacks, suppress recurrences and to terminate viral shedding (and hence transmission).

In primary episodes of genital herpes, all three preparations of acyclovir (topical, oral and intravenous) have been shown to be of clear benefit in reducing the severity of the local disease but the systemic symptoms will not respond to topical therapy. Furthermore, topical therapy is often impractical in women when many of the lesions are within the vagina or on the cervix. Out-patient therapy with oral acyclovir (200mg five times daily for 7–10 days) seems the best management for most patients, although for rectal infection a higher dose (400mg five times daily for 10 days) is recommended. The intravenous preparation can be reserved for those patients who need hospitalization because of severe symptoms or who develop complications such as urinary retention or nervous system involvement.

In recurrent herpes genitalis the clinical benefits of therapy are less dramatic. As with any infection, specific therapy should be started as soon as possible – the best results are obtained if the patient can initiate a 5-day course of oral acyclovir therapy as soon as he or she gets prodromal symptoms: a dose of 800mg taken twice daily is effective and may be more convenient for the patient than the traditional dose of 200mg taken 4-hourly. For the patient with recurrences every few weeks consideration may be given to prophylactic administration: optimal suppression can be achieved using acyclovir, 400mg twice daily.

SYPHILIS

The enormous increase in incidence of sexually transmitted disease of recent decades is related chiefly to gonorrhoea and non-specific genital infection. Notifications of new syphilis infections, after a great reduction in the years following the Second World War, began to rise again in Western countries in the mid 1960s: these infections were chiefly in homosexual and bisexual men. With the emergence of the AIDS epidemic, however, there was a change in sexual practices among these men and cases of syphilis also began to decline. In the developing world and in deprived communities in the West, however, syphilis still constitutes a major health problem.

The organism causing syphilis is *Treponema pallidum*, a spirochaete 6–14mm long and 0.5mm wide. The organism cannot be cultured *in vitro*. The major route of spread is by sexual contact, although transmission may occur *in utero* and via blood transfusions. The manifestations of syphilis are notoriously diverse. Early disease is divided into primary and secondary stages and is characterized by mucocutaneous lesions. There is then a period of latent infection followed by the tertiary stage, characterized by chronic progressive lesions of the nervous, cardiovascular and musculoskeletal systems.

Primary syphilis

After an incubation period of between 10 days and 3 months – the average is about 21 days – a lesion (usually single but occasionally multiple) appears at the site of treponemal inoculation. The primary lesion (the chancre) begins as a dull red papule which breaks down to form a well-defined indurated ulcer with a granulating or scabbed base (Fig. 7.27). Although most chancres are on the external genitalia, lesions may be within the urethra (Fig. 7.28), in the anorectal area (in both homosexuals and heterosexuals – Fig. 7.29), on the fingers (Fig. 7.30), in the oral cavity or on the lips (Fig. 7.31). Primary lesions in the female may also occur on any part of the external genitalia (Figs 7.32 & 7.33) and on the cervix uteri (Fig. 7.34).

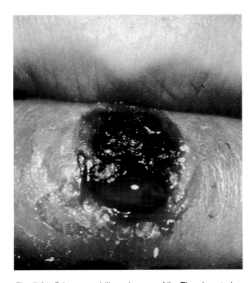

Fig. 7.31 Primary syphilis – chancre of lip. The ulcerated area is covered by a scab. By courtesy of Dr R. D. Catterall.

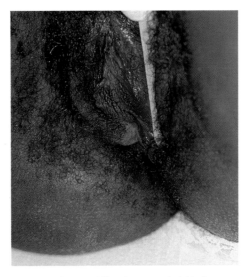

Fig. 7.32 Primary syphilis – chancre on the labia. By courtesy of Dr B. K. Fisher.

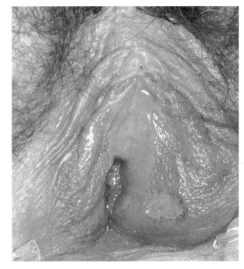

Fig. 7.33 Primary syphilis. A well-defined chancre seen on the labia minora. The base of the ulcer is clean with a shallow covering of slough. By courtesy of Dr R. D. Catterall.

Chancres at any site are usually painless and accompanied by discrete painless enlargement of the regional lymph nodes. The primary lesion heals slowly over 2–8 weeks if untreated. *T. pallidum* can be seen by dark ground examination (Fig. 7.35) of material from the chancre, which is highly infectious. Any suspicious lesion should be re-examined serially if the initial test is negative.

Secondary syphilis

The symptoms and signs of secondary syphilis appear 6–8 weeks after the appearance of the primary lesion, which may not have yet healed. They are caused by blood-borne dissemination of treponemes. The features are notoriously variable: most patients have non-specific systemic symptoms such as fever, aching limbs, anorexia, headache and (sometimes) meningism, arthritis and liver disease, but initial suspicion of the diagnosis rests largely on recognition of the mucocutaneous lesions. Most patients with secondary syphilis have a generalized rash (syphilide) and many have generalized lymphadenopathy, sometimes with mucosal lesions. Rashes vary greatly in their character but are generally widespread, including the palms and soles, non-irritant and slow in progression. The main vari-

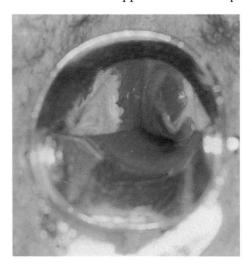

Fig. 7.34 Primary syphilis. View through vaginal speculum showing chancre on the cervix. By courtesy of Dr J. Clay.

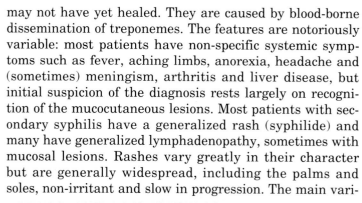

Fig. 7.35 Syphilis. Close coiled regular spirals characteristic of *Treponema pallidum*. Stained preparations are usually unsatisfactory for fresh specimens but silver impregnation methods can be used for tissue sections. By courtesy of Dr R.D. Catterall.

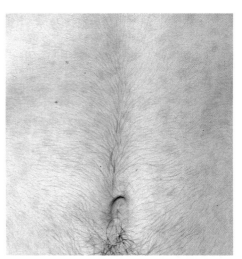

Fig. 7.36 Secondary syphilis – early erythematous macular rash. There are widespread non-irritant macules of varying size widely distributed over the body surface. By courtesy of Dr R. D. Catterall.

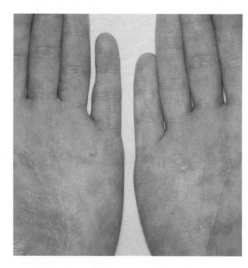

Fig. 7.37 Secondary syphilis. Macular lesions of palms. By courtesy of Dr R. D. Catterall.

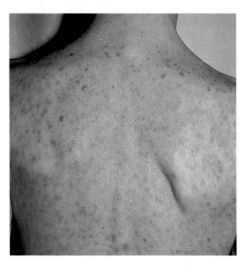

Fig. 7.38 Papular syphilide of secondary syphilis. The papules are widely distributed. Each lesion is rounded, discrete and slightly indurated. By courtesy of Dr B. K. Fisher.

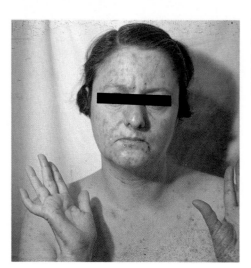

Fig. 7.39 Secondary syphilis. Papular rash showing lesions on palms. By courtesy of the late Dr B. Shaffer.

eties of secondary syphilitic rash and mucosal lesion are outlined below.

A macular or roseolar syphilide with discrete pinkish macules uniformly distributed over the trunk is the earliest of the eruptions of secondary syphilis (Figs 7.36 & 7.37). The common papular syphilides appear a little later with smallish discrete scaly papules, together with the dull red macules which precede them, widely distributed over the whole body including the head (Fig. 7.38). Lesions of the hands are often prominent (Fig. 7.39). Scaling is a common feature and in some patients becomes prominent enough to simulate psoriasis (Fig. 7.40). In the later stages of secondary syphilis some of the lesions may become necrotic, giving a pustular appearance (Fig. 7.41). Widespread pustular rashes (Fig. 7.42) are now rare; they are associated with heavy scarring and are seen especially on the face.

The mucosal lesion of secondary syphilis is the mucous patch: these oval, shallow erosions may be anywhere in the mouth or throat and the well-defined white or grey areas may become confluent (Fig. 7.43). When the slough disappears the well-known snail track ulcer is formed. Condylomata lata may be seen in any warm and moist area, especially round the anus (Figs 7.44, 7.45 & 7.46);

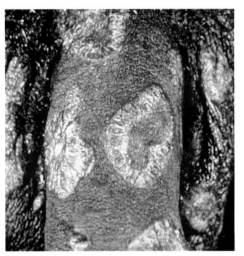

Fig. 7.40 Secondary syphilis. Three large papules on the penis and scrotum with waxy scaling. They look in many respects like psoriasis, which has suggested the name 'psoriasiform secondary syphilide'. By courtesy of Dr S. Olansky.

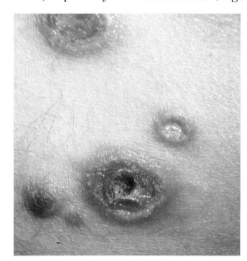

Fig. 7.41 Secondary syphilis. Lesions which have undergone central necrosis. By courtesy of Dr R. D. Catterall.

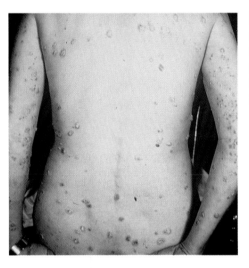

Fig. 7.42 Secondary syphilis. Pustular lesions may become extensively crusted; such lesions are called rupia. By courtesy of Dr S. Olansky.

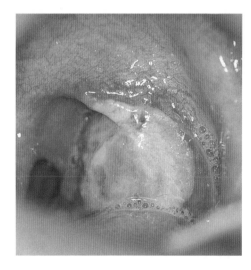

Fig. 7.43 Secondary syphilis. A large well-defined mucous patch on the fauces. By courtesy of Dr J. Clay.

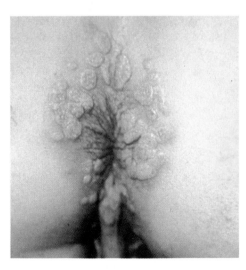

Fig. 7.44 Secondary syphilis. Condylomata lata of the perianal area. Large papular lesions with well-defined margins and pale irregular surfaces which tend to ulcerate. These lesions are swarming with spirochaetes and are highly infectious. By courtesy of Dr R. D. Catterall.

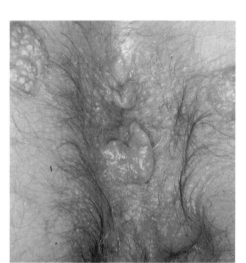

Fig. 7.45 Secondary syphilis – condylomata lata. By courtesy of Dr R. D. Catterall.

they consist of papular lesions which have enlarged to form flat-topped, often ulcerating masses.

In about 25% of cases of untreated secondary syphilis, secondary relapses with further highly infectious lesions occur within a few years of the initial infection.

Latent syphilis

Early syphilis, even if untreated, tends to resolve slowly after many weeks or months. Thereafter, infection remains latent and may be revealed only by a chance blood test, during pregnancy for example. The early latent period (4 years) is defined as the period during which relapses may occur. The late latent period is the subsequent period up to the development of tertiary disease.

Tertiary syphilis

Clinical tertiary lesions eventually appear in about one-third of patients with untreated latent syphilis. Almost every organ of the body can be affected by gummata (benign tertiary syphilis) but lesions are most often seen in skin, mucous membranes, bones and joints: with the longest latent period the cardiovascular and neurological complications of tertiary syphilis appear (See Chapters 3 and 9).

Late syphilitic skin lesions are nodular, asymmetrical, sometimes grouped and found anywhere on the skin with a slow cycle of healing, scarring and the development of new lesions (Figs 7.47 & 7.48). Scaly lesions may resemble psoriatic patches. Gummata may develop anywhere but are most frequently found in mucocutaneous or musculoskeletal sites (Fig. 7.49). They are subcutaneous in origin but gradually increase in size and become attached to skin. This eventually breaks down to give the well-known punched-out ulcer; either a clean granulating floor or the 'wash-leather' slough may be seen (Fig. 7.50). The same changes taking place in the tongue eventually lead to the

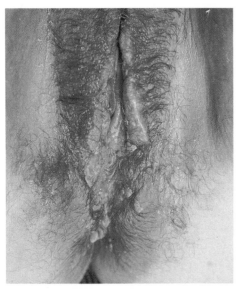

Fig. 7.46 Secondary syphilis. Condylomata lata of the vulval area. These lesions are most common during relapses of secondary syphilis. By courtesy of Dr J. Clay.

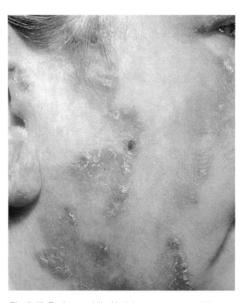

Fig. 7.47 Tertiary syphilis. Nodular cutaneous syphilitic lesions of the face: some show signs of healing, others have undergone central ulceration. By courtesy of Dr R. D. Catterall.

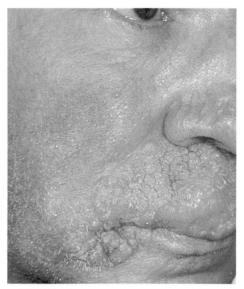

Fig. 7.48 Tertiary syphilis: nodular cutaneous syphilide with an almost confluent area of skin infiltration and nodules on the upper lip and cheek. By courtesy of Dr R.D. Catterall.

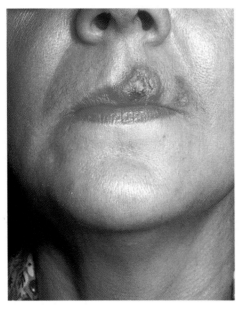

Fig. 7.49 Tertiary syphilis: gumma on the upper lip. By courtesy of the late Dr B. Shaffer.

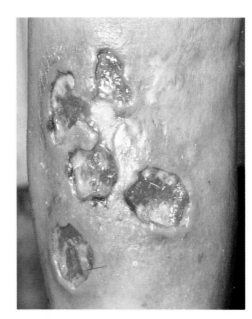

Fig. 7.50 Tertiary syphilis. Multiple gummata of the leg showing the typical punched-out appearance of the ulcers. Parts of the ulcer base are composed of clean granulation tissue, others of yellow slough. By courtesy of Dr R. D. Catterall.

appearance recognized as chronic superficial glossitis, a precancerous condition (Fig. 7.51).

Microscopically a gumma shows areas of central necrosis surrounded by granulation tissue with lymphocytes and plasma cells, often with perivascular accentuation. Fibroblasts are present in the periphery. Occasional epithelioid and giant cells are seen (Fig. 7.52). Details of cardiovascular syphilis and neurosyphilis are provided in Chapters 3 and 9.

Congenital syphilis

Congenital syphilis is now rare in developed countries and its various manifestations are not often seen. Nevertheless, routine serological testing and, if necessary, treatment for congenital syphilis should always be carried out during pregnancy. Serological screening should be repeated during the third trimester in those women at high risk of syphilitic infection. Transplacental spread of *T. pallidum* may result in fetal death, prematurity or congenital syphilis. Congenital syphilis occurs when *T. pallidum* spreads to the fetus after the first trimester of pregnancy. A woman with untreated early syphilis is unlikely to have a normal child. As with other disorders, it is the child born to a mother who has not received normal antenatal care who is most at risk.

The features of the early syndrome may not be present at birth, only developing during the subsequent 4 weeks. They are characterized by a generalized eruption that may be vesicular or bullous on palms and soles (Figs 7.53 & 7.54): the fluid within these lesions is heavily infected with *T. pallidum*. The rashes of congenital syphilis generally resemble those of acquired secondary syphilis as do the mucosal lesions, those of the nasal mucosa giving rise to syphilitic rhinitis. Hair and nails may be lost. Of the internal organs, enlargement of the liver, spleen and lymph nodes is most common but many other organs may be involved. Bone lesions, characterized by symmetrical

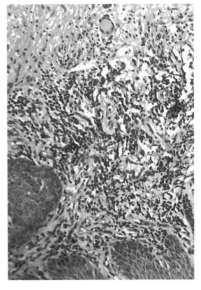

Fig. 7.51 Tertiary syphilis. Chronic superficial glossitis. The tongue is deeply fissured; some of the mucosal surface is quite smooth and white patches of leucoplakia are seen on the surface. By courtesy Dr J. Clay.

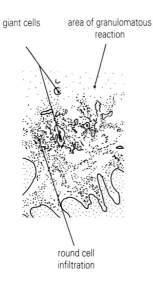

giant cells   area of granulomatous reaction

round cell infiltration

Fig. 7.52 Tertiary syphilis – histological appearance of skin lesion. The subepidermis is heavily infiltrated with small round cells. Beneath this is a gummatous reaction with granuloma-like changes including giant cells. H&E stain. By courtesy of Dr R. D. Catterall.

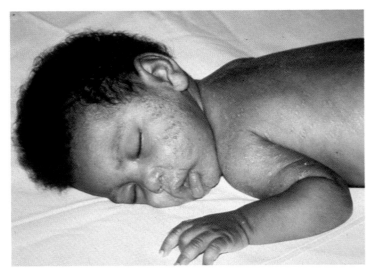

Fig. 7.53 Congenital syphilis. Generalized eruption in an otherwise well-looking child. By courtesy of Dr S. Olansky.

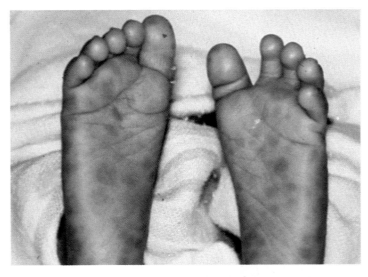

Fig. 7.54 Congenital syphilis. Discrete macular lesions on soles, similar to those seen in acquired secondary syphilis. By courtesy of Dr S. Olansky.

metaphyseal perichondritis and osteitis, appear at 1–3 months in most infected infants (Fig. 7.55). After a latent period late congenital syphilis may develop and involve the eyes giving interstitial keratitis (Fig. 7.56) as well as the skin, bones and joints (Fig. 7.57), ear and central nervous system.

The later development of congenital syphilis leaves residual stigmata many of which show characteristic signs. Hutchinson's teeth (Fig. 7.58) are abnormal permanent incisors, smaller than usual with the sides converging towards the cutting edge, which often shows a notch. Gummatous lesions of the nasal septum may lead to its destruction (Fig. 7.59). Syphilitic 'saddle nose' is a different deformity – a flattened bridge due to poor development resulting from syphilitic rhinitis.

The diagnosis of early syphilis is based upon clinical examination and demonstration in early infectious lesions of *T. pallidum* by dark ground examination, with or without serological tests. The latter are not of help in primary syphilis but are useful for the diagnosis of secondary, latent and tertiary disease and for the assessment of response to treatment. There are two types of tests:

• reagin tests, such as the VDRL (Venereal Disease Research Laboratory) or RPR (rapid plasma reagin) which are non-specific and employ a cardiolipin antigen;

• specific antitreponemal antibody tests, such as the *T. pallidum* haemagglutination test (TPHA), the fluorescent treponemal antibody absorption test (FTA-Abs) and the *T. pallidum* immobilization test (TPI).

The FTA-Abs is the standard specific test used. The rates of positive tests in untreated syphilis at various stages are summarized in Figure 7.60. Congenital syphilis may be diagnosed by finding passively transferred maternal serological reactivity or by measuring specific IgM by a modification of the FTA-Abs test.

The reaginic antibody tests are useful as screening tests or for measuring the response to treatment. There are however frequent false positive results, so any positive result requires confirmation. A positive VDRL from the CSF is diagnostic of neurosyphilis (see Chapter 3). A positive FTA-Abs is diagnostic of present or past infection – once a patient is positive for FTA-Abs, she or he remains so for life, with or without treatment – so it cannot be used to document the adequacy of therapy.

Penicillin remains the drug of choice for the treatment of all stages of syphilis. The recommended regimens and follow-up are summarized in Figure 7.61.

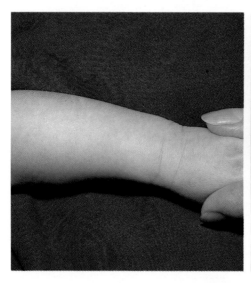

Fig. 7.55 Congenital syphilis. Left: Soft tissue swelling in an infant. Right: Radiograph showing the underlying periosteal reaction in the ulna. The pain caused by these lesions may lead to a pseudoparalysis of the limb (pseudoparalysis of Parrot). By courtesy of Dr M. J. Tarlow.

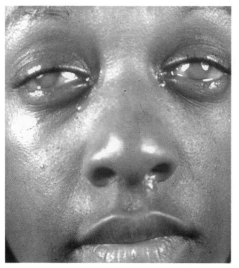

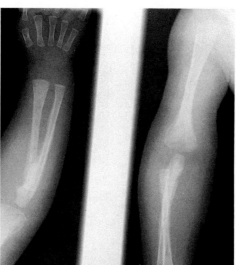

Fig. 7.56 Congenital syphilis. Interstitial keratitis develops at any age from a few years to young adult life. Vascularization of the cornea results in corneal scarring and opacity; there is often an associated iridocyclitis. This patient is blind. By courtesy of Dr S. Olansky.

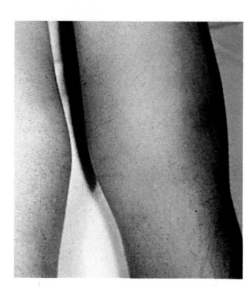

Fig. 7.57 Congenital syphilis. Clutton's joints, a painless chronic arthropathy developing in the second decade of life, with effusion into the joints but no bone change. The effusions tend to resolve slowly over a number of months. By courtesy of Dr S. Olansky.

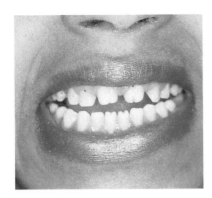

Fig. 7.58 Congenital syphilis. Hutchinson's teeth – the incisors are smaller than normal, with sloping sides and central semilunar notches. By courtesy of Dr J. Clay.

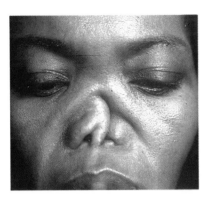

Fig. 7.59 Congenital syphilis. Gummatous infiltration of the nasal septum has led to its destruction with collapse of the nose. By courtesy of Dr S. Olansky.

Serological Tests for Syphilis		
	Rate of Positivity (%)	
Stage of Disease	**VDRL**	**FTA–Abs**
Primary	50–75	70–85
Secondary	99	99
Latent	75	98
Tertiary	70	98

Fig. 7.60 Table showing the rate of positivity (%) of the standard serological tests in various stages of syphilis.

Fig. 7.61 Table of recommended treatment and follow-up of syphilis.

Treatment and Follow–up of Syphilis		
Stage of Disease	**Treatment**	**Follow–up**
Primary, secondary or latent of less than 1 year duration	Benzathine penicillin 2.4 million units (1.44g) IM; or penicillin G 600 000 units (0.36g)/day for 10 days	1, 3, 6 and 12 months
Latent of more than 1 year duration or cardiovascular	Benzathine penicillin as above, weekly for 3 weeks	As above, then at 18 and 24 months
Neurosyphilis	Penicillin G, 12–24 million units (7.2–14.4g)/day IV for 10 days; or procaine penicillin 2–4 million units/day IM plus probenecid for 10 days. Either regimen to be followed by benzathine penicillin 2–4 million units IM weekly for 3 weeks	As above, then at 18 and 24 months
Congenital	Procaine penicillin 50,000 units/kg (30mg/kg) IM daily for 10 days or penicillin G 100 000–150 000 units/kg/day IV for 10–14 days	1, 3, 6 and 12 months
Penicillin–allergic patients		
Primary, secondary or latent of less than 1 year duration	Tetracycline or erythromycin 500mg PO, QID for 15 days	
Latent of more than 1 year duration or cardio–vascular	Tetracycline or erythromycin 500mg PO, QID for 30 days	
Neurosyphilis or congenital	Skin–testing with desensitization to penicillin recommended	

LYMPHOGRANULOMA VENEREUM

This condition is caused by the L-1, L-2, and L-3 serovars of *C. trachomatis* – different serological groups from those which cause non-specific urethritis and cervicitis. It is uncommon in the West – most cases arise in subtropical and tropical countries. The primary lesion is a painless non-indurated penile vesicle or papule which develops 1–4 weeks after infection but which is often unnoticed, since it heals quickly. Regional adenitis, with stretched and discoloured overlying skin (Figs 7.62 & 7.63), and constitutional symptoms follow 1–2 weeks later; the lymph nodes become matted and suppurate, with multiple abscess and sinus formation (Fig. 7.64). In males the inguinal glands are most commonly involved but in females and homosexual males the perirectal glands suppurate and may be associated with painful proctitis and bloody anal discharge.

Unless treated the inflammation becomes chronic leading to fibrosis and lymphatic obstruction. Rectal strictures, sometimes with the formation of perirectal abscesses and fistulas, and elephantiasis of the genitalia may follow (Fig. 7.65).

Diagnosis is usually made by serological means (complement fixation and microimmunofluorescence) but *C. tra-*

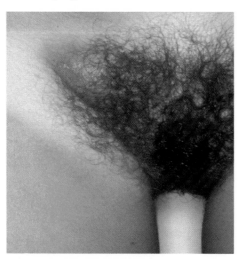

Fig. 7.62 Painful buboes in lymphogranuloma venereum. By courtesy of Dr J. Bingham.

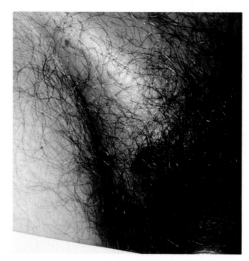

Fig. 7.63 Lymphogranuloma venereum. Inguinal adenitis. By courtesy of Dr J. Clay.

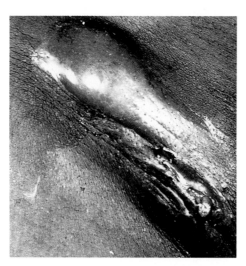

Fig. 7.64 Lymphogranuloma venereum. The bubo of chronic inguinal lymphadenopathy. The nodes are matted together by inflammatory periadenitis and a sinus is also visible. By courtesy of Dr S. Olansky

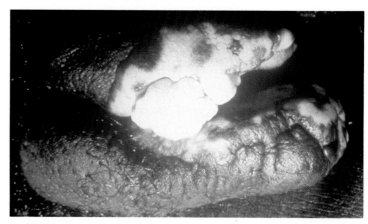

Fig. 7.65 Lymphogranuloma venereum. Vulval elephantiasis resulting from chronic infection. By courtesy of Dr J. Bingham.

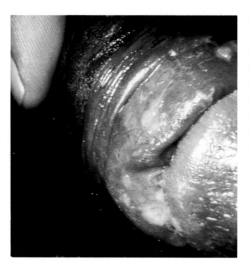

Fig. 7.66 Chancroid. Irregular ulcers extending along the coronal sulcus of the penis. They are irregular in shape, painful and not indurated, all points of distinction from syphilitic chancre. By courtesy of Dr S. Olansky.

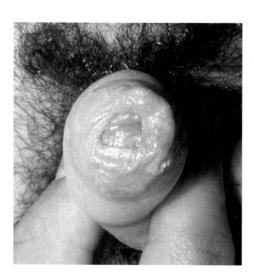

Fig. 7.67 Chancroid. Several irregular ulcers on the prepuce. By courtesy of Dr L. Parish.

chomatis can be cultured from aspirates of the suppurative lymph nodes or abscesses, if the necessary special facilities are available. The organism can now be detected in smears or other specimens by direct fluorescent tests with monoclonal antibodies. Treatment with tetracyclines or sulphonamides during the acute phase will prevent the subsequent chronic changes, but once these have developed antimicrobial agents have little effect.

CHANCROID

Now a rare disease in the Western World, chancroid or soft chancre is still frequently seen in southeast Asia, tropical Africa and South America. The causative organism is *Haemophilus ducreyi*, a fastidious Gram-negative aerobic rod. The incubation period is usually 4–10 days and then an erythematous genital papule appears which rapidly becomes pustular and breaks down to form a ragged ulcer. The ulcers often have a beefy, granular base and may be extremely painful. The lesion is usually single but sometimes multiple lesions are found which may merge together (Figs 7.66 & 7.67). In men ulcers on the prepuce are often accompanied by swelling and phimosis. Many patients with chancroid have unilateral or bilateral painful lymphadenopathy – without effective treatment buboes may occur and suppurate.

Haemophilus ducreyi can be seen in a Gram-stained smear of material from a genital lesion. Sometimes the organisms form long trails within strands of mucin, the so-called 'railroad tracks' (Fig. 7.68) and it may be possible to culture the organism on special media. Treatment with oral cotrimoxazole (960mg every 12 hours for 7 days), erythromycin (500mg every 6 hours for 7 days), a 4-quinolone such as ciprofloxacin (500mg every 12 hours for 3 days) or a single intramuscular dose of ceftriaxone (250mg) usually results in healing within one or two weeks. More prolonged courses may be needed for those with HIV infection.

GRANULOMA INGUINALE

This uncommon, sexually-transmitted condition is seen mainly in tropical and subtropical countries and is rare in the West. Small papular lesions appear 1–12 weeks after exposure on the genitalia, perineum, groin or occasionally at other sites; these break down into progressively enlarging ulcers (Fig. 7.69). The ulcers are elevated with a rolled edge and the raised friable granulomatous mass spreads and involves new areas of skin by contact. The slowly progressive destruction may cause considerable disfigurement (Figs 7.70, 7.71 & 7.72). Regional lymphadenopathy does not usually occur unless there is secondary infection (although the enlarging granulomatous process may mimic a bubo) and systemic symptoms are rare. Sequelae include stenosis of the urethral, vaginal or anal orifices, and massive elephantoid oedema. When there is a uterine lesion, associated metastatic lesions have occasionally been reported (Fig. 7.73).

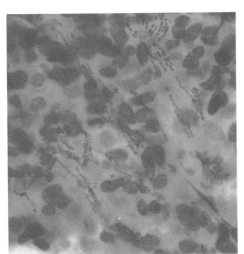

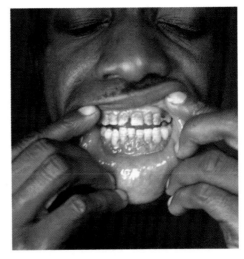

Fig. 7.68 Chancroid. Gram stain smear of exudate showing the 'railroad-track' appearance of *Haemophilus ducreyi*, the causal agent. By courtesy of Prof. G. R. Schmid, Dr W. O. Schalla and Dr W. E. DeWitt.

Fig. 7.69 Granuloma inguinale. Ulcerating lesions on gums. By courtesy of the late Dr B. Shaffer.

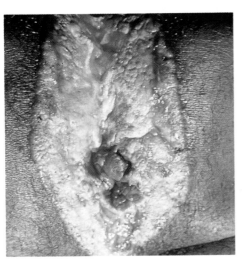

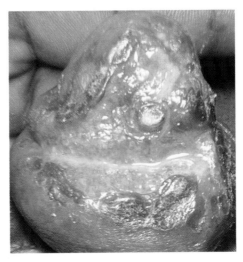

Fig. 7.70 Granuloma inguinale. A large area of ulceration in perianal area with a friable irregular granulomatous base. Some areas have bled and scabbed. By courtesy of Dr T. F. Sellers, Jr.

Fig. 7.71 Granuloma inguinale. A large area of ulceration on the penis, showing involvement of contiguous areas of the glans and shaft. By courtesy of Dr T. F. Sellers, Jr.

The causal organism, *Calymmatobacterium granulomatis*, is a nonmotile, gram-negative coccobacillus, often showing bipolar staining, that can not be cultured on ordinary laboratory media.

Diagnosis is confirmed by biopsy of a piece of granulation tissue from the edge of the lesion, crushing it between slides and staining the smear with Wright's, Giemsa or Warthin-Starry stain (Fig. 7.74). The Donovan bodies can be seen within the cytoplasm of large mononuclear cells: they have a 'closed safety-pin' appearance which is due to bipolar staining (Fig. 7.75). The drugs of choice for treatment are tetracycline or cotrimoxazole given until healing has occurred (usually 2–3 weeks). Patients should then be followed for several months to detect relapse or possible malignant change.

GENITAL WARTS

Genital and anal warts are caused by papillomaviruses and are nearly always spread by sexual contact. Human papillomaviruses (HPV) are non-capsulated DNA viruses approximately 50nm in diameter. There are at least 40 different HPV types, differentiated on the basis of analysis of their DNA. Some of these types are being increasingly linked to premalignant and malignant transformation of cervical, penile and anal cells.

Two types of genital warts are seen; condylomata acuminata and sessile warts. The former are fleshy soft growths that frequently coalesce into large masses, often affecting areas traumatized during intercourse (Figs 7.76, 7.77 & 7.78); sessile warts are only 1–2mm in diameter and affect

dry areas of skin, particularly the shaft of the penis. Genital warts may be solitary but are usually multiple; they may occur anywhere on the external genitalia, within the vagina and on the cervix. In men with penile lesions the urethra is commonly also involved, producing haematuria. Perianal warts are common in homosexual men and should always prompt a search for lesions within the anal canal or the rectum. Genital warts may be so profuse as to interfere with sexual intercourse (Fig. 7.79). It is now recognized that subclinical HPV infections of the cervix, penis, vulva and anus are common: lesions may be seen as white areas after the application of 5% acetic acid. Occult

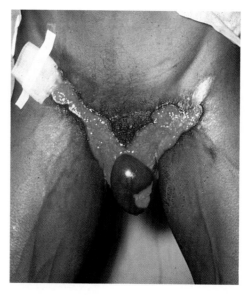

Fig. 7.72 Granuloma inguinale. Severe ulceration with granulomatous base in both groins. By courtesy of the late Dr B. Shaffer.

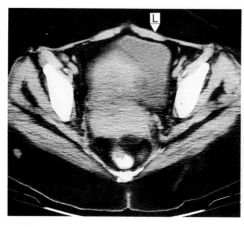
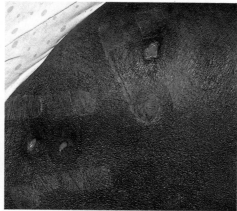

Fig. 7.73 Granuloma inguinale. CT scan of the pelvis (left) showing a uterine lesion (L) in a patient with biopsy-proven metastatic cutaneous lesions (right) of Donovanosis. By courtesy of Dr M. Wansborough Jones.

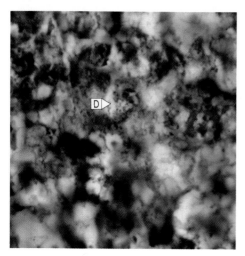

Fig. 7.74 Granuloma inguinale. Intracellular Donovan bodies (D) can be seen as small purple dots in this granulation tissue. Warthin–Starry stain.

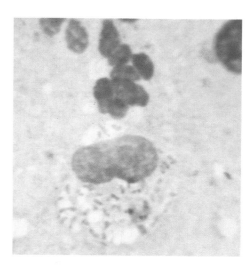

Fig. 7.75 Granuloma inguinale. Preparation of *Calymmatobacterium granulomatis* showing intracytoplasmic bipolar-stained bacilli within a large mononuclear cell. Giemsa stain. By courtesy of Dr T. F. Sellers, Jr.

anorectal HPV infection is also frequently discovered histologically. Cellular immunity is believed to play a role in the progression or resolution of genital warts: when cellular immunity is depressed (as in pregnancy or in HIV infection) condylomata acuminata proliferate.

HPV replicate in squamous epithelium and the histological features of condylomata acuminata are similar to those of other warts (Fig. 7.80). There is hyperplasia of the epithelium, and within the stratum granulosum there are large vacuolated cells whose nuclei contain inclusion bodies. In the cervix and within the anus HPV infection does not cause warts but leads to characteristic cellular changes (cells with hyperchromic nuclei surrounded by a clear, cytoplasmic halo, surrounded in turn by peripheral dark cytoplasm and called koilocytes – Fig. 7.81).

The association between HPV, particularly types 16 and 18, and cervical or vulval neoplasia has been much debated and there is now a suggestion of a similar association in the male genital tract and in the anus. HPV DNA sequences are associated with both cervical intra-epithelial neoplasia (CIN) and intra-epithelial neoplasia of the anus and the penis. HPV DNA is, however, also found in normal tissues from these sites – whether HPV has an oncogenic potential is still the subject of research.

Genital warts can be treated with a 10% or 25% solution of podophyllin resin in tincture of benzoin, applied to the lesions once or twice a week for 3 or 4 weeks. It should not be used for cervical or intra-anal warts as its effects can not be controlled at these sites. Alternative therapies with systemic or intralesional interferon or topical 5-fluorouracil cream are similarly successful. Physical therapies such as cautery, cryotherapy and diathermy or laser ther-

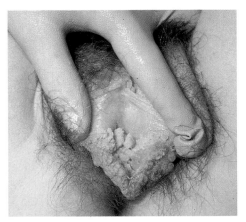

Fig. 7.76 Condylomata acuminata. Several large fleshy lesions around the anus of a homosexual male. It is important to examine the anal canal and lower rectum to determine the precise extent of the problem. By courtesy of Dr L. Parish.

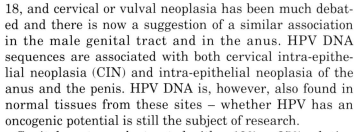

Fig. 7.77 Numerous condylomata acuminata affecting the glans and inner lining of the prepuce. By courtesy of Dr B. K.Fisher.

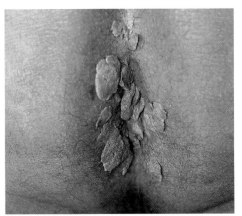

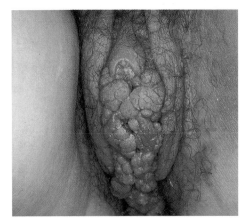

Fig. 7.78 Condylomata acuminata; fleshy viral warts on the introitus. By courtesy of Dr J. Clay

Fig. 7.79 Condylomata acuminata. Numerous fleshy lesions of the introitus causing severe sexual difficulties. By courtesy of Dr J. Clay.

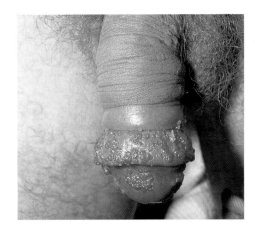

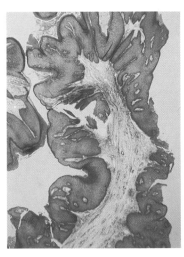
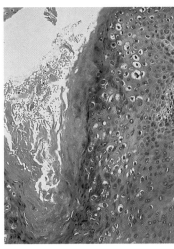

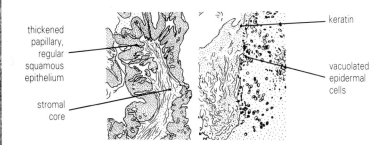

thickened papillary, regular squamous epithelium

stromal core

keratin

vacuolated epidermal cells

Fig. 7.80 Condylomata acuminata. Left: Histological appearance showing acanthosis (epithelial hyperplasia) and papillomatosis. ×5. Right: The high power view shows the characteristic cytoplasmic vacuolation. ×120. H & E stain. By courtesy of Mr J. P. S. Thomson and Dr I. Talbot.

apy (under general anaesthetic) are suitable for internal or extensive lesions.

OTHER GENITAL LESIONS

Many lesions may be seen on the genitalia which have to be considered in differential diagnosis. Some of these are sexually transmitted, such as scabies (Fig. 7.82) and crab lice (Fig. 7.83). Others are circinate balanitis in Reiter's syndrome (Fig. 7.84), various forms of pyogenic infection and allergic or vasculitic disorders such as Stevens-Johnson syndrome and Behçets syndrome (Fig. 7.85), and lichen planus, which is seen as papular or annular lesions on the genitalia (Fig. 7.86).

PELVIC INFLAMMATORY DISEASE

This term covers a spectrum of conditions, from limited acute salpingitis to abscesses involving the Fallopian tubes, ovaries and uterus and localized or generalized

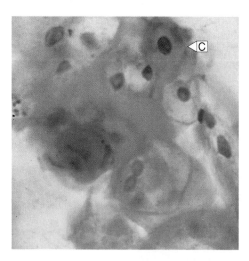

Fig. 7.81 Papillomavirus infections. Cervical cytology showing cell (C) with hyperchromic nucleus and perinuclear halo (koilocyte). By courtesy of Prof. A. A. Moreland, Dr K. Stone and Prof. B. Majmudar.

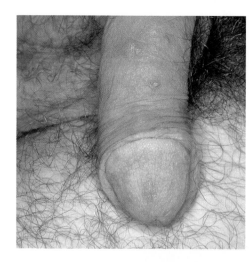

Fig. 7.82 Scabies. Papular lesions on the shaft of the penis. By courtesy of Dr B.K. Fisher.

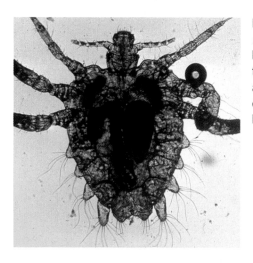

Fig. 7.83 Crab louse. *Phthirius pubis* is so called because of its resemblance to a crab 1–2mm long. The adult clings to hairs and the eggs adhere to hair shafts. By courtesy of Dr L. Parish.

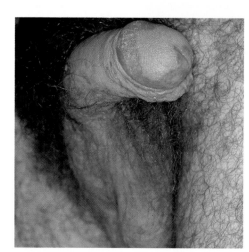

Fig. 7.84 Circinate balanitis. Shallow erosions on the glans have coalesced to give the circinate appearance. By courtesy of Dr B. K. Fisher.

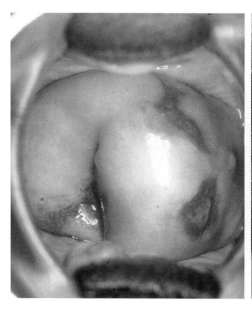

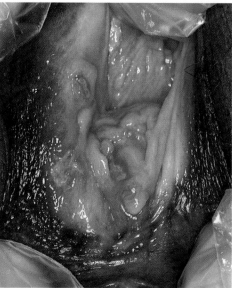

Fig. 7.85 Behçets syndrome. Superficial ulcers on the cervix (left) and vulva (right). by courtesy of Mr D. Sturdee.

peritonitis. Spread of infection to the liver capsule causes perihepatitis (Fitz-Hugh-Curtis syndrome). It is usually an ascending infection, caused by the normal aerobic or anaerobic bacterial flora of the vagina or a sexually transmitted organism. It is a common problem in young, sexually active women and there are a number of epidemiological factors associated with an increased risk (Fig. 7.87)

Acute salpingitis

Acute salpingitis may be caused by a number of different organisms which spread to the fallopian tubes via the cervix and the endometrium. A common cause is *N. gonorrhoeae* (see above); about 15% of women with untreated endocervical gonorrhoea will develop salpingitis. Other bacteria isolated from such infections include aerobic gram-negative rods (especially *E. coli*), aerobic streptococci, and a variety of anaerobic organisms such as *Bacteroides fragilis* and peptostreptococci. Indeed, anaerobic bacteria have been shown to be of major importance, being isolated alone or as part of a mixed culture in up to 80% of cases. Another organism of great importance is *C. trachomatis* (the serovars that cause NSU – see above). Salpingitis is more common in sexually active women aged 15–20, women using intrauterine contraceptive devices (IUCDs) and women with abnormal pelvic anatomy. The symptoms are lower abdominal pain, dysuria, fever and purulent vaginal discharge; the signs are those of lower abdominal guarding together with tenderness of the cervix or adnexae. In general, chlamydial PID is less clinically overt than gonococcal PID or that due to anaerobic organisms. These features are not very specific and the diagnosis of acute salpingitis should be confirmed by isolation of pathogens from specimens taken at laparoscopy (Fig. 7.88) or culdocentesis. Cervical swabs for detection of chlamydia and gonococci (see above) should also be taken.

Initial therapy should be aimed at the likely pathogens but there is no consensus as to the optimal regimen. For the less severely ill woman, a single high dose of oral amoxicillin (3g) or intramuscular cefoxitin (2g) followed by 10–14 days of a tetracycline (except in pregnancy) with or without metronidazole is suitable. For the hospitalized patient, a number of treatments are available: high dose penicillin, gentamicin and metronidazole followed by tetracycline; doxycycline and cefoxitin; or clindamycin and gentamicin, followed by a tetracycline. Total treatment should last for 14 days. With the use of such therapy the complications of salpingitis, such as infertility (Fig. 7.89), ectopic pregnancy and pelvic adhesions can be reduced.

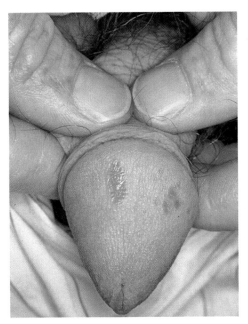

Fig. 7.86 Lichen planus. Characteristic itchy shiny papules on the glans penis. They may be accompanied by similar lesions on the limbs and in the mouth. By courtesy of Dr S. Olansky.

Factors Increasing the Risk of Pelvic Inflammatory Disease
Early age of onset of sexual activity
Multiple sexual partners
Recent change of sexual partner
Lower socioeconomic class
Previous pelvic inflammatory disease
Previous sexually transmitted disease
Use of IUCD
Recent pregnancy
Recent gynaecological surgery

Fig. 7.87 Table of factors associated with an increased risk of pelvic inflammatory disease

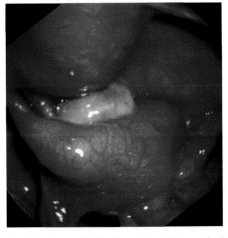

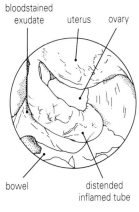

bloodstained exudate · uterus · ovary
bowel · distended inflamed tube

Fig. 7.88 Acute salpingitis. The tube is red, haemorrhagic and oedematous.

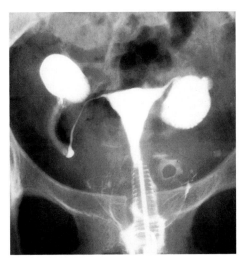

Fig. 7.89 Hydrosalpinx secondary to previous pelvic inflammatory disease. Hysterosalpingogram with contrast material filling the uterine cavity and fallopian tubes, with dilatation of the ampullary portions of both tubes and no free intraperitoneal spillage of contrast material.

Tubo-ovarian Abscesses

These are usually the result of recurrent episodes of acute salpingitis but may also occur without prior pelvic infection, especially if an IUCD is used. The organisms responsible are similar to those causing salpingitis with the exception of the gonococcus and chlamydia, which are only rarely isolated from abscesses. The symptoms and signs are similar to those of salpingitis with the addition that a mass is often found on pelvic examination. If the abscess ruptures then acute peritonitis and shock develop very rapidly. The diagnosis may be confirmed by pelvic ultrasonography (Fig. 7.90) and/or computerized tomography. Therapy needs to be individualized and often involves both broad spectrum antibiotics and surgical drainage of pus.

Perihepatitis

Acute perihepatitis (Fitz-Hugh-Curtis syndrome) develops as a result of gonococcal or chlamydial infection spreading through the peritoneum to the liver capsule. The symptoms are right upper quadrant pain, liver tenderness and signs of localized peritonitis. Laparoscopy shows adhesions between the liver capsulae and the parietal peritoneum (Fig. 7.91). Recognition of the syndrome and appropriate antibiotic therapy prevents an unnecessary laparotomy.

Pelvic Actinomycosis

Pelvic actinomycosis is associated with the use of IUCDs which provide a portal of entry for the organism from the lower genital tract. Colonies of the organism have been found on IUCDs removed from women with this infection (Fig. 7.92). Sulphur granules are sometimes found in Pap smears from women using IUCDs and many authorities recommend removal of the IUCD in these cases to prevent development of pelvic infection.

Tuberculosis

Tuberculous epididymitis is dealt with in Chapter 6. Female genital tuberculosis is, however, the result not of local spread but of haematogenous dissemination. The Fallopian tubes are most commonly involved (Fig. 7.93). Constitutional symptoms are not prominent and most patients are diagnosed as a result of investigation for infertility or menstrual disorders. Endometrial curettage taken in the second half of the menstrual cycle may show granulomata (Fig. 7.94).

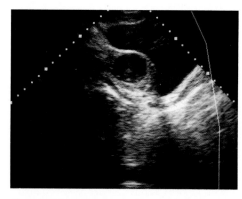

Fig. 7.90 Tuboovarian abscess. Ultrasound study of left sagittal section of the pelvis showing a complex thick-walled cystic left adnexal man with internal septations.

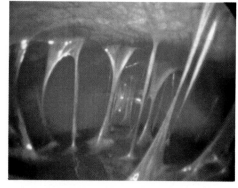

Fig. 7.91 Laparoscopic view of 'violin-string' adhesions between parietal peritoneum and hepatic capsule in a patient with perihepatitis (Fitz-Hugh-Curtis syndrome).

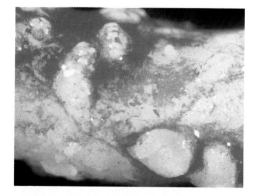

Fig. 7.92 Pelvic actinomycosis. Portion of an intrauterine contraceptive device (Lippes loop) studded with 'molar-tooth' colonies of *Actinomyces israelii*. By courtesy of A. E. Prevost.

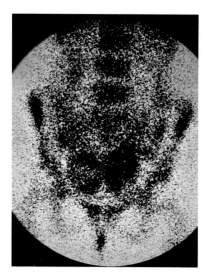

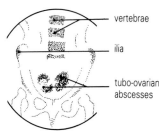

Fig. 7.93 Genital tuberculosis. [67]Gallium-scan at 48 hours in a 13-year-old girl showing large bilateral tubo-ovarian abscesses. The patient had received treatment for tuberculosis several years earlier. By courtesy of Dr C. S. Hicks.

vertebrae

ilia

tubo-ovarian abscesses

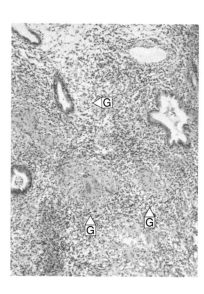

Fig. 7.94 Tuberculous endometritis (curettage preparation). The granulomata (G), being shed monthly at an early stage of their development, do not show caseation. H&E stain.

8

BONES AND JOINTS

OSTEOMYELITIS

Acute Osteomyelitis

Depending upon the pathogenic mechanism responsible, three different types of osteomyelitis are recognized: haematogenous, resulting from bacteraemia, contiguous, when it is secondary to infection in adjacent structures, and that associated with peripheral vascular disease. Haematogenous osteomyelitis is still the most common type, but the other two forms are increasing in frequency.

Haematogenous osteomyelitis occurs most frequently in rapidly growing bone, particularly in children. Although any bone may be infected, the highly vascular metaphyses of long bones are the most common sites for initial localization of infection. Here the capillaries loop and enter into a system of sluggishly flowing sinusoidal veins which drain into the medullary vessels (Fig. 8.1). Once bacterial infection becomes established in and around the capillaries (Fig. 8.2), the slow blood flow and the essentially end-artery nature of the capillary loops encourage spread by direct extension of the suppurative process and also because of ischaemic necrosis of bone produced by plugging of the blood vessels. The subsequent route of spread of infection depends upon whether there are anastomatic channels between the metaphyseal and epiphyseal circulations. In neonates such channels exist and infection can spread rapidly to involve the adjacent joint. In older children the epiphyseal growth plate prevents such anastomoses and the infection tracks laterally through the cortex into the sub-periosteal space. The loose periosteum is stripped off the cortex and new bone is laid down beneath the elevated periosteum: when this is circumferential it is termed an involucrum. After some time the increase in pressure leads to vascular obstruction, and segments of avascular dead bone (sequestra) may be formed. In this age group spread to adjacent joints only occurs where the metaphysis is intra-capsular, as in the hip and the shoulder. When the infection breaks through the cortex to form a sinus tract, the hole in the bone is termed a cloaca (Fig. 8.3). In adults the growth plate has been resorbed and spread of infection from the metaphysis to the joint is again possible. In older adults, however, many cases of haematogenous osteomyelitis involve the vertebrae. Blood-borne bacteria localize first in the well-vascularized end plate adjacent to the disc space and then spread to the disc and to the next vertebral body (Figs. 8.4, 8.5). In drug addicts the vertebrae, pelvic bones and clavicles are also frequently the sites of osteomyelitis.

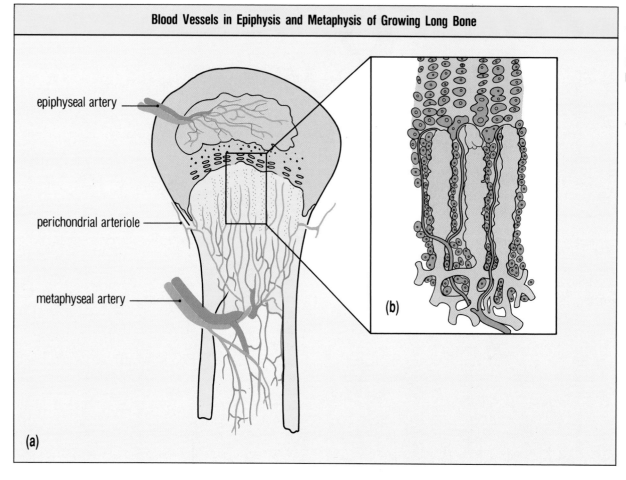

Blood Vessels in Epiphysis and Metaphysis of Growing Long Bone

epiphyseal artery

perichondrial arteriole

metaphyseal artery

(b)

(a)

Fig. 8.1 (a) Diagram of blood vessels in epiphysis and metaphysis of growing long bone. (b) Close up of area highlighted in (a) showing metaphyseal capillary 'end–artery' loops draining into venous sinuses.

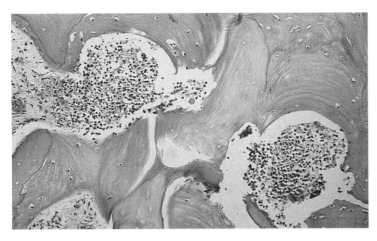
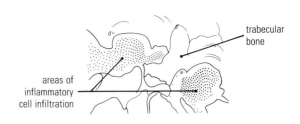

trabecular bone

areas of inflammatory cell infiltration

Fig. 8.2 Acute osteomyelitis. Section of trabecular bone showing infiltration with acute inflammatory cells. Haematoxylin and eosin stain. By courtesy of Dr C.W. Edwards.

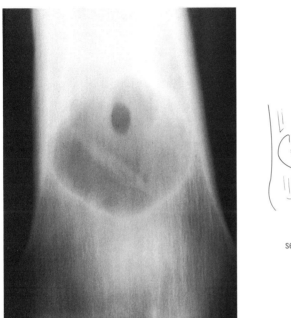
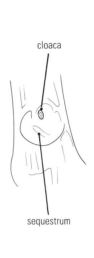

cloaca

sequestrum

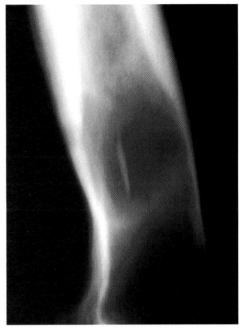
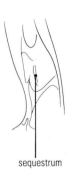

sequestrum

Fig. 8.3 Acute osteomyelitis. Antero–posterior (left) and lateral (right) tomograms of osteomyelitis of femur, showing an area of bone destruction containing sequestrum. There is a cloaca situated posteriorly. By courtesy of Dr D.C. Tudway.

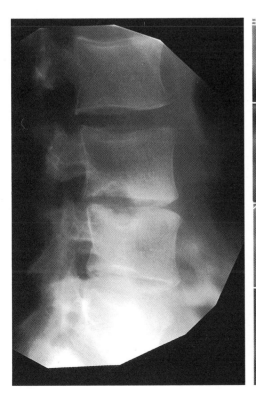
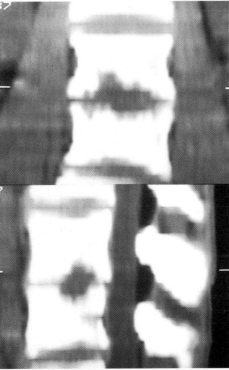

Fig. 8.4 Vertebral osteomyelitis. Lateral radiograph of the lumbar spine (left), and lateral (bottom right) and antero–posterior (top right) CT scan reconstructions showing narrowing of the disc space and early destruction of the end–plates of two adjacent vertebrae. By courtesy of Mr R.J. Cherry.

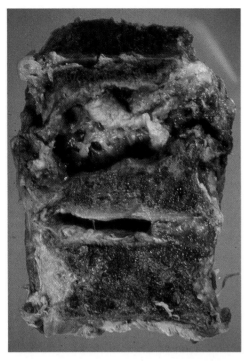

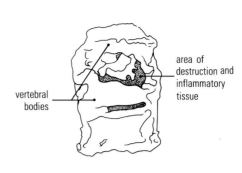

vertebral bodies

area of destruction and inflammatory tissue

Fig. 8.5 Vertebral osteomyelitis. Postmortem specimen showing extensive destruction of an intervertebral disc and two adjacent vertebral bodies by inflammatory tissue. By courtesy of Dr C.W. Edwards.

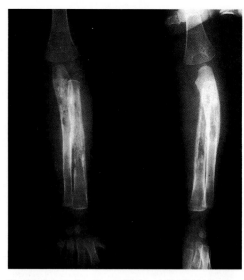

Fig. 8.6 Salmonella osteomyelitis in a child with sickle cell disease. Radiographs of swollen left forearm show extensive osteomyelitis of the radius and ulna. The causal organism was *Salmonella paratyphi B*.

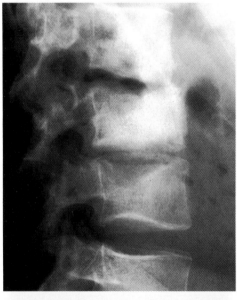

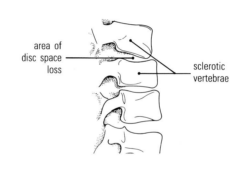

area of disc space loss

sclerotic vertebrae

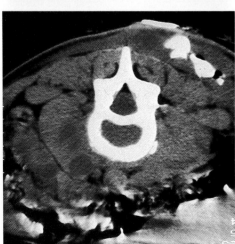

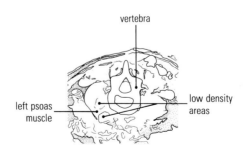

vertebra

left psoas muscle

low density areas

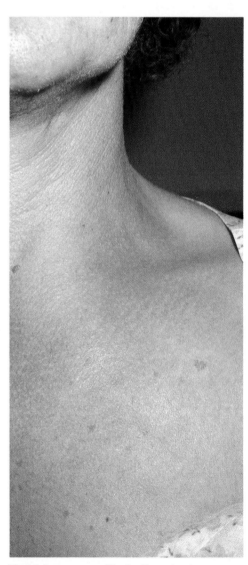

Fig. 8.7 Salmonella osteomyelitis. Radiograph (top) showing disc space loss at L2/3 and sclerosis of adjacent vertebral bodies in a 24–year–old man with HbSC disease and *Salmonella hadar* vertebral osteomyelitis. A CT scan of the same patient at L3/4 (bottom) shows several focal low density areas in the left psoas muscle. There is packing material in a large abscess cavity in the right flank which had been drained surgically.

Fig. 8.8 Acute osteomyelitis. Swelling and erythema over the medial end of the left clavicle of a 45–year–old woman who complained of local pain and tenderness and who was pyrexial. *Staphylococcus aureus* was isolated from blood cultures.

Staphylococcus aureus is the most common aetiologic agent of acute osteomyelitis in children, but in certain patient groups other bacteria must be considered. In neonates Group B streptococci and *Enterobacteriaceae* are particularly common, and in children between 6 months and 6 years old *Haemophilus influenzae* must be considered. Patients with sickle cell anaemia and other major haemoglobinopathies are especially prone to development of osteomyelitis due to *Salmonella* organisms, a disease found very rarely in patients with normal haemoglobin (Figs. 8.6, 8.7). Various Gram-negative bacilli cause nearly half the cases in persons with chronic renal disease, malignancy and other debilitating diseases, and they are the dominant organisms in osteomyelitis in intravenous drug abusers.

The classical presentation of acute haematogenous osteomyelitis is with high fever, severe local pain, with limitation of movement if a limb is affected, and signs of erythema, swelling and tenderness associated with subperiosteal abscess formation (Fig. 8.8). In such cases the diagnosis of osteomyelitis is readily suspected. In adults, however, the history may be less acute and the signs are often much less florid. Neonatal osteomyelitis is also characterized by few systemic signs, and the diagnosis requires a high index of suspicion (Fig. 8.9). Similarly insidious, and difficult to diagnose, is vertebral osteomyelitis in adults. Dull nagging back pain, sometimes with referred pain from nerve root irritation, and often only a low-grade fever are the only symptoms, and hence such infections may remain unsuspected for a long period, perhaps only becoming considered when signs of cord compression develop. When infection involves the cervical vertebrae (Fig. 8.10), persistent fever and torticollis are the warning signals.

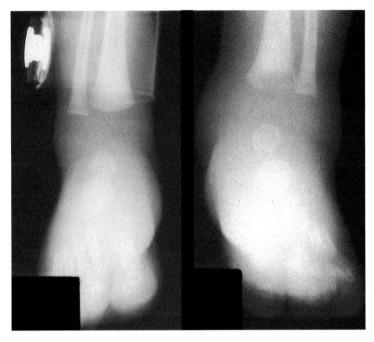

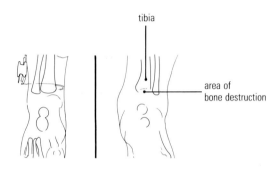

Fig. 8.9 Neonatal osteomyelitis. A one–month–old baby who developed osteomyelitis at the distal end of the right tibia. She had had a Group B streptococcal septicaemia following delivery but the only signs of osteomyelitis were failure to thrive and swelling of the right ankle. By courtesy of Dr G.S. Jones.

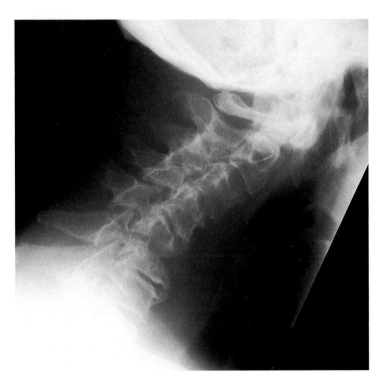

Fig. 8.10 Cervical osteomyelitis. Erosion and collapse of C5/6 due to osteomyelitis in a 74–year–old woman. There is an associated soft–tissue swelling anterior to the cervical spine. By courtesy of Dr D.C. Tudway.

The second form of osteomyelitis occurs when there is a contiguous focus of infection, often related to surgical procedure or trauma in older patients. The precipitating event is often the open reduction of a fracture, although cases are also seen after puncture wounds of the hands or feet. Infected teeth, sinuses (Fig. 8.11) or decubitus ulcers (Fig. 8.12) may also be an underlying factor. The site of the osteomyelitis is determined by the preceding surgery, trauma or soft tissue infection.

Again *Staph. aureus* is the most common aetiological agent, but mixed infections are frequently found. Certain bacteria are particularly likely in certain circumstances. *Staphylococcus epidermidis* must be considered in infection associated with prosthetic joints, *Pasteurella multocida* after dog or cat bites, *Pseudomonas aeruginosa* is associated with osteomyelitis secondary to puncture wounds of the feet and with infection after sternum-splitting for open heart surgery (Fig. 8.13), and anaerobes are increasingly recog-

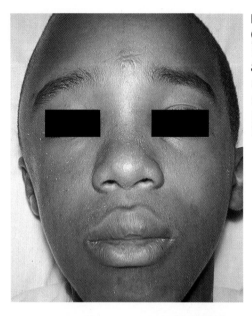

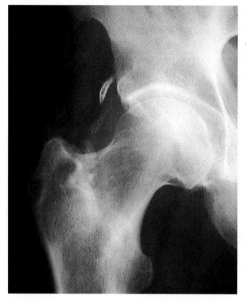

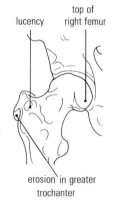

Fig. 8.11 Acute osteomyeltis. Osteomyelitis of the right frontal bone due to *Staphylococcus aureus*, secondary to infection in the right frontal sinus ('Pott's puffy tumour'). By courtesy of Dr T.F. Sellers, Jr.

Fig. 8.12 Contiguous osteomyelitis. Erosion of the greater trochanter underlying a chronic decubitus ulcer in an elderly man. By courtesy of Dr A.M. Davies.

lucency

top of right femur

erosion in greater trochanter

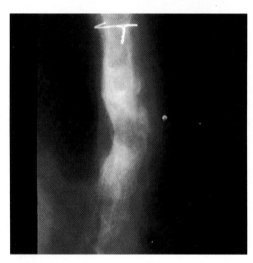

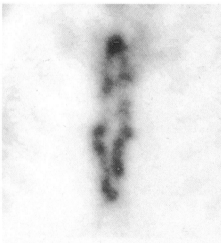

Fig. 8.13 Psuedomonas osteomyelitis. Lateral tomogram of the sternum (left) showing areas of lucency and sclerosis with periosteal new bone formation in osteomyelitis following open heart surgery in a 69–year–old man. A technetium scan (right) in the same patient showed irregular high activity along the sternal margin. *Pseudomonas aeruginosa* was isolated.

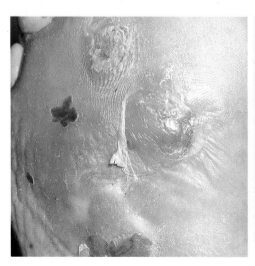

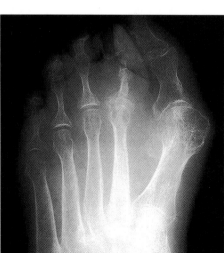

Fig. 8.14 Osteomyelitis due to peripheral vascular disease. Plantar surface of the right foot of a 78–year–old diabetic woman, showing multiple draining sinuses (left). A radiograph of the same foot (right) showed destruction of head of 2nd metatarsal and base of proximal phalanx due to osteomyelitis.

nized as the cause of osteomyelitis secondary to human bites, decubitus ulcers, infected teeth or sinuses.

Older individuals with peripheral vascular disease, especially that associated with diabetes, may develop osteomyelitis involving the toes or other bones of the feet. Many of these patients have diabetic neuropathy and deep chronic draining ulcers on the plantar surface of the foot (Fig. 8.14). Fever and systemic symptoms are rare. The infections are almost always due to a mixture of Gram-positive bacteria (staphylococci and streptococci), *Enterobacteriaceae* and anaerobes, and bone biopsy and culture are often needed to determine the exact aetiology.

In the early stages of osteomyelitis X-rays are often normal. After 10–14 days periosteal elevation and new bone formation may be seen, and lytic changes develop between 2 and 6 weeks after the onset (Fig. 8.15). Sclerotic changes take even longer to appear (Fig. 8.16), and the characteristic appearance of involucra and sequestra denotes a long-standing osteomyelitis. Spinal X-rays are essential if vertebral osteomyelitis is suspected. Changes primarily affect-

ing the intervertebral disc suggest infection rather than tumour. Radionuclide scanning with ^{99m} technetium diphosphonate, which localizes in areas of accelerated bone turnover, is useful in the early stages of osteomyelitis (Fig. 8.17), and it may reveal positive features within 24–48h of the onset of symptoms. Technetium scans unfortunately are not specific for osteomyelitis and give false-positive results in other inflammatory processes such as cellulitis, infarction and synovitis. They are especially difficult to interpret in osteomyelitis associated with a contiguous focus of infection or with peripheral vascular disease. Scans with gallium citrate may help distinguish the false-positive technetium scan, and these are also useful for demonstrating recrudescence of activity in cases of prior chronic osteomyelitis. Computed tomographic (CT) scans (Figs. 8.4 right, 8.7 bottom) and magnetic resonance imaging (MRI) of infected areas (Fig. 8.18) enable the areas of bone destruction and soft tissue collections of pus to be clearly delineated, and, where available, MRI is the imaging method of choice in the diagnosis of osteomyelitis.

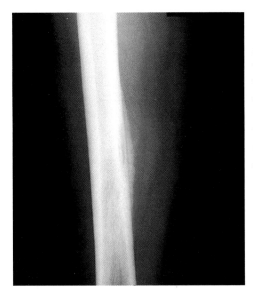

Fig. 8.15 Acute osteomyelitis Radiograph of early staphylococcal osteomyelitis in the femur of a 24–year–old woman. There is a well defined periosteal reaction in relation to the midshaft of the femur and an underlying lucency. By courtesy of Dr A.M. Davies.

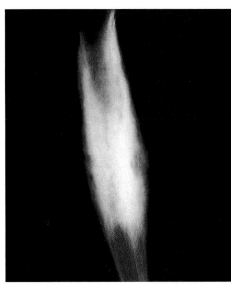

Fig. 8.16 Acute osteomyelitis. Marked new bone formation with extensive sclerosis and patchy lucencies in the left femur of a 21–year–old woman. By courtesy of Dr A.M Davies.

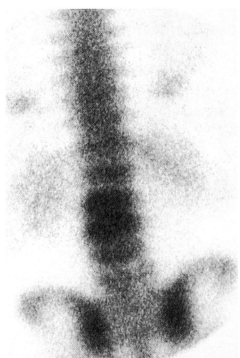

Fig. 8.17 ^{99m}Technetium bone scan showing high uptake in lumbar vertebrae. This is same patient as in Fig. 8.4.

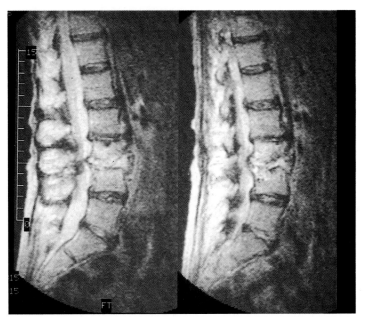

Fig. 8.18 Magnetic resonance image of lumbar spine showing destruction of L3 and L4 due to active tuberculous osteomyelitis. The intervertebral disc is particularly involved and there is indentation of the theca at the L3/L4 level. The patient presented with tuberculous meningitis.

In all cases of osteomyelitis attempts should be made to isolate the aetiological agent. Blood cultures are often positive in neonatal osteomyelitis and in haematogenous osteomyelitis, but they are less useful in the other types of bone infection. Needle aspiration of the lesion is the optimal method for determining the aetiology. It is particularly important in vertebral osteomyelitis and in non-haematogenous osteomyelitis, but it should be undertaken in any form of osteomyelitis that is not responding to initial therapy. Open biopsy should also be undertaken if the aetiology is in any doubt and especially if tuberculosis or fungal infection is suspected.

The mainstay of treatment for acute osteomyelitis is antibiotic therapy, but the penetration of most agents into bone is low and the usual practice is to give parenteral agents in high doses. The period of treatment is generally 3 or 4 weeks for haematogenous osteomyelitis affecting long bones, and providing sufficiently high doses are administered for this time, there is no advantage in prolonging therapy. There have been a number of studies suggesting that for this form

Initial Empirical Therapy for Acute Osteomyelitis		
Patient age	Likely aetiology	Therapy
Infants less than 2 months old	Staph. aureus Group B streptococci Gram-negative bacilli	Penicillinase-resistant semisynthetic penicillin (PRSP) and an aminoglycoside
Children under 6 years old	Staph. aureus and H. influenzae	PRSP and ampicillin or a third-generation cephalosporin
Children with haemoglobinopathy	Staph. aureus and Salmonella spp.	PRSP and ampicillin or a third-generation cephalosporin
Normal adults	Staph. aureus	PRSP
High-risk adults (Chronic renal failure, debilitating diseases, drug addicts, diabetics)	Staph. aureus and Gram-negative bacilli	PRSP and an aminoglycoside, or a third-generation cephalosporin

Fig. 8.19 Therapy for acute osteomyelitis in patients of different ages

Optimal Therapy for Osteomyelitis due to Specific Pathogens		
Pathogen	First Choice antibiotic	Alternatives
Staph aureus	Penicillinase-resistant semisynthetic penicillin	Cefazolin, cephalothin or clindamycin
Group B streptococci	Penicillin G	As above
H. influenzae	Ampicillin*	Chloramphenicol or a third generation cephalosporin
Salmonella spp.	Ampicillin	Co-trimoxazole or chloramphenicol
Enterobacteriaceae	Third-generation cephalosporin	Aminoglycoside
Pseudomonas aeruginosa	Aminoglycoside and ticarcillin, piperacillin or azlocillin	
Bacteroides spp.	Clindamycin	Metronidazole
Anaerobic streptococci	Penicillin G	Clindamycin
* If strain is beta-lactamase-positive use one of the alternative agents		

Fig. 8.20 The choice of therapy for osteomyelitis caused by different pathogens

of osteomyelitis oral antibiotics may be used after a few days of intravenous therapy, and providing that patient compliance is good and that the antibiotic chosen achieves adequate blood and bone levels, the results seem encouraging. For vertebral osteomyelitis, contiguous focus osteomyelitis, and that associated with prostheses or peripheral vascular disease, longer periods of parenteral therapy are indicated. The empirical therapy of osteomyelitis and the optimal treatment for specific pathogens are given in Figs. 8.19 and 8.20.

Surgery is usually not needed for the treatment of acute haematogenous osteomyelitis of long bones. It is, however, sometimes required for diagnostic purposes, if there are neurological complications of vertebral infection, or if sequestra are present. Surgery is also needed for many cases of osteomyelitis associated with peripheral vascular disease, where antibiotic therapy is notoriously unsatisfactory. The prognosis for acute haematogenous osteomyelitis is good, with a 10–20% risk of recurrence.

Chronic Osteomyelitis

Chronic focal osteomyelitis (Brodie's abscess) usually follows acute haematogenous osteomyelitis in teenagers. It arises when infection is contained but not eradicated. Typically it occurs in the metaphysis of a bone in the leg, usually the tibia. The acute episode settles but is followed by a focus of chronic infection that may persist for several years. Pain is the predominant symptom and radiologically there is irregular destruction with an intense sclerotic response (Fig. 8.21), but sequestra are not seen. Treatment is a combination of surgery and antibiotics.

Recurrent osteomyelitis at the same site as an earlier episode poses a very different problem from the acute forms. Both local and systemic clinical manifestations are much less florid, and it is sometimes difficult to determine whether active disease is present since blood cultures are unlikely to be positive and radiological changes present problems of interpretation in the presence of old disease. Gallium scans are more useful than technetium studies (Fig. 8.22). It is easier to recognize when there are draining sinuses, but cultures from the tracts are notoriously inaccurate when it comes to determining the aetiology and bone biopsy is mandatory. Adequate surgical debridement is essential and antibiotic therapy needs to be prolonged.

Squamous-cell carcinoma is a late complication of chronic osteomyelitis, most cases occurring in the legs. Amyloidosis no longer seems a problem of chronic bone infections.

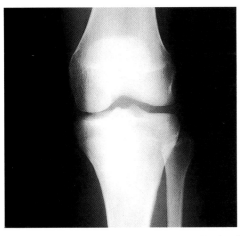
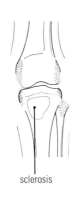
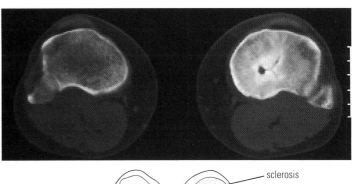
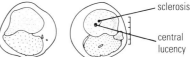

Fig. 8.21 Brodie's abscess. Radiograph of the tibia of a girl with pain in the knee (left) showing a poorly defined area of sclerosis. The central lucency and surrounding sclerosis are shown more clearly on the CT scan (right). By courtesy of Dr A. M. Davies.

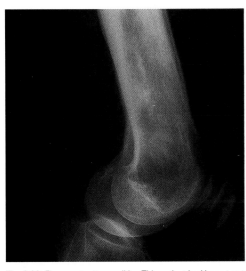
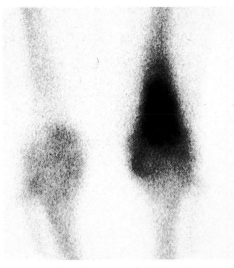
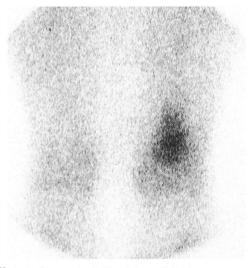

Fig. 8.22 Recurrent osteomyelitis. This patient had been treated for osteomyelitis of the distal left femur ten years previously. She then complained of fresh pain at the site and the radiograph showed periosteal reaction and an area of sclerosis containing irregular lucencies (left). The high uptake on a ^{99m} technetium scan (centre) is not diagnostic but the positive gallium scan (right) suggests active disease. By courtesy of Dr G.S. Jones.

FUNGAL INFECTIONS

Most fungal bone infections are secondary to haematogenous spread and are associated with disseminated disease (Fig. 8.23). Patients who are severely immunocompromised or who have had long intravenous catheters in situ for prolonged periods are particularly likely to get osteomyelitis with *Candida* or *Aspergillus* species. Candida osteomyelitis is also likely to affect intravenous drug addicts. Blastomycosis and cryptococcosis (Fig. 8.24) are both accompanied relatively frequently by skeletal involvement with osteomyelitis of the vertebrae, skull or long bones. There are no distinctive features of fungal osteomyelitis and diagnosis rests upon obtaining and examining biopsy material. Fungal osteomyelitis is usually treated with amphotericin B, although newer agents, such as fluconazole, show some promise.

MYCETOMA (MADURA FOOT)

This is a localized, chronic, progressive destructive infection involving the skin, subcutaneous tissues, muscles and bone. In tropical countries a large number of fungi and actinomycetes may be involved as aetiologic agents, but in temperate areas most cases are due to *Petriellidium (Allescheria) boydii*, *Nocardia asteroides* and *Nocardia braziliensis*. Organisms from the soil enter the tissues, usually of the foot or hand, following local trauma. The infection spreads through skin and subcutaneous tissue, eventually involving the bone. Gradually the granulomatous process completely destroys the architecture of the tissues involved (Fig. 8.25), and leads to production of deep abscesses and multiple draining fistulous tracts from which granules, which are actually colonies of the causative organism, can be obtained (Fig. 8.26). Amputation is often required because most

Fig. 8.23 African histoplasmosis. Chronic draining sinus on the shoulder secondary to chronic osteomyelitis due to *Histoplasma duboisii*. By courtesy of Dr W.M. Rambo.

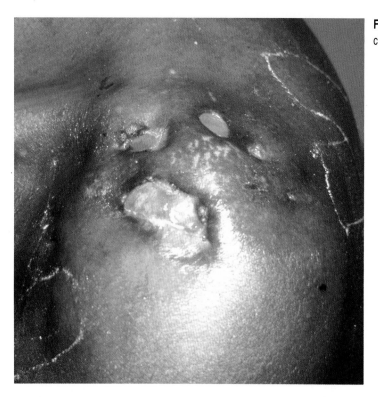

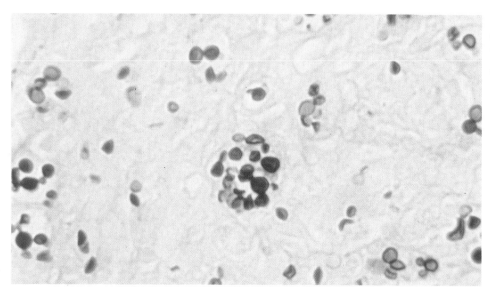

Fig. 8.24 Disseminated cryptococcosis. Many yeast cells of *Cryptococcus neoformans* in a biopsy specimen from the femur. Gomori–methenamine silver stain. By courtesy of A. E. Provost.

of the causative organisms are not very susceptible to chemotherapeutic agents, and the foot is often irreparably damaged by the time the patient is first seen.

INFECTIVE ARTHRITIS

Septic Arthritis

Bacterial infection of the joint space usually occurs because of the spread of organisms from a distant site by the haematogenous route, but occasionally it can result from direct inoculation from a penetrating wound or bite, from contiguous osteomyelitis, prosthetic joint surgery, or when intra-articular injections of corticosteroids are given. Recent joint trauma and underlying joint diseases such as rheumatoid or osteoarthritis are predisposing factors, as are chronic debility, immunosuppressive therapy and intravenous drug abuse.

Upon reaching a joint bacteria localize in the synovium and the subsequent inflammatory response leads to destruction of the cartilage. The initial step in this is the release of proteolytic enzymes from activated polymorphonuclear leucocytes, and the removal of these cells by repeated aspiration of infected joints is an important part of the management of septic arthritis.

The predominant bacterial aetiology of septic arthritis varies with the age of the patient. Group B streptococci, various Gram-negative bacilli and *Staph. aureus* are common in neonates, *H. influenzae* type b predominates between the ages of 1 month and 2 years, and *Staph. aureus* is found most frequently in older children. In sexually active young adults gonococcal infection is the most likely form of septic arthritis, but in older adults *Staph. aureus*, *Streptococcus pneumoniae* and other streptococci are the chief pathogens. As is the case for osteomyelitis, Gram-negative bacteria need to be considered in those with malignancy, other

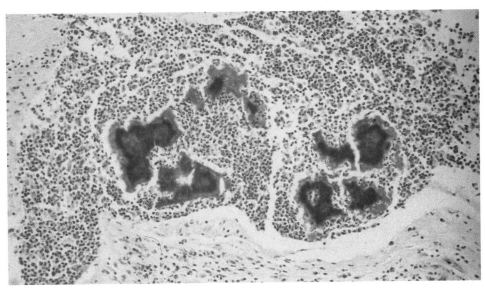

Fig. 8.25 Madura foot. A 58–year–old African with chronic swelling of the right foot and discharging sinuses on the sole and dorsum. The radiograph shows dissolution of the distal halves of the 4th and 5th metatarsals. The bases of the proximal phalanges are also affected.

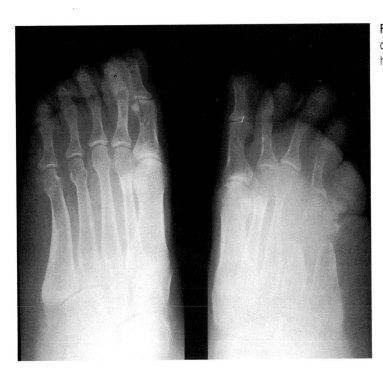

Fig. 8.26 Madura foot. An Asian man with a chronically swollen foot. Radiographs showed soft–tissue swelling, sclerosis and destruction of the calcaneum and mid–tarsal bones. Biopsy of the tissues shows colonies of a *Nocardia* species and a mixed inflammatory infiltrate surrounded by fibrous tissue. Haematoxylin and eosin stain. By courtesy of Dr J. Newman.

debitating diseases or medical immunosuppression, and in intravenous drug abusers. Prosthetic joints are particularly likely to be infected by *Staph. epidermidis*. There are major differences between the features of arthritis caused by gonococci and those of that due to other bacteria.

Nongonococcal arthritis

Bacterial arthritis is usually monarticular and the joints most frequently affected are the knee, ankle, elbow, hip, shoulder and wrist joints. Occasionally oligo- and polyarticular forms occur. The presentation is usually acute with pain, swelling, erythema and tenderness in the affected joint (Figs. 8.27, 8.28). Most patients have a fever, although this may be minimal in those who have rheumatoid arthritis or who are receiving steroid therapy. Rigors and chills are uncommon. A marked limitation in the range of joint mobility is the normal finding in infected natural joints, but in prosthetic joint infections pain may be the only symptom.

Gonococcal Arthritis

Gonococcal joint involvement may occur in either of two clinical forms. The most common manifestation of disseminated gonococcal infection is an initial migratory polyarthritis (Fig. 8.29) accompanied by marked systemic symptoms with fever, tenosynovitis (Fig. 8.30) and characteristic skin lesions which are often pustular with a necrotic centre and maximal on the hands or feet (Fig. 8.31). Blood culture is usually positive and although Gram-negative diplococci may be seen on a Gram stain smear of material from a skin lesion, bacteria are usually not found in joint fluid. The joint effusions associated with this syndrome are believed to involve immune or hypersensitivity reactions.

The other type of patient presents with suppurative monarticular arthritis, with bacteria recoverable from the pus in the joint space (Figs. 8.32, 8.33). Such patients often exhibit little evidence of systemic illness, and blood cultures are usually negative.

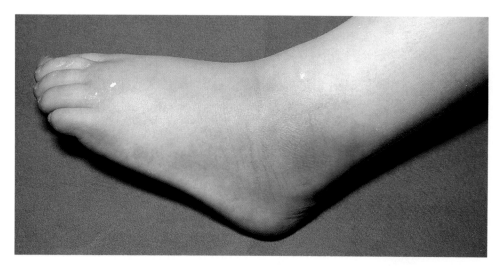

Fig. 8.27 Septic arthritis. Erythema and swelling of the left ankle joint in a young girl with staphylococcal sepsis (see also Fig. 8.34). By courtesy of Mr N. St. J. P. Dwyer.

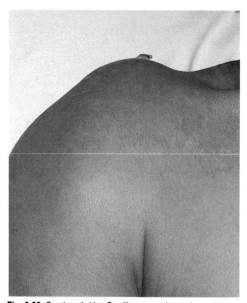
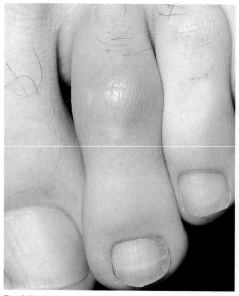
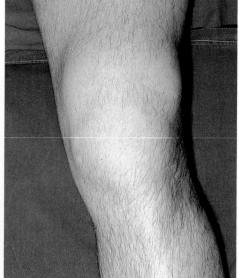

Fig. 8.28 Septic arthritis. Swellings superior and anterior to the right acrominoclavicular joint in a 48–year–old labourer who had blamed his shoulder pain upon trauma at work. *Staphylococcus aureus* was isolated from the aspirated synovial fluid.

Fig. 8.29 Acute gonococcal arthritis. Acute joint swelling in the proximal interphalangeal joint (left) and the knee (right) in a young man with disseminated gonococcal infection. Culture of the synovial fluid was negative.

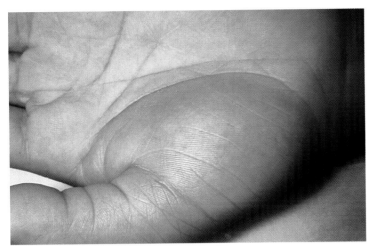

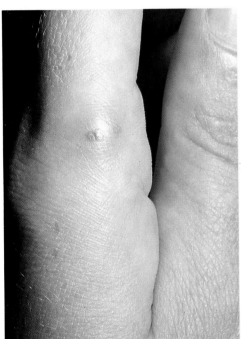
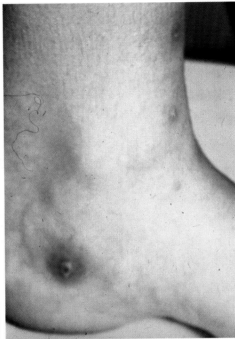

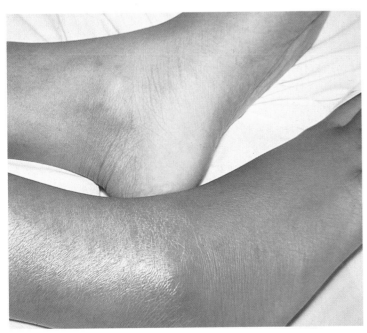

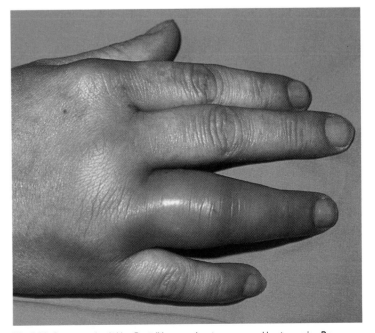

Fig. 8.30 Gonococcal tenosynovitis of the left thumb secondary to gonococcal bacteraemia. Note the erythema and swelling of thenar eminence. By courtesy of Dr T.F. Sellers, Jr.

Fig. 8.31 Gonococcal septicaemia. Typical skin lesions of disseminated gonococcal infection on the hand (left) and ankle (right). By courtesy of Prof. A. M. Geddes.

Fig. 8.32 Gonococcal septic arthritis. Arthritis due to *Neisseria gonorrhoeae* in a 24–year–old woman, showing marked erythema and swelling of the right ankle and leg. By courtesy of Dr T.F. Sellers, Jr.

Fig. 8.33 Gonococcal arthritis. Dactylitis secondary to gonococcal bacteraemia. By courtesy of Dr S. E. Thompson.

The diagnosis of bacterial arthritis depends upon examination of aspirated joint fluid, which should be carefully examined. The fluid should be sent for Gram stain, culture, crystal analysis, white cell count and differential, and glucose estimation. The fluid is often purulent and usually there is a marked increase in the total white cell count (often above 100 000/mm^3), with polymorphonuclear cells predominating. The glucose levels are reduced and Gram stains are positive in about two-thirds of cases (Fig. 8.34). Blood cultures should always be taken, along with cultures of the urethra, cervix, rectum and pharynx if gonococcal infection is likely.

Radiographic investigations are not very helpful in the early stages of septic arthritis except as a means of determining the presence of a synovial effusion in the hip joint (Fig. 8.35), or of revealing evidence of prosthetic joint loosening (Fig. 8.36). Later they may show loss of cartilage, periarticular osteoporosis and bone destruction (Fig. 8.37).

If bacterial arthritis remains untreated, destruction of articular cartilage and spread to adjacent bone eventually occur. Therapy involves adequate drainage of the joint and appropriate antibacterial therapy. Drainage is needed to relieve the symptoms, to remove toxic products of inflammation that damage the cartilage and to monitor the response to therapy. Drainage can be via repeated needle aspiration or by surgical procedures. Surgery is needed for prosthetic joints, or if needle aspiration is impossible due to loculation of the fluid or inaccessibility of the joint. Infected prosthetic joints may need to be removed and replaced.

Antibiotic therapy is given parenterally and the agents most commonly used (an exception is erythromycin) will penetrate adequately into synovial fluid. The optimal antibiotics for individual organisms are identical to those used in osteomyelitis and shown in Fig. 8.20. For gonococcal septic monarthritis high dose penicillin followed by oral amoxycillin for a total of 7 days is adequate; cephalosporins or quinolones are suitable for penicillinase-producing organisms. For the dermatitis/arthritis syndrome associated with gonococci, however, high dose ampicillin and probenecid is the initial therapy. Nongonococcal forms of bacterial arthritis require 2–4 weeks of treatment.

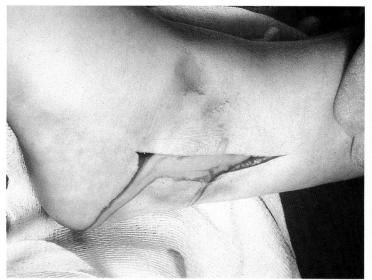
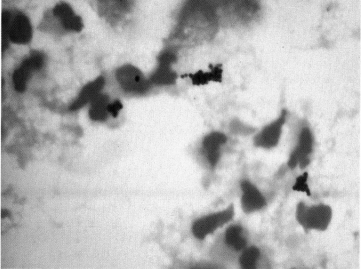

Fig. 8.34 Septic arthritis. Release of pus from ankle joint at arthrotomy (left). Numerous polymorphonuclear cells and clumps of staphylococci can be seen on Gram stain (right). Same case as Fig. 8.27. By courtesy of Mr N. St. J. P. Dwyer and Dr J.G.P. Hutchison.

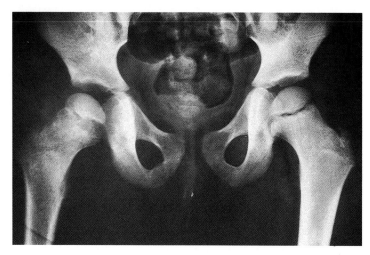

Fig. 8.35 Acute infective arthritis of the right hip. The joint space is widened with lateral displacement of the femoral head and there is periarticular osteoporosis in a young girl who developed a severe febrile illness and painful limited mobility of the right hip.

Chronic Arthritis

Chronic granulomatous arthritis may be produced by *Mycobacterium tuberculosis* or atypical mycobacteria (see below), or by a number of fungi (Fig. 8.38). The joint is usually infected from adjacent osteomyelitis, but blood-borne spread from another focus may occur.

Sporothrix shenckii is the fungus which most commonly infects the joints. It is usually, but not always, secondary to local cutaneous inoculation and particularly affects the wrist, elbows or knees.

Lyme disease

Lyme disease is an infection caused by the spirochaete *Borrelia burgdorferi*, which is transmitted to man by tick vectors, most commonly *Ixodes dammini*. These ticks are widely distributed in North America and Europe.

The disease occurs in three stages and begins when, 3 to 21 days after being bitten by an infected tick, some persons develop a characteristic rash, known as erythema chronicum migrans (ECM) (see Chapter 11) at the site of the tick bite (Stage 1). Stage 2 of the infection may follow some

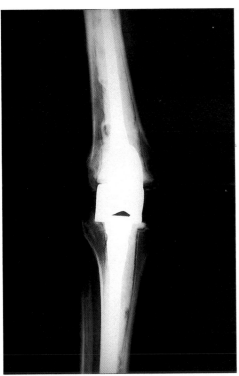
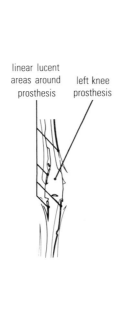
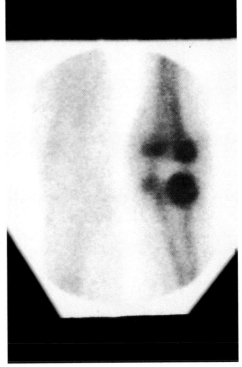
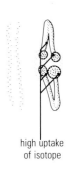

linear lucent areas around prosthesis

left knee prosthesis

high uptake of isotope

Fig. 8.36 Prosthetic joint infection. Radiograph of a total knee replacement that had become painful (left). There is an area of lucency around the prosthesis. There was a delayed blood pool image and high uptake around the prosthesis on isotope scanning (right) suggestive of infection rather that just loosening of the prosthesis. By courtesy of Dr G.S. Jones.

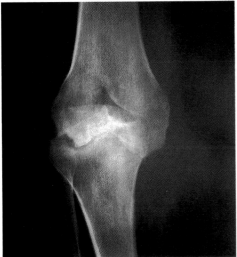

Fig. 8.37 Septic arthritis. Radiograph of right knee showing loss of joint space, soft tissue swelling, bony sclerosis and destruction of articular surfaces of femur and tibia with subluxation anteromedially. By courtesy of Dr A. M. Davies.

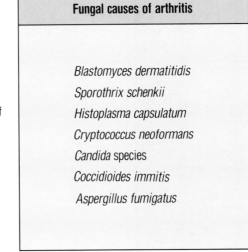

Fungal causes of arthritis
Blastomyces dermatitidis
Sporothrix schenkii
Histoplasma capsulatum
Cryptococcus neoformans
Candida species
Coccidioides immitis
Aspergillus fumigatus

Fig. 8.38 Fungal species commonly causative of arthritis

weeks later and consists of neurological (see Chapter 3) or cardiac abnormalities. In about two-thirds of patients arthritis (Stage 3) occurs some months or years later (the mean period being 4 weeks): a monarticular or oligoarticular arthritis that is often recurrent develops, the patient suffering intermittent joint swelling and pain for several years. In about 10% of cases the arthritis is sustained, leading to a proliferative, erosive synovitis similar to that seen in rheumatoid arthritis.

The diagnosis is readily confirmed by serology since all patients with arthritis have high levels of specific IgG. Occasionally spirochaetes can be seen or cultured from the synovium. Treatment with high dose penicillin or ceftriaxone, given for at least 10 days, reduces the severity and frequency of recurrent arthritis.

Viral Arthritis

A number of viruses, particularly rubella, parvovirus B19, hepatitis B virus, mumps and varicella may cause an acute arthritis.

Rubella arthritis principally affects women within three days of the onset of the rash. Usually the small joints of the hand are affected, although sometimes larger joints are also involved. The synovial fluid shows increased numbers of mononuclear cells, and the virus can sometimes be cultured. The arthritis may take several weeks to resolve, but sequelae are rare. Immunization with rubella virus may also be followed by arthritis. Children of both sexes are affected, and arthralgias are noted in up to 40% of adult women given the vaccine.

Arthritis following chickenpox (Fig. 8.39) tends to affect large joints and appears during the first week of the illness. It is probably due to viral invasion, unlike the arthritis that occurs during the incubation period of hepatitis B infection, which is presumed to be part of serum-sickness-like illness.

Parvovirus B19 (see Chapter 11) is now recognized as the cause of erythema infectiosum. As part of this illness up to 10% of children, and up to 80% of adults, develop arthralgia or arthritis. It tends to affect the peripheral joints symmetrically and follows the rash by a few days. The symptoms usually resolve within a month, but occasionally they persist for much longer.

In some parts of the world arbovirus infections are a common cause of arthritis as part of a more generalized infection.

Reiter's Syndrome

It is presumed that Reiter's syndrome is initiated by infection. In temperate climates it usually appears as a sequel to nonspecific urethritis, and the arthritis is assumed to be triggered by the same agent that initiates this. An identical syndrome, with conjunctivitis or iritis and polyarthritis, may follow infections of the gastrointestinal tract by various organisms including *Shigella*, *Salmonella*, *Campylobacter*, and *Yersinia* species. Predisposition to Reiter's syndrome is strongly associated with the HLA-B27 antigen.

Conjunctivitis is a common feature. Anterior uveitis may occasionally develop during the acute episode, but more commonly this follows as a late sequel. The skin lesions of Reiter's syndrome include circinate balanitis, and more general rashes. Keratoderma blennorrhagica first affects the soles of the feet, but sometimes the hands, limbs, trunk and scalp may be involved. The nails too may be affected, and painless ulcers of the buccal mucosa are seen in a minority of patients.

The joint lesions begin as transient episodes affecting predominantly the knees, ankles, wrists and feet in an asymmetric manner. Spondylitis and sacroiliitis may also occur during the acute phase. New attacks may develop following bouts of nonspecific urethritis (or diarrhoea), and

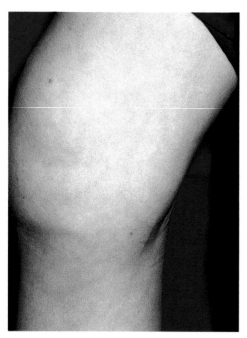

Fig. 8.39 Varicella arthritis. Acute effusion in the knee of a 13-year-old boy suffering from varicella. Note the healing skin lesions of chickenpox above and medial to the knee.

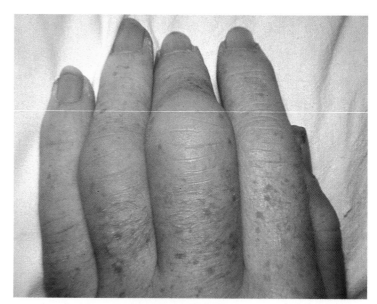

Fig. 8.40 Reiter's syndrome. Severe chronic swelling of the metacarpophalangeal and interphalangeal joints. By courtesy of Dr T.F. Sellers, Jr.

a substantial proportion of patients may be left with a chronic deforming arthropathy (Fig. 8.40). Inflammatory lesions at tendon and fascial attachments, particularly painful calcaneal spurs (Fig. 8.41), tenosynovitis and bursitis are also common.

SEPTIC BURSITIS

Infection of the prepatellar or olecranon bursa usually occurs within the context of trauma or sustained pressure to the bursa incurred as part of particular occupations such as carpet layer, gardener, bricklayer or plumber. It is therefore a disease of young or middle-aged men. Pain, redness, tenderness and swelling of the bursa (Fig. 8.42), sometimes accompanied by fever, may mistakenly suggest septic arthritis. Whilst septic arthritis causes pain upon joint movement, in bursitis movement of the joint is painless. The aetiological agent (almost always *Staph. aureus* or

Strep. pyogenes) is determined by aspiration, Gram stain and culture of the bursa fluid.

Adequate drainage, either by serial needle aspiration or by surgery, is essential, together with systemic antibiotics for 2–3 weeks. The less ill patient can be treated with oral antibiotics, but those with systemic symptoms or underlying disease should be given parenteral agents.

TUBERCULOSIS

Mycobacterium tuberculosis reaches bones and joints by haematogenous spread during the primary infection, but it takes a variable time, anything from less than a year to many decades, before presentation of the infection. It is a common form of extrapulmonary tuberculosis. Any bone may be involved, although in adults about half the cases involve the vertebrae (Fig. 8.43) and many of the remainder involve the bones around the large joints: extension into

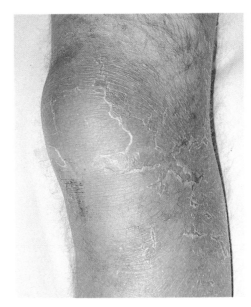

Fig. 8.42 Acute septic bursitis: prepatellar bursitis with associated cellulitis in a carpet layer. *Streptococcus pyogenes* was cultured from the bursal fluid.

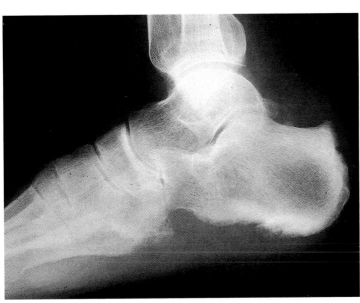

Fig. 8.41 Reiter's syndrome. Radiograph of foot showing calcaneal spurs with characteristic 'fluffy' appearance. The posterior and inferior surface of the os calcis is affected. By courtesy of Dr S. Olansky.

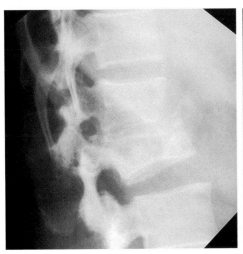
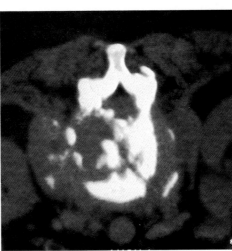

Fig. 8.43 Spinal tuberculosis. Radiograph showing loss of disc space and partial collapse of adjacent vertebral bodies with calcification anterior to vertebra (left). A CT scan (right) shows destruction of vertebral body, soft–tissue swelling and calcification. By courtesy of Dr A. M. Davies.

the joint is common. Multiple sites may be involved. The granulomatous inflammatory process erodes and destroys cartilage and bone, often causing marked deformity, and the bone or joint infection may be associated with much adjacent caseation (Fig. 8.44). Cold abscesses may form, and these may provide the presenting sign (Figs. 8.45, 8.46). Sometimes the pus may track along fascial planes for some distance before reaching the surface. Chronically discharging sinuses over the infected site are also common.

Tuberculous osteomyelitis may be asymptomatic or present as a pyrexia of undetermined origin, but usually there is local pain, and in general progression of the illness is slow and insidious. Weight loss is common. With increasing vertebral destruction, angulation of the spine to

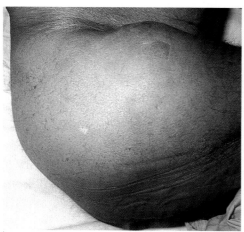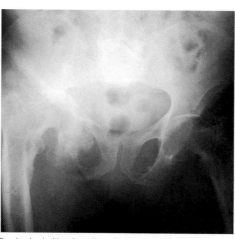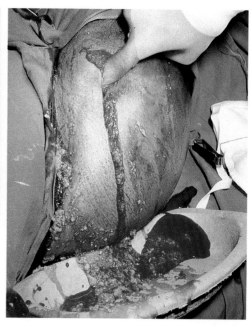

Fig. 8.44 Tuberculosis of the hip. This Asian man had been confined to bed with pain and swelling around his right hip for at least one year. There was a large soft–tissue swelling around the hip (left) and radiographs (centre) showed total destruction of the acetabulum and head of the femur, with calcification in the soft–tissue mass. At surgical drainage large quantities of pus and caseous material (right) were removed. *Mycobacterium tuberculosis* was isolated from this material.

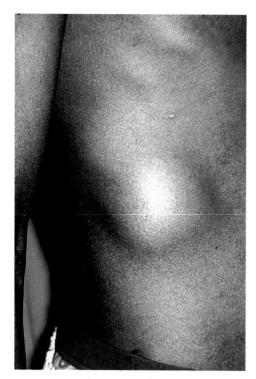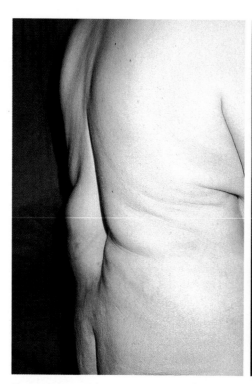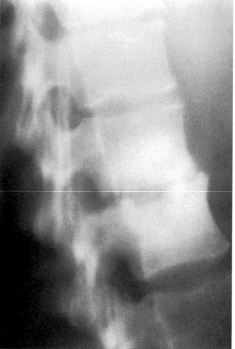

Fig. 8.45 Cold abscess of chest wall. This painless indolent swelling had been present for several months. Radiographs showed tuberculosis of the underlying ribs.

Fig. 8.46 Cold abscess in the left lumbar region of a 45–year–old woman. The abscess (left) appeared while she was receiving antituberculous therapy for tuberculous meningitis diagnosed six months previously. Radiographs (right) showed spondylitis at L1/2, and *Mycobacterium tuberculosis* (sensitive to the drugs she had been receiving) was isolated from the abscess.

form a kyphus, or neurological symptoms due to spinal cord or nerve root compression appear. Typically, tuberculous arthritis involves a weight-bearing joint with swelling and limited movement but little erythema (Fig. 8.47). A 'classical', but now rarely seen, manifestation of tuberculous osteitis is dactylitis in young children (Fig. 8.48).

Radiological changes may not be seen for weeks or months after the onset of symptoms, although radioisotopic bone scanning is more sensitive in the detection of single or multiple foci of tuberculous infection. Common changes in tuberculous osteitis of the spine include erosion of the vertebral body and diminution of the disc space (Figs. 8.43, 8.46), and often the soft tissue shadow of a paravertebral abscess may be detected (Fig. 8.49). Destruction of bone increases with time (Fig. 8.50).

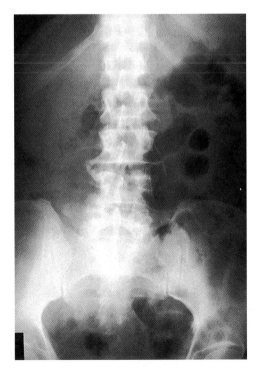

Fig. 8.47 Tuberculosis of the knee. The patient was a 27–year–old Asian man whose knee had been swollen for 18 months and who had miliary shadowing on chest X–ray. *Mycobacterium tuberculosis* was isolated from synovial fluid.

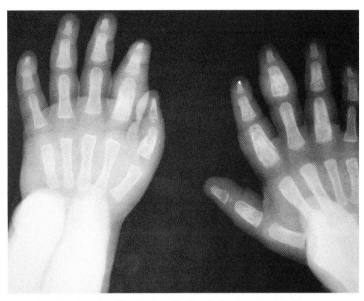

Fig. 8.48 Tuberculous dactylitis. Radiograph of hands showing several phalanges with multiple erosions; the affected bones are expanded.

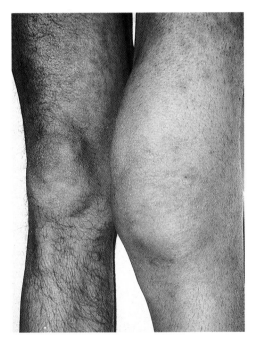

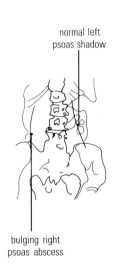

normal left psoas shadow

bulging right psoas abscess

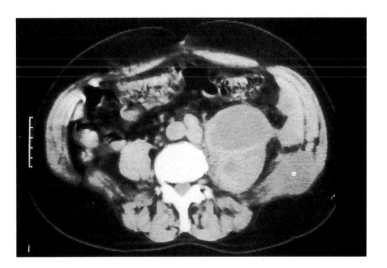

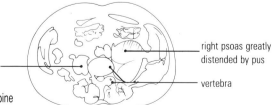

normal left psoas muscle

right psoas greatly distended by pus

vertebra

Fig. 8.49 Tuberculous psoas abscess. This patient had been treated for tuberculous spondylitis of the lower thoracic spine several years previously. He re–presented with a fluctuant swelling in his right groin and a plain abdominal radiograph (left) showed a bulging psoas which was confirmed on CT scan (right).

In tuberculous osteomyelitis needle or open biopsy is essential (Fig. 8.51). The organism may be seen in the joint fluid in cases of arthritis, but if this is unsuccessful, synovial biopsy can be diagnostic. Treatment is with standard anti-tuberculous chemotherapy, and surgical intervention is rarely required.

BRUCELLOSIS

Brucellosis (see Chapter 13) may affect the bones and joints in a number of ways. During the acute illness the symptoms may vary from the mild to the severe, but they are often nonspecific. Many patients have arthralgias, which may be monarticular, and some have a more severe arthritis of

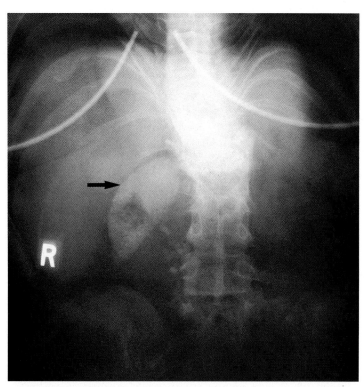

Fig. 8.50 Spinal tuberculosis. Radiograph of Pott's disease of the spine with gross vertebral destruction and deformity. There is soft tissue calcification and a calcified psoas abscess.

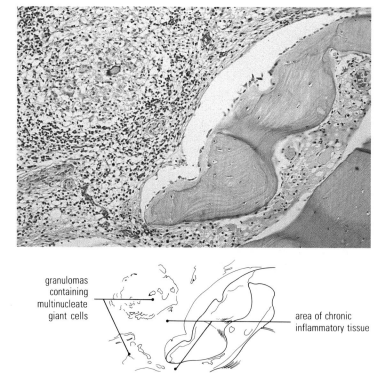

granulomas containing multinucleate giant cells

area of chronic inflammatory tissue

Fig. 8.51 Tuberculous osteomyelitis. Giant cell granulomas in bone biopsy from a patient with vertebral osteomyelitis. By courtesy of Dr C.W. Edwards.

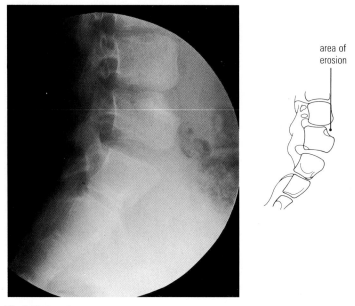

area of erosion

Fig. 8.52 Brucella osteomyelitis. Erosion of the anterior vertebral plate. By courtesy of Mr N. St. P. J. Dwyer.

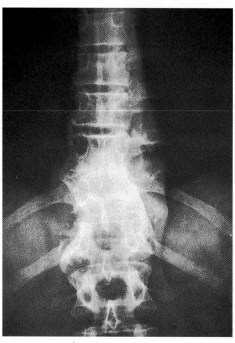

Fig. 8.53 Brucellosis. Radiograph of the spine with destruction of the intervertebral disc showing fusion of vertebral bodies and a large paravertebral abscess containing areas of calcification.

the knee or hip, which is believed to be due to immune complexes. *Brucella melitensis* is the species most likely to cause localized, chronic skeletal infection, often affecting the vertebrae. Such purulent Brucella spondylitis typically affects elderly males, involving the lumbo-sacral area and producing back pain which is often relieved by rest. The earliest radiological changes are osteoporosis of the involved vertebrae, followed by erosion of the anterior vertebral plates (Fig. 8.52). Periosteal thickening and paravertebral abscesses may also be seen (Fig. 8.53). When the lesion heals a rim of dense sclerosis is found, with prominent anterior ('parrot beak') osteophytic projections. Osteomyelitis may occur, albeit rarely, in long bones, skull or ribs, and chronic arthritis is also occasionally seen.

The diagnosis must be confirmed by culture of blood or tissue, or from serological findings. Treatment is with tetracyclines and rifampicin, sometimes combined with cotrimoxazole or streptomycin.

SYPHILIS

Syphilitic bone and joint disease is now rarely seen. In the acquired disease arthritis, osteitis and periosteitis, typically presenting with nocturnal pains that are helped by movement, are uncommon features of secondary disease; late benign disease (gumma) is rare in the penicillin era. If gummas do occur they lead to local destruction of bone and hence to fractures or joint destruction.

The loss of deep pain and temperature sensation in tabes dorsalis may lead to trophic degenerative joint disease (Charcot's joints) of the lower limbs (Figs. 8.54, 8.55).

Congenital syphilis (see Chapter 7) may be accompanied by a generalized osteochondritis that affects the entire skeletal system, particularly the nose (saddle nose) or the tibia (sabre shin), and by recurrent arthropathy and effusions in both knees (Clutton's joints).

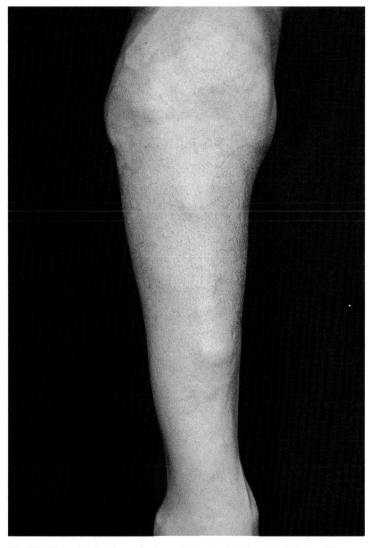

Fig. 8.54 Charcot's joint. Gross swelling and deformity of the knee joint in late syphilis. Swelling on the tibia at sites of healed spontaneous fractures are also seen.

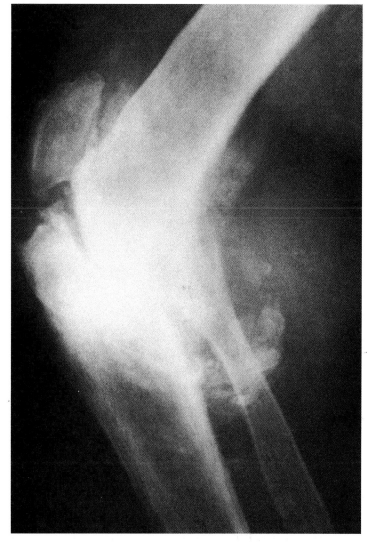

Fig. 8.55 Charcot's joint. Radiograph showing misshapen sclerotic joint surfaces and loose bodies in the joint cavity.

LEPROSY

The neuropathy of leprosy may lead to clumsiness and anaesthesia of the hands and feet, which become extremely susceptible to damage from repeated trauma and infection. This eventually leads to severe deformity from chronic ulceration and resorption of the bones of the digits (Fig. 8.56).

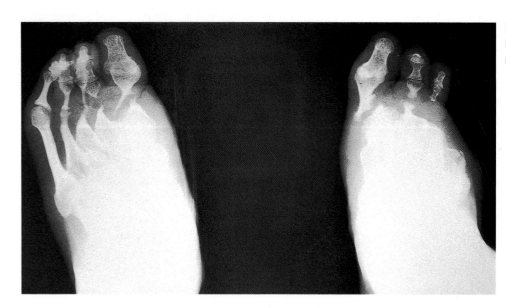

Fig. 8.56 Leprosy. Radiograph of foot in lepromatous leprosy showing gross destruction and pencilling of the metatarsals and phalanges.

THE CARDIOVASCULAR SYSTEM

9

ENDOCARDITIS

Infective endocarditis (IE) involves infection of the endothelial surfaces of the valves and chambers of the heart, major blood vessels and congenital cardiac and large vessel defects. The spectrum of clinical presentation ranges from rapidly progressive and destructive disease associated with *Staphylococcus aureus* (Fig. 9.1), to more indolent (sub-acute) or chronic infections. Describing such polar groups is helpful in overview; however, in the individual case it is more pertinent to look for the presence of underlying disease or predisposition to endocarditis, for evidence of the microorganism involved, and manifestations of complications. These latter are the major factors governing management.

The incidence of IE, approximately 0.1% of hospital admissions, has not significantly decreased during the antibiotic era. The age of patients with endocarditis has steadily increased; the number of patients with non-rheumatic valve disease and congenital abnormalities has increased; and the contribution from nosocomial endo-carditis relating to the increased use of prolonged venous access has increased. The overall mortality has not improved, in part the result of the increasing average age.

The development of endocarditis involves a sequence of three processes: endothelial damage, colonization and amplification (Fig. 9.2).

The endocardial surface may be damaged due to haemodynamic abnormalities. Relatively high pressure jets of regurgitant blood flow impinging on small areas of endocardium have a greater potential for promoting endocarditis than low pressure turbulence affecting a large area. IE is thus much more common on the left side of the heart than on the right (Fig. 9.3).

Intracardiac catheterization, acute febrile diseases and chronic wasting disorders may all contribute to endothelial susceptibility. Such surface damage is associated with platelet and fibrin deposition, often referred to as non-bacterial thrombotic endocarditis (Figs 9.4 & 9.5).

The next factor required is bacteraemia. The common sources of organisms include oral (Fig. 9.6), respiratory, gastrointestinal, gynaecological, urological and skin sites of primary infection or colonization. Small numbers of bacteria from these sites may gain access to the circulation spontaneously or as a result of such minor trauma as brushing the teeth. More significant bacteraemia is usually provoked by surgical procedures or instrumentation involving colonized surfaces.

The spectrum of bacteria involved reflect the resident flora of colonized surface sources and the pathogenic factors contributed by individual bacterial species. Thus, the efficiency of adherence and colonization is greatest with *Streptococcus viridans* and *S. aureus*; both these organisms produce dextran, which experimentally increases colonization.

Amplification or growth of bacteria on the colonized valve endothelium may be promoted by microbial stimulation and platelet aggregation (Fig. 9.7). The immune responses may be diminished by the platelet layers obstructing access or by interference with anti-bacterial activity (as with the rheumatoid factors impairing bacterial opsonization).

The age, presence of underlying congenital or acquired valve disease and other structural defects, the presence of

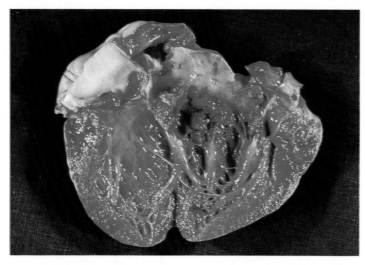

Fig. 9.1 Bacterial endocarditis. Acute endocarditis due to *Staphylococcus aureus* showing virtually complete destruction of the mitral valve.

Pathomechanisms in Endocarditis	
Endothelial Damage	Haemodynamic trauma Intracardiac catheter Acute systemic illness Chronic wasting disease
Platelet/fibrin Deposition	Increased platelet aggregation
Bacterial Colonization	Bacteraemia (Sources: dental, skin, gut, gynae, respiratory) Bacterial virulence adherance factors Impaired antibacterial defences

Fig. 9.2 Endocarditis. Pathomechanisms in endocarditis.

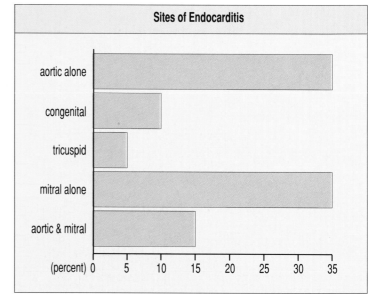

Fig. 9.3 Endocarditis. Sites of endocarditis.

prosthetic valves, acquired immune deficiencies and exposure to contaminated intravenous injections all influence the susceptibility to a broad spectrum of microbes that are potentially pathogenic (Fig. 9.8).

The group of organisms referred to as the viridans streptococci consists of the following species: *S. bovis*, *S. sanguis*, *S. mitior* and *S. mutans*. These organisms do not usually carry Lancefield antigens. Another large group of Lancefield group D streptococci are involved; they are often referred to as the enterococci, in view of their usual origin. *S. faecalis* and *S. faecium* are amongst this group. *S. milleri* and *S. bovis* are non-group D enteric organisms rarely associated with the disease. *S. pneumoniae* is capable of causing acute endocarditis but is relatively rare. The streptococci on the whole account for almost one-half of the organisms responsible.

S. aureus, the next most common cause, accounts for one-fifth of all organisms and the majority of acute endocarditis. The ability of this organism to colonize an undamaged endocardium and the relative speed and destructiveness of

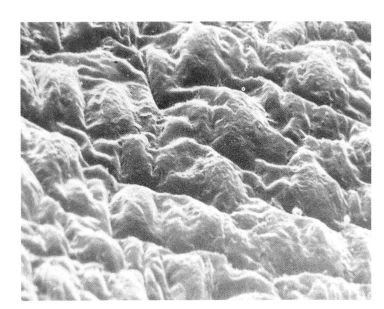

Fig. 9.4 Normal rabbit aortic valve. Scanning electron micrograph. By courtesy of W.M. Scheld *in* Sande, Kaye and Root (1984) *Contemporary Issues in Infectious Diseases*, **2**.

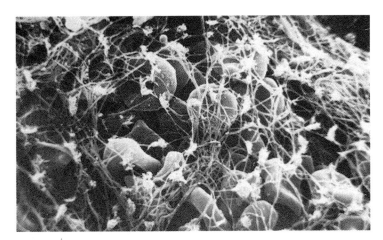

Fig. 9.5 Non-bacterial endocarditis. Traumatized rabbit aortic valve, 30 minutes after catheter trauma. Fibrin platelet deposition on the denuded epithelium. Scanning electron micrograph. By courtesy of W.M. Scheld *in* Sande, Kaye and Root (1984) *Contemporary Issues in Infectious Diseases*, **2**.

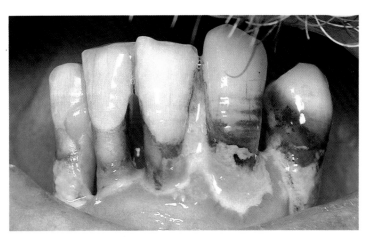

Fig. 9.6 Bacterial endocarditis. Peridontal disease in a patient with *Streptococcus viridans* endocarditis.

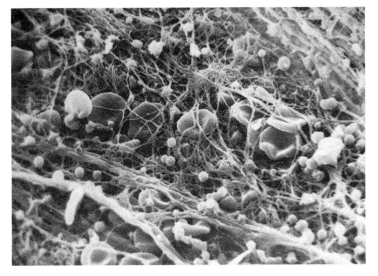

Fig. 9.7 Endocarditis. Traumatized rabbit aortic valve following intravenous inoculation of *Candida albicans* (10^6 cfu), showing yeast cells adherent to the fibrin–platelet areas. By courtesy of W.M. Scheld *in* Sande, Kaye and Root (1984) *Contemporary Issues in Infectious Diseases*, **2**.

Microbes in Infective Endocarditis	
Organism	**Occurrence (%)**
Streptococci	60–80
Viridans	30–40
Enterococci	5–18
Others	15–25
Staphylococci	20–35
S. aureus	10–27
S. epidermidis	1–3
Gram-negative bacilli	2–13
Fungi	2–4
Others	0–5
Culture negative	5–24

Fig. 9.8 Infective endocarditis. Microbes in infective endocarditis.

the infection accounts for a higher mortality. Although *Staphylococcus epidermidis* is a common cause of endocarditis in patients with prosthetic heart valves, the relatively slow onset, the confusion over the significance of finding these organisms in blood cultures and the unpredictable antibiotic sensitivities makes this a difficult group.

Although gram-negative organisms are a frequent cause of bacteraemia, they are a relatively poor source of endocarditis. The incidence of gram-negative endocarditis is greatest in early prosthetic valve endocarditis and with drug addicts. *Escherichia coli* and species of *Klebsiella*, *Proteus* and *Serratia,* are the most commonly involved. *Pseudomonas aeruginosa* is a rare but increasing pathogen, mainly amongst drug addicts, causing local destruction and embolization. *Salmonella typhimurium* and other subspecies are uncommon. *Haemophilus influenzae* and *H. parainfluenzae* are occasional causes. Endocarditis may occur as part of a systemic brucella infection. Of the gram-negative organisms the majority arise from intestinal, urinary and gynaecological tracts, although they may be acquired from intravenous drug injection or at the time of cardiac surgery.

A large number of other organisms can occasionally cause endocarditis. Classically, *Coxiella burnetti* endocarditis can complicate Q-fever; *Candida albicans* and Aspergillus cause prosthetic valve infections; and *Candida parapsilosis* is important in drug addicts. The latter diagnoses are often difficult and may first present with complications or embolization of the large vegetations.

Neisseria gonorrhoeae was previously a cause of acute and sub-acute endocarditis, but this is now rarely the case. *Neisseria meningitidis* is also an unusual acute aetiology.

Listeria monocytogenes may cause endocarditis as part of a systemic listeriosis. *Erysipelothrix rhusiopthiae* may be acquired from handling marine or terrestrial animals and endocarditis is a recognized complication. In rat-bite fever *Strepobacillus moniliformis* can cause endocarditis. *Nocardia asteroides* (usually occurring in imunocompromized patients) can cause endocarditis.

The changing epidemiology is reflected in the proportions of differing background pathologies. Currently just under half of the patients have background rheumatic valve disease and the remainder split fairly equally between congenital valve disease and endocarditis occurring in the absence of established pathology. Infection of prosthetic valves is a small but significant group.

Of those with rheumatic valve disease the mitral valve is involved in more than three-quarters and the aortic valve in half, with a minority experiencing dual involvement.

Congenital heart disease accounts for the majority of children with infective endocarditis and the risk increases as these patients age. More than 10% suffer infection of an uncorrected ventricular septal defect at some stage (Fig. 9.9). Incomplete correction of complicated defects may increase the risk of endocarditis; this tends to parallel the post-correction rise in left-sided pressures, increasing any regurgitant jet-stream.

Those patients who lack evidence of rheumatic or congenital valve diseases form an increasing proportion of the enlarging group of elderly patients with endocarditis. Atherosclerosis, endocardial damage accompanying myocardial infarcts, and calcific mitral and degenerative aortic valve pathologies are prominent in this group.

The primary pathology of IE involves vegetations (Figs 9.10, 9.11 & 9.12). There may be considerable secondary cardiac pathology. Vegetations which have been built up of platelets, fibrin, bacteria and inflammatory cells vary in size (0.1–2cm). The valve may be obstructed, incompetent or perforated; the chordae tendineae and muscles may be damaged, aneurysms may involve the sinus of Valsalva; and valve ring abscesses and pancarditis may occur.

Embolization may be local, causing myocardial infarction, or systemic. The larger acute vegetations tend to

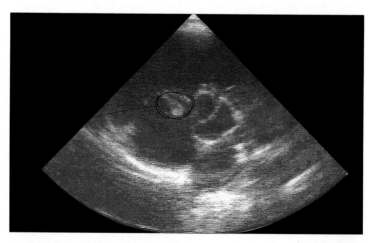

Fig. 9.9 Endocarditis. Echocardiogram showing endocarditis at the site of a high stream jet from a ventricular septal defect impinging on the tricuspid valve.

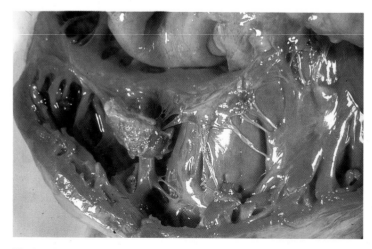

Fig. 9.10 Endocarditis. Mitral valve vegetation due to *S. aureus* endocarditis.

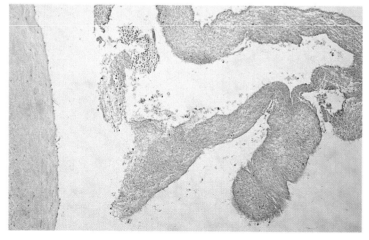

Fig. 9.11 Endocarditis. Mitral valve vegetation with *S. aureus* present.

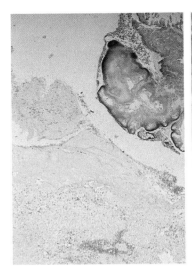
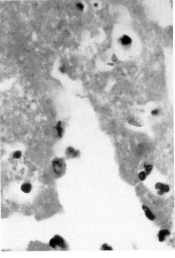

Fig. 9.12 Bacterial endocarditis. Left: Section of heart valve from an infection due to β-haemolytic streptococci showing cellular infiltration of the valve leaflet, deposition of fibrin and inflammatory cells on the surface and, in the upper right-hand corner, a vegetation containing enormous numbers of bacteria. Right: Section of a vegetation from a valve leaflet in a case of acute bacterial endocarditis due to *Neisseria gonorrhoeae* showing enormous numbers of pale-staining diplococci. The larger purple structures are the nuclei of inflammatory cells. H & E stain. By courtesy of Dr J. F. John, Jr.

Physical Findings in Endocarditis	
Finding	Occurrence (%)
Fever	89
Cardiac murmur	86
Varying murmurs	7
New murmur	4
Embolization	50
Skin features	35
Splenomegaly	24
Septic complications	19
Mycotic aneurysms	18
Clubbing	32
Retinal lesion	7
Renal failure features	12

Fig. 9.13 Endocarditis. Physical findings in endocarditis.

embolize, particularly with *Candida albicans*. These emboli may cause large or small vessel occlusions, mycotic aneurysms and abscess formation. Mycotic aneurysms are most common in cerebral vessels and may rupture.

The brain may be involved with cerebral embolization, leading to infarction, infection with abscess formation or mycotic aneurysms with secondary haemorrhage. Meningeal involvement is relatively rare.

The lung is most commonly involved with right–sided endocarditis – embolization results in infarction, abscess, effusion and empyema.

Chronic stimulation of B lymphocytes occuring in endocarditis results in hypergammaglobulinaemia. Persistent circulation of immune complexes is associated with vascular damage to small vessels in organs and the peripheries.

The hypergammaglobulinaemia is in part antigen-specific, relating to microbial antigens but also to host IgG antigens. The latter are rheumatoid factors which can be detected in the majority of patients with established subacute endocarditis. In addition there is a polyclonal activation of B cells producing antibodies to unrelated microbes and tissue antigens, with the formation of circulating immune complexes and auto-antibodies. Immune complex levels correlate with low complement levels and extracardiac manifestations in the more persistent infections; successful treatment reverses these abnormalities.

Physical findings in endocarditis are shown in Fig. 9.13. Febrile symptoms and fever occur in the majority of patients (80–90%) and usually start within three weeks of the provoking event.

Dyspnoea is common, whereas chest pain is a relatively rare cardiac symptom. Heart murmurs are present in 85% of patients with new or changing murmurs occurring in 15%. Clinical evidence of heart failure is a serious complication which may result from deteriorating left-sided valve regurgitation or infarction. A pericardial rub may be the result of pancarditis, valve ring sepsis or myocardial abscess/infarction.

One or more of the endocarditis stigmata occur in 50–80% of patients, the type depending upon the nature and duration of the infection. Many of the cutaneous features – splinter haemorrhages, petechiae (Fig. 9.14), Osler's nodes (Fig. 9.15), livedo-reticularis (see Fig. 9.16),

Fig. 9.14 Endocarditis. Splinter haemorrhages and petechial lesions.

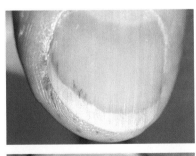
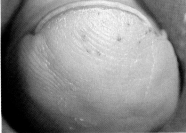

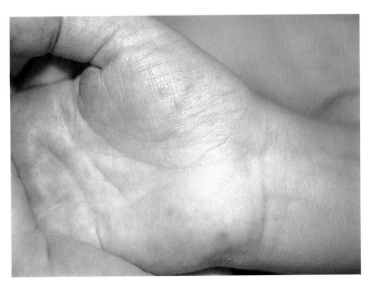

Fig. 9.15 Endocarditis. Tender Osler's nodes on palm.

purpura (Fig. 9.17) and a vasculitic rash (Fig. 9.18) – are variously due to immune complex-mediated vasculitis, focal platelet aggregation and vascular permeability. Osler's nodes are tender, nodular and erythematous with some central pallor, and affect the fingertips and the palms. Janeway lesions (Fig. 9.19) are due to microemboli and are macular, ecchymotic and painless. They tend to occur on the feet, particularly the toes and plantar aspects. Janeway lesions are common in acute endocarditis, whereas Osler's nodes are rare. Petechiae may occur on the skin of the distal limbs or conjunctivae. Finger clubbing (Fig. 9.20) may occur in longstanding IE.

The involvement of immune mechanisms in the retinal haemorrhage (Roth spots – see Fig. 9.26) and frequent joint and muscle symptoms is uncertain. Immune complexes are responsible for a focal and a diffuse glomerulonephritis. It is postulated that the physical differences in immune complex size may be a factor in determining the site of immune complex deposition. In addition to focal glomerulonephritis, diffuse proliferative glomerulonephritis and a range of membranoproliferative disorders, there may be renal micro-infarcts. The majority of patients with sub-acute disease have glomerular changes; infarctions are found in most patients with acute infections.

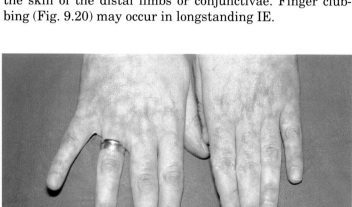

Fig. 9.16 Endocarditis. Livedo reticularis in infective endocarditis.

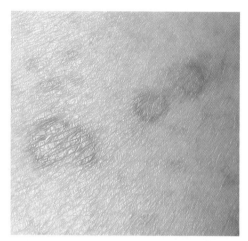

Fig. 9.17 Endocarditis. Vasculitic immune complex rash in subacute bacterial endocarditis.

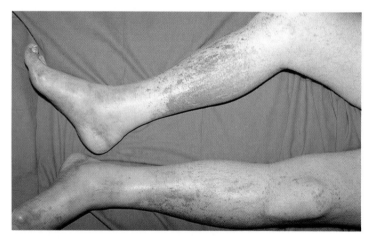

Fig. 9.18 Endocarditis. Vasculitic rash in late persistent infective endocarditis.

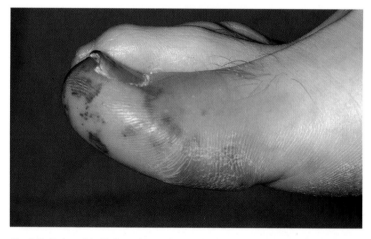

Fig. 9.19 Endocarditis. Ecchymotic embolic Janeway lesions in *S. aureus* endocarditis.

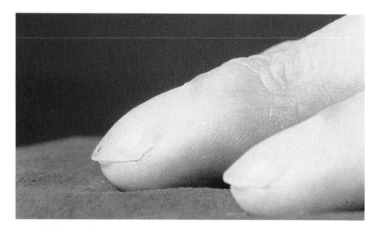

Fig. 9.20 Bacterial endocarditis. Clubbing of the fingers in long-standing subacute bacterial endocarditis.

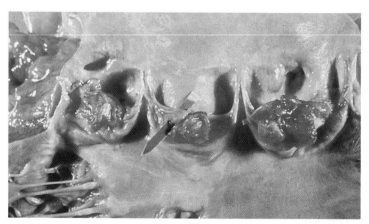

Fig. 9.21 Endocarditis. Aortic valve endocarditis with rupture of the non-coronary cusp.

Patients may present with complications which include heart failure, embolic occlusive complications and embolic septic phenomena.

Cardiac decompensation most commonly results from acute endocarditis involving aortic valve regurgitation, and least commonly as a result of a *Streptoccocus viridans* infection of congenital heart disease; it rarely occurs later than six months. Besides aortic valve destruction, acute deterioration may result from rupture of valve cusps (Fig. 9.21) or chordae tendineae (Fig. 9.22) and also from ischaemia. Ventricular septal defects, aneurysms of the sinus of Valsalva, and fistulae may develop.

Extension of the infection beyond the valves is most common with *S. aureus* (Fig. 9.23); valve ring abscesses are the most frequent site (Fig. 9.24). Involvement of the intraventricular septum and occasionally pericarditis may occur. Infected micro-emboli may produce cardiac muscle abscesses (Fig. 9.25) and may be involved in the development of myocarditis.

Embolization occurs in one-third of patients and, besides involving the coronary vessels, there may be retinal (Fig. 9.26), cerebral (Fig. 9.27), renal or splenic involvement (see Fig. 9.28). Patients may present with cerebral infarction as the first clinical feature of endocarditis (see Fig. 9.29).

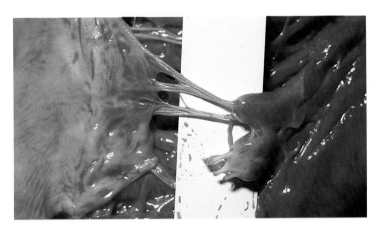

Fig. 9.22 Ruptured chordae tendineae.

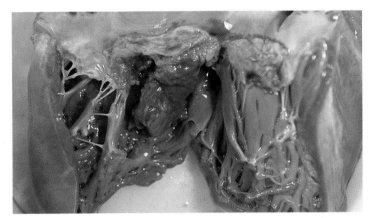

Fig. 9.23 Endocarditis. Extension of *S. aureus* endocarditis beyond the aortic valve. By courtesy of Dr G. Griffin.

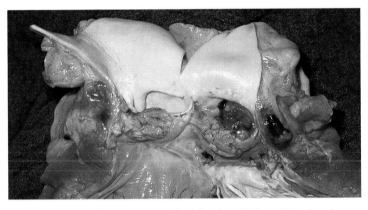

Fig. 9.24 Endocarditis. *Staphylococcus epidermidis* endocarditis in a patient with aortic stenosis. The initial bacteraemia occurred at the time of acute toxic epidermal necrolysis 7 months previously. The patient presented with left ventricular failure. A valve ring abscess is present.

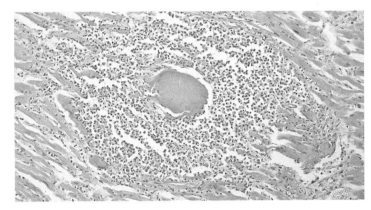

Fig. 9.25 Endocarditis. Myocardial abscess in *S. aureus* endocarditis.

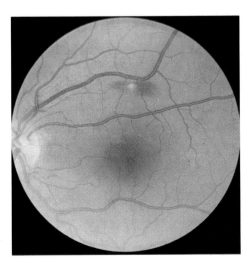

Fig. 9.26 Roth spot in endocarditis. Fundus photograph showing haemorrhage with a white centre in a patient with infective endocarditis.

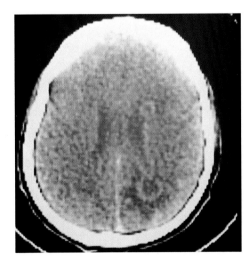

Fig. 9.27 *Streptococcus viridans* aortic valve endocarditis. CT scan of head showing multiple cerebral abscesses.

Such emboli, whether large or small, may give rise to metastatic infection – this is most common with *S. aureus*. Besides major organ involvement, small emboli may damage the vessels supplying arteries with the consequent formation of mycotic aneurysms (Fig. 9.30).

Muscle pain and, occasionally, evidence of synovitis may develop; acute arthritis is uncommon except in infections with either *N. gonorrhoeae* or *N. meningitidis*.

Being alert to prediposing pathology may afford an early diagnosis at a time when there are few clinical features. The mortality rises abruptly with delay in treatment.

Endocarditis involving prosthetic heart valves

Although the incidence of prosthetic valve endocarditis has fallen, the mortality and morbidity remain high. The interval after valve replacement or exposure to bacteraemia, the spectrum of organisms involved and the mortality, all separate prosthetic valve endocarditis into two groups: early and late.

Early endocarditis, occuring within 2 months of valve surgery, usually results from perioperative bacteraemia. *Staphylococcus epidermidis*, gram-negative bacilli and diphtheroids predominate. The mortality is high.

In endocarditis occurring beyond 2 months *Streptococcus viridans* and other streptococci predominate, although *S. epidermidis* and *S. aureus* are still frequent pathogens. The mortality is moderate. In either situation the infection may lead to disruption of the prosthetic valve anchorage with perivalvular regurgitation and heart failure.

The systemic features are otherwise similar to that of non-prosthetic valve endocarditis, but the clinical setting adds the further differential diagnosis of the post-cardiotomy syndrome and transfusion-associated infections.

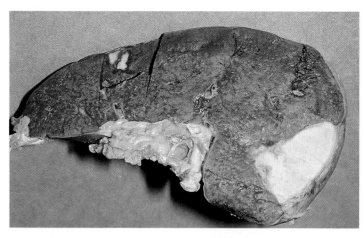

Fig. 9.28 Splenic infarcts following *Candidia albicans* endocarditis. By courtesy of Prof. R. Y. Cartwright.

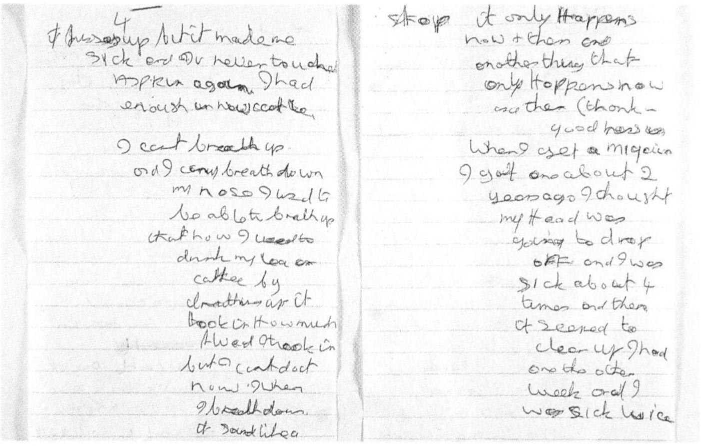

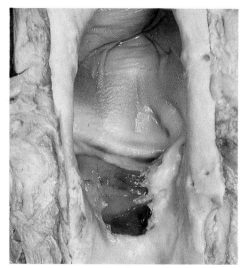

Fig. 9.30 Bacterial endocarditis. Mycotic aneurysm of the aorta in a case of pneumococcal endocarditis. The aorta has been opened and the view is down into the cavity of the aneurysm.

Fig. 9.29 Presentation with complication. *Streptococcus viridans* endocarditis presenting with homonymous hemianopia following cerebral embolization.

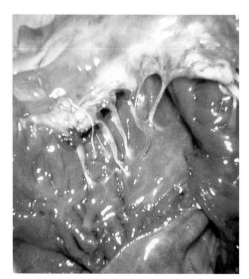

Fig. 9.31 Bacterial endocarditis. Acute right-sided *S. aureus* endocarditis in a 24-year-old heroin addict. Marked thickening and distortion of the tricuspid valve can be seen. By courtesy of Dr T. F. Sellers, Jr.

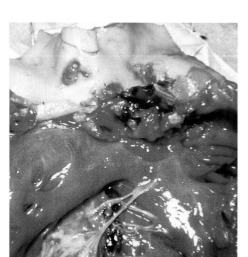

Fig. 9.32 Bacterial endocarditis. Same patient as Fig. 9.31, showing destructive vegetations on the pulmonary valve. By courtesy of Dr T. F. Sellers, Jr.

Drug addicts

Poor general health and frequent injection of contaminants provide the initial right heart endothelial damage preceding IE. Only a small proportion have existing congenital or rheumatic valve disease.

The infections are predominantly right-sided (Figs 9.31 & 9.32) with the tricuspid being involved in more than half of the patients; mitral involvement is relatively uncommon. *S. aureus* predominates and is presumed to arise from the frequent skin sepsis. The traditional streptococci are the next most common organism with *Candida parapsilosis* and *C. albicans* important occasional pathogens.

With the tricuspid valve being predominantly involved and *S. aureus* the common pathogen, the infection tends to be acute and severe with chest features a prominent clinical component. Signs of tricuspid valve incompetence should be sought; the chest x-ray may show infiltrates, abscesses or effusions. An isolate may be achieved from right-heart sampling if peripheral cultures are negative.

Underlying congenital heart disease

Congenital abnormalities of the heart and great vessels predispose children to endocarditis but the risk to the individual increases rather than decreases with age. Persistent ductus, ventricular septal defect, Fallot's tetralogy and stenosis of the aortic or pulmonary valves are the most frequent conditions. Infection usually occurs later in childhood and the clinical presentation is similar to that in adults. Acute endocarditis in infants and neonates may be due to septicaemia; this combination has a high mortality.

Laboratory and other investigations

There are a number of abnormal laboratory findings in IE. A normochromic normocytic anaemia occurring in the absence of any haematinic deficiency is common and the white cell count may be normal, mildy diminished or prominently raised. The erythrocyte sedimentation rate is usually elevated and may be grossly raised. The renal function may be normal or indicate functional impairment associated with renal complications.

Blood cultures play a central role in diagnosis and are positive in at least 88%. In acute endocarditis the bacteraemia is fairly consistent, and 3–5 cultures taken shortly after admission would be adequate before initiating treatment. With less urgent situations the cultures may be taken over a period. One advantage of taking multiple cultures is that contaminants can be more easily differentiated. Right-sided endocarditis is best identified from right heart catheter specimens, but peripheral venous samples may be positive following secondary pulmonary infection. Negative cultures may be the result of prior antibiotic treatment, difficult or unculturable organisms, right-sided infection, late disease, non-bacterial thrombotic endocarditis (Fig. 9.33), or misdiagnosis.

Echocardiography (Figs 9.34 & 9.35) now provides evidence of vegetations in three-quarters of patients; additional transoesophageal echocardiography and colour flow doppler techniques increase the figure to 90%, with vegetations as small as 2mm being shown. Valuable information concerning the presence of valvular pathology and congenital abnormalities is also provided. With prosthetic mechanical valves the echoimages are more difficult to interpret.

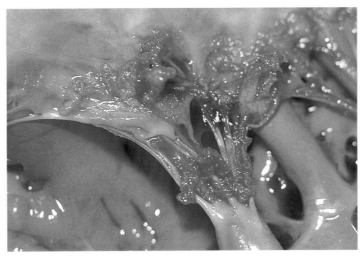

Fig. 9.33 Endocarditis. Non-bacterial thrombotic vegetations in a young woman with severe varicella and protracted complications.

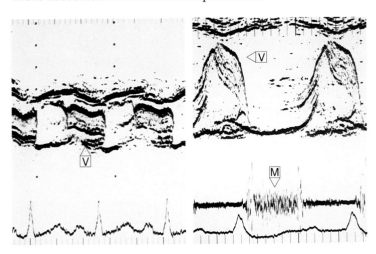

Fig. 9.34 Bacterial endocarditis. Echocardiogram showing echoes suggestive of vegetations (V) on the aortic valve (left), and on the anterior leaflet of the mitral valve (right). Posterior motion during systole suggests a 'floppy' valve. A pan-systolic murmur (M) can be seen on the right. By courtesy of Mr G. J. Leech.

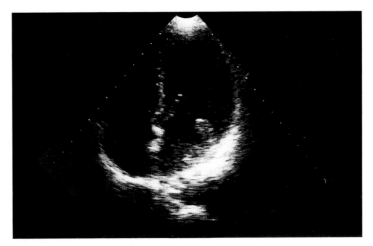

Fig. 9.35 Endocarditis. Echocardiogram showing vegetations of the mitral valve. *Streptococcus mitis* was isolated.

Serial ECGs may provide evidence of coronary embolization and valve ring extension.

Serology in the culture-negative group should include antibody titres for *Coxiella burneti*, *Chlamydia psittaci* and *Candida* species. Patients have an elevation of acute phase reactants including C-reactive protein and there may be false positive syphilitic serology. The development of IgM antibodies to IgG is common and these rheumatoid factors may be detected in more than 70% after 5 weeks of infection. The development of immune complexes is reflected in complement levels. Microscopic haematuria is frequently the result of renal micro-infarcts.

The duration of treatment and the need for prolonged parenteral treatment is continually debated. On the whole, sensitive *Streptococcus viridans* infections are most amenable to shorter courses and an early switch to oral antibiotics. At the other end of the spectrum, some cases of fungal infection and prosthetic valve infection may require more long term suppressive antimicrobial treatment.

A prolonged course of highly active bactericidal drugs, in high dose and synergistic combination, is required. Initial treatment is usually given parenterally. A detailed profile of the organism's sensitivity to single and combined antibiotics (in terms of mean inhibitory concentration and mean bacteriocidal concentration) should be obtained at the outset. The levels of antibiotics achieved during the peaks and troughs of treatment should be estimated and back-titrations against the organism may be undertaken (detecting the highest dilution at which bactericidal and inhibitory actions are maintained). Although Fig. 9.36 gives brief details of the common antibiotics used to treat endocarditis, a detailed description of therapy is beyond the scope of this account.

Surgical intervention in patients with progressive aortic or mitral regurgitation has to be timed to avoid the rising surgical risks which parallel increasing heart failure. With one-third of patients developing significant embolic pathology, particularly cerebral infarction, those at higher risk of embolization may be considered for valve replacement. Occasionally, clearance of infection can only be achieved by valve replacement. Awareness of the endocarditis risk associated with mechanical prosthetic valves has increased interest in techniques of valve repair and debridement.

MYOCARDITIS

Microbial involvement of heart muscle may be the result of cellular invasion by viruses, functional depression by toxins or as a component of a microbe-provoked immune response involving the myocardium (Fig. 9.37).

The majority of cases of myocarditis are viral and involve the Coxsackie, mumps, influenza and Epstein–Barr viruses.

Both myocardium and pericardium are commonly affected, the cellular necrosis may be diffuse, localized or patchy and the severity may be mild or transmural. Severe disease is associated with ventricular dilatation. The myocardial biopsy shows focal infiltration with acute and chronic inflammatory cells causing broadening of the interstitium (Fig. 9.38).

Suggested Therapy for Endocarditis	
Streptococcus viridans	Benzyl penicillin alone (4 weeks) Benzyl penicillin + aminoglycoside (2 weeks)
Streptococcus faecalis	Ampicillin + gentamicin
Staphylococcus aureus	Nafcillin or cloxacillin
Staphylococcus epidermidis	Nafcillin or cloxacillin + gentamicin or rifampicin (6–8 weeks)
Gram-negative bacilli	β-lactam + aminoglycoside (6 weeks) * choice depends on sensitivity of organisms
Fungi	Amphotericin B, fluconaxole + flucytosine combinations (6–8 weeks)*
Coxiella burnetii	Tetracycline + cotrimoxazole (6 weeks)
* Surgery is often needed to effect a cure	

Fig. 9.36 Suggested therapy for endocarditis.

Principal Microbial Causes of Myocarditis
Viruses
Coxsackie A & B
Mumps
Influenza
Epstein–Barr
Echo
Measles
Polio
Bacteria
Corynebacterium diptheriae
Streptococcus pyogenes
Clostridium perfringens
Others
Rickettsia rickettsii
Rickettsia typhi
Mycoplasma pneumoniae
Chlamydia psittaci
Coxiella burnetii
Toxoplasma gondii
Trypanosoma cruzi
Trichinella spiralis
Candida
Aspergillus

Fig. 9.37 Principal microbial causes of myocarditis.

Myocarditis often starts with an acute febrile illness with non-specific systemic symptoms (often generalized myalgia), then progresses to breathlessness, palpitations and possibly retrosternal pain. The symptoms and signs of heart failure may develop with increasing dyspnoea, tachycardia, paradoxical pulse, rising jugular venous pressure, diminished heart sounds (associated pericardial effusion) and dysrhythmias.

The characteristic clinical features of a specific infection (Fig. 9.39) may be present and help to identify infections such as mumps, varicella and meningococcus. Elevation of enzymes such as glutamic oxaloacetic transaminase and creatine phosphokinase indicate myocardial necrosis.

The ECG may be relatively normal or show ST segment changes, pericarditis, dysrhythmias and conduction disturbances.

The chest x-ray may show progressive cardiac enlargement. The echocardiogram may confirm dilatation, focal damage, abnormal contraction patterns and pericardial effusion. Direct cultures or pericardial, myocardial, faecal and throat specimens may provide a viral isolation.

Most patients with viral myocarditis recover fully. Progression of the acute phase of myocarditis may involve heart failure, dilatation, infarction and dysrhythmia. Associated effusions may cause early tamponade or later constriction. A chronic cardiomyopathy may continue in the long term. Death due to arhythmia may occur in the covalescent phase of a specific viral illness in which no myocarditic features had been recognized.

There is no specific therapy for most forms of infectious myocarditis, and treatment is largely supportive. Bed rest, adequate oxygen therapy and cardiac monitoring are all important. For nonviral forms of myocarditis there may be specific antimicrobial therapy available. Glucocorticoids are often given but in animal models, these and other forms of immunosuppresive therapy are harmful.

Diphtheria

Corynebacterium diphtheriae may carry a toxin-producing phage. Beside promoting membrane formation and peripheral neuropathy, the toxins may cause acute degeneration of myocardial cells and invoke interstitial inflammatory changes. The conduction system may be involved.

Clinically the patient's condition deteriorates in the first 1–2 weeks with signs of cardiac failure. The ECG may confirm conduction defects and supraventricular or ventricular rhythm disturbance. Anti-toxin given at the time of diagnosis may prevent or ameliorate toxigenic cardiac involvement. Benzylpencillin is the most appropriate treatment of the primary infections.

Rheumatic fever

Rheumatic fever may occur two weeks after a group A β-haemolytic streptococcal throat infection. The precise pathomechanism is uncertain but involves an abnormal immune response to streptococcal products; this causes pancarditis, erythema marginatum, subcutaneous nodules, chorea and polyarthritis. A characteristic histological feature, the Aschoff nodule (Fig. 9.40), involves inflammatory necrosis surrounding a central vessel; around this are epithelioid cells and then a perimeter of lymphocyte infiltration.

Fig. 9.38 Acute Coxsackie B myocarditis. Inflammatory cell infiltrate, widening of the interstitium and some hypertrophy and malalignment of the myocardial fibres. By courtesy of Dr C. Edwards.

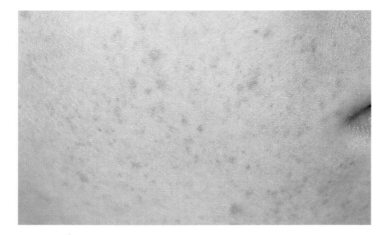

Fig. 9.39 Myocarditis. Punctate erythematous rash in a patient with acute Coxsackie B myocarditis.

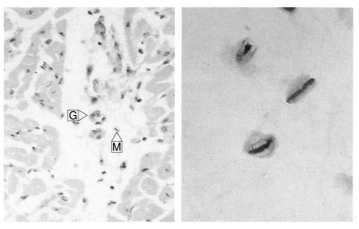

Fig. 9.40 Acute rheumatic fever. Left: Aschoff's body (proliferative stage) in myocardium showing central fibrinoid necrosis, giant cells (G) and Anitschkow myocytes (M). Right: Anitschkow myocytes showing central nuclei with condensation of chromatin in a wavy 'caterpillar' pattern. H & E stains.

Rheumatic fever commonly involves children in the 5–15 year age group, 1–4 weeks after a sore throat. Arthritis in rheumatic fever affects knees, ankles, wrists and elbows and is migratory. Pancarditis usually appears in the first few weeks: endocarditis favours the mitral valve (Fig. 9.41) and may cause a diastolic Carey–Coombes murmur and later mitral regurgitation. Subcutaneous, painless nodules up to 1 cm in diameter appear over bony prominences, often in conjunction with carditis. Erythema marginatum, an enlarging serpiginous rash on the trunk and limbs (Fig. 9.42), can also occur.

Chagas' disease

Chagas' disease occurs in South and Central America. It is caused by *Trypanosoma cruzi*, a protozoan transmitted from animals to man by triatomid bugs. *T. cruzi* has a variety of mammalian hosts, including rodents and

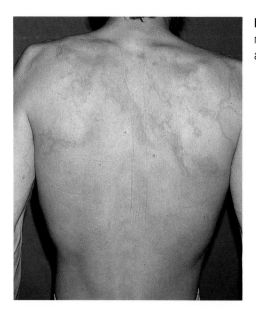

Fig. 9.42 Erythema marginatum in a patient with acute rheumatic fever.

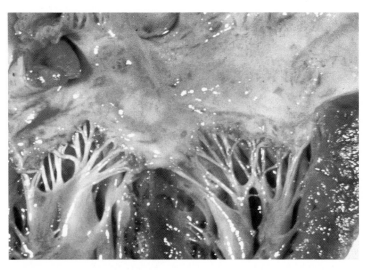

Fig. 9.41 Acute rheumatic fever. Mitral valvulitis showing thickening of chordae tendineae and valve leaflets, with small verrucae along the line of valve closure.

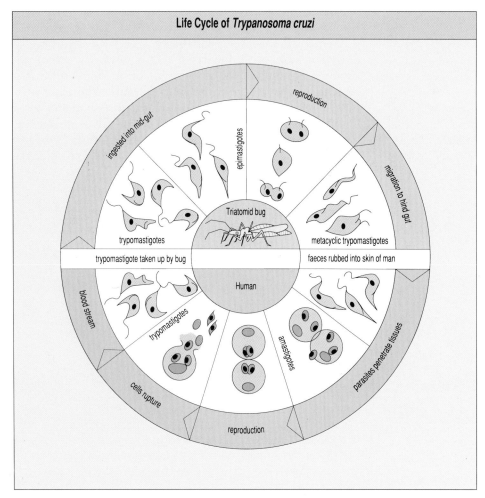

Fig. 9.43 Life cycle of *Trypanosoma cruzi*.

Life Cycle of *Trypanosoma cruzi*

reproduction

ingested into mid-gut

epimastigotes

migration to hind gut

trypomastigotes

metacyclic trypomastigotes

Triatomid bug

trypomastigote taken up by bug

faeces rubbed into skin of man

Human

blood stream

trypomastigotes

amastigotes

parasites penetrate tissues

cells rupture

reproduction

armadillos, which form an animal reservoir (Fig. 9.43). As the bug feeds it defaecates on the skin; the organisms are inoculated as the host scratches the site of the bite (Fig. 9.44). Transmission to man occurs predominantly where triatomid bugs inhabit poorly constructed housing in close association with reservoir animals. It is estimated that more than 10 million people are infected with the parasite.

The parasite in the blood has a flagellate form (the trypomastigote – Fig. 9.45); the tissue form (the amastigote – Fig. 9.46), has no flagellum.

During the acute phase the trypanosomes parasitize muscles, including the myocardium (Fig. 9.47); in chronic Chagas' disease the heart is the organ chiefly affected. The ventricles and atria dilate, aneurysms may develop at the apex of the ventricles and mural thromboses may form with subsequent embolization. Microscopically, the amastigotes multiply to form pseudocysts within the myocardium, provoking a lymphocytic reaction with granuloma formation. The muscle fibres of the heart are damaged, there is diffuse and focal lymphocyte infiltration and also fibrosis. The conducting system shows disruption, fibrosis and atrophy. In chronic Chagas' disease the oesophagus and colon are also affected and hugely dilated. Histologically there is a reduction in the number of parasympathetic neurones and focal inflammation. The pathogenesis of the cardiac and gastrointestinal lesions of chronic Chagas' disease is not known but is believed to be either autoimmune damage, or due to damage to the autonomic nervous system that occurs during the acute phase.

The clinical features of acute Chagas' disease involve local inflammation at the site of infection, fever and generalized or local lymphadenopathy 2–4 weeks after infection. During this phase trypanosomes may be found in the blood along with a lymphocytosis. Any myocarditis that develops during this phase is usually not severe. The acute illness then settles spontaneously and many years later the cardiomyopathy and megadisease of the oesophagus and colon become apparent. Death is usually due to complications of one or other of these manifestations.

In acute Chagas' disease trypanosomes may be found in the blood using concentration techniques. Zenodiagnosis (a triatomid bug is fed on the patient's blood and the bug faeces are examined for *T. cruzi*), is also sometimes used. Serological methods (see Fig. 9.48) are used for the diagnosis of chronic Chagas' disease.

No fully satisfactory treatment for American trypanosomiasis has been found, although nifurtimox and benznidazole are currently in use.

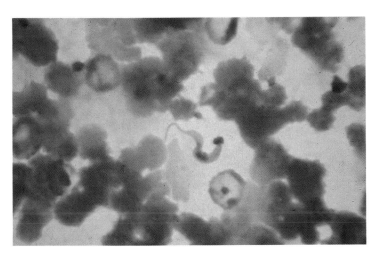

Fig. 9.44 Chagas' disease. *T. cruzi* in the blood.

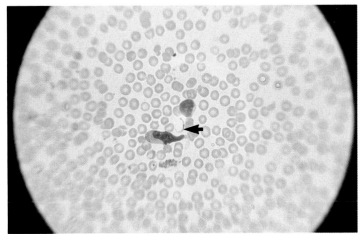

Fig. 9.45 *Trypanosoma cruzi.* Trypomastigote in blood smear.

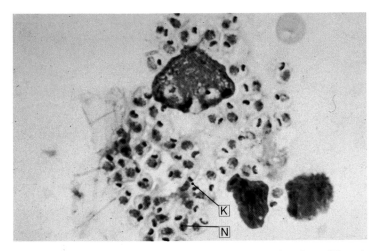

Fig. 9.46 Chagas' disease. Macrophage containing numerous amastigote forms of *T. cruzi*. Note the prominent kinetoplast (K) and nucleus (N) in each organism. Giemsa stain. By courtesy of Dr I. G. Kagan.

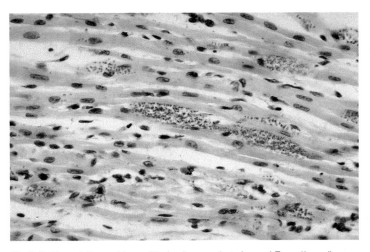

Fig. 9.47 Chagas' disease. Myocarditis showing amastigote forms of *T. cruzi* in cardiac muscle. H & E stain.

Myocardial involvement with other systemic protozoan infections

Toxoplasmosis may involve the myocardium in congenital infections, occasionally in healthy primary infections and as recrudescent disease in immunocompromised patients. Sarcocystis hominis is a zoonotic infection acquired from eating undercooked beef (Fig. 9.49).

Cardiovascular syphilis

Aortitis leading to aneurysm, aortic valvular incompetence and coronary artery stenosis, is a feature of late syphilis. As a result of inflammatory changes in the vasa vasorum of the aortic wall there is damage to the smooth muscle and elastic fibres which cause irregular thickening and localized weakness with aneurysm formation and dilatation (Fig. 9.50).

Dilatation of the first part of the aortic arch results in aortic regurgitation. Scarring of the intima of the coronary ostia may cause stenosis (Fig. 9.51).

Clinically early aneurysms are asymptomatic but later cause pressure phenomena in the mediastinum (Fig. 9.52)

and subsequent rupture. Coronary ostial stenosis may present as angina. The aortic regurgitation may have an associated ejection click.

The presence of late syphilitic features elsewhere may give an important clue to the aetiology of cardiovascular features. Specific serological tests are positive though the non-specific serology may be negative (see Chapter 7).

Penicillin is the drug of choice (see Chapter 7) – it only rarely provokes a significant Jarisch–Hercheimer reaction in cases of late syphilis.

PERICARDITIS

Most of the viruses associated with myocarditis will also cause pericarditis. Coxsackie viruses predominate. However, the spectrum of bacteria involved with pericarditis differs from that of bacterial myocarditis. This is because many of the bacteria involved in purulent pericarditis, especially *S. pneumoniae* and *S. aureus*, primarily cause pulmonary infection – the pericarditis results from a complication of the adjacent lung sepsis. Other bacterial pericarditic infections are associated with septicaemia due

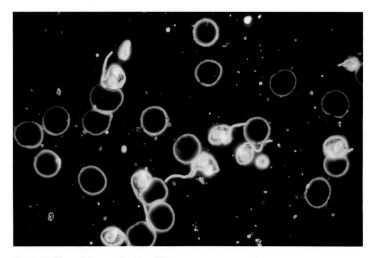

Fig. 9.48 Chagas' disease. Positive IFT test.

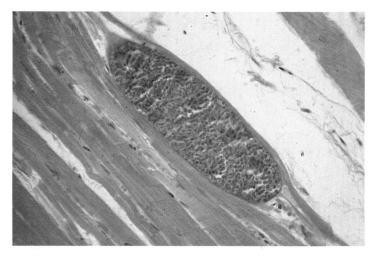

Fig. 9.49 Sarcocystis hominis. Sarcocyst in heart muscle.

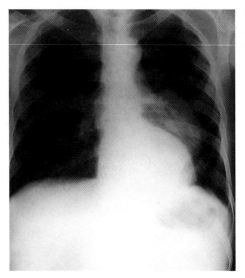

Fig. 9.50 Syphillis. Aortic aneurysm in a patient with tertiary syphilis.

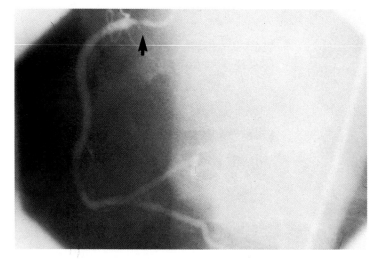

Fig. 9.51 Syphillis. Coronary ostial occlusion in tertiary syphilis.

to enteric gram-negative rods, *H. influenzae* (in children) and meningococci. Tuberculosis is still an important cause. In immunocompromised patients *Cryptococcus neoformans* and other fungi are important. Fungal pericarditis is also seen following cardiac surgery.

Morphologically, in acute pericarditis there is typically a shaggy, fibrinous exudate covering the pericardium (Figs

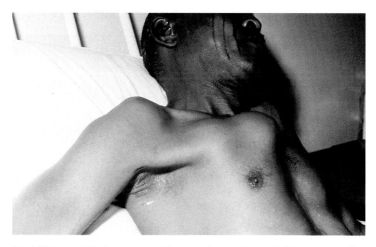

Fig. 9.52 Late syphilis. An aneurysm of the ascending aorta has eroded the sternum and is bulging through the anterior chest wall as a pulsating mass.

9.53 & 9.54), with a small or large amount of pericardial effusion. Microscopically there is deposition of fibrin with infiltration by inflammatory cells.

In acute viral pericarditis the presenting feature is often continuous retrosternal chest pain which may be exacerbated by either respiratory or trunk movements. A concurrent 'flu-like illness' is often present. The pericardial rub may vary with the cardiac cycle, respiration and position; the rub diminishes with the accumulation of fluid. In bacterial pericarditis chest pain and a pericardial rub are infrequent: the patient is usually severely unwell with high fever and signs of concomitant systemic infection.

The ECG is abnormal in most patients. The ST segment is initially elevated, with subsequent return to baseline and inversion of the T waves, and there may be supra-ventricular rhythm disturbances. The chest x-ray may show evidence of pericardial effusion, but the cardiac shadow may not be enlarged even with more than 200ml of pericardial fluid. The echocardiogram will give precise indications of pericardial fluid and pericardial thickness.

Increasing pericardial effusion impairs ventricular filling (Figs 9.55 & 9.56). A compensatory tachycardia and a rise in atrial pressures may maintain an adequate cardiac output despite a small stroke volume until a point of decompensation. Clinically there is tachycardia, pulsus

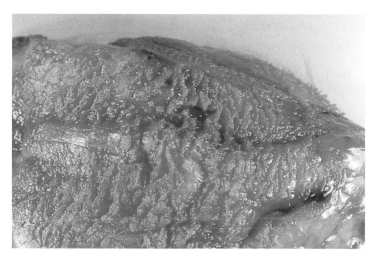

Fig. 9.53 Acute fibrinous pericarditis. Unfixed specimen of the heart showing beefy-red, granular, shaggy appearance of surface of the heart.

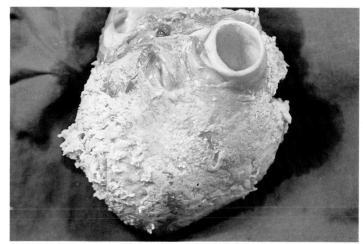

Fig. 9.54 Acute fibrinous pericarditis. Gross specimen of heart (formalin fixed) showing shaggy latex-like appearance of exudate covering the surface of the heart.

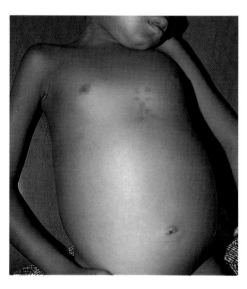

Fig. 9.55 Pericarditis. Congestive cardiac failure (ascites and raised jugular venous pressure) in a child with pericardial effusion and tamponade.

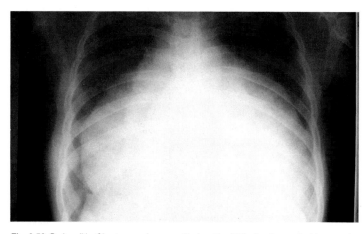

Fig. 9.56 Pericarditis. Chest x-ray of same patient as Fig. 9.55, showing marked increase in cardiac diameter due to a large pericardial effusion.

paradoxus (an unusually prominent fall in arterial pressure during inspiration, greater than 10mmHg). The central venous pressure may be raised and there may be signs of peripheral arterial shut down despite an apparently adequate systolic pressure. The heart sounds may be diminished. The ECG may show low voltage, the chest x-ray prominent cardiac diameter and the ECG, once again, should confirm the diagnosis.

Constrictive pericarditis

Constrictive pericarditis is a late complication of viral (rarely) and tuberculous pericarditis. There is prominent thickening of the parietal pericardium, dense fibrous tissue and adhesion to the ventricular wall, obliteration of the pericardial space and, sometimes, calcification (Fig. 9.57). The stroke volume is fixed, possibly reduced, the central venous pressure raised, and, as with tamponade, a tachycardia may sustain or increase cardiac output.

Clinically the jugular venous pressure is raised and may have abnormal features. There may be hepatomegaly with ascites and peripheral oedema, and a pericardial knock in early diastole may be present. The ECG is variable and may show atrial dysrythmia, right ventricular hypertrophy and other non-specific features. There may be pericardial calcification and the cardiac diameter may be increased. The echocardiogram may show the thickening of pericardium.

With acute pericarditis the management of possible bacterial or purulent pericarditis involves pericardiocentesis, appropriate antimicrobial medication and occasionally surgical drainage. Pain is controlled with non-steroidal anti-inflammatory medication. Steroids may reduce the incidence of constriction following mycobacterial infection but otherwise their use is limited by the adverse effects they might have on concurrent viral myocarditis.

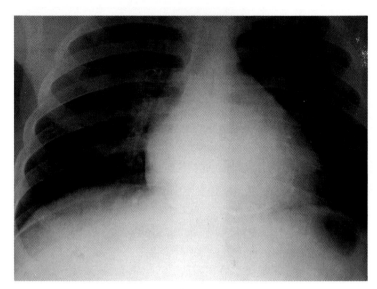

Fig. 9.57 Constrictive pericarditis. Calcification of the pericardium.

10

SKIN AND SOFT TISSUE
BACTERIAL, PROTOZOAL AND HELMINTH INFECTIONS

BACTERIAL INFECTIONS

Folliculitis

Folliculitis is an infection of the hair follicles and produces a number of small erythematous or pustular lesions (Fig. 10.1). It is usually caused by *Staphylococcus aureus*. Extensive folliculitis of the beard area is called sycosis barbae. Local warm compresses and topical antibiotics are all that is needed as therapy.

A particular form of folliculitis occurs in persons who have bathed in swimming pools or whirlpool baths contaminated by *Pseudomonas aeruginosa* (Fig. 10.2). A pruritic papulopustular rash, particularly affecting areas of moisture or those covered by a bathing suit (the buttocks, hips, axillae and the lateral side of the trunk), develops within a day or two of exposure. *P. aeruginosa* may be isolated from the lesions but no therapy is required and topical steroids should be avoided.

Furunculosis

A furuncle (boil) is a *S. aureus* infection of an obstructed hair follicle (Fig. 10.3). It begins as a red, tender, inflammatory nodule on the face, neck, axilla or other area of hairy skin; over the next few days this becomes fluctuant and usually spontaneously discharges a quantity of yellowish pus. Constitutional symptoms and fever are not common. Antibiotic therapy is not usually necessary; surgical drainage or the application of warm soaks is all that is normally required.

Patients with diabetes, poor hygiene and excessive sweating may suffer from recurrent furuncles. It can be difficult to control this problem, which is often due to nasal staphylococcal carriage in the patient or other family members. Antibiotic ointment to the nares and/or the use of systemic rifampicin may eradicate carriage.

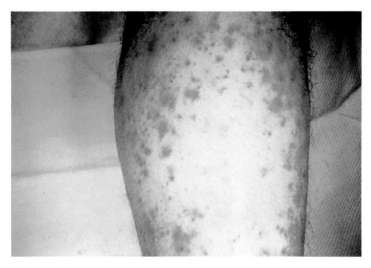

Fig. 10.1 Folliculitis. Small red raised lesions, each associated with a hair follicle and caused by *Staphylococcus aureus*. By courtesy of Dr. Eleanor Sahn.

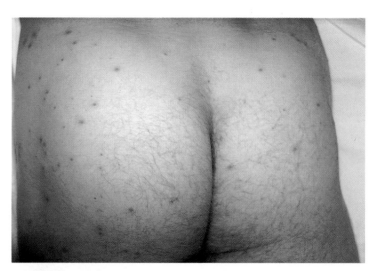

Fig. 10.2 Pseudomonas folliculitis. Papulopustular rash over the buttocks and thighs following use of a spa pool.

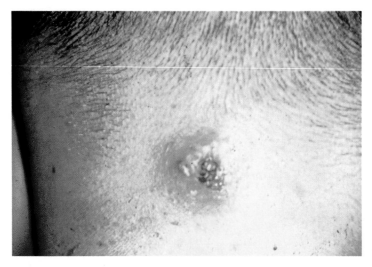

Fig. 10.3 Furuncle. Small cutaneous abscess associated with hair follicle on back of neck. By courtesy of Department of Dermatology, Medical University of South Carolina.

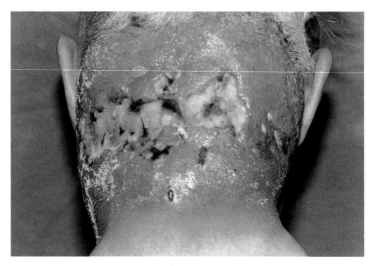

Fig. 10.4 Carbuncle. A huge area of induration of the neck with multiple discharging follicular abscesses.

Carbuncle

A carbuncle is a larger abscess (almost always staphylococcal) extending from an infected follicle into the subcutaneous fat. It is often seen at the nape of the neck (Fig. 10.4), or on the back. There are constitutional signs of infection and as the abscess extends there are multiple points of drainage from infected follicles. Bacteraemia and spread of infection to metastatic foci is not uncommon. Carbuncles require surgical drainage and treatment with an anti-staphylococcal antibiotic.

Hydradenitis suppurativa

This indolent, chronic, suppurative infection of apocrine sweat glands is fortunately rare. It is often due to *S. aureus*, and occurs principally in adults. It results in recurrent crops of abscesses, leading to sinus formation and extensive scarring in the axillary, perineal and/or genital areas (Fig. 10.5). Oral anti-staphylococcal therapy combined with moist compresses and drainage of fluctuant lesions is usually effective.

Impetigo

Impetigo is a superficial streptococcal or staphylococcal infection of the skin, almost exclusively affecting young children in warm weather. It is highly communicable; transmission is enhanced by low socioeconomic status with its associated poor living conditions and hygiene. The organisms probably cannot invade intact skin – infection occurs through minor abrasions, insect bites, etc. The infection often spreads rapidly to other sites, presumably by scratching and autoinoculation. It may also complicate eczema (Fig. 10.6) or varicella. All impetigo is initially vesicular, later becoming crusted; the characteristic features of the infection depend on whether the aetiological agent is *Streptococcus pyogenes* or *S. aureus* . The vesicles in streptococcal impetigo very rapidly rupture and are often missed (Fig. 10.7). After rupture, the discharge dries to form characteristic thick, adherent, golden-yellow crusts (see Figs 10.8, 10.9 & 10.10). Staphylococcal impetigo, on the other hand, typically produces more long-lived bullae (see Fig. 10.11) and thin, light brown crusts (described as 'varnish-like'). It tends to occur in younger

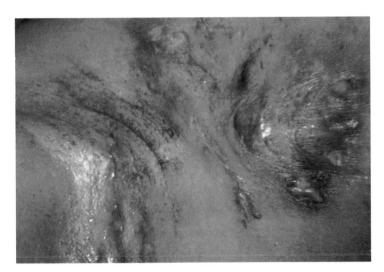

Fig. 10.5 Hydradenitis suppurativa. Extensive scarring with multiple sinuses in and around the axilla. By courtesy of Dr K. A. Riley.

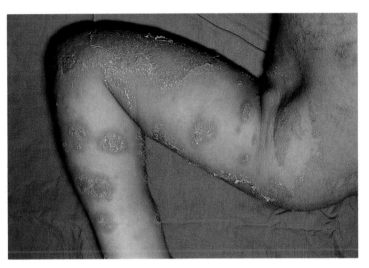

Fig. 10.6 Impetigenized eczema. Young Asian child with severe atopic eczema secondarily infected with impetigo.

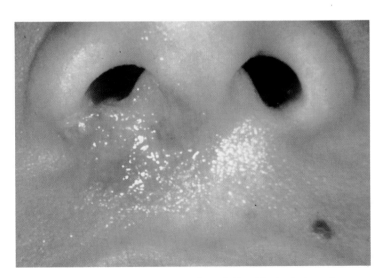

Fig. 10.7 Streptococcal impetigo. The cluster of superficial vesicles has broken to form a raw weeping surface, soon to be covered by a yellow crust.

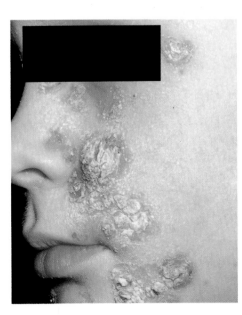

Fig. 10.8 Impetigo. These characteristic yellow crusts are often the main feature on presentation.

children and is a reaction to the exfoliative toxins of *S. aureus* that are also responsible for the scalded skin syndrome (see below). The cause of impetigo can be determined by Gram stain or by culture of the exudate beneath the crust. Anti-DNAase B and anti-hyaluronidase titres usually rise after streptococcal skin infection, but the anti-streptolysin O (ASO) titre often does not.

Certain strains of β-haemolytic streptococci – the so-called nephritogenic strains – may give rise to immunologically-mediated acute post-streptococcal nephritis after skin infection, especially in tropical countries, but rheumatic fever does not follow streptococcal pyoderma.

There are two approaches to the antibiotic treatment of impetigo. One is to use penicillin alone (or erythromycin in the penicillin-allergic individual), given the primary role of streptococci in this condition. The other approach is to use an anti-staphylococcal antibiotic to deal with both of the common pathogens. Bullous impetigo should certainly be treated as a staphylococcal infection. Systemic antibiotics are more effective than topical therapy, as they are superior at preventing transmission. If appropriate treatment is not given, the lesions may slowly enlarge and multiply over weeks or months. Injudicious treatment with steroid skin creams removes the crusts but promotes spread of the infection, with numerous red raw lesions (Fig. 10.12).

Ecthyma

Ecthyma occurs when infection with Group A streptococci spreads through the epidermis to cause 'punched out' ulcers that extend into the dermis. The lesions have raised margins and are covered in yellowish crusts. They are usually on the lower limbs (Fig. 10.13) but may be found elsewhere (Fig. 10.14). Treatment is the same as for impetigo.

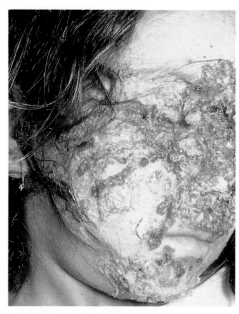

Fig. 10.9 Impetigo. Severe streptococcal impetigo crusts over the face of a young girl. Courtesy of Prof. A. M. Geddes.

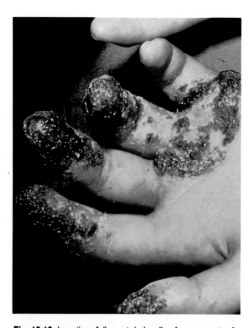

Fig. 10.10 Impetigo. Adherent dark yellow/brown crusts of impetigo on fingers. By courtesy of Dr. E. Sahn.

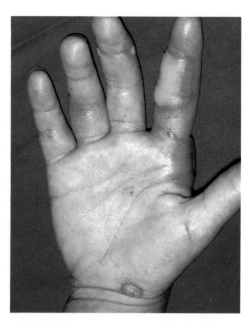

Fig. 10.11 Bullous impetigo. Lesions on finger and wrist. By courtesy of Dr. E. Sahn.

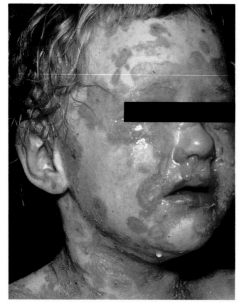

Fig. 10.12 Impetigo. Multiple raw areas following incorrect treatment of the initial areas with steroid-containing cream. By courtesy of Prof. A. M. Geddes.

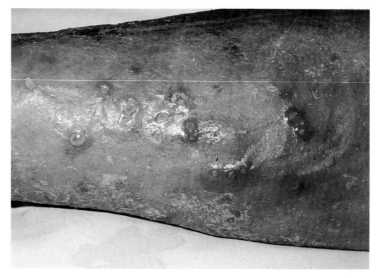

Fig. 10.13 Ecthyma. Small punched out lesions over the shin of an elderly woman. Group A streptococci were isolated.

Cellulitis

Cellulitis is a spreading superficial infection of the skin. A number of different bacteria can be responsible but the vast majority of cases are due to streptococci (usually group A β-haemolytic streptococci but occasionally other groups) or *S. aureus*. Infection can occur at any age and, although it often develops at a site of previous trauma or skin lesion, the entry site may be unapparent. Patients frequently have an abrupt onset of malaise, fever, chills and headache and the involved skin becomes tender, red, warm and swollen (Fig. 10.15). The inflammation spreads with poorly defined margins (compare with erysipelas – see below) and may be accompanied by lymphangitis (see below) and lymphadenopathy. Streptococcal cellulitis occasionally becomes bullous (Figs 10.16 & 10.17).

The diagnosis of cellulitis is usually a clinical one, but there is often no way of clinically distinguishing between streptococcal and staphylococcal cellulitis – differentiation requires a Gram stain (Fig. 10.18) or culture of material

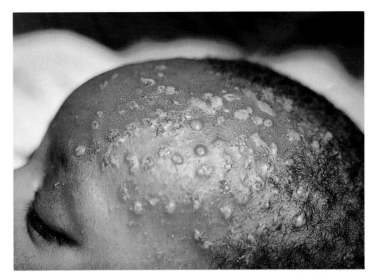

Fig. 10.14 Ecthyma. Lesions due to streptococcal infection over the scalp of an African child.

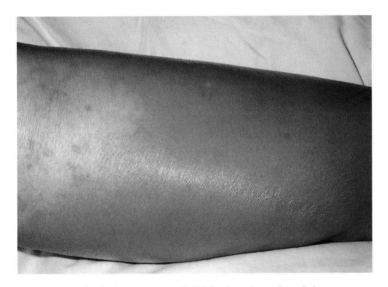

Fig. 10.15 Cellulitis. Erythematous area with ill-defined margin over lower limb.

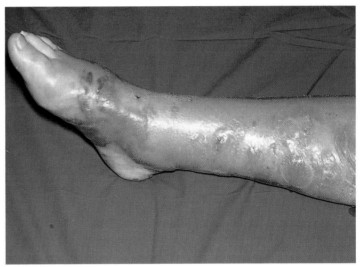

Fig. 10.16 Cellulitis. A severe, rapidly developing infection of the subcutaneous tissues of the leg with large bullae and scabs.

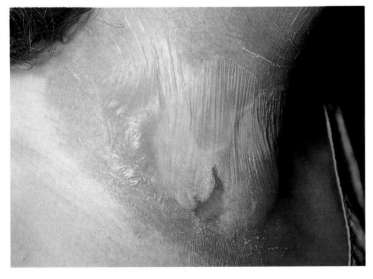

Fig. 10.17 Cellulitis. Large bullae in an area of cellulitis of the neck caused by *Streptococcus pyogenes*.

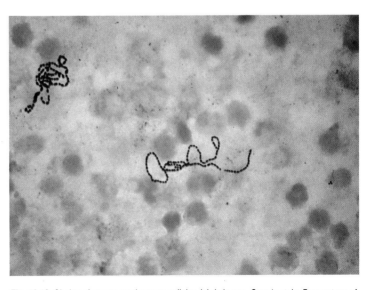

Fig. 10.18 Chains of streptococci among cellular debris in pus. Gram's stain. By courtesy of Dr I. Farrell.

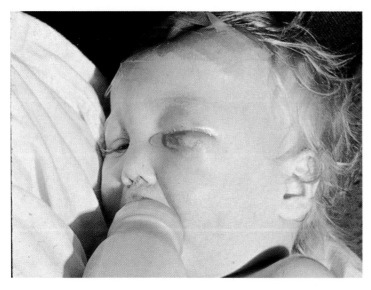

Fig. 10.19 Cellulitis due to *Haemophilus influenzae* of the cheek and preorbit. By courtesy of Dr. R. B. Turner

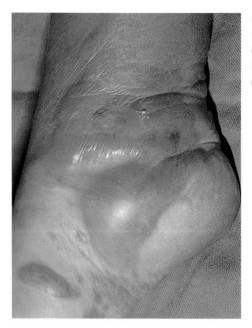

Fig. 10.20 Cellulitis. Severe infection with bullous lesions due to *Vibrio vulnificans* infection following immersion of leg in brackish water.

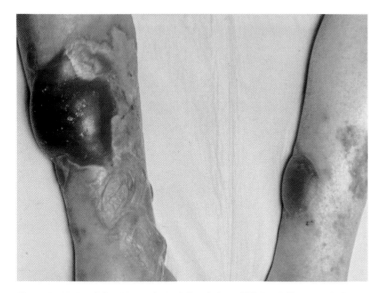

Fig. 10.21 Vibrio cellulitis. Haemorrhagic, bullous lesions of *Vibrio vulnificans* sepsis. By courtesy of Dr J. R. Cantey.

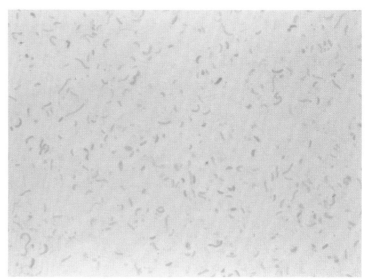

Fig. 10.22 Vibrio cellulitis. Comma-shaped cells of *Vibrio vulnificans*. Gram's stain. By courtesy of Dr J. R. Cantey.

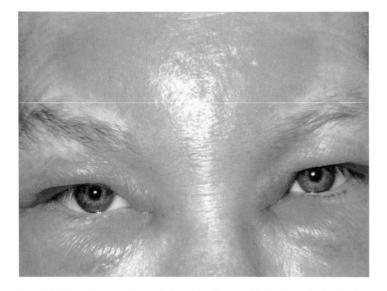

Fig. 10.23 Erysipelas. Well demarcated area of erythema and induration on the forehead.

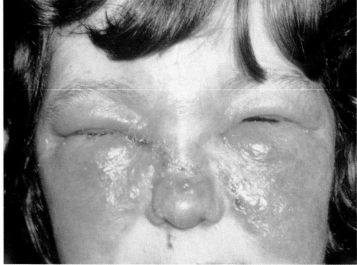

Fig. 10.24 Erysipelas. A typical butterfly-wing rash on the cheeks. Both eyes are closed by oedema of the lids.

aspirated from the leading edge of the cellulitis. Therapy should be based upon bacteriological results if available, but if there are no initial clues to the aetiology then a penicillinase-resistant penicillin should be given (e.g. flucloxacillin 0.5–1.0g orally every 6 hours). For the more severely ill patient parenteral therapy may be needed and for the penicillin-allergic individual, erythromycin or clindamycin would be suitable.

A number of other distinctive forms of cellulitis are also seen. In children an unusual form of cellulitis may be caused by *Haemophilus influenzae* type b. It is commonly seen on the cheek and produces a purple-red, bruised appearance (Fig. 10.19). This colour distinguishes it from other forms of cellulitis and the indistinct margin differentiates it from erysipelas. Following laceration or trauma during swimming in fresh water, cellulitis may be caused by *Aeromonas hydrophila*, an environmental gram-negative bacillus. After contamination of wounds by seawater, a severe form of cellulitis, often complicated by necrosis and bacteraemia, is caused by *Vibrio vulnificans* and other *Vibrio* species (Figs 10.20, 10.21 & 10.22).

Erysipelas

Erysipelas is a characteristic variant of cellulitis, almost always caused exclusively by *S. pyogenes*. It is a painful, bright red, shiny lesion with a raised, sharply demarcated, advancing edge (Fig. 10.23). It is most common on the legs or face and often spreads across the nose to involve both cheeks (the 'butterfly-wing' rash – fig 10.24).

There is much systemic upset with high fever and rigors and a leucocytosis is common. Erysipelas is treated with penicillin, given parenterally in the more severe cases.

Erysipeloid

Erysipeloid is an occupational disease of people handling fish and meat, as the organism (a gram-positive rod, *Erysipelothrix rhusiopathiae*) is found in many wild and domestic animals. The infection develops as an indolent, purple, swollen, non-purulent area at the site of inoculation, which spreads slowly outwards (Fig. 10.25). New purple areas may develop locally and systemic infection with endocarditis is an occasional complication. Penicillin is the antibiotic of choice.

Lymphangitis

Acute lymphangitis is particularly likely to complicate group A streptococcal infection of the skin of a limb. It is usually accompanied by the signs of the cutaneous infection but occasionally lymphangitis can appear before the skin infection is apparent. The clinical signs are red lines of inflammation (Fig. 10.26) corresponding to the lymphatic channels, extending to the regional lymph nodes. The lymph nodes themselves are tender and swollen and oedema of the limb may develop. Fever is common. Untreated lymphangitis is likely to lead to bacteraemia and antibiotic therapy should be started promptly. Parenteral penicillin is the empirical therapy of choice.

Other bacteria, notably *S. aureus* and *Pasteurella multocida* (often complicating cat or dog bites) are rarer causes of acute lymphangitis. In the tropics, filariasis due to *Wuchereria bancrofti* (see Chapter 13) may also warrant consideration.

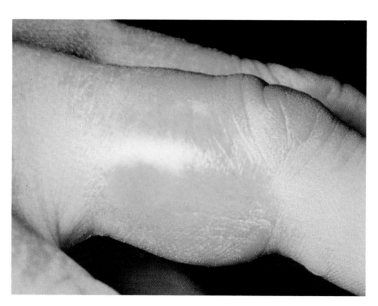

Fig. 10.25 Erysipeloid. Characteristic indolent, purple, non-purulent swelling of the finger, one of the most common sites of infection.

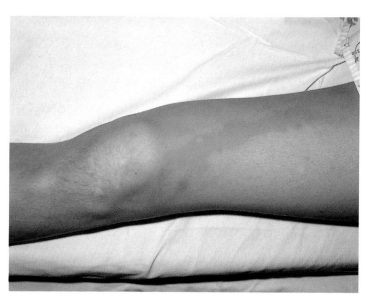

Fig. 10.26 Lymphangitis. Inflamed lymphatic channels extending up the thigh to regional lymph nodes from an area of cellulitis of lower leg.

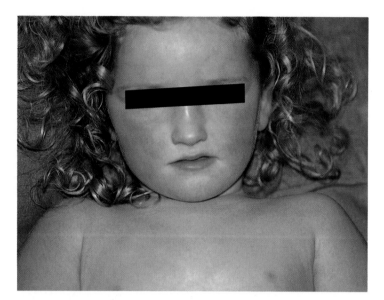

Fig. 10.27 Scarlatina. The face appears flushed with circumoral pallor.

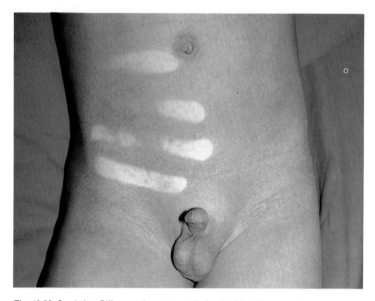

Fig. 10.28 Scarlatina. Diffuse erythematous rash showing blanching where finger pressure has been applied to the abdomen.

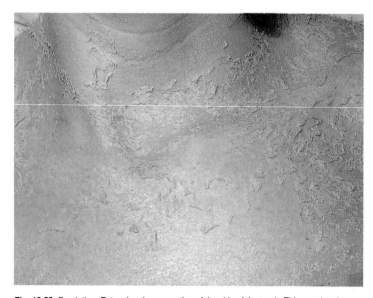

Fig. 10.29 Scarlatina. Extensive desquamation of the skin of the trunk. This may last for several weeks.

Scarlet fever (scarlatina)

Some group A haemolytic streptococci produce an erythrogenic toxin causing the characteristic rash of scarlet fever. Infection is usually of the pharynx or tonsils (see Chapter 1) although streptococcal skin or wound infection can also be associated with scarlet fever. The rash of scarlet fever begins on the face (Fig. 10.27), neck and upper chest, spreading to the abdomen and extremities: it consists of a diffuse scarlet erythema with almost confluent punctate papules. This is called punctate erythema. There is often also slight prominence of the hair follicles, giving a sand-paper-like texture to the skin. The rash blanches upon pressure (Fig. 10.28). The erythema often spares the area around the mouth but is accentuated in the creases of the elbows, groin and axillary folds (Pastia's lines). The tongue is at first furred with prominent papillae (the 'white strawberry' tongue). After about 4 days there is extensive desquamation of the skin which may continue for 2 weeks or more (Fig 10.29). Desquamation of the tongue also occurs leaving a raw, red tongue with prominent papillae ('red-strawberry' tongue).

Culture of a swab from the throat or from the infected wound will demonstrate group A β-haemolytic streptococci. The condition is treated with penicillin.

Toxic shock syndrome

Toxic shock syndrome (TSS) is mediated by one or more of the exotoxins produced by *S. aureus*. It occurs predominantly in menstruating females using tampons (the

---

Toxic Shock Syndrome criteria

Temperature >38.9°C

Systolic blood pressure <90mmHg

Rash with subsequent desquamation

Involvement of 3 or more of the following organ systems:

    Gastrointestinal: vomiting; diarrhoea

    Mucous membrane hyperaemia

    Renal insufficiency; creatinine more than twice upper limit of normal

    Liver: hepatitis

    Blood: thrombocytopenia <100 000mm³

    Muscle: severe myalgia

    CNS: disorientation without focal signs

No other cause for symptoms

Fig. 10.30 Criteria for the diagnosis of toxic shock syndrome.

staphylococcus colonizes the vagina or cervix – the tampon probably promotes superficial ulceration and easy entry for the toxin) but can occur with staphylococcal infection at other sites and in males or children. TSS has many features, but there are certain clinical manifestations that are necessary criteria for the diagnosis (Fig. 10.30). The rash is a diffuse, blanching, macular erythema (Fig. 10.31), particularly affecting the hands and feet, which desquamates 1–2 weeks after it appears (Fig. 10.32).

The diagnosis of TSS is clinical and the isolation of *S. aureus* is not necessary. Attempts should be made to isolate the organism from the vagina, nares, sites of superficial sepsis etc. Bacteraemia is not a feature and indeed makes the diagnosis difficult to consider.

The initial treatment should be with aggressive supportive care. Intravenous anti-staphylococcal antibiotics are also given but, as the disease is toxin-mediated, this may not modify the initial course. Antibiotic therapy is usually given for 10–14 days (the latter half of the course can be administered orally). Women who have had TSS should not use tampons again.

Scalded skin syndrome

Certain strains of *S. aureus* of phage group II produce an exfoliative exotoxin, release of which may cause a syndrome termed staphylococcal scalded skin syndrome (SSSS), or Ritter's disease. In neonates it is also termed pemphigus neonatorum. It usually occurs in children and starts with fever and a tender scarlatiniform rash. Within a day or two, large flaccid, clear bullae develop and exfoliation of sheets of skin (resembling cigarette paper) occurs, leaving a red, denuded base (Figs 10.33, 10.34 & 10.35). Lateral traction of the skin causes it to wrinkle and be dis-

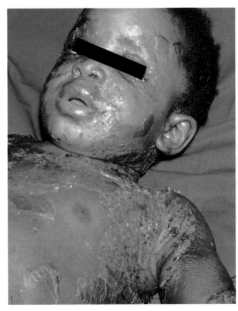

Fig. 10.31 Toxic shock syndrome. Typical sunburn-like rash over face and trunk. Note the dryness and hyperaemia of the lips.

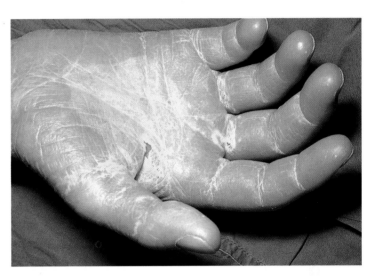

Fig. 10.32 Toxic shock syndrome. Desquamation of the skin, particularly of the palms and soles, occurs with recovery.

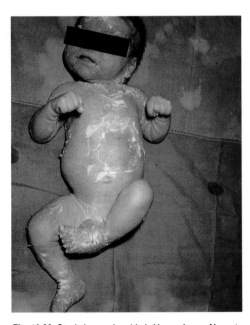

Fig. 10.33 Staphylococcal scalded skin syndrome. Neonate with large denuded areas of skin where bullae have burst. By courtesy of Dr L. Brown.

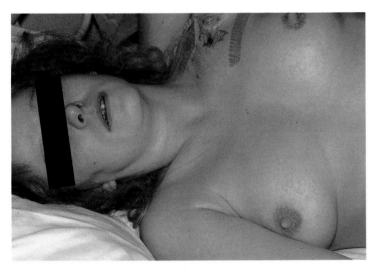

Fig. 10.34 Staphylococcal scalded skin syndrome. Large areas of epidermal loss, with some bullae still intact.

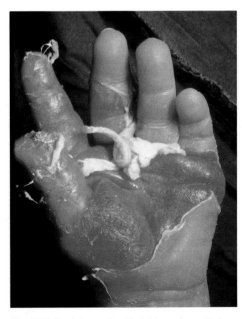

Fig. 10.35 Staphylococcal scalded skin syndrome. Red raw denuded area where skin has sloughed off. Courtesy of Dr M. H. Winterborn.

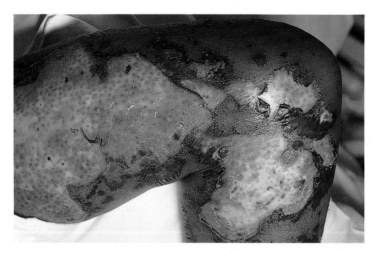

Fig. 10.36 Toxic epidermal necrolysis (Lyell's syndrome). Loss of epidermis in a black child associated with sulphonamide therapy.

placed (a positive Nikolsky's sign). The peeling is caused by the toxin which produces a cleavage plane high in the epidermis at the stratum granulosum level. The site of this cleavage distinguishes SSSS from toxic epidermal necrolysis (see below) where the splitting is at the dermoepidermal junction. As the areas of exfoliation dry, a flaky desquamation and then replacement with new epidermis occurs within two weeks. SSSS is treated with a penicillinase-resistant penicillin, given intravenously, together with measures to counter hypovolaemia.

A clinically identical syndrome to SSSS, termed toxic epidermal necrolysis or Lyell's syndrome, is seen in older children or adults as a manifestation of drug allergy (particularly to sulphonamides) or viral infections (Fig. 10.36). It differs in the plane of the skin splitting (see above) and is often a more severe and prolonged illness which may lead to scarring. Many advocate the use of high-dose corti-

Criteria for Kawasaki disease
Fever of more than 5 days duration
Four of the following five features:
dry, fissured lips
injected lips
injected pharynx
strawberry tongue
peripheral erythema
peripheral oedema
desquamation
nonvesicular rash
cervical lymphadenopathy

Fig. 10.37 Criteria for the diagnosis of Kawasaki disease.

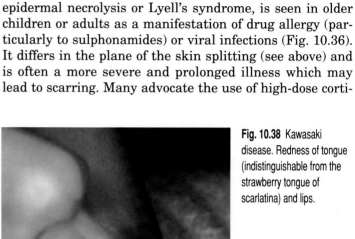

Fig. 10.38 Kawasaki disease. Redness of tongue (indistinguishable from the strawberry tongue of scarlatina) and lips.

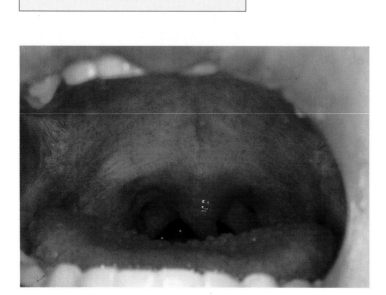

Fig. 10.39 Kawasaki disease. Pharyngeal and palatal injection in a Japanese child.

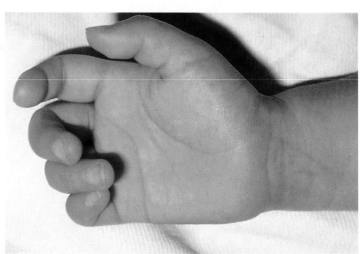

Fig. 10.40 Kawasaki disease. Erythematous rash on hand and wrist of child with mucocutaneous lymph node syndrome.

costeroids for the treatment of toxic epidermal necrolysis, so differentiation from SSSS by means of a skin biopsy is important.

Kawasaki disease

The aetiology of Kawasaki syndrome (or mucocutaneous lymph node syndrome) is unknown. It usually occurs in children less than five years old and is rare in adults. It is particularly common in children of Japanese extraction. The clinical diagnosis depends upon the presence of five of the six criteria listed in Fig. 10.37. There is lymphadenopathy, fever, strawberry tongue (Fig 10.38), redness of the mucous membranes (Fig. 10.39), a morbilliform or scarlatiniform eruption, particularly on the trunk and extremities (Fig. 10.40), and induration or swelling of the hands and feet (Fig. 10.41). Later, the extremities desquamate (Fig. 10.42). In addition to the features already noted (see Fig. 10.37) there may be gastrointestinal symptoms such as diarrhoea and abdominal pain, arthritis, aseptic meningitis and cardiac problems. It is the latter that are the most dangerous complications. Pericardial effusions, myocarditis and aneurysms of the coronary arteries (Fig. 10.43) are seen in 20% of cases. These should be sought by echocardiography in any child with suspected Kawasaki disease and repeat examinations should be done about two weeks, two months and one year after the onset.

Kawasaki disease is treated with intravenous immunoglobulin and aspirin, administered as soon as possible in order to prevent cardiac complications. Those who have coronary artery changes require specialist care from a paediatric cardiologist.

Anaerobic bacterial infections

Anaerobic infections are caused either by anaerobic bacteria alone or, more often, by a mixture of anaerobic and aerobic organisms. They are particularly likely to develop in patients with vascular insufficiency or diabetes mellitus, and in tissues which are ischaemic as a result of disease, trauma or surgical intervention. There are a number of different clinically distinct syndromes, depending upon the anatomic site of infection and the specific causative organisms. All types are distinguished by rapid spread of the infection along anatomic planes and by the presence of either crepitus in the tissues or a putrid exudate.

Bacterial synergistic gangrene

This usually follows infection at an abdominal wound (especially when metal sutures have been used) or a colostomy. It begins as an area of erythema and tenderness that ulcerates and gradually enlarges. There is a margin of gangrenous skin surrounded by a violaceous zone (Fig. 10.44). *Staphylococcus aureus* is present in the ulcerated area and anaerobic or microaerophilic streptococci can be recovered from aspirates of the advancing edge. Therapy is with parenteral penicillin and another antibiotic chosen on the basis of the organisms identified from the lesion, together with wide excision of the necrotic tissue.

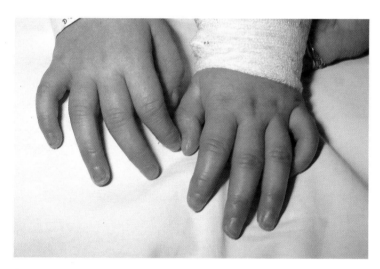

Fig. 10.41 Kawasaki disease. Swelling of the fingers and hands in a young child who satisfied the other criteria for the diagnosis of Kawasaki disease.

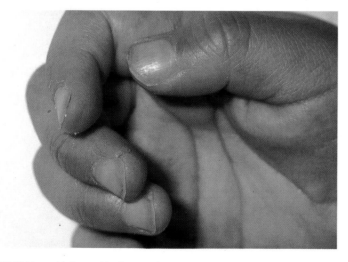

Fig. 10.42 Kawasaki disease. Membranous desquamation of fingertips begining in the periungual region. This occurs in almost all children during the subacute phase of Kawasaki disease.

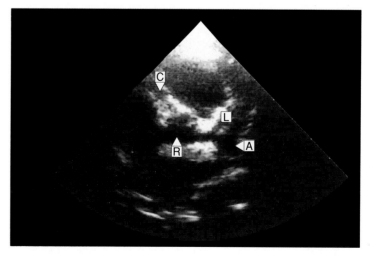

Fig. 10.43 Kawasaki disease. Echocardiogram in 7-month old showing giant aneurysm (A) of circumflex coronary artery. R = aorta. C = right coronary artery. L = left anterior descending coronary artery. By courtesy of Dr J. Wright.

Anaerobic cellulitis

This is a necrotizing infection of subcutaneous tissues usually occurring as a result of trauma or operations in the perineum, abdomen or lower extremities. It may be caused (alone or in combination) by clostridial species (usually *C. perfringens* or *C. septicum*), a variety of other, non-sporing anaerobic bacteria, and sometimes by aerobic bacteria such as streptococci, staphylococci and coliforms. There is a gradual onset of swelling and erythema and frank crepitus in the involved area (Figs 10.45, 10.46 & 10.47). There is little pain and the systemic toxicity of gas gangrene (see below) is absent. There may be a foul smelling discharge from the wound. In clostridial anaerobic cellulitis the discharge is thin and dishwater-like; in non-clostridial infection it is thicker and darker in colour. Radiology may show gas in the tissues (Fig. 10.48). Exploration of the wound should be performed to ensure that there is no myonecrosis. Treatment consists of surgi-

cal debridement and parenteral antibiotic therapy. In the patient shown in Fig. 10.49 for example, although *C. perfringens* had been grown from the wound, there was no involvement of muscle. Following debridement of the necrotic tissue and antibiotic therapy (given on the basis of the findings of gram-stained smears of the exudate) the patient made a good recovery.

Necrotizing fasciitis

Necrotizing fasciitis is a severe infection of the subcutaneous tissues and the superficial fascia. It is most commonly seen on the legs, the abdominal wall and the perineum. The infection either arises as a result of trauma or surgery in the presence of faecal soiling, or spreads from a perirectal abscess. The patient is often diabetic or alcoholic. The skin becomes inflamed and extremely tender and the changes progress rapidly over a few days. The skin becomes discoloured and bullae form, filled with

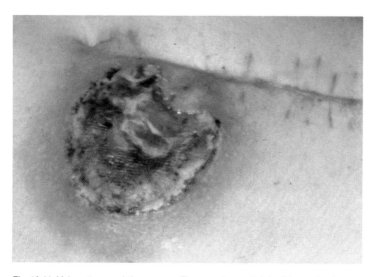

Fig. 10.44 Meleney's synergistic gangrene. The area of necrosis is begining to slough, revealing a granulomatous base. The surrounding area of erythema is quite narrow.

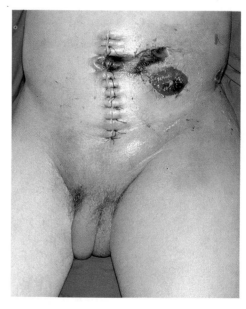

Fig. 10.45 Anaerobic cellulitis. Note the areas of cutaneous necrosis and the very extensive erythema and oedema extending upwards to the chest wall and downwards over the thigh.

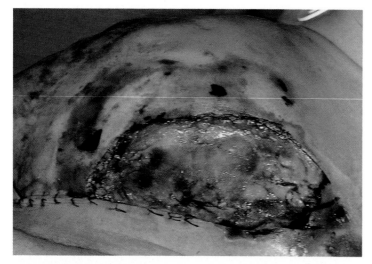

Fig. 10.46 Postoperative gangrenous cellulitis. A huge area of ulceration filled with gangrenous skin and slough lies adjacent to the wound. There is surrounding cellulitis and a further area of necrotic skin in the flank.

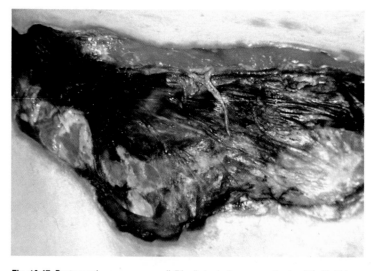

Fig. 10.47 Postoperative gangrenous cellulitis. (Later in the same patient as Fig. 10.46.) The cellulitis has resolved and the ulcerated area is filled with black necrotic tissue.

serosanguinous fluid (Fig. 10.50). As the infection spreads along fascial planes there is destruction of cutaneous nerves, leading to anaesthesia of the skin together with thrombosis of small vessels and the skin ultimately leading to gangrene. There is marked systemic toxicity. Subcutaneous gas is seen on radiography (see Fig. 10.50). Gram-stained smears usually reveal a mixture of peptostreptococci, *Bacteroides* species and a facultative anaerobe, such as one of the Enterobacteriaceae or a streptococcus.

Fournier's gangrene is a form of necrotizing fasciitis affecting the male genitals. It starts with scrotal swelling followed by progressive necrosis of the scrotal skin, the penis, the perineum and the lower abdominal wall (Fig. 10.51). The testes have their own blood supply and are almost never involved.

Therapy of necrotizing fasciitis must be prompt, with immediate surgical debridement of all necrotic tissue. Empirical antibiotic therapy should include agents directed at anaerobes, Enterobacteriaceae and streptococci and can be modified after bacteriological data are available.

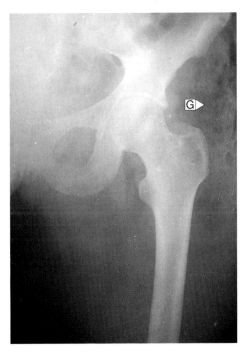

Fig. 10.48 Anaerobic cellulitis. Considerable amounts of gas (G) in the tissues of the thigh of a patient with anaerobic infection following intravenous drug abuse.

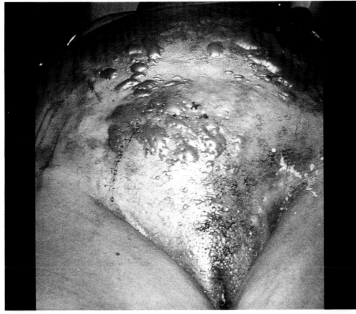

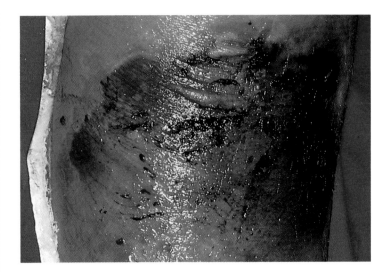

Fig. 10.49 Clostridial cellulitis, following a compound fracture of the tibia. Crepitus was noted on examination and the presence of gas was confirmed radiologically.

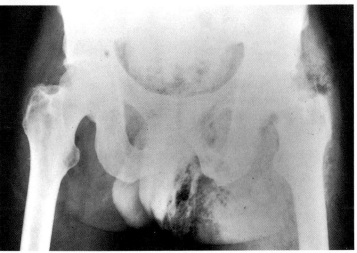

Fig. 10.50 Necrotizing fasciitis of the abdominal wall. Top: Multiple bullae and blackened areas of skin. Bottom: A soft tissue radiograph of the same patient shows gas in the tissues. By courtesy of Dr W. M. Rambo.

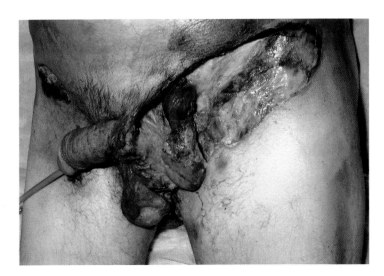

Fig. 10.51 Fournier's gangrene. Extensive necrosis of the skin and subcutaneous tissues of the scrotum and abdominal wall in a diabetic man. The presence of necrosis extending beyond the upper margin of the wound shows that insufficient debridement has been performed and further surgery is necessary.

Gas gangrene

Gas gangrene (clostridial myonecrosis) is a fulminant life-threatening infection of skeletal muscle caused by *C. perfringens* (Fig. 10.52). It follows the contamination of wounds with spores of the organism, which is a normal constituent of the faecal flora. *C. perfringens* produces a number of powerful toxins; of these, it is the α-toxin which is associated with the severe toxicity, haemolysis and myositis of gas gangrene. The incubation period is 1–4 days and the earliest symptom is severe pain at the site of the wound. The skin is pale and then assumes a bronze discolouration, followed by the appearance of haemorrhagic bullae (Fig. 10.53). There is often a distinctive, sweetish odour to the serosanguinous discharge.

There are often profound systemic features. Tachycardia and apprehension are prominent and there may be haemolysis and renal failure. In suspected cases it is imperative to examine the muscles for myonecrosis, the widespread coagulation necrosis of the muscle fibres and destruction of the connective tissues produced by α-toxin.

A Gram stain of the exudate or the muscle will show numerous gram-positive bacteria, but this finding does not determine the need for treatment. Affected muscles initially are pale and fail to bleed or contract on electrical stimulation (Fig. 10.54): later they become beefy red and then gangrenous and friable. If myonecrosis is present then immediate, extensive surgical debridement of involved muscles and fasciotomy to decompress the oedema is the only hope. Penicillin, chloramphenicol or metronidazole, gas gangrene antitoxin and hyperbaric oxygen are of help but must be regarded as of secondary importance to emergency surgery.

Animal bites

Bites from domestic dogs and cats are frequent and range from the trivial to the life-threatening. Infections are caused by the animals' oral bacterial flora. The most important organism in both dog and cat bites is *Pasteurella multocida*, a small gram-negative coccobacillus. Staphylococci, streptococci and anaerobic bacteria are

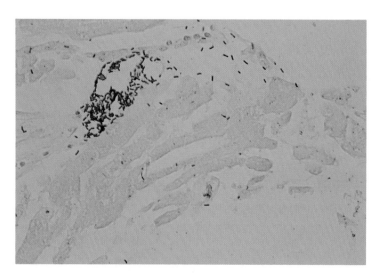

Fig. 10.52 Gas gangrene. Histology showing typical 'box-car' appearance of *C perfringens* in necrotic tissue. Spores are rarely seen in clinical specimens. Gram's stain. By courtesy of Dr J. Newman.

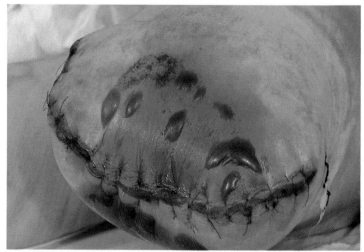

Fig. 10.53 Gas gangrene. Amputation stump with discolouration of skin and haemorrhagic bullae typical of gas gangrene. By courtesy of Dr J. Newman.

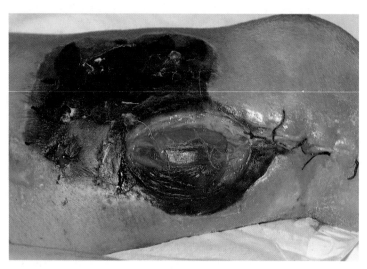

Fig. 10.54 Gas gangrene. There is a serosanguinous discharge from the lower end of the surgical wound and the affected muscles show pallor and failure to bleed. By courtesy of Mr E. Taylor.

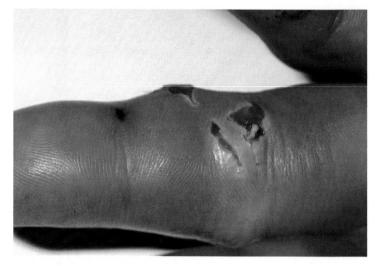

Fig. 10.55 Animal bite. Infected wound of finger following bite of domestic cat. *Pasteurella multocida* was isolated from the wound.

the other common pathogens. An infected animal bite usually presents with a localized cellulitis, a malodorous wound exudate and a low-grade fever (Fig. 10.55). Many bites occur close to bones or joints and septic arthritis, tendonitis and osteomyelitis sometimes occur. Antibiotic therapy for animal bites should include an agent active against *P. multocida*. Penicillin or ampicillin is very suitable but erythromycin and the penicillinase-resistant penicillins are less effective. Amoxicillin/clavulanic acid will cover all the likely pathogens and tetracycline can be used in the penicillin-allergic individual. Tetanus and/or rabies prophylaxis should also be considered.

Human bites

The normal human oral flora is capable of causing severe infections, either as a result of bites or in clenched fist injuries (lacerations that result from one individual striking another in the mouth with a clenched fist). The organisms responsible are α-haemolytic streptococci and various anaerobes including *Fusobacterium* spp. *Bacteroides* spp.

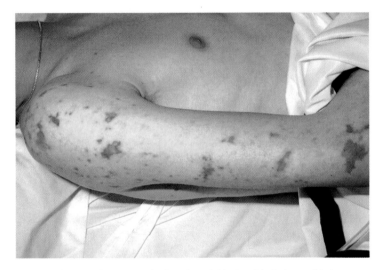

Fig. 10.56 Acute meningococcaemia. Note the variable size of the lesions and their peripheral distribution. Some of the lesions are obviously purpuric, others macular or papular.

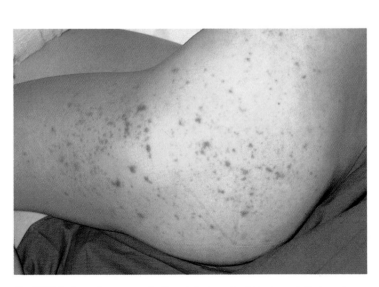

Fig. 10.57 Acute meningococcaemia. Purpuric lesions of variable size on buttocks and thighs.

and *Eikenella corrodens*. The latter is particularly important as it often produces an indolent infection and is resistant to clindamycin, metronidazole, penicillinase-resistant penicillins and some cephalosporins. Human bites and clenched fist injuries should probably not be managed with primary closure but require irrigation, debridement, immobilization, elevation and close observation. Penicillin plus a penicillinase-resistant penicillin or amoxicillin/clavulanic acid are the drugs of choice.

Pyomyositis

This is an acute bacterial infection of skeletal muscle that is characterized by intramuscular pus and is predominantly caused by *S. aureus*. Most cases occur in the tropics and it is often referred to as tropical myositis. It is not secondary to septicaemia and occurs in the absence of a penetrating wound. Why it occurs is far from clear. There is often a history of trauma followed a few days later by a subacute onset of pain, tenderness and swelling. The muscles chiefly involved are those of the legs or buttocks. Fever, chills and malaise follow. Initially the muscles may feel woody: only later does fluctuation appear. The diagnosis may be suggested by ultrasound or CT scanning but ultimately microbiological diagnosis rests upon aspiration or drainage of pus. In conjunction with drainage, a suitable anti-staphylococcal antibiotic is the suggested (empirical) therapy.

Meningococcaemia

The rash of meningococcal septicaemia varies a good deal in distribution and extent, as well as in the character of the individual lesions. The lesions of acute meningococcaemia in its most florid form are easily identified and virtually pathognomonic, with a mixed petechial and maculopapular rash most prevalent on the extremities and extensor surfaces (Figs 10.56 & 10.57). The rash starts as erythematous macules that are at first not purpuric, although their nature is revealed after a short while by their brown-stained appearance. Purpuric lesions vary in size between petechiae (Fig. 10.58) and ecchymoses of up

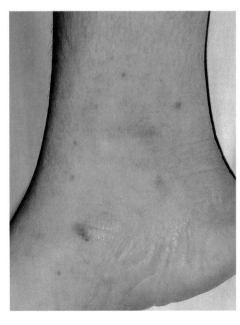

Fig. 10.58 Meningococcaemia. Petechiae on the ankle of a young child with meningococcaemia.

to several centrimetres in diameter with an irregular edge (Fig. 10.59). Petechiae may also be seen in the conjunctivae (Fig. 10.60). The central part of the skin lesions can undergo necrosis and extensive grey, haemorrhagic, necrotic patches may develop by confluence of several lesions (Fig. 10.61). Clinical meningitis is common (see Chapter 3) and the organism is often seen in the cerebrospinal fluid deposit. Gram-negative diplococci can occasionally be seen on smears obtained from the skin lesions of acute meningococcaemia. In the most severe form of meningococcal septicaemia, accompanied by hypotension and disseminated intravascular coagulation (see Chapter 13), peripheral gangrene and purpura fulminans occur (Figs 10.62 & 10.63).

Chronic meningococcaemia is an infrequent syndrome of recurrent episodes of fever, arthralgia and rash occurring over a few weeks. The rash coincides with the fever and occurs in crops of individual lesions, particularly on the extremities. The lesions may be maculopapular (Fig. 10.64), petechial, vesicular or pustular (Fig. 10.65) and are similar to those seen in gonococcaemia (see Chapter 7).

Rocky Mountain spotted fever

Rickettsiae are obligate intracellular bacteria with a cell wall similar to that of gram-negative bacilli. They may appear as small cocci or as rods. The diseases caused by the typhus and scrub typhus groups of rickettsiae are described in Chapter 13; the diseases caused by the spotted fever group, Rocky Mountain spotted fever (RMSF) being the most important, are detailed here.

RMSF is caused by *Rickettsia rickettsii,* which is transmitted to humans by the bite of an infected tick (either the dog tick *Dermacentor variabilis* or the wood tick *D. ander-*

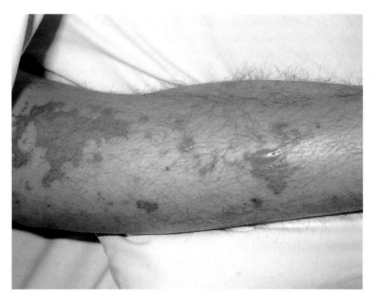

Fig. 10.59 Acute meningococcaemia. Large ecchymoses of variable size and with an irregular edge.

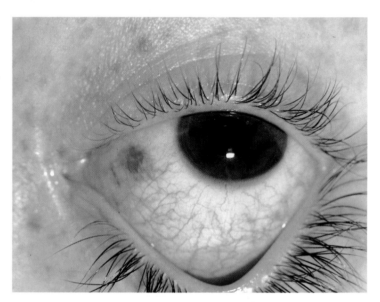

Fig. 10.60 Acute meningococcaemia. Petechia on bulbar conjunctiva.

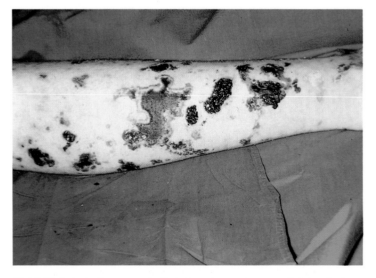

Fig. 10.61 Acute meningococcaemia. Ecchymoses have undergone central ulceration in the aftermath of the acute illness with subsequent skin necrosis. Skin grafting was required.

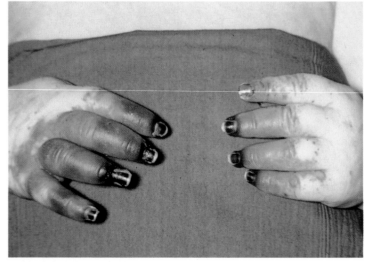

Fig. 10.62 Acute meningococcaemia. Gangrene of the extremities following a near-fatal illness with hypotension.

soni). It is not limited to the Rocky Mountain states of the USA and the vast majority of cases are now acquired in the central and southern Atlantic seaboard states and in the south-west central region (Fig. 10.66). Most cases occur in children, presumably reflecting close contact with the families' pet dogs.

Rickettsiae infect vascular endothelium and proliferate intracellularly. Vasculitis injury leads to increased vascular permeability and this results in oedema in various organs and hypovolaemia. The incubation period is about one week and the onset is usually sudden with fever, chills, myalgia and headache. The distinctive rash usually appears within 3–5 days of the fever and is seen in about 90% of all cases. Initial lesions are maculopapular, erythematous and on the extremities, especially around the wrists and ankles (Fig. 10.67). It rapidly spreads to the

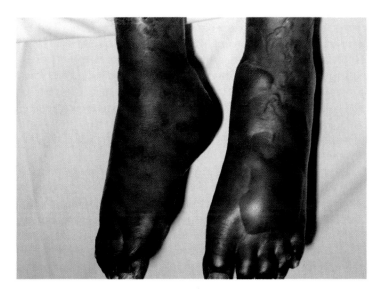

Fig. 10.63 Acute meningococcaemia. Gangrene of both legs in a black man with acute meningococcal infection. Bilateral below-knee amputations were later required.

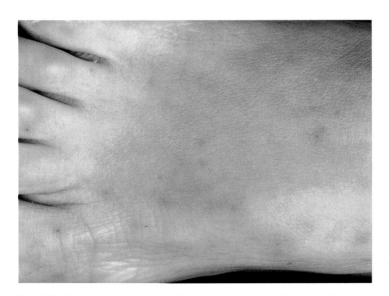

Fig. 10.64 Chronic meningococcaemia. Maculopapular lesions over the dorsum of the foot of a young woman with recurrent arthralgia and fever. *Neisseria meningitidis* was isolated from blood culture.

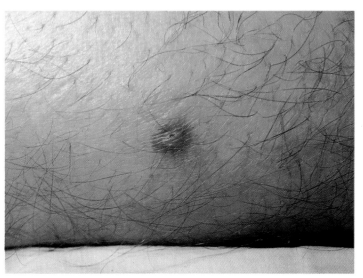

Fig. 10.65 Chronic meningococcaemia. Vesiculopustular lesion on the leg of a homosexual man with *N. meningitidis* bacteraemia. The lesion is similar to that seen in gonococcal septicaemia, which was the initial clinical diagnosis in this man.

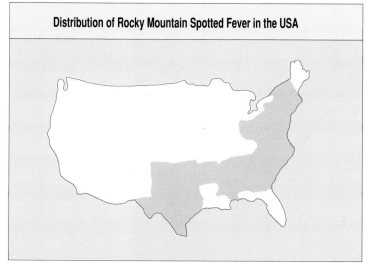

Distribution of Rocky Mountain Spotted Fever in the USA

Fig. 10.66 Map showing the area of the USA where most cases of Rocky Mountain spotted fever occur. Isolated cases occur almost anywhere else on the continental United States.

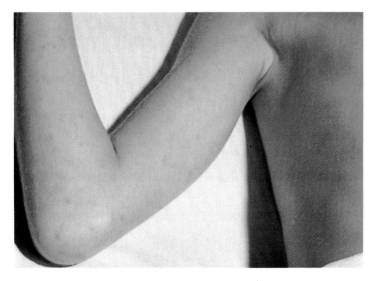

Fig. 10.67 Rocky Mountain spotted fever. A relatively sparse rash, first evident peripherally and spreading centripetally, in a 12-year-old boy. This picture was taken on the fifth day of illness. By courtesy of Dr T. F. Sellers, Jr.

trunk and becomes petechial and purpuric (Fig. 10.68). Involvement of the palms and soles is characteristic (Fig. 10.69). The most severe eruptions later resemble fulminant meningococcaemia with peripheral gangrene. Neurological manifestations are common (see Chapter 3) and renal failure and pulmonary oedema are also frequently seen. Death occurs in about 5% of cases but depends upon the speed with which appropriate antibiotic treatment is commenced.

Diagnosis during the acute phase must normally be clinical although direct immunofluoresence of skin biopsies from the rash can be undertaken at reference laboratories. Serological methods can be used for retrospective confirmation of the diagnosis. RMSF responds to oral tetracycline, doxycycline or chloramphenicol therapy given for about 7 days. The response is usually rapid and relapses are rare.

Other tick-borne spotted fevers

There are a variety of other tick-borne rickettsial illnesses in the Eastern hemisphere. Their names reflect the geographical areas where the disease is prevalent: Marseilles fever, South African tick typhus and Mediterranean fever (*fièvre boutonneuse*) are all caused by varieties of *R. conori*; Asian tick typhus by *R. siberica*; and Queensland tick typhus by *R. australis*. In most clinical and therapeutic respects these illnesses resemble RMSF. An important feature, however, is the presence of an eschar or *tache noire* at the site of the tick bite. This is a small painless ulcer with a central black necrotic area resulting from the endothelial damage caused by the rickettsiae (Figs 10.70 & 10.71). The rash is usually seen on the trunk, face and extremities (Figs 10.72 & 10.73).

Tropical ulcer

A form of chronic ulcer known as tropical ulcer is widespread in tropical Africa, Southeast Asia and South America. It starts as a painful swelling following minor injury or an insect bite and rapidly vesiculates and bursts to form a rapidly enlarging, painful ulcer. The lower half

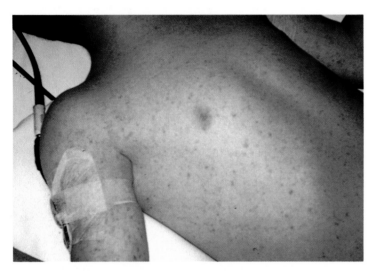

Fig. 10.68 Rocky Mountain spotted fever. Seventh day of illness in a small boy. A moderately severe eruption with macular and petechial elements of various size. By courtesy of Dr T. F. Sellers, Jr.

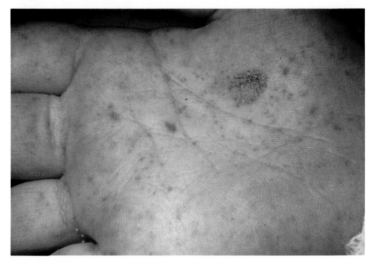

Fig. 10.69 Rocky Mountain spotted fever. Hand of the same patient (see Fig.10.68) on seventh day of illness. By courtesy of Dr T. F. Sellers, Jr.

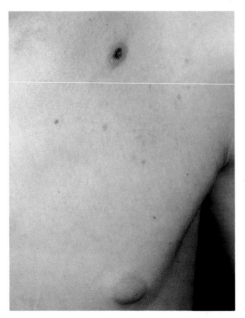

Fig. 10.70 South African tick typhus. Eschar (*tache noire*) at the site of the initial tick bite on the thorax. Sometimes this is not noticed by the patient but its presence may be suspected from regional lymphadenopathy. There is also a discrete macular rash over the thorax.

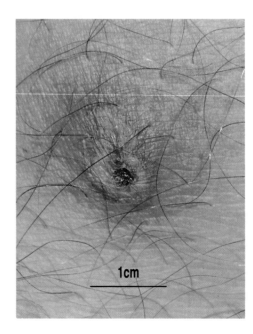

Fig. 10.71 Spotted fever. Close-up of an early eschar, showing a necrotic centre with surrounding erythema.

1cm

of the leg is the usual site. The floor of the ulcer is puru-lent and the edge of the lesion is typically slightly raised but not undermined (Fig. 10.74): the surrounding tissues are acutely inflamed. The exact aetiology of the condition is still unclear but recent evidence implicates dual infec-tion with *Fusobacterium fusiformis* and the spirochaete *Borrelia vincenti*. Treatment consists of a course of peni-cillin and wet dressings.

Cutaneous diphtheria

Diphtheritic infection of the skin may occur in the tropics and has also been seen in the USA among native Americans and homeless men. In hot, arid areas chronic ulceration is characteristic (veldt sore). The lesion proba-bly starts with contamination of an abrasion by organisms already present on the skin. The initial vesicle is painful and bursts to reveal a punched-out ulcer with grey slough at its base, which may persist for months. *Corynebacterium diphtheriae* is usually isolated in associ-ation with other bacteria. Wound infections and other forms of cutaneous diphtheria indistinguishable from impetigo may also occur. Although diphtheria exotoxin is secreted, paralysis and cardiac toxicity are rare.

Leprosy

Leprosy is still one of the most important infectious dis-eases, affecting many millions of persons worldwide. The organism responsible, *Mycobacterium leprae*, cannot be grown in tissue culture or synthetic media but is cultured in the footpads of mice or in armadillos. The organism invades skin and peripheral nerves and is probably spread by nasal secretions of patients with very bacilliferous forms of the disease (see below).

The spectrum of cutaneous lesions of leprosy is too wide to be fully represented here. Essentially, the clinical pre-sentation of leprosy depends on the host's immune response to infection with *M. leprae*. The form of disease determines infectivity and the likelihood of neurological damage. The type of disease can be assessed by clinical and histological evaluation.

In the lepromatous form of the disease (designated LL), the individual's cellular immune response is not activated. Lepromatous disease is characterized by widespread skin lesions and by the presence of abundant organisms. The latter can be demonstrated in preparations of nasal smears (Fig. 10.75), or in biopsy specimens taken even

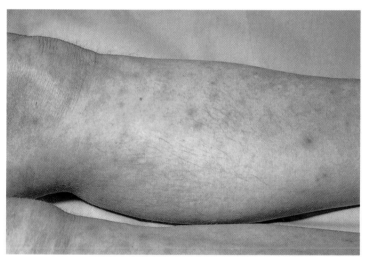

Fig. 10.72 Tick typhus; maculopapular rash over legs. By courtesy of Dr G. Wyatt.

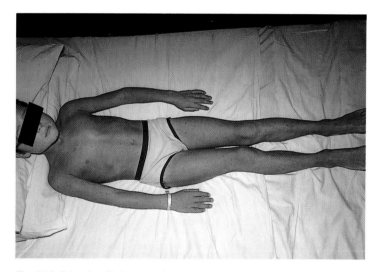

Fig. 10.73 Tick typhus. Rash over trunk and extremities in a child with *fièvre boutonneuse* due to *R. conori*.

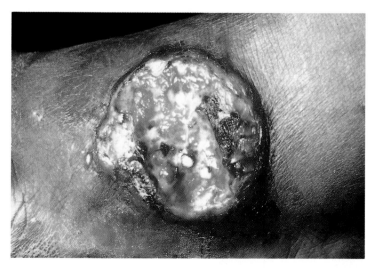

Fig. 10.74 Tropical ulcer. A typical lesion with a slightly raised edge on the foot of a patient from Africa. By courtesy of Prof. A. M. Geddes.

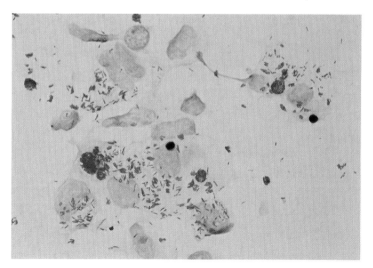

Fig. 10.75 Lepromatous leprosy. Smear from nasal mucosa showing numerous acid-fast bacilli. Ziehl–Neelson stain. By courtesy of Dr I. Farrell.

from apparently intact skin (Fig. 10.76). Patients with lepromatous disease may present with a widespread, discrete, erythematous or brown, papular or nodular eruption (Fig. 10.77). The lesions are not anaesthetic. As the disease extends the skin becomes thickened, producing a typical leonine facies (Fig. 10.78) with deeply wrinkled, thickened skin and thickened nose and ear lobes (Fig. 10.79). Loss of eyebrows, atrophic rhinitis, testicular atrophy and ocular damage are common.

Patients with tuberculoid leprosy (designated TT) have a more effective cellular immune response to *M. leprae*; they have fewer skin lesions, but are subject to damage to peripheral nerves mediated by delayed-type hypersensitivity reactions to mycobacterial antigen located in the sheaths and fibres (see also Chapter 3). Tuberculoid leprosy is characterized by a limited number of erythematous or hypopigmented skin lesions which may be macular or annular with a raised edge and an anaesthetic, dry and hairless centre (Fig. 10.80). Certain 'nerves of predilection' – the ulnar, median, radial, lateral popliteal and great auricular – are particularly likely to be damaged and

these nerves feel thickened (Fig. 10.81). The neuropathy of leprosy leads to specific palsies (Fig. 10.82); the anaesthesia leads to ulceration and loss of tissue (Fig. 10.83). Occasionally skin lesions are absent altogether – this pure neural leprosy presents as a mononeuritis multiplex involving one or more nerves of predilection which are characteristically thickened and, during states of heightened immune reactivity, tender. Histology of the skin in tuberculoid leprosy shows granulomata and absent or scanty bacilli (Fig. 10.84).

Borderline leprosy (designated BB) occupies a halfway position between TT and LL forms. (Intermediate forms are designated BT and BL.) It tends to be clinically unstable and patients usually move towards one of the polar forms of the disease. The skin lesions of borderline leprosy are variable in size, shape and marginal definition (Fig. 10.85). Nodules do not occur. Nerve thickening and widespread severe neuropathy is common.

The myriad complications of leprosy, and the detailed management that this infection requires, are beyond the scope of this account; however, the principles of therapy

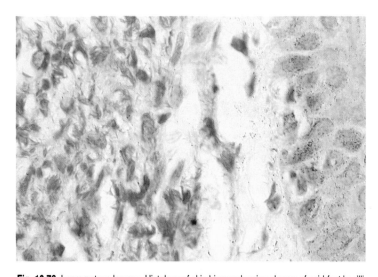

Fig. 10.76 Lepromatous leprosy. Histology of skin biopsy showing clumps of acid-fast bacilli (stained red) in the dermis. Ziehl-Neelsen stain. By courtesy of Dr C. J. Ellis.

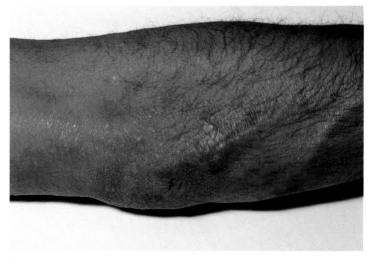

Fig. 10.77 Lepromatous leprosy. Papular and nodular lesions are visible in skin over the elbow.

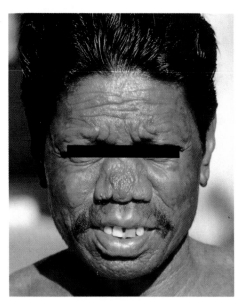

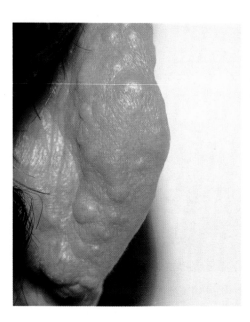

Fig. 10.78 Lepromatous leprosy. Typical 'leonine' facies with thickened infiltrated skin, widened nose and loss of eyebrows. By courtesy of Dr D. A. Lewis.

Fig. 10.79 Lepromatous leprosy. Numerous nodular skin lesions and thickening of pinna of patient with LL disease.

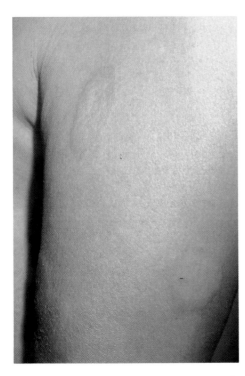

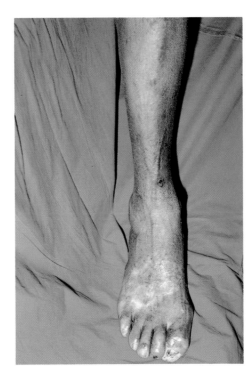

Fig. 10.80 Leprosy. Skin lesions of borderline tuberculoid (BT) leprosy showing raised erythematous margin. The centre of the lesion was anaesthetic. A similar solitary lesion is typical of tuberculoid (TT) disease. By courtesy of Dr C. J. Ellis.

Fig. 10.81 Tuberculoid leprosy. Thickened lateral perineal nerve over the ankle and foot. The depigmented lesion on the foot is a burn as a result of anaesthesia. By courtesy of Dr. C. J. Ellis.

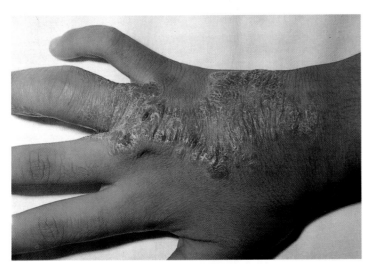

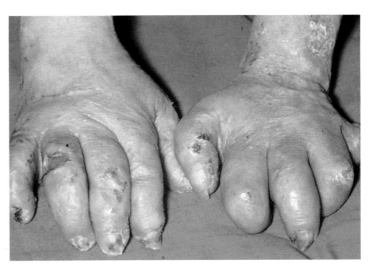

Fig. 10.82 Leprosy. Weakness of the small muscles of the right hand with early clawing of the ring and little finger, due to an ulnar nerve lesion. The skin lesion has a raised edge and anaesthetic centre. By courtesy of Dr. C. J. Ellis.

Fig. 10.83 Leprosy. Hands in advanced untreated leprosy showing gross deformity and loss of tissue.

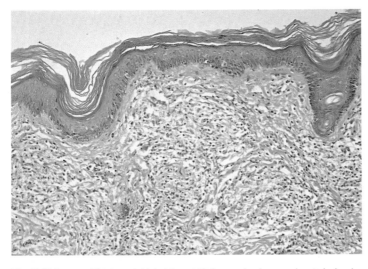

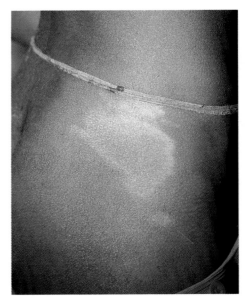

Fig. 10.84 Leprosy. Histology of skin in tuberculoid disease showing granulomata in dermis. By courtesy of Dr C. J. Edwards.

Fig. 10.85 Skin lesion of borderline leprosy over buttock of an African patient. This is a typical site. The skin is hypopigmented and anaesthetic. By courtesy of Dr D. A. Lewis.

are to render the patient non-infectious, to prevent further bacterial multiplication and to avoid or treat complications and reactions. Triple agent therapy with rifampicin, dapsone and clofazimine is recommended for multi-bacillary disease (LL, BL, or BB); dapsone and monthly rifampicin is given for pauci-bacillary forms (BT or TT). Contacts of highly infective LL or BL cases are given prophylaxis with dapsone.

Tuberculosis of skin

Although uncommon, cutaneous tuberculosis may display a variety of forms, depending on the pathogenesis. Skin lesions can be caused by bacterial replication at the site; others do not contain organisms, and are regarded (on the basis of histology) as an allergic reaction to tuberculosis infection elsewhere in the body: these latter conditions are called tuberculids.

Primary infection resulting from inoculation of the skin causes an indolent, shallow ulcer with an irregular base, and regional lymphadenopathy. Cutaneous infection may also arise as a result of acute generalized haematogenous dissemination from a site of tuberculosis elsewhere and cause cutaneous miliary disease, with pinhead lesions covering the entire body surface. More frequently, haematogenous spread to the skin from a distant site causes localized disease, termed lupus vulgaris (Fig. 10.86). This produces soft, rounded, brown or red papules, usually on the face or neck. Pressure upon the papule with a glass slide causes the lesions to turn an 'apple-jelly' colour. The plaques extend over a period of months and eventually scarring, contraction and destruction of tissue results (Fig. 10.87). Squamous cell carcinoma may develop as a complication. Organisms can be cultured from the skin. The condition is treated with a standard regimen of anti-tuberculosis therapy.

The tuberculids are classified in various ways, but the best recognized descriptions are the papulonecrotic tuberculid and lichen scrofulosorum. The former presents with crops of dusky red papules on the extremities (Fig. 10.88). Lichen scrofulosorum (Fig. 10.89) is sometimes seen in children or young adults with disseminated forms of tuberculosis. The lesions are not very prominent, consisting of groups of lichenoid papules often showing a perifol-

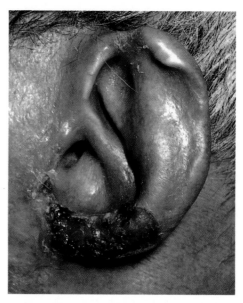

Fig. 10.87 Lupus vulgaris. Biopsy-proven cutaneous tuberculosis causing destruction of the pinna. By courtesy of Dr C. J. Ellis.

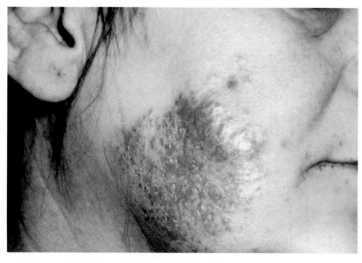

Fig. 10.86 Lupus vulgaris. An indolent, slowly spreading, reddish-brown plaque-like lesion characteristic of tuberculosis of the skin.

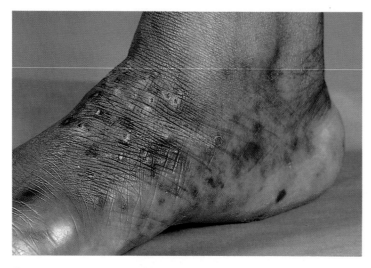

Fig. 10.88 Papulonecrotic tuberculid. Lesions on foot.

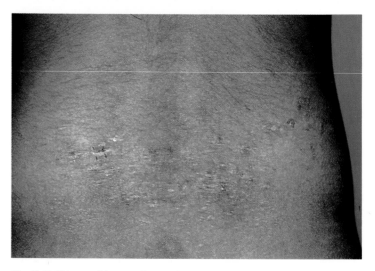

Fig. 10.89 Lichen scrofulosorum. Groups of very small lichenoid lesions on the trunk of a young adult with lymph node tuberculosis. The site of skin biopsy is visible.

licular distribution, usually seen on the trunk. These gradually regress over a period of months.

The nodular tuberculids are, in effect, forms of cutaneous vasculitis found in association with tuberculous infection. Erythema induratum (Bazin's disease) is found exclusively in women. Lumpy indurated lesions, very dark in colour, develop around the ankles and legs (Fig. 10.90) and may break down into ragged-edged shallow ulcers with a notably indolent course. Although evidence of tuberculosis elsewhere in the body is lacking, the patients show a high degree of tuberculin sensitivity and the lesions respond to treatment with antituberculous drugs. Less clinically-specific forms of cutaneous vasculitis are also sometimes associated with mycobacterial infection (Fig. 10.91).

Atypical mycobacteria

Mycobacteria other than *M. tuberculosis* and *M. leprae* can also cause skin diseases. Most result from inoculation of organisms from a natural reservoir and the characteristics are variable depending upon the organism involved.

Infection with *M. marinum*, an organism that inhabits water or marine organisms, causes swimming pool granuloma. Inoculation occurs in swimming pools, salt water and fishtanks. After an incubation period of several weeks, slowly enlarging, blue-purple papules develop, usually on the extremities (Fig. 10.92). Sporotrichoid spread with satellite lesions along lymphatics may occur. Therapy should be guided by sensitivity testing, as organisms vary in their susceptibility to antibiotics.

Infection with *M. avium–intracellulare* is one of the most common complications of AIDS and maculonodular cutaneous lesions may develop as part of the disseminated disease.

Rapidly growing mycobacteria such as *M. chelonae* cause skin lesions that may resemble pyogenic abscesses (Fig. 10.93).

Infection with *M. ulcerans* causes a chronic cutaneous lesion called Buruli ulcer. It is found in localized foci in Uganda, Nigeria, New Guinea and elsewhere. It spreads more slowly than a tropical ulcer (see above) and is characterized by undermining of subcutaneous tissue far beyond the limits of the obvious ulcer.

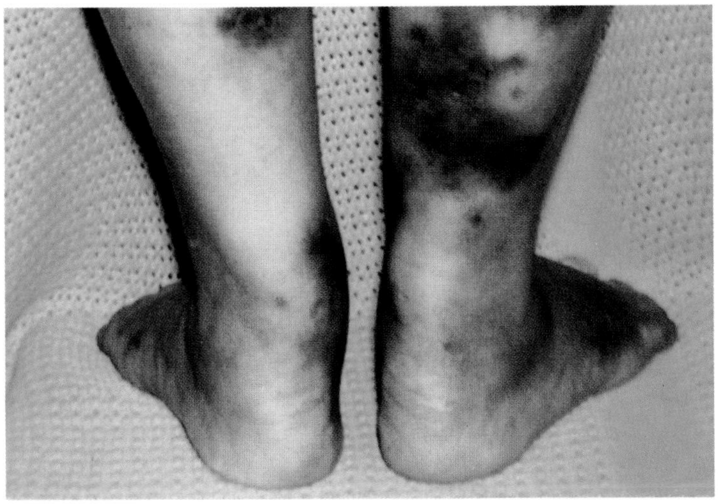

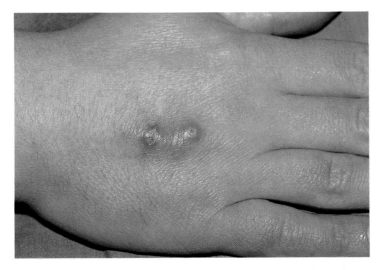

Fig. 10.90 Erythema induratum (Bazin's disease). Indurated nodular lesions in both legs. The skin is very dark and discoloured. The lesions may ulcerate.

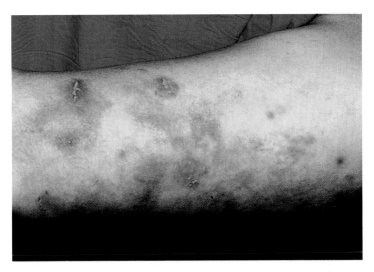

Fig. 10.91 Cutaneous vasculitis in atypical mycobacteriosis. There is irregular scarring, telangiectasis and nodular thickening. The patient was highly sensitive to tuberculin and developed an axillary abscess from which *Mycobacterium gordonae* was grown.

Fig. 10.92 Atypical mycobacteriosis. Fish tank granuloma due to *Mycobacterium marinum* over the dorsum of the wrist.

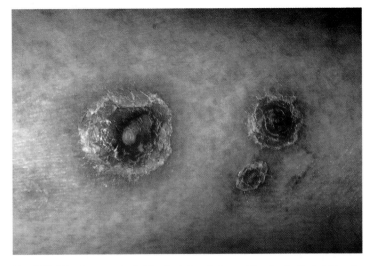

Fig. 10.93 Skin abscesses due to *Mycobacterium chelonae* at the site of self-administered insulin injections in the thigh of a diabetic patient. The syringe was not sterilized adequately.

Anthrax

Bacillus anthracis is a gram-positive spore-forming bacterium (Fig. 10.94) that primarily infects animals. Anthrax in humans occurs when persons come into contact with animals dying of anthrax, or wool and other products contaminated with the bacterial spores. Cutaneous anthrax develops when the spores are inoculated into a minor abrasion, usually on the face, neck or arms. The cutaneous lesion begins, 1–3 days later, as a small papule and is soon surrounded by vesicles. The central area becomes ulcerated and then dries to form the characteristic brown or black eschar, which slowly enlarges to cover the previously vesicular area. There is a wide area of surrounding non-pitting, gelatinous oedema but pus is not formed (Figs 10.95, 10.96 & 10.97). The lesion is painless and systemic symptoms are not prominent.

Fluid from the vesicles or from beneath the eschar show gram-positive bacilli, often in chains. The organisms can be seen in blood smears in occasional patients with bacteraemic dissemination. Treatment is with parenteral peni-cillin or tetracycline until the oedema settles; oral therapy is given for a further 5–7 days. Incision and drainage should not be performed.

Yaws

The classification of the treponemes that infect man is based upon the diseases they cause in man and in experimental animals. The species *Treponema pallidum* causes a variety of conditions and on the basis of these is divided into three subspecies. *T. pallidum* subspecies *pallidum* causes syphilis. Another subspecies, *T. pallidum* subspecies *pertenue*, causes yaws, a non-venereal disease that occurs in humid tropical countries. It is spread from skin to skin in children living in unhygienic conditions.

The early lesions occur about one month after infection and consist of papillomatous skin lesions that superficially erode and then heal spontaneously after a few months (Fig. 10.98). Some weeks or months later there are similar, but generalized lesions; these continue to reappear at intervals for several years. Osteitis and periostitis also

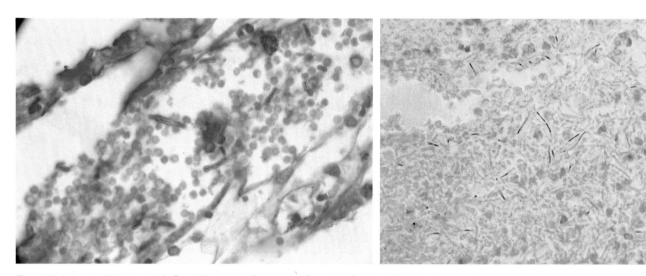

Fig. 10.94 Anthrax bacilli in tissues.Left: Gram/Wiegert stain. Right: Hucker/Conn stain. Courtesy of Dr I. Farrell.

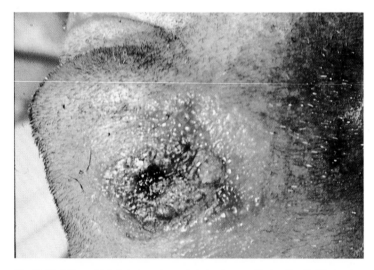

Fig. 10.95 Anthrax. Clinical photograph on admission (same patient as Fig. 10.96), showing characteristic black eschar surrounded by a ring of vesiculation. There is much oedema of the neck and face. By courtesy of Dr F. J. Nye.

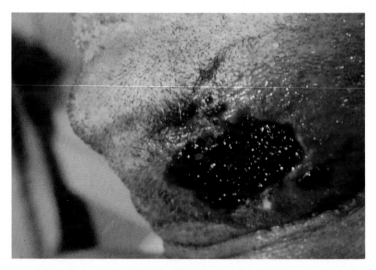

Fig. 10.96 Anthrax. Eight days after Fig. 10.95 was taken, the eschar has enlarged to cover the previously vesicular area, and the surrounding oedema has diminished. By courtesy of Dr F. J. Nye.

occur during the secondary stage (Fig. 10.99). In the late stage of yaws there are hyperkeratoses of the palms and soles and gummatous lesions in the bones. Yaws can be diagnosed by dark-ground microscopy or by serological testing for treponemal antibodies. Treatment with a single injection of benzathine penicillin usually leads to improvement within 2 weeks.

Pinta

Pinta is a non-venereal treponemal infection caused by *T. carateum* and occurring in Central America and Colombia. Transmission is similar to that for yaws. The primary lesions, however, are small pruritic papules on the face or trunk which then enlarge and coalesce. They may take several years to heal (Fig. 10.100). At the same time disseminated lesions, known as pintids, appear. As the

lesions heal they become depigmented (Figs 10.101 & 10.102). Diagnosis and treatment is similar to that for yaws, although it may take several months for the lesions to heal.

Lyme disease

Lyme disease (see also Chapters 3 and 8) is a multisystem disorder that is now known to be caused by the tick-transmitted spirochaete *Borrelia burgdorferi*. The infection occurs in many parts of the world and affects all age groups. Tick bites usually occur in the summer and autumn months and the onset of the illness is generally between May and November. The illness begins with a characteristic skin rash called erythema chronicum migrans (ECM) which begins within a few weeks at the site of the tick bite. ECM starts as a small indurated red

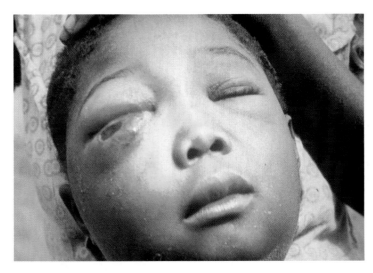

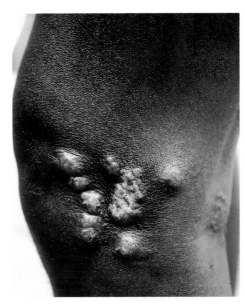

Fig. 10.98 Yaws. Papillomatous lesions on the knee. By courtesy of Dr P. J. Cooper.

Fig. 10.97 Anthrax. The eschar can be seen on the lower eyelid and there is extensive oedema of the face. By courtesy of Dr T. F. Sellers, Jr.

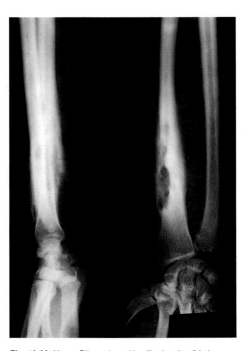

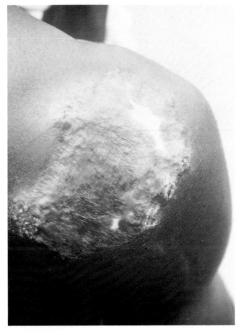

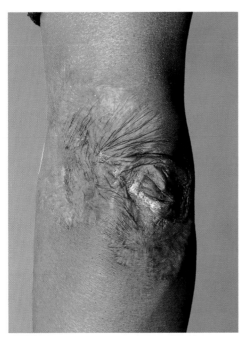

Fig. 10.99 Yaws. Bilateral osteitis affecting the tibia in secondary yaws. Courtesy of Dr A. M. Davies.

Fig. 10.100 Pinta. Primary lesion over shoulder. Courtesy of Dr G. Griffin.

Fig. 10.101 Pinta. Depigmented late lesion of yaws on elbow. By courtesy of Dr J. Clay.

macule or papule that progresses to form an annular plaque with a clear centre and a red-blue outer border (Fig. 10.103). This primary ECM lesion may be 50–60cm in diameter (Fig 10.104). In the USA secondary lesions appear within a few days in a significant number of individuals, although such lesions are uncommon in European cases. These secondary lesions are similar, but smaller than the primary one. During this first stage of Lyme disease, patients may also have fever, headache, stiff neck and meningism, musculoskeletal pains, fatigue and malaise, often intermittent and changing. The skin lesions tend to last for several weeks although the dermatological manifestations of Lyme disease may recur.

The later musculoskeletal, cardiac and neurological stages of Lyme disease are described elsewhere in the relevant chapters.

The diagnosis of Lyme disease presently relies upon serological techniques, although the optimal test is still to be determined. IgM titres rise within two and six weeks whereas IgG titres may take months to peak. The initial antibody response seems to be directed at one of the flagellar antigens of the spirochaete. Later responses are to other components of the organism.

The best treatment for ECM and the early stages of Lyme disease is probably amoxycillin and probenecid, or doxycycline, for at least 10 days. These seem to offer theoretical advantages over tetracycline or penicillin and may be more effective at preventing the later neurological and musculoskeletal stages of Lyme disease.

Erythema nodosum

This condition consists of red, raised, painful, tender, discrete yet ill-defined nodules (Fig. 10.105), usually occurring on the shins (Fig. 10.106), but less commonly on the upper limbs and face. The lesions are usually symmetrical. They progress over days or weeks to a more indolent purple-brown appearance before gradually subsiding. Fever, malaise and painful swelling of the ankles are common accompaniments. Erythema nodosum is a form of cutaneous vasculitis that represents a hypersensitivity reaction with numerous clinical associations. The most frequent are sarcoidosis, primary tuberculosis, β-haemolytic streptococcal infections, leprosy, yersiniosis, coccidioidomycosis and histoplasmosis. It may also be precipitated by drugs, inflammatory bowel disease and cer-

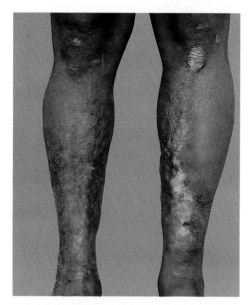

Fig. 10.102 Pinta. Depigmented lesions of late pinta. By courtesy of Dr J. Clay.

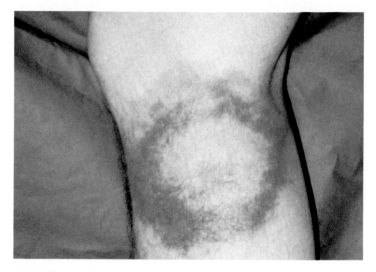

Fig. 10.103 Lyme disease. Rash of erythema chronicum migrans on leg. By courtesy of Dr E. Sahn.

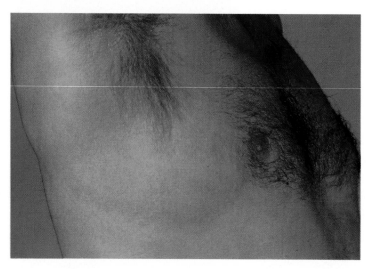

Fig. 10.104 Lyme disease. Margin of large erythema chronicum migrans lesion extending over chest wall and around axilla. By courtesy of Dr V. E. Del Bene.

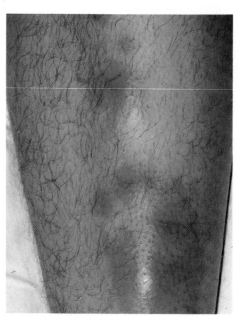

Fig. 10.105 Erythema nodosum; close-up of purple-red nodular lesions on shins. By courtesy of Prof. A. M. Geddes.

tain collagen diseases. Rarely, the following infections have also been associated with erythema nodosum: orf, cat-scratch disease, psittacosis, other chlamydial infections and measles.

Therapy should be directed at eliminating the underlying cause. Symptoms are treated with aspirin or anti-inflammatory therapy.

Erythema multiforme

Erythema multiforme is a hypersensitivity reaction that develops in response to an infection (often seemingly banal and unidentified) or to drugs or other chemicals. The skin lesions appear suddenly over any body area, including the palms and soles. As its name implies, the lesions of erythema multiforme vary greatly; maculopapular, petechial and vesicular elements may all be seen, but the characteristic element is the target lesion, in which the initial lesion spreads in an annular fashion, followed by the development of a new spot in the middle of the ring (Figs 10.107, 10.108 & 10.109). Usually only the skin is affected but inflammation and sometimes ulceration of the oral, ocular and genital mucosal surfaces may also occur: it is then termed the Stevens–Johnson syndrome (see Figs 10.110 & 10.111; see Chapters 1 & 12).

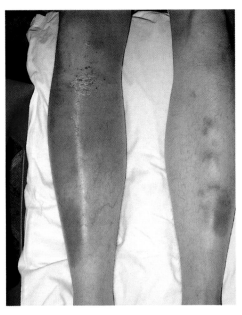

Fig. 10.106 Erythema nodosum. Lesions are typically symmetrical over lower legs. By courtesy of Prof. A. M. Geddes.

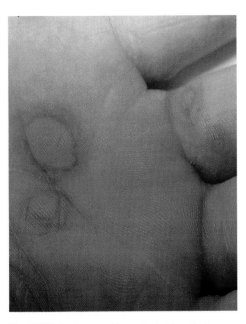

Fig. 10.107 Erythema multiforme. Typical target lesions on the palm.

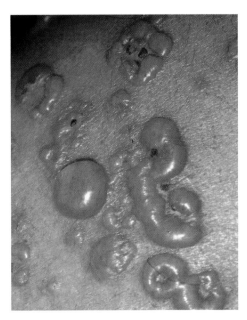

Fig. 10.108 Erythema multiforme. Annular target-like vesicular lesions.

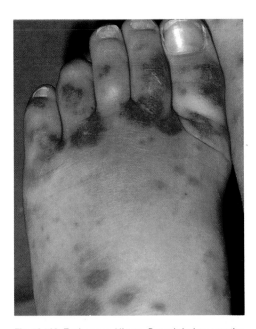

Fig. 10.109 Erythema multiforme. Purpuric lesions over the foot. Although these lesions are not as typical as those shown above, the target-like configuration of some of these lesions can still be discerned.

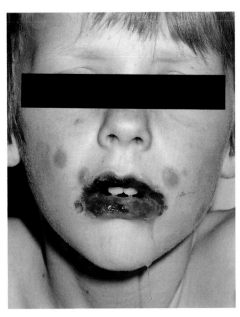

Fig. 10.110 Stevens–Johnson syndrome. Lesions of erythema multiforme can be seen on the face, together with involvement of the mouth.

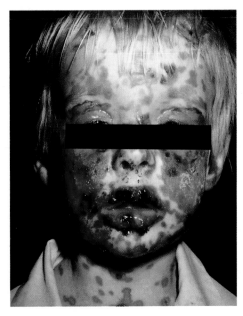

Fig. 10.111 Stevens–Johnson syndrome. Severe illness with marked cutaneous and mucous membrane lesions of erythema multiforme.

The best established infective associations of erythema multiforme are herpes simplex and *Mycoplasma pneumoniae*; others include histoplasmosis, coccidioidomycosis and infections caused by coxsackie virus B5, adenoviruses, *Salmonella*, *Yersinia* and *Mycobacterium* species. The other well established association is drug exposure, notably to sulphonamides and phenylbutazone.

Toxic erythema

Other less severe forms of toxic erythema are fairly common and enter into the differential diagnosis of infectious diseases affecting the skin. Some may develop as a form of allergy to antimicrobial or other drugs (Figs 10.112, 10.113 & 10.114).

PROTOZOAL AND HELMINTH INFECTIONS

Leishmaniasis

Leishmaniasis is caused by protozoa of the genus *Leishmania*. It is a zoonosis with animal reservoirs in rodents, dogs and other canines and other mammals. Sandflies feed on the infected mammal and ingest amastigote forms of Leishmania. Within the fly's gut the parasites become promastigotes, replicate and are then inoculated into another host (sometimes human) when the sandfly next feeds.

Leishmania are the cause of a wide spectrum of human disease. Visceral leishmaniasis (*Kala azar*) is caused when *Leishmania donovani* infects the entire reticuloendothelial system and is described in Chapter 13. The other species of *Leishmania* have mainly dermal or mucosal manifestations. In the Old World three distinct species of *Leishmania* can be distinguished by isoenzyme analysis, monoclonal antibodies or DNA analysis: *L. tropica*, *L. major* and *L. aethiopica*. In the New World there are two main species complexes: *L. mexicana* and *L. braziliensis*.

Old World cutaneous leishmaniasis is prevalent in Mediterranean countries, the Middle East through to North Eastern India, in the Congo basin and in China.

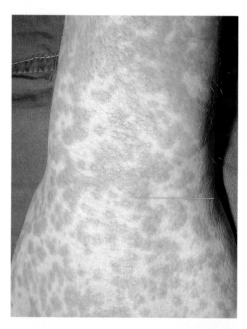

Fig. 10.112 Toxic erythema. Typical toxic rash following ampicillin therapy.

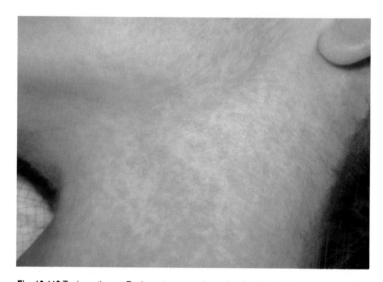

Fig. 10.113 Toxic erythema. Erythematous macular rash, allergic in origin. Measles, rubella and scarlatina have to be considered in the differential diagnosis. By courtesy of Dr T. F. Sellers, Jr.

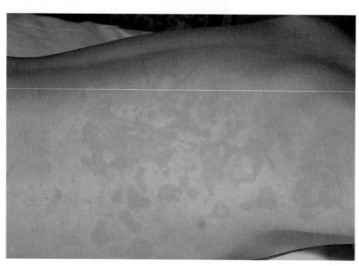

Fig. 10.114 Toxic erythema. Urticarial plaques in a young man with drug allergy. Some of the plaques have cleared centrally to form annular lesions.

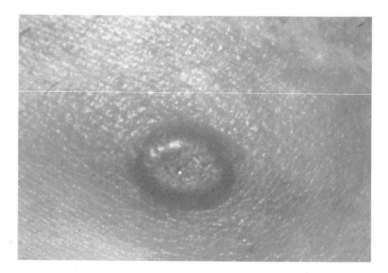

Fig. 10.115 Cutaneous leishmaniasis. Early stage of *Leishmania tropica* infection showing local lesion with erythematous surround at site of sandfly bite.

The rural form is caused by *L. major* which has a reservoir in gerbils and other rodents; the urban form, due to *L. tropica*, infects dogs and humans. After an incubation period ranging from 2 weeks to several months, an itchy red papule appears at the site of the sandfly bite (Fig. 10.115). The papule develops into a shallow ulcer which slowly enlarges with a well-marked edge and a base of granulation tissue (the oriental sore or Delhi boil – Fig. 10.116). The granulating base of the ulcer may contain a hard excrescence. Lesions of *L. tropica* are usually single and take many months to heal, while *L. major* usually gives rise to multiple lesions and heals more quickly. After healing there is a flat, atrophic, depigmented scar (Fig. 10.117).

New World cutaneous leishmaniasis is widespread in South and Central America. The manifestations range from small, dry cutaneous lesions to a progressive mutilat-ing mucosal infection. The infection is most common in persons who work at the edge of the forest which is the natural habitat of the sandflies. The localized cutaneous disease is similar to that caused in the Old World, ranging from dry lesions (Fig. 10.118) to large deep ulcers (Fig. 10.119). In some patients with *L. braziliensis* infection, however, mucous membrane involvement (espundia) develops some months after the cutaneous lesions have healed. The process often starts in the septum of the nose and may extend to destroy the whole of the front of the face, the process taking months or many years. The definitive diagnosis of leishmaniasis depends upon the demonstration of amastigotes in smears or aspirates taken from a lesion (Fig. 10.120).

Large or potentially disfiguring lesions are usually treated. The drugs used are pentavalent antimonials; the optimal treatment regimens are a matter for expert opinion.

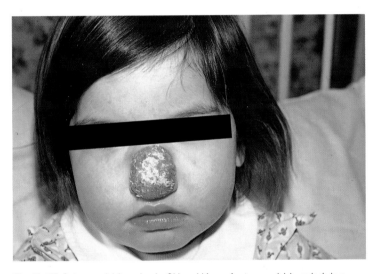

Fig. 10.116 Cutaneous leishmanisasis. Old-world form of cutaneous leishmaniasis in a young child from the Middle East.

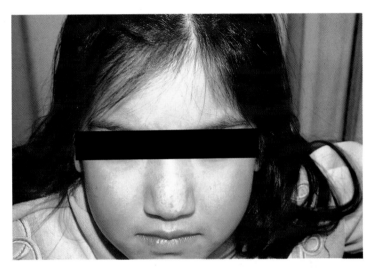

Fig. 10.117 Cutaneous leishmaniasis. Scarring on nose of child (see Fig. 10.116) after healing.

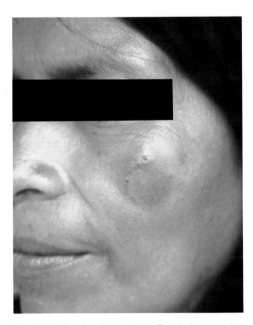

Fig. 10.118 American leishmaniasis. Early lesion caused by *L. braziliensis* on the face of young woman. By courtesy of Dr P. J. Cooper.

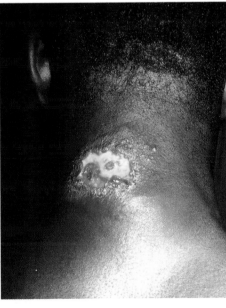

Fig. 10.119 American leishmaniasis. Cutaneous ulcer on neck caused by *L. braziliensis*. By courtesy of Dr P. J. Cooper.

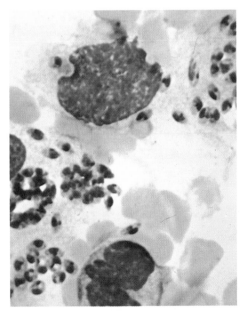

Fig. 10.120 American leishmaniasis. Leishmanial organisms within macrophages in aspirate from lesion of Old World leishmaniasis.

Trichinosis

Trichinosis is a ubiquitous disease of man and animals acquired by eating raw or undercooked meat containing encysted larvae of the roundworm, *Trichinella spiralis*. In most cases the meat is pork or wild boar, but recently a number of cases have been traced to bear or walrus meat and even (occasionally) horsemeat. Following ingestion, the cyst walls are digested in the stomach and the viable larvae pass into the small intestine. They attach to the mucosal lining and develop into adult worms. Each fertilized female releases several hundred larvae over a period of about two weeks before she dies. The newborn larvae burrow into the intestinal lymphatics, then move via the thoracic duct to the general circulation, by which means they are distributed throughout the body. In most tissues they are killed by the inflammatory response which they

elicit, but in skeletal muscle (particularly in the diaphragm, chest wall, biceps and gastrocnemius) they become encysted (Figs 10.121, 10.122, 10.123 & 10.124) and remain viable and infectious. After many years they die and the lesions eventually calcify.

Most infections are asymptomatic but heavy exposure may cause diarrhoea or an illness characterized by fever, muscle pain, and periorbital oedema. Diarrhoea and abdominal pain is caused by the adult worms in the intestine and is usually seen only in the first few days after ingestion. The other symptoms are associated with the burden of larvae in the muscles. Occasionally conjunctivitis (Fig. 10.125) and haemorrhages in the conjunctivae and nail beds (Fig. 10.126) are present. In extremely heavy infections a fatal myocarditis or encephalitis may occur. The systemic symptoms are usually maximal after 2–3 weeks and then subside slowly.

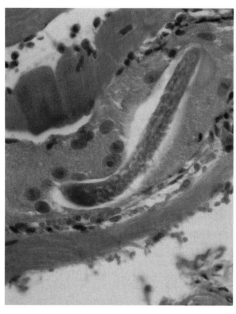

Fig. 10.121 Trichinosis. Early stage of infection showing larva of *Trichinella spiralis* in skeletal muscle before encystment. By courtesy of Dr I. G. Kagan.

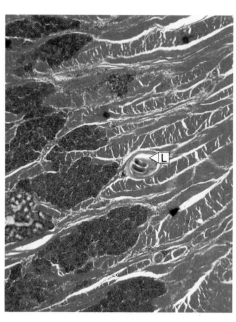

Fig. 10.122 Trichinosis. Coiled encysted larva of *T. spiralis* (L) in muscle of tongue. H & E stain.

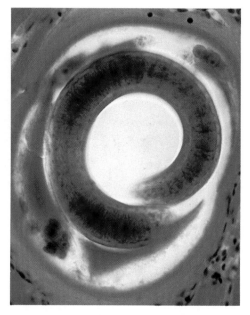

Fig. 10.123 Trichinosis. High power view of coiled larva of *T. spiralis* in fully formed cyst within striated muscle of tongue, showing hyaline capsule of the cyst. H & E stain.

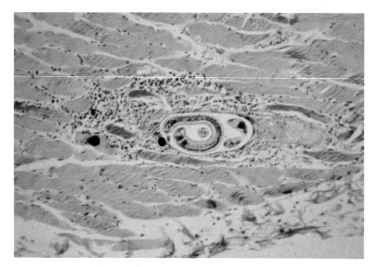

Fig. 10.124 Trichinosis. Coiled encysted larva of *T. spiralis* in striated muscle showing intense inflammatory reaction around cyst. Trichrome stain. By courtesy of Dr I. G. Kagan.

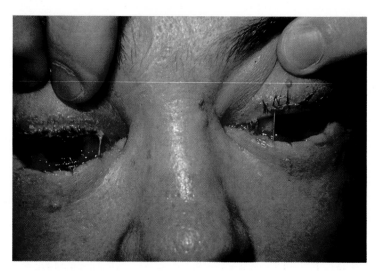

Fig. 10.125 Trichinosis. Oedema of eyelids and intense conjunctivitis with conjunctival haemorrhages in a comatose patient with trichinosis. By courtesy of Dr T.F. Sellers, Jr.

The diagnosis is suspected on finding an impressive eosinophilia and elevated muscle enzyme levels, and confirmed by finding the larvae in a fresh specimen of muscle pressed between two glass slides (Fig. 10.127). When larvae are not seen a rise in antibody titre may substantiate the diagnosis, although antibodies are not detectable until three or more weeks after infection. The bentonite flocculation test is the most reliable and widely used test.

There is no satisfactory treatment for trichinosis: thiabendazole is effective against the adult worms but it does not kill the larva in muscle. Hence it can only be used in individuals known to have ingested contaminated meat but who have not yet developed symptoms. Mebendazole may be more effective against the larvae. Corticosteroids may have some value in suppressing the intense inflammatory reaction in vital organs in critically ill patients. Trichinosis is best prevented by proper cooking of meat (until there is no trace of pink flesh). Smoking and salting of meat is not reliable.

Cysticercosis

Infection with the larvae of *Taenia solium* (cysticercosis) most often produces symptoms referable to the central nervous system (see Chapter 3), but the larvae may also develop in skeletal muscle (Fig. 10.128). After a few years the organism dies and the wall of the cyst eventually calcifies. The condition is usually clinically silent and is generally only recognised when soft tissue x-rays are taken in asymptomatic patients with other conditions and the characteristic calcified cysts are seen (Fig. 10.129).

The larval forms of the fish tapeworm (*Diphyllobothrium latum*) may also affect man. The intermediate forms of this tapeworm are found in certain amphibians or reptiles; humans may become infected by eating raw snakes or frogs (a delicacy in China and other parts of the Far East). The larvae migrate to subcutaneous tissues or muscles and may produce lumps over the surface of the body. This larval stage is termed a sparganum and the disease is called sparginosis.

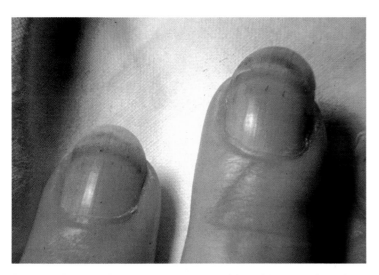

Fig. 10.126 Trichinosis. Splinter haemorrhages in the nail beds of the same patient as in Figure 10.125. By courtesy of Dr T. F. Sellers, Jr.

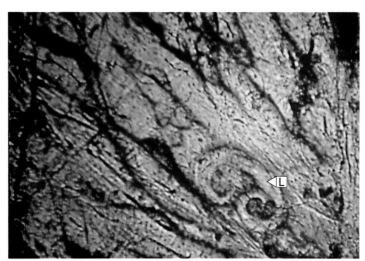

Fig. 10.127 Trichinosis. Coiled larva of *T. spiralis* (L) seen in a fresh specimen of muscle (taken from the same patient as in Figure 10.125) pressed between two glass slides. By courtesy of Dr T. F. Sellers, Jr.

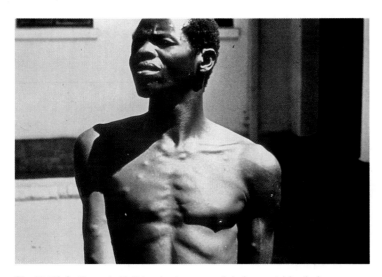

Fig. 10.128 Cysticercosis. Multiple subcutaneous cystic lesions containing the larvae, which are known as *Cysticercus cellulosae*. By courtesy of Dr. M. G. Schultz.

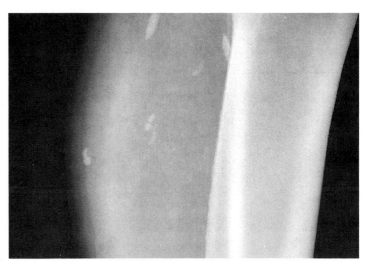

Fig. 10.129 Cysticercosis. Radiograph of leg showing characteristic elongated calcified cysts of *T. solium*. At this site they produce no symptoms.

Onchocerciasis

Onchocerciasis is a filarial infection caused by *Onchocerca volvulus* which is prevalent in tropical Africa and parts of South America. The life cycle is simple, involving only man. The larval filaria, known as microfilariae, are transmitted by blackfly bites. They mature into adult worms located free in the dermis, or in tangled groups which give rise to nodules in the skin overlying bony prominences. The resulting microfilariae migrate through the dermis (Fig. 10.130) and cornea, provoking an inflammatory reaction. The cycle is completed when they are taken up by blackflies and transmitted to new hosts. The flies breed in fast flowing water and feed on the human population living and farming on river banks. When onchocerciasis is prevalent such prime land is rendered uninhabitable. The eye changes are described in Chapter 12.

The main symptom of the dermatitis an intense itching, usually most severe in areas of the skin in which nodules of up to 5cm in diameter can be palpated (Fig. 10.131). In time the dermis becomes thickened and leathery with loss of pigmentation (Figs 10.132 & 10.133). This is often most evident on the shins, the main target for blackfly bites. A chronic regional lymphadenitis ensues.

Diagnosis is established by microscopic examination of excised nodules in which tangles of adult filariae are seen (Figs 10.134 & 10.135) or, more simply, by examination of 'skin snips'. These are obtained by piercing the skin with a fine needle, raising the needle tip to form a 'tent' of skin, and slicing off a tiny piece. Snips are placed on a microscopic slide in a drop of saline and examined under low power after about half an hour. If the skin is infected, microfilariae are seen wriggling in the saline (Fig. 10.136). Treatment is with diethylcarbamazine which, however, evokes active itching and conjunctivitis with visual deterioration. Ivermectin, a newer microfilaricide, has the advantage of not provoking host reactions. Nodules containing adult worms can be removed surgically (Fig. 10.137).

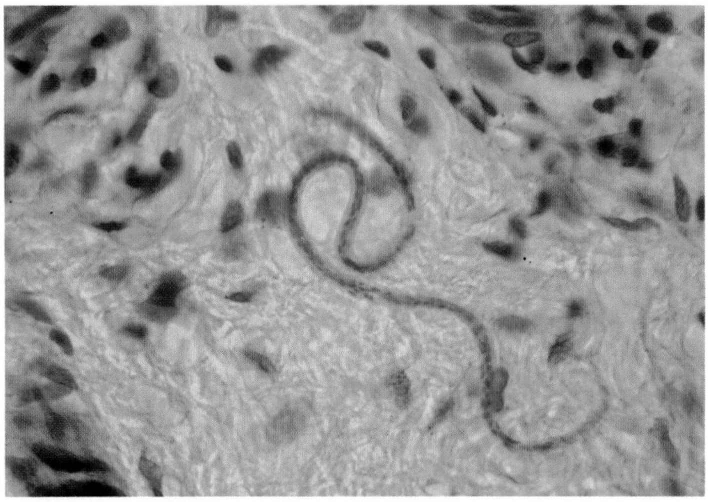

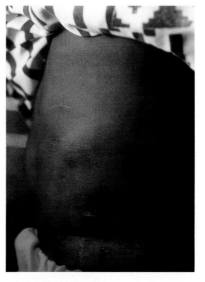

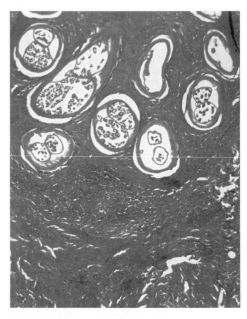

Fig. 10.131 Onchocerciasis. Nodule containing adult worm over abdominal wall. By courtesy of Dr P. J. Cooper.

Fig. 10. 130 Onchocerciasis. Microfilaria in cutaneous tissues.

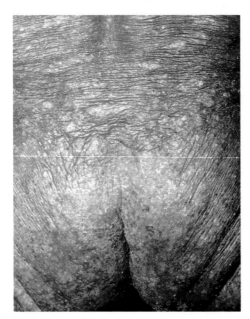

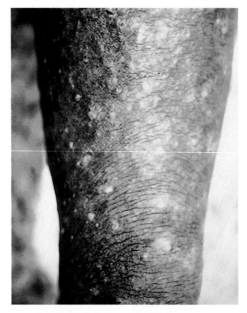

Fig. 10.132 Onchocerciasis. Thickened leathery skin over lower back and buttocks of 50-year-old man. By courtesy of Dr P. J. Cooper.

Fig. 10.133 Onchocerciasis. Thickened leathery skin with patchy depigmentation on the thighs of an African man. By courtesy of Dr C. J. Ellis.

Fig. 10.134 Onchocerciasis. Section through a subcutanous nodule showing a granulomatous lesion containing numerous adult forms of *Onchocerca volvulus*. H & E stain.

Cutaneous larva migrans

Also known as creeping eruption, this lesion consists of a migrating serpiginous eruption which is intensely itchy. A patient may have a single lesion or they may be very numerous. They develop as a result of infestation with larval nematodes of various species, usually dog or cat hookworms of low human pathogenicity, but sometimes from human nematode species. The animal hookworms produce eggs which are then shed with the animal's faeces, often on beaches or other sandy areas. The larvae hatch and are able to penetrate human skin, but lack the enzyme necessary for them to leave the epidermis. The track marks the route of the parasite as it wanders aimlessly in the skin (Figs 10.138 & 10.139). Although the lesions gradually disappear without treatment, topical or systemic thiabendazole leads to more rapid resolution.

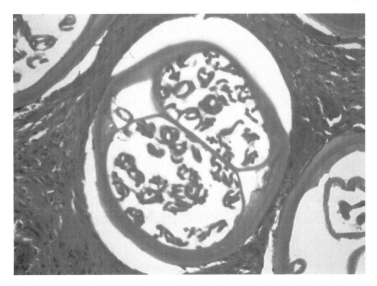

Fig. 10.135 Onchocerciasis. Higher power of section through female *O. volvulus* showing numerous immature microfilariae within the uterus.

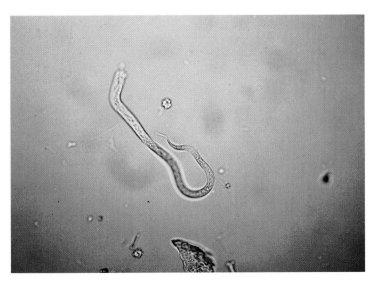

Fig. 10.136 Onchocerciasis. Microfilaria obtained after immersing skin snip from infected individual in saline solution.

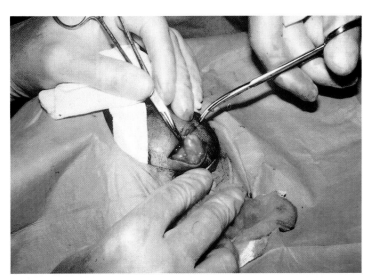

Fig. 10.137 Onchocerciasis. Nodule containing adult worm being surgically removed. By courtesy of Dr P. J. Cooper.

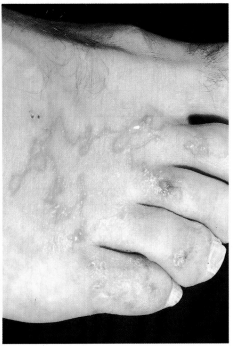

Fig. 10.139 Cutaneous larva migrans. Track of larval migration on dorsum of foot.

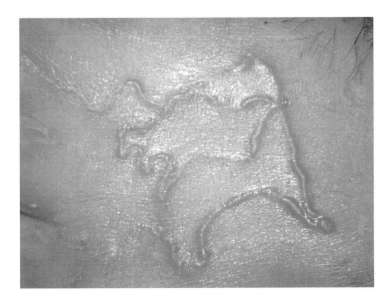

Fig. 10.138 Cutaneous larva migrans. Creeping eruption with characteristic serpiginous raised lesion. By courtesy of Dr K. A. Riley.

Dracunculiasis (Guinea worm infection)

Estimates of the number of people infected with *Dracunculus medinensis* in Africa, the Middle East, India and other tropical areas range from 50–150 million. It has been estimated that the number of people at risk from unsafe drinking water may be as high as 800 million. Infection is acquired by ingesting water containing infected crustaceans (copepods), primarily of the genus *Cyclops*. The larvae are released in the stomach, pass into the small intestine and penetrate the mucosa to reach the retroperitoneal space, where they complete their maturation and mate. The female worm slowly migrates, over a period of about a year, to the subcutaneous tissues (Fig. 10.140), usually in the legs. A painful papule develops at the site which eventually ulcerates, exposing a portion of the worm (Figs 10.141 & 10.142). When this area comes in contact with water, large numbers of larvae (Fig. 10.143) are released from the uterus of the worm. They are then ingested by copepods to complete the life cycle.

At the time of the larvae are released, the patient may develop a systemic illness with allergic symptoms, and secondary bacterial infection of the ulcers is common. Treatment with niridazole or thiabendazole reduces the inflammation and enables the worm to be removed by gently rolling it around a small stick.

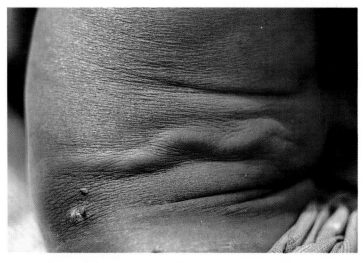

Fig. 10.140 Dracunculiasis. Subcutaneous female worm beneath skin of lateral aspect of trunk.

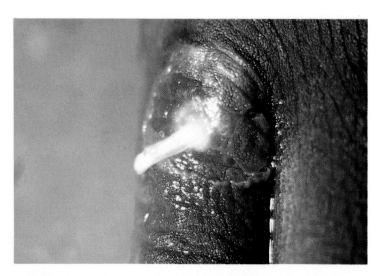

Fig. 10.141 Dracunculiasis. Female guinea worm being extruded from skin of finger.

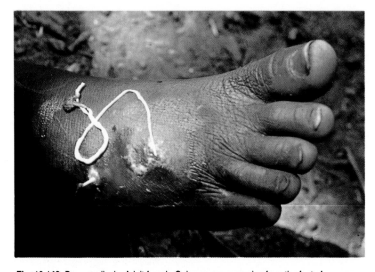

Fig. 10.142 Dracunculiasis. Adult female Guinea worm emerging from the foot of a young child. The foot is swollen and there is cellulitis due to secondary bacterial infection along the track of the worm. By courtesy of Dr R. Muller.

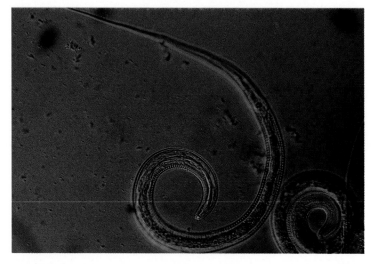

Fig. 10.143 Dracunculiasis. First stage larvae of *D. medinensis* living in water. By courtesy of Dr R. Muller.

11

SKIN AND SOFT TISSUE

VIRAL, FUNGAL AND ECTOPARASITIC INFECTIONS

VIRUSES

Measles (Rubeola)

Humans are the only natural host for measles virus, an RNA containing, pleomorphic, enveloped paramyxovirus with a worldwide distribution. The virus remains infective for several hours in droplet form and measles is spread by direct contact with droplets of respiratory secretions. The disease is very readily communicable and epidemics tend to occur in young children every 2–5 years in countries where the use of measles vaccine is not widespread.

The incubation period of measles is 10 to 14 days and is followed by a prodromal phase that corresponds to the secondary viraemia. The prodromal symptoms are cough, coryza, conjunctivitis, fever and anorexia and normally last for 2–4 days. During this period the epithelium of the entire respiratory tract is inflamed and reddened and patients are at their most infectious: croup, bronchiolitis

and viral pneumonitis (characterized by multinucleate Warthin–Finkeldey giant cells – see Fig. 2.12) may occur.

Koplik's spots (see Figs 11.1 & 1.19) are to be found towards the end of the prodrome and can still be seen during the first two days of the skin eruption. Koplik, writing in 1896, was the first to observe this pathognomonic sign of measles; the enanthem he described can be seen as minute bluish white spots on an erythematous base, varying in number from a few to hundreds. The spots are best seen in the buccal groove at the level of the lower premolars but extend upwards on the mucous membrane of both gum and cheek; they can sometimes be seen in the conjunctiva.

The measles rash appears first on the temples and behind the ears (Fig. 11.2) then spreads rapidly over the face (Fig. 11.3) and down the body to involve the trunk and limbs (including the palms and soles). It is generalized, maculopapular, erythematous and often somewhat purplish in tinge. Individual spots are irregular in shape

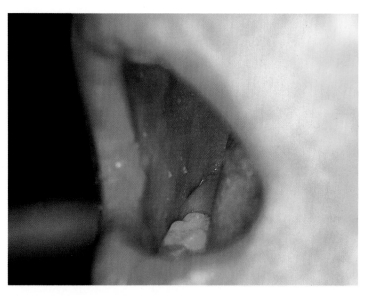

Fig. 11.1 Measles (rubeola). The minute white dots seen on the inflamed buccal mucosa are Koplik's spots.

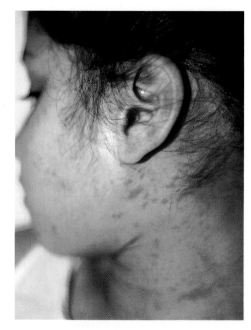

Fig. 11.2 Measles (rubeola). The rash often begins behind the ears. Koplik's spots were visible on the buccal mucosa of this Asian child.

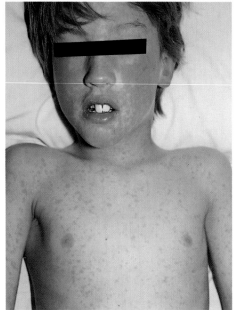

Fig. 11.3 Measles (rubeola). The rash is already prominent on the face and is spreading down the body onto the trunk and extremities.

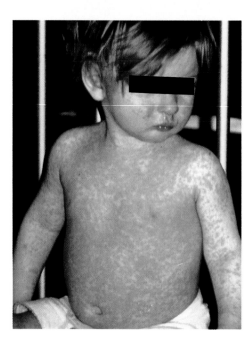

Fig. 11.4 Measles (rubeola). Blotchy purplish generalized rash in a child with a runny nose and sore eyes.

and of variable size. As it progresses, the rash often becomes confluent on the face and upper trunk (Figs 11.4 & 11.5). In black skins the appearance may be deceptive, with paler follicular dots on a dark background (Fig. 11.6). The rash is believed to represent cell-mediated hypersensitivity to the measles virus and the appearance of the rash coincides with the development of serum antibody and the end of communicability of the infection.

After a few days of uncomplicated measles, fever subsides and the rash fades at the same time. Capillary leakage at the height of the illness is revealed by transient purpura (post-measles staining) in the distribution of the rash (Fig. 11.7). The common complications of measles are secondary bacterial infections of the respiratory tract (particularly pneumonia and otitis media) and a form of post-infectious hypersensitivity encephalitis (see Chapter 3). Malnourished children in the tropics often develop very severe measles, which is frequently complicated by secondary herpes simplex infection (Fig. 11.8). In patients with defective cellular immunity, measles can be a very severe illness: giant cell pneumonia may develop without any evidence of a rash.

Atypical measles

An unusual form of measles has been seen in patients infected by measles virus several years after receiving killed measles vaccine. The immunity induced by this vaccine is partial and does not include antibodies against the viral protein that enables the measles virus to penetrate into cells. The rash, which often starts peripherally and may be vesicular, urticarial or haemorrhagic, is accompanied by interstitial pneumonitis and the illness may be more prolonged and severe than typical measles. It is recommended that those who have received killed vaccine and who may be exposed to wild virus should be re-immunized with live vaccine (even though this may produce severe local reactions in such persons).

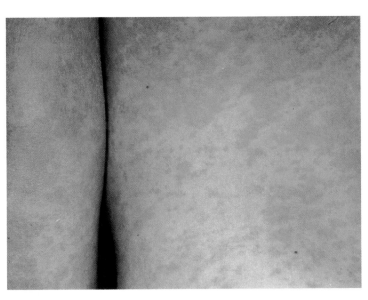

Fig. 11.5 Measles (rubeola). The rash is irregular, with some small discrete lesions and other blotchy confluent areas.

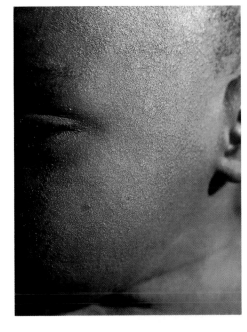

Fig. 11.6 Measles (rubeola) rash on a black child, merely showing slight follicular swelling on a darker background.

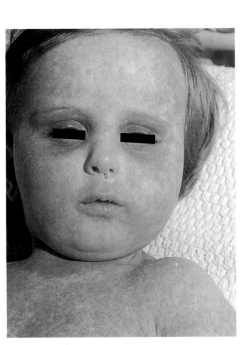

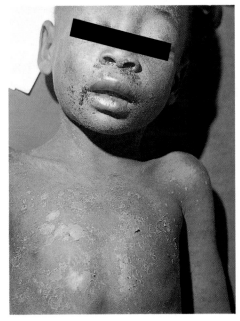

Fig. 11.7 Measles. During the healing phase, a transient brown staining of the skin may be apparent in white children.

Fig. 11.8 Severe measles with desquamating skin rash and herpes simplex stomatitis and rhinitis in an African child. The child died from respiratory complications.

Classic measles is usually easy to diagnose clinically but laboratory methods may be needed for atypical cases. A rapid diagnosis can be made by the immunofluorescent detection of measles antigens in nasopharyngeal cells but the usual laboratory method is the demonstration of measles antibody by a haemagglutination inhibition test.

No specific treatment for measles is available but active immunization with live vaccine confers immunity which is probably lifelong. It is usually given as part of the MMR (measles, mumps and rubella) vaccine at 15–18 months of age. Passive immunization with immune globulin is recommended for those who are susceptible to measles and who are at high risk of severe or fatal infection (children with cell-mediated immunity defects or malignancy). The immune globulin should be given within 6 days of exposure to measles.

Rubella (German measles)

Rubella virus, an enveloped RNA virus in the Togaviridae family, is moderately infectious and spread by droplets of respiratory secretions. It is most frequently seen in primary school children and cases are most numerous during the spring. The large epidemics of infection that previously occurred every 5–10 years have been prevented in countries where vaccination is widespread.

The incubation period of rubella averages 18 days with a range of 12–23 days. The clinical features of rubella (notoriously) vary from patient to patient. Children tend to have milder disease than adults and do not usually have prodromal symptoms: adults may have several days of malaise and fever before adenopathy and rash appear.

The lymphadenopathy may be generalized, but the posterior cervical and suboccipital lymph nodes are characteristically enlarged. It may last for several weeks. The exanthem of rubella is a discrete, pink, diffuse, macular rash which is most marked upon the face and trunk on the first day (Figs 11.9, 11.10 & 11.11), then spreads peripherally along the limbs on the second day before disappearing on the third and fourth day. In black children the rash is extremely difficult to detect (Fig. 11.12).

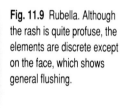

Fig. 11.9 Rubella. Although the rash is quite profuse, the elements are discrete except on the face, which shows general flushing.

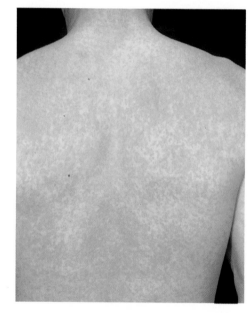

Fig. 11.10 Rubella. A typical diffuse macular rash over the trunk.

Fig. 11.11 Rubella. Close up of the rash in Fig. 11.10.

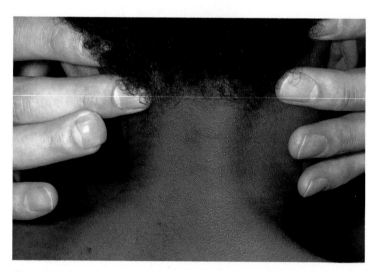

Fig. 11.12 Rubella. This young black child has occipital and posterior cervical lymphadenopathy, serologically confirmed to be due to rubella. The skin changes are limited to slight prominence of the follicles.

Other common features of rubella are mild conjunctival injection (Fig. 11.13), pharyngeal injection and petechial lesions (Forscheimer spots) on the palate (Fig. 11.14). Subclinical infection is common, and the rash and lymphadenopathy may be so trivial and transient that many cases escape diagnosis. Even when a rash is evident it may easily be mistaken for mild measles, scarlatina, parvovirus infection, secondary syphilis, or an enterovirus eruption (see Chapter 7 and below); the rash of infectious mononucleosis is also very similar (Fig. 11.15) but this infection can usually be differentiated by its associated clinical and haematological features (see Chapter 1).

The diagnosis of rubella is confirmed serologically. The haemagglutination–inhibition (HAI) technique was widely used but has now been superseded by several simpler methods, including passive latex agglutination, enzyme-linked immunosorbent assay (ELISA) and radial haemolysis. IgG and IgM antibodies to rubella can be distinguished and an acute infection diagnosed within a few hours.

The most common complication of postnatal rubella is arthritis due to the virus itself; this occurs in adult women more frequently than in children or adult men (see Chapter 8). Thrombocytopenia is occasionally seen in children with rubella (Fig. 11.16). The effects of rubella upon the fetus are described in Chapter 3.

There is no specific therapy for rubella. Live vaccines are used in an attempt to prevent congenital rubella. The USA and the UK vaccinate young children and susceptible women just after delivery of an infant. Other countries vaccinate girls as they approach puberty. Despite specific immunity, reinfection with rubella virus is now known to occur. Although most such reinfections are asymptomatic, viraemia (and hence clinical illness and transmission of virus to the fetus) can occur.

Roseola infantum (exanthem subitum)

This disease of infants aged 6 months to 3 years is now believed to be caused by primary infection with the recently discovered human herpes virus type 6 (see Figs 11.17 & 11.18). The incubation period is 10–15 days and there is not usually any prodromal illness. The usual first symptom

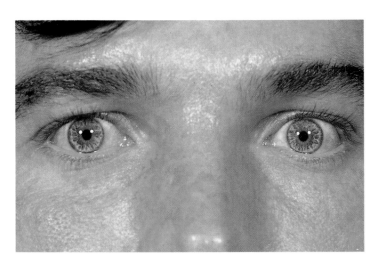

Fig. 11.13 Rubella. Mild conjunctivitis sometimes occurs but it is not usually as severe as that seen in measles.

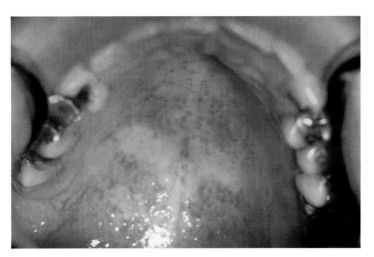

Fig. 11.14 Rubella. Petechial lesions (Forscheimer spots) on the palate. These are not diagnostic for rubella and in this case are exceptionally profuse.

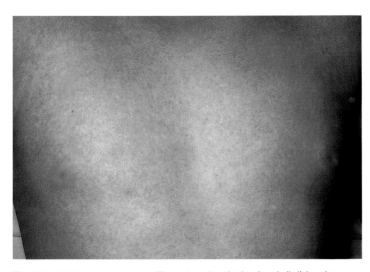

Fig. 11.15 Infectious mononucleosis. The rash can be mistaken for rubella if the other features are not prominent.

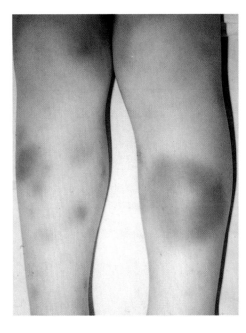

Fig. 11.16 Rubella. Thrombocytopenia following rubella caused petechiae and ecchymoses in this child. By courtesy of Prof. A. M. Geddes.

is high fever, sometimes with lymphadenopathy, and this lasts for a few days during which the child appears quite well. As the fever resolves it is followed by a maculopapular rash of central distribution which itself lasts for a few hours to a few days (Fig. 11.19). Apart from occasional febrile convulsions, complications are most unusual and immunity to infection appears lifelong.

Erythema infectiosum (Fifth disease)

Although the cause of this illness was long assumed to be a viral infection, the discovery that the aetiological agent was parvovirus type B19 was only made in 1984. This is a small (22–23nm diameter) DNA-virus (Fig. 11.20) that causes a biphasic illness in susceptible volunteers. About one week after infection there is a viraemia for a few days. At this time there are non-specific symptoms but 7–10 days later there is rash and arthralgia. At the same time there is a fall in haemoglobin concentration.

Fifth disease is seen usually in school-age children, sometimes in small epidemics during the winter or spring. The incubation period is 4–14 days and infection is probably spread by droplets. A short prodrome of fever may occur in adults but is rare in children in whom the rash is often the only feature. The rash has three stages; the first is the 'slapped cheeks' appearance (Fig. 11.21). A variable, often reticular rash on the limbs (Fig. 11.22) appears a day or so later. During the third stage, this peripheral rash may appear to settle, only to reappear with temperature, exercise or emotion. Some patients have systemic features with fever, adenopathy and gastrointestinal symptoms. Arthralgia and arthritis are particularly likely to occur in adults with parvovirus B19 infection and may occur in the absence of a rash. Parvovirus-specific IgM can

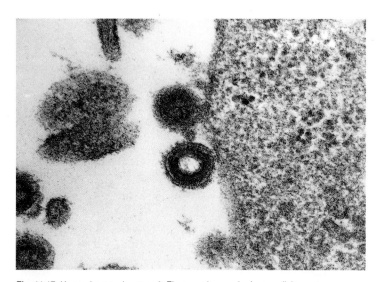

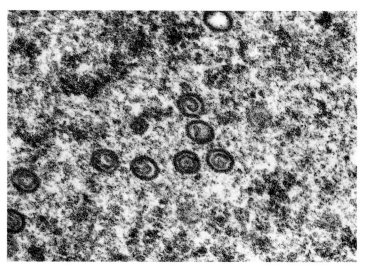

Fig. 11.17 Human herpes virus type 6. Electron micrograph of extracellular, mature, enveloped HHV-6 virus budding from a cell. Negatively stained. By courtesy of Dr D. Robertson.

Fig. 11.18 Human herpes virus type 6. Electron micrograph of HHV-6 capsids in a cell nucleus. By courtesy of Dr D. Robertson.

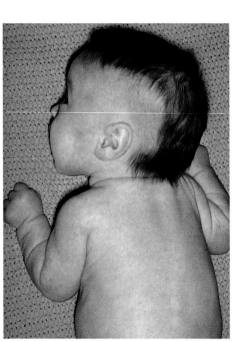

Fig. 11.19 Roseola infantum. The rather non-specific maculopapular rash with a central distribution developed as fever, subsiding on the third day of illness.

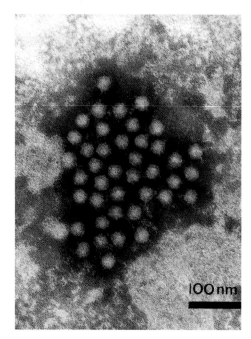

Fig. 11.20 Erythema infectiosum. Immuno-electron micrograph of parvovirus B19 virions in the blood. By courtesy of Regional Virus Laboratory, East Birmingham Hospital.

100 nm

be detected and used as a diagnostic test. After acute infections adults are likely to remain fatigued and depressed for several weeks. It is also recognised that parvovirus infection may affect the fetus and lead to spontaneous abortion or hydrops fetalis.

In patients with certain kinds of chronic haemolytic anaemia, infection with parvovirus B19 causes aplastic crises. This is due to an inhibition of the bone marrow erythroid precursors by the virus. Cytotoxic effects of the virus can be seen in the erythroid precursor cells.

Herpes simplex

The herpes viruses are all large DNA viruses and herpes simplex virus (HSV) is typical in that it consists of a nucleocapsid containing the viral genome, outside which there is a protein tegument and then a trilaminar outer envelope (Fig. 11.23). The virus is unable to survive for long in the environment and does not penetrate intact keratinized skin. Transmission is principally by intimate contact. HSV has a worldwide distribution and causes a variety of different mucocutaneous clinical illnesses. Following primary infection, the virus induces lifelong latent infection in sensory nerve ganglia. Recurrent infection occurs frequently. The factors that precipitate recurrences differ between individuals but include menstruation, fever, UV light, trauma, emotional stress, and menstruation. HSV infections of the mouth, nervous system, genital tract and eyes are described in Chapters 1, 3, 7 and 12 respectively. Only the cutaneous manifestations of herpes simplex infection will be described here.

Primary HSV skin infections may occur at any site as a result of direct inoculation of the virus through traumatised skin. This may occur as a result of wrestling (herpes gladiatorum) or other contact sports such as rugby football (Fig. 11.24) or by transfer of infection from oral sites to

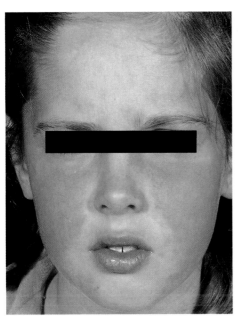

Fig. 11.21 Erythema infectiosum. The rash on the face is frequently described as having a 'slapped-cheeks' appearance.

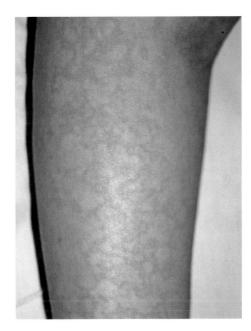

Fig. 11.22 Erythema infectiosum. The rash on the extremities often clears centrally to produce a lace-like appearance.

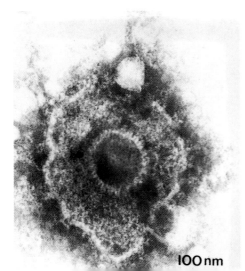

Fig. 11.23 Herpes simplex virus. Electron micrograph of HSV from vesicle fluid. Negatively stained. By courtesy of Regional Virus Laboratory, East Birmingham Hospital.

100 nm

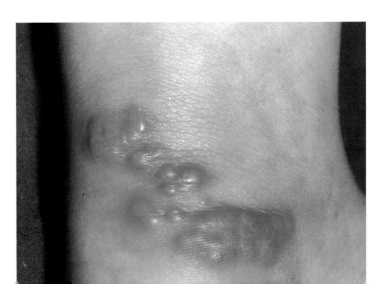

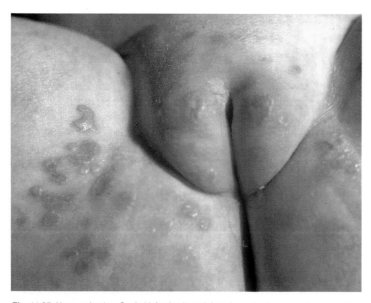

Fig. 11.25 Herpes simplex. Genital infection in an infant due to implantation of virus carried on the hand from primary herpetic stomatitis.

other areas via the fingers (Fig. 11.25). Recurrent cutaneous HSV may also occur at any site and then may mimic herpes zoster (see below) (Fig. 11.26). Although there may be some prodromal symptoms of tingling or itching, systemic symptoms are not usually seen and the rash does not usually have a clear dermatomal distribution.

Primary infections of the finger (herpetic whitlow) are to be seen after accidental inoculation with the virus. Thumb- or finger-sucking children sometimes develop herpetic whitlow at the time of their primary oral infection (Fig. 11.27). Usually only one finger is involved, with pain and one or more deeply situated vesicles (Fig. 11.28). The appearances may erroneously suggest bacterial infection and prompt incision. HSV, but not bacteria, can be grown from the pustular fluid. Medical, paramedical or dental personnel may get lesions as a result of carrying out procedures with ungloved hands: in these instances the whitlows is generally caused by HSV-1. In the adult general population, however, whitlows often result from sexual contact and are then usually caused by HSV-2.

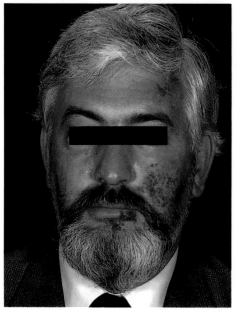

Fig. 11.26 Herpes simplex. Recurrent infection in a zoster-like distribution over the face.

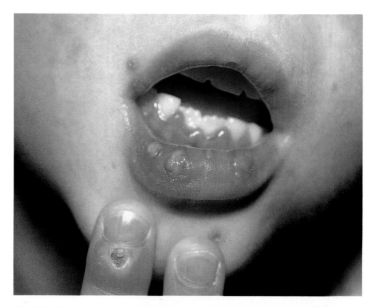

Fig. 11.27 Herpes simplex. In children, herpetic whitlows often accompany stomatitis.

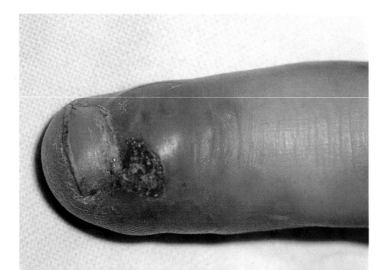

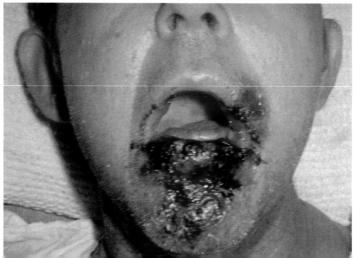

Although there have been no formal double-blind trials, anecdotal reports suggest that cutaneous HSV infections can be treated successfully with oral acyclovir – the doses used range from 1000–1600mg/day.

Patients whose cellular immunity is compromised by disease or immunosuppression are at increased risk of severe HSV infections. Thus, patients with haematological or lymphoreticular malignancies, those who have received organ or bone-marrow transplants and patients with AIDS are at particular risk of severe and persistent cutaneous disease due to HSV (Fig. 11.29). The other group who develop severe HSV skin infection are patients with certain skin disorders or burn wounds. Patients with eczema, pemphigus or Darier's disease, for instance, are unable to localize their infection, especially if they have been using topical steroid preparations. The result is widespread cutaneous HSV – a condition termed Kaposi's varicelliform eruption or eczema herpeticum (Figs 11.30, 11.31 & 11.32). The severity can range from localized and mild, to disseminated and fatal. Secondary bacterial infections and septicaemia may follow. For the mild case, oral acyclovir is recommended, but the more severe forms should be treated with intravenous acyclovir and antistaphylococcal antibiotics.

The diagnosis of HSV infections of the skin can usually be made upon clinical grounds. If there is any doubt, vesicle fluid can be examined for virus particles by electron microscopy (Fig. 11.23), or scrapings from the floor of suspect lesions can be examined by the Tzanck test (Fig. 11.33). Neither of these techniques will distinguish HSV from varicella–zoster virus infection, for which monoclonal antibodies or viral culture are needed.

A small number of patients have recurrent attacks of erythema multiforme (see Chapter 10) following a week or two after attacks of recurrent HSV. The erythema multiforme can be abolished by acyclovir administered prophylactically for the HSV.

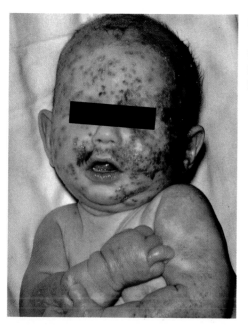

Fig. 11.30 Herpes simplex. Eczema herpeticum may follow primary infection with the virus in infancy as well as in adult life.

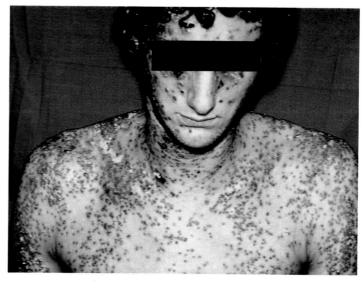

Fig. 11.31 Herpes simplex. The lesions of herpes simplex spread widely in patients with eczema (eczema herpeticum).

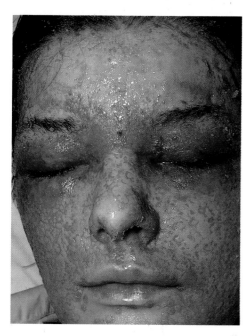

Fig. 11.32 Eczema herpeticum. Although the rash is almost confluent over the face of this young woman, the typical individual lesions of herpes simplex can still be seen around the mouth. By courtesy of Prof. A. M. Geddes.

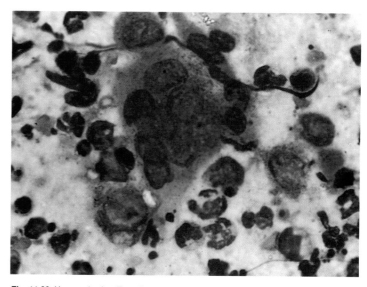

Fig. 11.33 Herpes simplex. Tzanck test preparation showing multinucleate giant cell. Wright's stain. By courtesy of Dr H. P. Holley, Jr.

Varicella (chicken pox)

Varicella–zoster virus (VZV) (Fig. 11.34) is morphologically indistinguishable from herpes simplex virus. It is transmitted from person to person by the respiratory route and the virus may arise either from the oropharynx of a patient late in the prodrome of the illness or from vesicular fluid during the first 3–4 days of each skin lesion. It is a very communicable disease with more than 95% of susceptible household contacts of an index case developing chicken pox.

The incubation period of varicella is usually 14 or 15 days with a range of 11–20 days. In children there is rarely any prodromal illness; fever and rash are the initial manifestations of infection. Adults more commonly have myalgia, arthralgia, fever and chills for 2–3 days before the rash appears. The eruption of chicken pox is discrete, varying in severity from a few spots to a very profuse rash. Each lesion starts as a tiny macule which rapidly becomes papular and then vesiculopustular (Figs 11.35 & 11.36). The rash often starts on the scalp. The vesicles are very superficial and there is little or no induration around the lesion. After a few hours to a few days, the lesion is scratched or becomes inspissated: in either case the fluid is replaced by a central scab (Fig. 11.37). Within a few more days the scabs separate, leaving small often oval

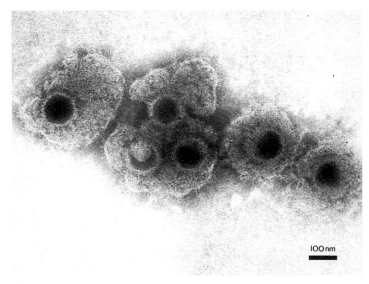

Fig. 11.34 Varicella-zoster virus. Electron micrograph of enveloped virus particles from vesicle fluid. The nucleocapsids, surrounded by tegument and envelope, are clearly seen. Negatively stained. By courtesy of Regional Virus Laboratory, East Birmingham Hospital.

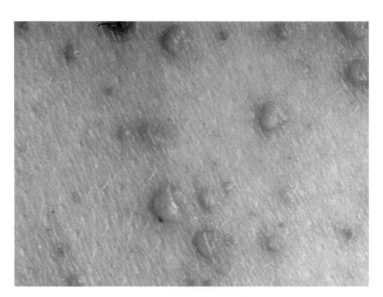

Fig. 11.35 Varicella (chicken pox). Early rash with macules, papules and superficial vesicles, some beginning to inspissate.

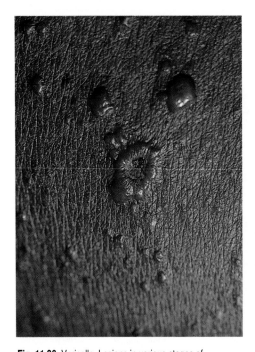

Fig. 11.36 Varicella. Lesions in various stages of development on black skin.

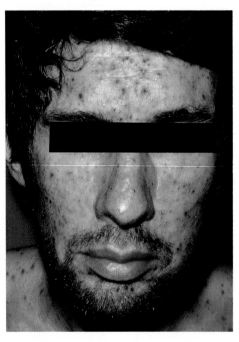

Fig. 11.37 Varicella. Within a few days of the early rash, most of the lesions have become scabs of varying size.

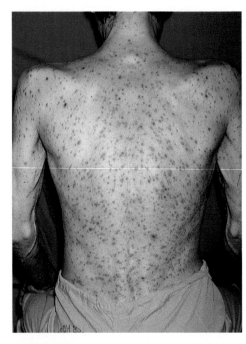

Fig. 11.38 Varicella. General view of severe rash showing characteristic distribution of lesions with lesions most numerous centrally.

scars, and in dark skins, temporary depigmentation at the site of each lesion. It is characteristic of varicella that the eruption appears in crops over a period of about 4 days, so that lesions of different ages and different stages of evolution are to be seen in any one region of the body.

The distribution of chicken pox is central, that is, the rash is more dense on trunk and face and becomes less so peripherally (Fig. 11.38). Lesions are often found on the mucous membranes of the conjunctivae or mouth (see Figs 1.16 and 11.39). The varicella skin lesions may be more numerous on an area of skin that has been subject to sunburn, irritation or mechanical trauma (Fig. 11.40). In the normal individual secondary infection of the lesions with staphylococci or streptococci (Fig. 11.41) is the only frequent complication although haemorrhagic chickenpox with disseminated intravascular coagulation (Fig. 11.42) and pneumonitis occasionally occur. Cerebellar ataxia and other neurological complications are dealt with in Chapter 3.

In the immunocompromised individual (usually a child), varicella may be more severe and prolonged. In these cases the rash is more extensive and may be prominent on the extremities (Fig. 11.43): the individual lesions are often haemorrhagic and necrotic (see Figs 11.44 & 11.45). The lesions continue to appear for more than one week and visceral involvement (particularly of the lungs, liver and central nervous system) is frequently found. Varicella

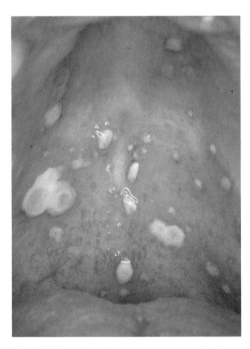

Fig. 11.39 Varicella. Lesions commonly occur within the mouth.

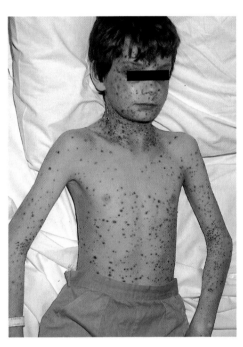

Fig. 11.40 Varicella (chickenpox). In this young boy the lesions are more confluent in the antecubital fossae and over the neck – areas where he had previously suffered from atopic eczema.

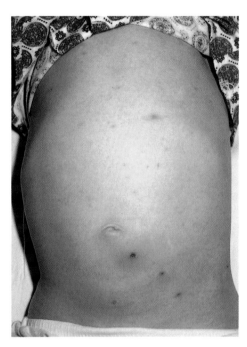

Fig. 11.41 Varicella. Scratching of the lesions not infrequently leads to secondary infection with streptococci or staphylococci and hence cellulitis around individual lesions.

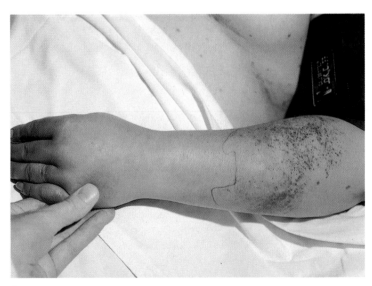

Fig. 11.42 Varicella. Purpura fulminans and disseminated intravascular coagulation complicating chickenpox in an immunocompetent adult woman.

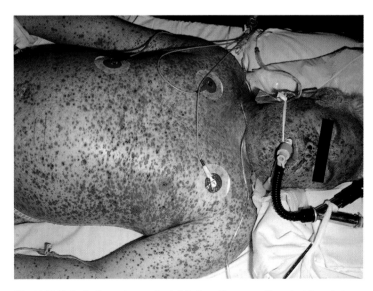

Fig. 11.43 Varicella. Severe haemorrhagic infection with pneumonitis and adult respiratory distress syndrome in a man with lymphoma. By courtesy of Prof. A. M. Geddes.

may also be particularly severe in the perinatal period. Neonatal varicella (Figs 11.46 & 11.47) is a rare condition as most women of childbearing age possess immunity against the virus. Its severity is related to the timing of maternal disease; if the baby is born within five days of the onset of varicella in the mother, the attack tends to be severe, because maternal antibody has not yet developed in sufficient quantity to provide passive protection for the infant. Severe varicella in the immunocompromised individual should be treated with parenteral vidarabine or acyclovir.

Congenital varicella infection resulting from maternal chickenpox during the first trimester of pregnancy is uncommon but results in skin scarring (often of a dermatomal distribution), eye abnormalities, hypoplastic limbs and neurological damage (Fig. 11.48).

The clinical diagnosis of varicella is usually not difficult; if laboratory assistance is required then it can be done by finding typical herpes virus particles in the vesicular fluid by electron microscopy (see Fig. 11.34). The appearances are identical to those of HSV and only culture will distinguish between the different herpes viruses. In the normal individual the virus is present in the vesicle for about 3 days but this may be prolonged for 10 days or more in the immunocompromised. Serological diagnosis is by the complement fixation test, but the transitory nature of this antibody means that other tests have to be used to determine immune status. The tests used for this are the determination of antibody against the membrane antigen by fluorescence microscopy (FAMA) or ELISA.

A live attenuated vaccine for varicella is now available. The Oka strain vaccine has been shown to be immunogenic and safe in both normal and immunocompromised individuals and may well become widely used to prevent chickenpox in Western nations. The treatment of varicella infection is with acyclovir. Parenteral acyclovir has been

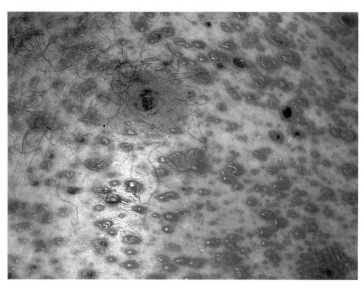

Fig. 11.44 Varicella. Close-up of haemorrhagic lesions shown in Fig. 11.43. By courtesy of Prof. A. M. Geddes.

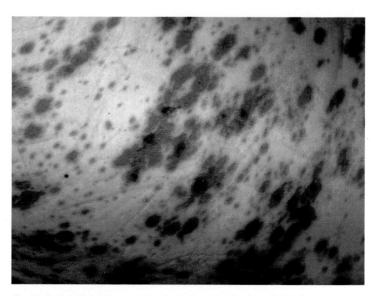

Fig. 11.45 Varicella (chicken pox). Trunk of patient with chronic myeloid leukaemia and chickenpox showing purpuric confluent lesions. By courtesy of Dr G. D. W. McKendrick.

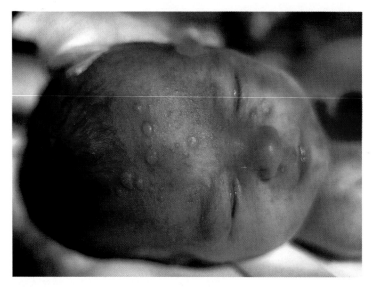

Fig. 11.46 Neonatal chickenpox. Severe varicella occurs in the infant when maternal disease develops between 5 days before delivery and 2 days postpartum.

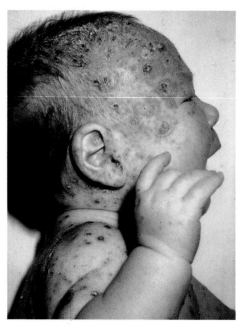

Fig. 11.47 Varicella. Pleomorphic lesions in a neonate. By courtesy of Dr M. H. Winterborn.

clearly shown to be of benefit in preventing the serious consequences of varicella in the immunosuppressed individual and in the treatment of those normal hosts who develop varicella pneumonitis. Whether the slight clinical benefits produced by the use of oral acyclovir in the normal child with chickenpox are cost-beneficial is still a matter of debate.

Herpes zoster (shingles)

Following the initial infection with VZV, the virus, as for other herpesviruses, persists in the individual in a latent form. VZV remains in the dorsal root ganglia but the exact nature of the latent state is unknown. It seems likely that the cellular immune system is chiefly responsible for maintaining the virus in the latent state as anything that depresses this form of immunity is associated with a more frequent reactivation of VZV. Zoster is much more common in patients with lymphoma or after transplantation and is being seen increasingly in young persons infected with HIV, especially in Africa.

Zoster can occur at any age but in normal individuals is much more likely to be seen in individuals beyond the age of 50 years. It has been estimated that about 20% of the population will suffer from an attack of shingles at some time in their lives. When it is seen in a young child who has never suffered from varicella (Fig. 11.49), the virus will have been transmitted *in utero* from the mother who had chickenpox during pregnancy. Following reactivation of virus there is degeneration of the cells of the dorsal root ganglion and the virus then affects the area of skin supplied by the sensory nerves from that ganglion (Figs 11.50 & 11.51).

The resultant illness usually begins with pain in the areas of distribution of the affected posterior nerve root(s), followed by the rash. The rash is unilateral and involves

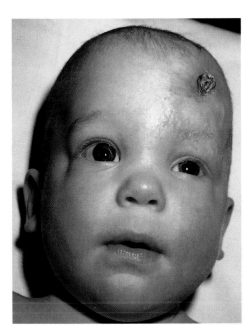

Fig. 11.48 Congenital varicella syndrome. This infant has skin scarring in the area supplied by the ophthalmic division of the left trigeminal nerve and a hypoplastic left eye. His mother suffered from varicella during the first weeks of her pregnancy.

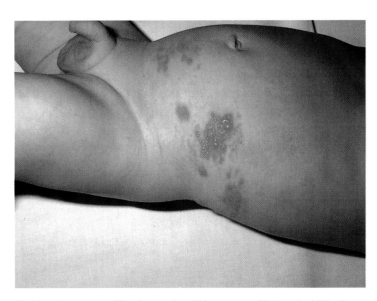

Fig 11.49 Herpes zoster. When it occurs in a child as young as this 8-month-old it is often as result of primary infection *in utero*.

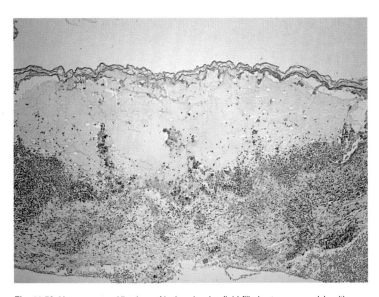

Fig. 11.50 Herpes zoster. Histology of lesion showing fluid-filled cutaneous vesicle with inflammation at its base. By courtesy of Dr J. Newman.

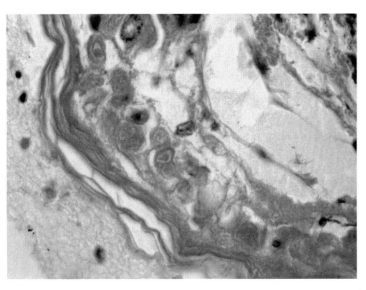

Fig. 11.51 Herpes zoster. Higher power view of base of vesicle seen in Fig. 11.50, showing inclusion bodies. By courtesy of Dr J. Newman.

1–3 adjacent dermatomes. There is often a faint erythema (Fig. 11.52) before the typical vesiculopustular eruption (Fig. 11.53). Any dermatome(s) may be involved although the thoracic dermatomes are affected in about half the cases. The single most commonly involved dermatome is that of the trigeminal nerve. The ophthalmic branch is most commonly affected (Fig. 11.54) but shingles in the distribution of the maxillary (see Figs. 11.55 & 1.17) or mandibular branch (Fig. 11.56) is occasionally seen. New lesions appear within the affected dermatome for several days and the eruption gradually scabs. The scabs separate after a week or two, the whole eruption generally lasting for 2–3 weeks. After the eruption has healed the skin may appear normal or atrophic and, occasionally, keloidal scarring follows (Fig. 11.57). The clinical features of herpes zoster are often much more severe in the immunosuppressed individual, the rash persisting for several weeks and often becoming haemorrhagic and leaving more severe scars (Fig. 11.58).

It is not uncommon to find several varicella-type skin lesions outside the primary dermatome in zoster, but in both normal and immunosuppressed patients more widespread dissemination may occur (Figs 11.58 & 11.59). This typically occurs about a week after the rash appears and, in the immunocompromised individual, may include visceral as well as cutaneous involvement. The complications of herpes zoster include Ramsay–Hunt syndrome (see Chapter 1), a variety of other neurological complications (see Chapter 3), and ocular problems after trigeminal involvement (see Chapter 12). The most frequent problem is, however, post-herpetic neuralgia which is more common in the elderly.

Herpes zoster in the immunocompromised individual is treated with parenteral acyclovir. In the normal host acyclovir, given either parenterally or in high doses orally, reduces the severity of the acute illness, but has not yet been clearly shown to be beneficial in preventing post-herpetic neuralgia, often the most troublesome feature of her-

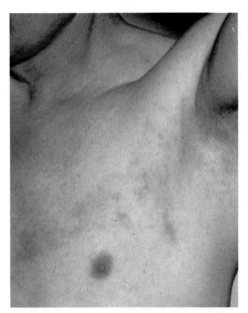

Fig. 11.52 Herpes zoster (shingles). A band of faint erythema in the distribution of an intercostal nerve, the first physical sign of shingles, can be seen. The patient had been in pain for several days.

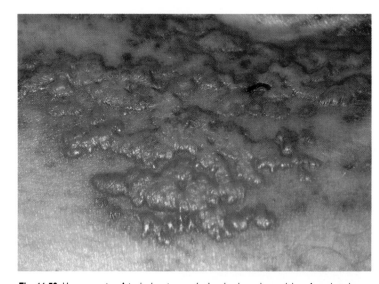

Fig. 11.53 Herpes zoster. A typical mature rash showing irregular vesicles of varying size on an erythematous base.

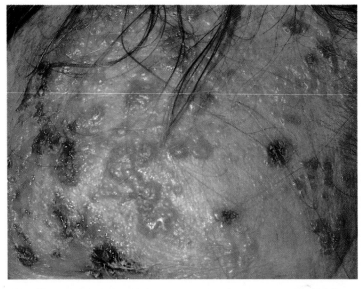

Fig. 11.54 Herpes zoster. The most frequently affected dermatome is that of the ophthalmic division of the trigeminal nerve.

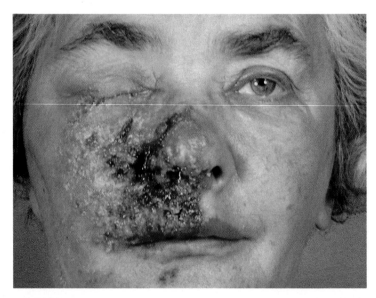

Fig. 11.55 Herpes zoster. Lesions in the distribution of the maxillary division of the trigeminal nerve.

pes zoster. Whether the use of varicella vaccine in the elderly will reduce the frequency or severity of zoster has also not been determined.

Enteroviral rashes

Rashes are a common feature of enteroviral infection, especially in childhood. Some types, such as echoviruses 9, 16 and 4 and Coxsackie viruses A9 and A16, are especially important in this respect.

The most common form of rash resembles that of rubella (Fig. 11.60). It is fine and pink, begins simultaneously with fever and always affects the face (where the rash may sometimes be more blotchy than rubella); lymphadenopathy is most unusual and this, together with its summer occurrence, is useful in distinguishing it from true rubella. Another form of enteroviral rash appears in young children and is characteristic in that it appears as the fever settles. This illness is typically caused by

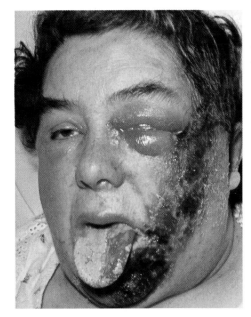

Fig. 11.56 Herpes zoster. Lesions in the distribution of the mandibular division of the trigeminal nerve. By courtesy of Dr G. D. W. McKendrick.

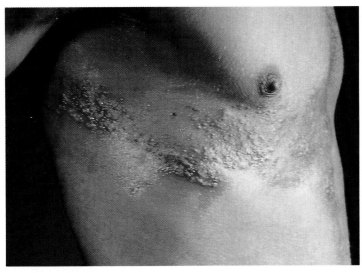

Fig. 11.57 Herpes zoster. Although most lesions heal uneventfully, scarring in the affected areas is not uncommon and the scars may become keloidal. By courtesy of Dr J. F. John, Jr.

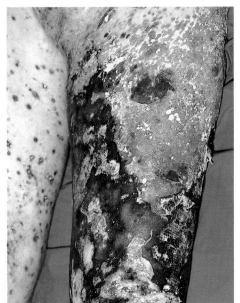

Fig. 11.58 Herpes zoster. Severe zoster with skin necrosis and disseminated varicella lesions in an immunosuppressed woman.

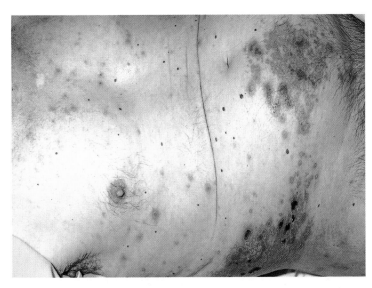

Fig. 11.59 Herpes zoster. Dermatomal rash in right T11 distribution with disseminated chicken pox lesions, in a patient with chronic lymphatic leukaemia.

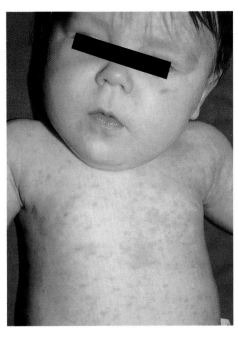

Fig. 11.60 Enteroviruses. Typical macular rash on forehead and trunk in a child with echovirus infection.

echovirus 16 and is sometimes called the 'Boston exanthem'. The rash consists of large (about 1cm diameter), discrete maculopapules that last for a few days (Fig. 11.61).

Hand, foot and mouth disease, usually caused by Coxsackie A16 (occasionally by A5 and A10) is characterized by small, lax vesicles within an erythematous margin on the hands (Figs 11.62 & 11.63) and feet (Fig. 11.64) together with vesicles within the oral cavity (see Figure 1.21). It is usually seen in children under 10 years old and is accompanied by fever and sore throat. Less commonly, there is an associated maculopapular rash on the buttocks and thighs (Fig. 11.65).

There is great variety of other rashes associated with enteroviral infections: petechial, purpuric, vesicular (Fig. 11.66), bullous, and even urticarial appearances are sometimes observed

Molluscum contagiosum

Molluscum contagiosum is a benign disease caused by an unclassified member of the poxvirus family (Fig. 11.67)

and spread by close human contact. The lesions are characteristic firm white nodules which vary greatly in number (Fig. 11.68) and tend to persist for a period of a few weeks to a few months. Sometimes they may be found in clusters along a scar. The lesions often become umbilicated (Fig. 11.69) and may discharge their contents. In patients with AIDS, the lesions may not resolve but continue to spread and enlarge: the correct diagnosis may be made by biopsy or electron microscopy.

Orf

Orf virus is a poxvirus of sheep and goats which accidentally infects humans at the site of an abrasion or bite. Most of those infected are farmers, veterinarians or butchers, who have come into contact with goats or sheep, especially lambs (Fig. 11.70).

The lesions may be single or multiple. Each begins as a reddish papule that becomes a large haemorrhagic pustule on a red base (see Figs 11.71 & 11.72). Lymphadenopathy may be present. The lesions are usually, but not always

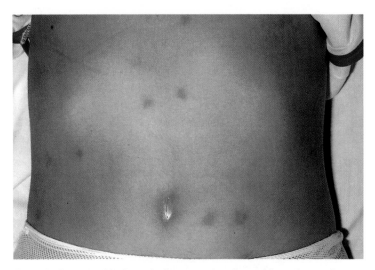

Fig. 11.61 Enterovirus infections – the Boston exanthem. Large pink macules over the trunk of a child with aseptic meningitis. Echovirus type 16 was isolated from the cerebrospinal fluid.

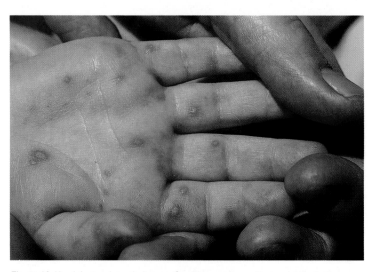

Fig. 11.62 Hand, foot and mouth disease. Small lax vesicles on the hand. Usually there are fewer lesions than this.

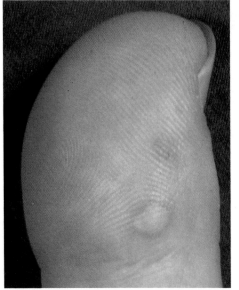

Fig. 11.63 Hand, foot and mouth disease. Lesions on the thumb clearly showing a vesicle with an erythematous base.

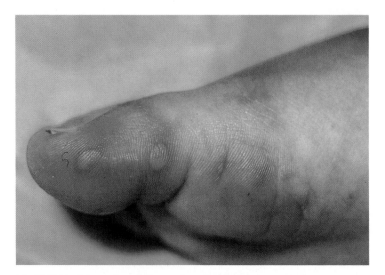

Fig. 11.64 Hand, foot and mouth disease. Several vesicular lesions on the foot.

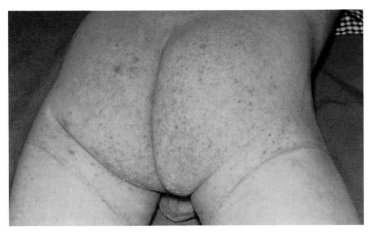

Fig. 11.65 Hand, foot and mouth disease. There may be a macular or petechial rash on the buttocks and thighs.

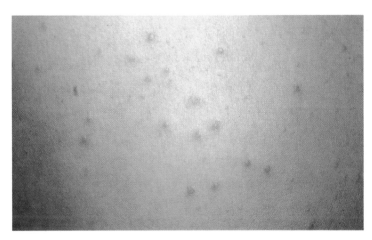

Fig. 11.66 Enteroviruses. Small vesicular lesions on trunk in a child with echovirus infection.

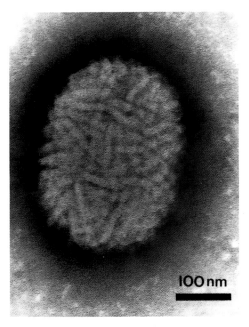

Fig. 11.67 Electron micrograph of virus responsible for molluscum contagiosum. The virus particle appears as a cylindrical shape with rounded ends and a criss-cross pattern of nucleoprotein strands. By courtesy of Regional Virus Laboratory, East Birmingham Hospital.

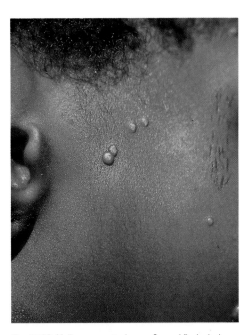

Fig. 11.68 Molluscum contagiosum. Several fleshy lesions with umbilicated centres on the face. They tend to regress and disappear after some months.

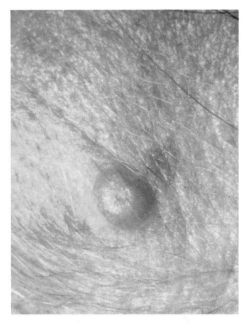

Fig. 11.69 Molluscum contagiosum. Single umbilicated lesion.

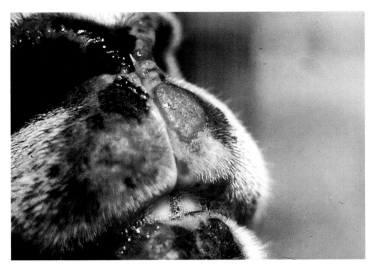

Fig. 11.70 Orf. Lesions on the lip and nose of a lamb. This is the source of infection in those working with animals.

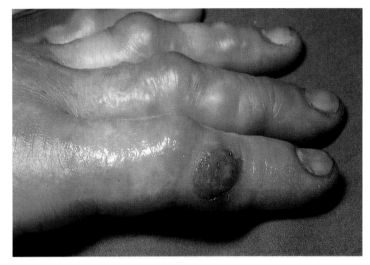

Fig. 11.71 Orf. Papular lesions on the hand of a farmer's wife. She also had severe erythema multiforme with arthritis. The proximal interphalangeal joints can be seen to be swollen.

(Fig. 11.73), on the hands. The pustule may become umbilicated and then rupture to leave an ulcerated nodule with a grey crust. Erythema multiforme may occur after a week or two (see Fig. 11.71).

The diagnosis is usually made clinically but can be confirmed if necessary by electron microscopy, which reveals the large, ovoid virus particles.

Warts

Papilloma viruses, which produce human warts, are small DNA viruses (Fig. 11.74). There are more than 50 different types of human papilloma virus (HPV) and each is associated to a large extent with one of the four clinically distinct types of wart; common warts (verrucae vulgaris), plantar warts (verrucae plantaris), flat or planar warts (verrucae plana) and condylomata acuminata (see Chapter 7). Following direct inoculation of the virus, epithelial cells are stimulated to divide and the period before lesions become visible is several months.

Histologically there is proliferation of all layers of the epidermis except the basal layer. The prickle cell layer of the epidermis contains large vacuolated cells with a shrunken nucleus, called koilocytes.

Most common warts (Fig. 11.75) are 2–10mm in diameter (although they may coalesce to larger masses), flesh-coloured or brown, keratotic papules with a rough surface. When they are pared, there is a speckled surface (due to thrombosed capillaries). On mucosal surfaces the warts may be filiform with a narrow base and finger-like projections. Flat warts ares smaller, flat topped, non-scaling, skin-coloured papules and seen especially in groups upon the hands, neck or face (Fig. 11.76).

Plantar warts (Fig. 11.77) are different in that they grow inwards and are more painful. They are particularly common in adolescents and children and can be differentiated from callouses by planing which reveals their speckled surface. Condylomata acuminata are dealt with in Chapter 7.

Warts are particularly common in immunodeficient persons and may spontaneously regress with immunostimu-

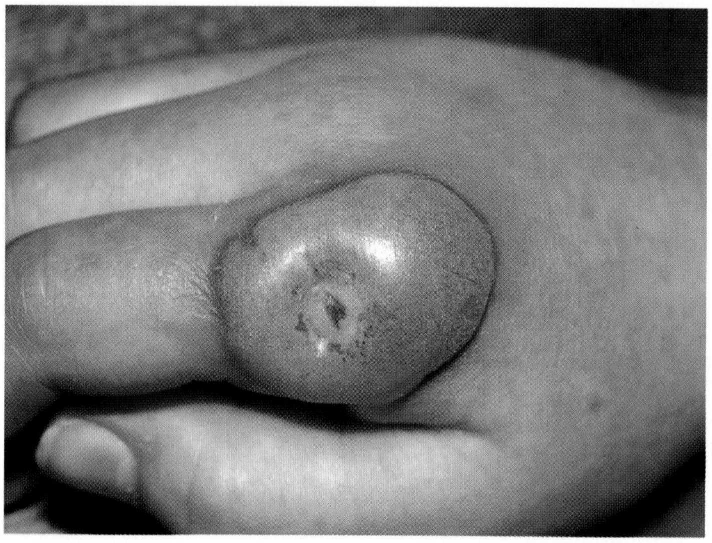

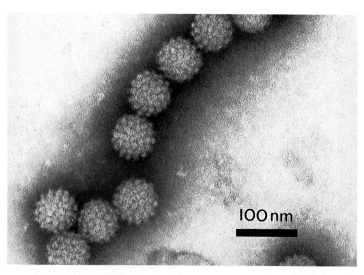

Fig. 11.72 Orf. Large pustular lesion on the hand of a farmworker. The diagnosis can be confirmed if necessary by electron microscopic examination of fluid from the lesion.

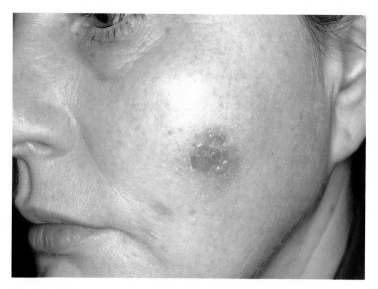

Fig. 11.73 Orf. Early lesion on the face.

Fig. 11.74 Electron micrograph showing papilloma virus. This member of the papovavirus group is the cause of human warts. By courtesy of Regional Virus Laboratory, East Birmingham Hospital.

100 nm

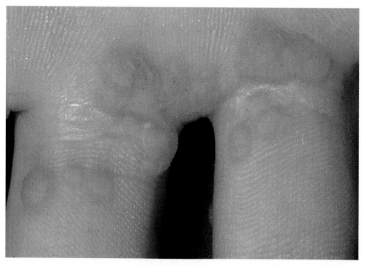

Fig. 11.75 Common warts. The hands and fingers are a common site.

lation. Treatment with cryosurgery or with topical lactic and salicylic acid paint is used for common or flat warts.

FUNGI

Tinea versicolor

Tinea (or pityriasis) versicolor is a superficial dermatomycosis caused by the lipophilic yeast, *Malassezia furfur*. The organism is a normal commensal of skin and what triggers transformation into hyphal forms and infection is not clear. Infection is most common in teenagers and young adults and is more likely in hot weather. The asymptomatic lesions are irregular, hypo- or hyper-pigmented, and may be circumscribed or diffuse (Figs. 11.78 & 11.79). They have a dust-like scale but are not itchy. They usually occur on the trunk or proximal aspects of the limbs, but occasionally affect other areas of the skin. The organisms may be identified in direct preparations of material scraped from the lesions or removed with sticky tape and

stained with methylene blue (the so called 'spaghetti and meatballs' appearance) (Fig. 11.80). Culture is difficult and is usually not attempted. Treatment for several weeks

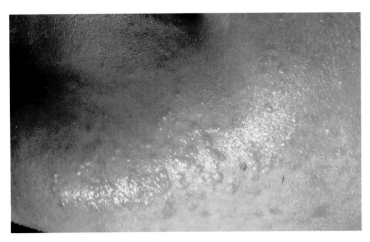

Fig. 11.76 Flat warts. Numerous small lesions on face. By courtesy of Dr E. Sahn.

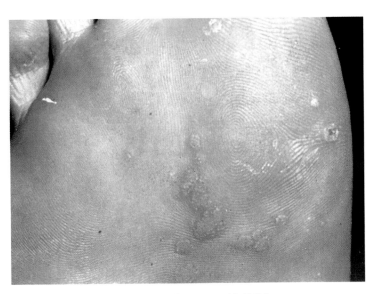

Fig. 11.77 Plantar warts in an adolescent. By courtesy of Dr E. Sahn.

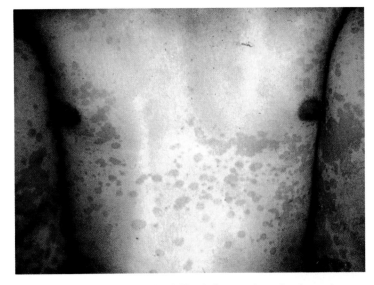

Fig. 11.78 Tinea versicolor. Brownish-red diffuse lesions over the trunk and arms of a young man. By courtesy of Dr E. Sahn.

Fig. 11.79 Tinea versicolor. Superficial, diffuse, brownish-red lesions over the back of a young man. By courtesy of Dr M. H. Winterborn.

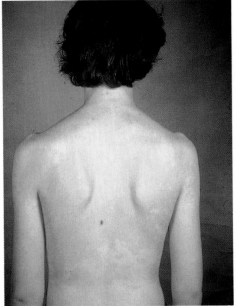

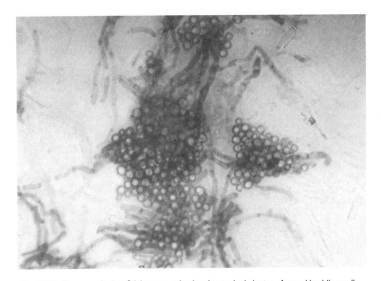

Fig. 11.80 Tinea versicolor. Sticky tape strip showing typical cluster of round budding cells and mycelial elements of *Malassezia furfur*. Methylene blue stain. By courtesy of A. E. Prevost.

with local application of selenium sulphide suspension or a topical azole antifungal cream is effective.

Dermatomycoses

The dermatomycoses are a group of fungal infections of the skin caused by organisms (the dermatophytes) which invade only the superficial stratum corneum of the skin and other keratinized tissues such as hair and nails.

Tinea corporis (ringworm of the body) is most often seen in children and is caused by various species of the genera *Trichophyton* (Fig. 11.81), *Epidermophyton* and *Microsporum*. Some of these species, such as *T. rubrum,* are exclusively human pathogens, transmitted through infected skin squames, and some, such as *M. canis,* are transmitted to humans from animals (in this case cats or dogs). The lesions are often found on the trunk or legs and usually have a prominent edge with a central scaly area – tinea circinata (Figs 11.82 & 11.83) – although granulomata involving deeper layers may also be seen (Fig. 11.84).

Tinea barbae (barber's itch) is a chronic infection of the beard area of the face and neck, with both superficial lesions and deeper lesions involving the hair follicles (Fig. 11.85).

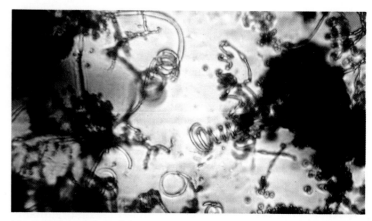

Fig. 11.81 Dermatophytes. Spiral hyphae of *Trichophyton mentagrophytes.* By courtesy of Prof. R. Y. Cartwright.

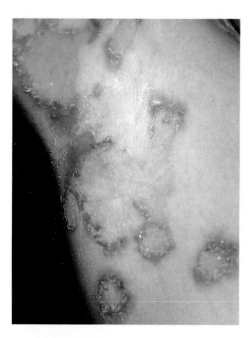

Fig. 11.82 Dermatophyte. Typical lesions of tinea circinata, with margins more inflamed than the centres.

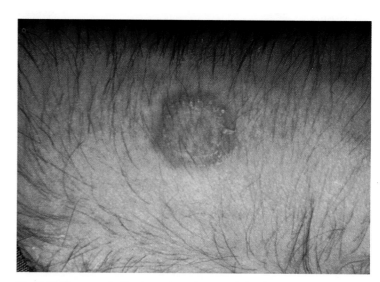

Fig. 11.83 Tinea corporis. Classic annular erythematous lesion due to *Microsporum* species showing an advancing active periphery and scaling in the central area. By courtesy of A. E. Prevost.

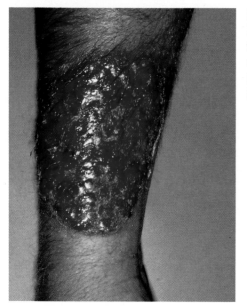

Fig. 11.84 Dermatophyte. Inflammatory infection due to the zoophilic fungus *T. mentagrophytes* in a farmer. By courtesy of Prof. R. Y. Cartwright.

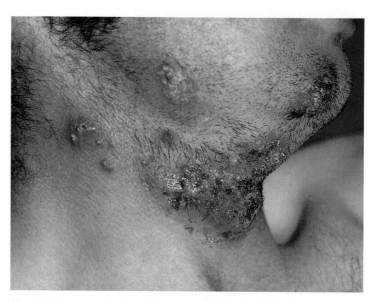

Fig. 11.85 Tinea barbae (barber's itch). Dermatophytic infection of beard area.

Tinea pedis (athlete's foot) is a chronic fungus infection of the feet, involving particularly the toes, toe webs, and soles (Fig. 11.86) usually caused by *T. rubrum* or *E. flocco-sum*. The intertriginous areas of the toe web usually show the most severe involvement with cracking and severe maceration of the skin. The major symptom is itching. Treatment involves careful drying of the feet after bathing, followed by application of various topical antifungal agents. The same two dermatophytes are the usual cause of infection in the groin (tinea cruris) and similar symptoms occur. Unlike candidal groin infection, dermatophytes tend to spare the scrotum (Fig. 11.87). Dermatophytes can be diagnosed by the examination of KOH preparations of skin scrapings (Fig. 11.88).

Most cases of dermatophyte infections respond readily to topical agents, either keratolytic agents such as salicylic and benzoic acid compound (Whitfield's ointment) or antifungal agents such as the imidazoles, given for 2–4 weeks. Very occasionally, chronic dermatophyte infections can cause scarring with keloid formation (Fig. 11.89).

Tinea capitis (ringworm of the scalp) is chiefly a disease of children and is also caused by *Trichophyton* or *Microsporum* species. It causes scaly erythematous scalp lesions with loss of hair (Fig. 11.90). Different species may

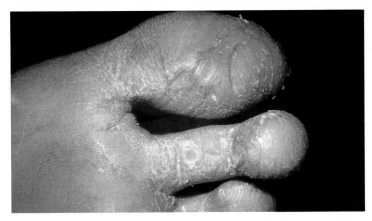

Fig. 11.86 Tinea pedis (athlete's foot). Scaling erythematous pruritic patches in the characteristic location involving the toes, toe webs and sole of the foot. By courtesy of A. E. Prevost.

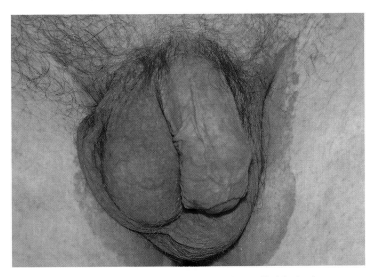

Fig. 11.87 Tinea cruris. Scaling rash over the thighs. Unlike candida infection the scrotum is usually spared.

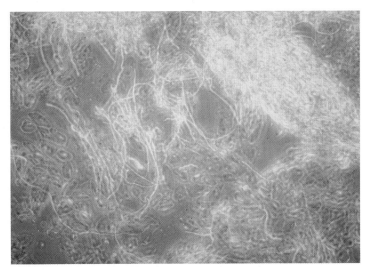

Fig. 11.88 Dermatophytes. The laboratory diagnosis can be made by softening skin scrapings in 10–20% KOH and examining under the microscope for fungal hypae. By courtesy of Prof. R.Y. Cartwright.

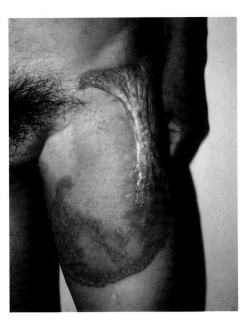

Fig. 11.89 Dermatophytes. Keloidal scarring on the thigh as a result of chronic tinea corporis in a South American man. By courtesy of Dr P. J. Cooper.

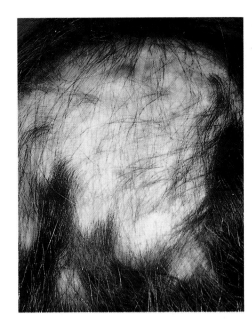

Fig. 11.90 Tinea capitis. Scaling of scalp and hair loss due to infection with *Microsporum canis*. By courtesy of Dr M. H. Winterborn.

produce arthrospores within the hair shaft (endothrix infections) (Figs 11.91 & 11.92) or on the outside of the hair shaft (ectothrix infections). There are variable degrees of inflammation present: cases acquired from cattle and due to *T. verrucosum* often are very inflammatory and form large pustular lesions called kerions (Fig. 11.93). Infection due to *T. schoenleinii* causes a condition called favus (Fig. 11.94). Here the hairs are infected but not structurally damaged or shed until late into the disease. This produces a marked inflammatory crust with matted hairs over the scalp. Diagnosis of *Microsporum* infection may be suspected by demonstration of green fluorescent hairs under Wood's light, but hairs infected by *T. tonsurans* do not exhibit fluorescence. Fungus can be detected by microscopic examination of the hair (preferably a broken stub) in KOH preparations. Scalp infections do not respond to topical therapy and are usually treated with 6–12 weeks of oral griseofulvin.

Onychomycosis (tinea unguium) is a chronic fungal infection of the nails, usually associated with infection of the adjacent skin due to *T. rubrum* (Fig. 11.95). There is thickening of the nail which becomes white, brown or yellow. The presence of heaped-up debris containing the organism under the nail differentiates onychomycosis due to dermatophytes from that due to chronic candida infection of the nails (Fig. 11.96). Treatment involves the removal of as much of the infected nail as possible and long term (6–12 months) systemic therapy with griseofulvin, but the infection is extremely difficult to eradicate and more than 50% relapse.

Candidiasis

Candida organisms are small budding yeasts that cause various conditions in humans (Fig. 11.97). The organisms are normal commensals of humans but are capable of causing infections whenever the normal defense mechanisms are interrupted. For the prevention of cutaneous candida infection, the most important defense mechanism is an intact integument. Any factor that causes maceration of the skin predisposes to candida invasion, as does diabetes mellitus.

The most common form of cutaneous candidiasis is spread of vaginal infection to the perineum (Fig. 11.98). The vulva and labia are red and intensely pruritic and there are usually irregular patches of affected skin, often

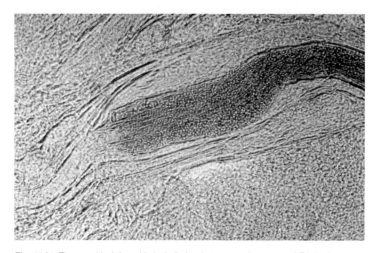

Fig. 11.91 Tinea capitis. Infected hair shaft showing many arthrospores of *Trichophyton tonsurans*. By courtesy of A. E. Prevost.

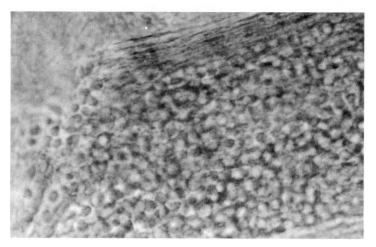

Fig. 11.92 Tinea capitis. High power view of endothrix infection due to *T. tonsurans* showing morphology of the arthrospores. By courtesy of A. E. Prevost.

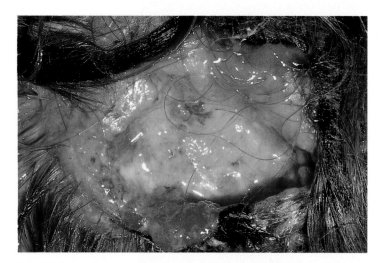

Fig. 11.93 Kerion. In some forms of tinea capitis there is severe inflammation causing a pustular lesion with an exudative crust. By courtesy of Prof. A. M. Geddes.

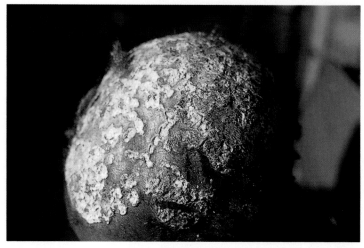

Fig. 11.94 Favus. An inflammatory response develops around individual hairs and the scalp appears to be covered with a thick crust. This is caused by *T. schoenleinii*.

with much scaling and spread to adjacent areas. In infants, the wearing of wet nappies (diapers) causes maceration of the skin: candida infection produces a similar appearance termed napkin (diaper) rash (Fig. 11.99). The perianal skin is another site (Fig. 11.100) and candidal intertrigo is often seen in moist sites where skin surfaces

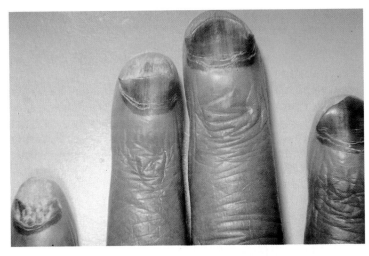

Fig. 11.95 Onychomycosis. Chronic infection with *Trichophyton rubrum* in a diabetic patient, showing brittle, discoloured nail with separation of nail bed by fungus-containing debris. By courtesy of A. E. Prevost.

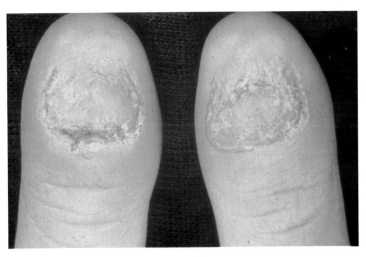

Fig. 11.96 Onychomycosis. Deformity and ridging of nails due to candida infection. By courtesy of Prof. R. Y. Cartwright.

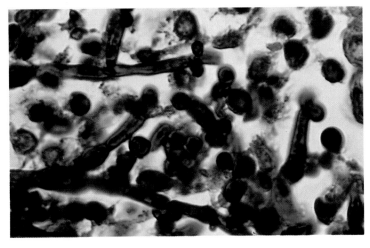

Fig. 11.97 *Candida* species. Both yeast and mycelial forms can be seen here.

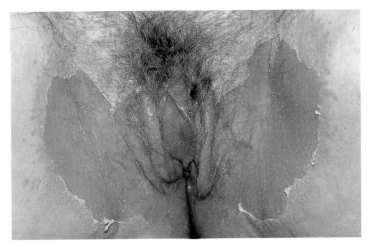

Fig. 11.98 Candidiasis of the perineum. Large areas of denuded skin with rather well-defined edges and some scaling. Satellite lesions are visible beyond the edges. This is often associated with vaginal candidiasis.

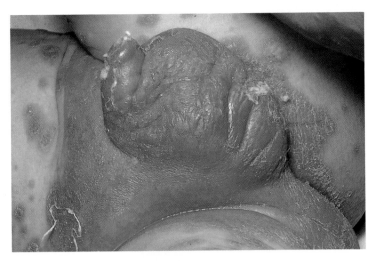

Fig. 11.99 Candida napkin rash. Inflammation affecting the napkin areas, including the scrotum with prominent satellite pustules.

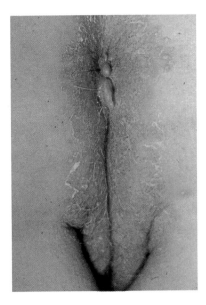

Fig. 11.100 Perineal candidiasis. A common distribution spreading from the perianal area along the perineum. By courtesy of the Institute of Dermatology.

are adjacent, as under the breasts or in the groin. Candida is a common cause of paronychia (Fig. 11.101). The acute phase of inflammation is followed by discolouration, ridging and thickening of the nail. Paronychia are more common in those whose hands are frequently immersed in water and, as for many of the other manifestations of cutaneous candidiasis, in diabetic patients.

Generalized acute cutaneous candidiasis is sometimes seen, even in patients without overt evidence of immunodeficiency and who do not develop chronic mucocutaneous candidiasis. Irregular red or brownish-red patches may be quite widespread (Fig. 11.102). In infants, a generalized rash of this type may begin with a napkin (diaper) rash.

All the above mild or moderate forms of cutaneous candidiasis are treatable topically with nystatin or imidazoles such as clotrimazole or miconazole.

Chronic mucocutaneous candidiasis is a persistent infection of the mucous membranes, skin, hair and nails associated with a number of immune defects, mainly of T-cell function. Some patients also have associated endocrine disorders, especially hyperparathyroidism or Addison's disease. The clinical illness usually begins in childhood with oral candidiasis but subsequent syndromes vary greatly from mild but chronic infections, for example, candidal paronychia and angular stomatitis (Fig. 11.103), to severe disfiguring granulomatous lesions (Fig. 11.104). Treatment with a variety of immunostimulants has been of limited success and the treatment of choice now appears to be long term ketoconazole or fluconazole.

Disseminated candidiasis, which tends to occur in the immunocompromised or those with candida endocarditis, can be associated with cutaneous lesions. These are typi-

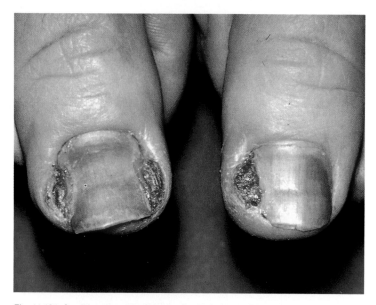

Fig. 11.101 Candida paroncyhia. Ridged nails with indolent inflammatory tissue lateral to the nails.

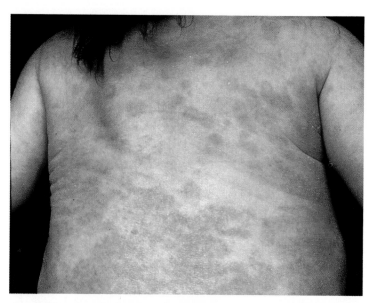

Fig. 11.102 Generalized acute cutaneous candidiasis. Rounded, slightly raised erythematous patches of various size developing as a generalized eruption following a napkin (diaper) rash. By courtesy of the Institute of Dermatology.

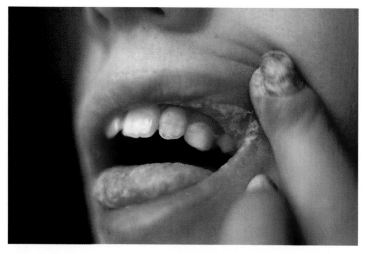

Fig. 11.103 Chronic mucocutaneous candidiasis. Chronic angular stomatitis and onychomycosis due to candida in a 12-year-old child with impaired T-cell response to candida antigens.

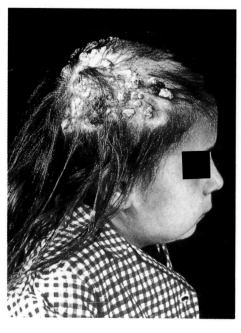

Fig. 11.104 Chronic mucocutaneous candidiasis. Chronic disfiguring candida infection of the scalp in a child. By courtesy of Dr. E. Sahn.

cally pink to red macronodules, up to 1cm in diameter, and can be single (Fig. 11.105) or multiple.

Sporotrichosis

This chronic infection is caused by *Sporothrix schenckii*, a widely distributed saprophytic fungus (Fig. 11.106). Most cases of infection in man are the result of minor trauma and inoculation of the organism through the skin. At the site of entry (often on the hands) a small, painless, pink or purple, verrucous, nodular or ulcerative cutaneous lesion develops anything from 1 week to several months later (Fig. 11.107). In 75% of cases the chronic primary inoculation lesion is associated with multiple painless nodules distributed along the lymphatic vessels draining the pri-

mary lesion (Fig. 11.108). Sometimes these lesions ulcerate. No constitutional symptoms develop unless secondary bacterial infection develops. The organism is readily cultured from purulent exudate or biopsy material placed on Sabouraud's medium, but is rarely seen on direct examination of the tissue. The histopathological response to sporotrichosis involves granulomas and microabscesses. Pseudoepitheliomatous hyperplasia may be present. Lymphocutaneous and cutaneous sporotrichosis usually responds to oral therapy with potassium iodide (3–4ml every 8 hours until the skin lesions disappear), but occasional cases require systemic treatment with amphotericin B, especially when deeper tissues are involved. Preliminary reports suggest that itraconazole may also be effective. Relapse is very rare.

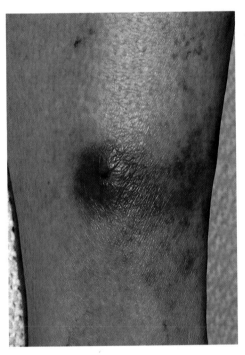

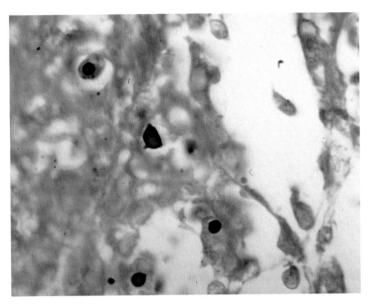

Fig. 11.105 Disseminated candidiasis. The typical skin lesions are pinkish-red nodules, here seen on the ankle of a patient with acute leukaemia. Candida can be visualized in punch biopsies.

Fig. 11.106 Sporotrichosis. Histological section showing small yeast-like organisms of *Sporothrix schenckii*. Gomori-methenamine silver stain. By courtesy of Dr R. D. Johnson.

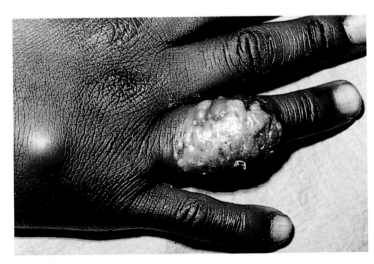

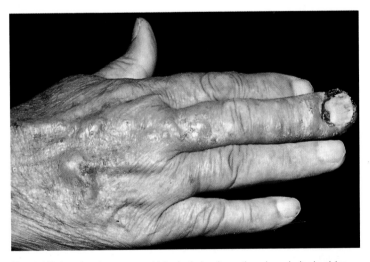

Fig. 11.107 Lymphocutaneous sporotrichosis. A large, verrucous and ulcerative lesion on the dorsal surface of the fourth finger. A single satellite lesion is present on the dorsum of the hand, probably along a lymphatic vessel draining the primary lesion. By courtesy of Dr K. A. Riley.

Fig. 11.108 Lymphocutaneous sporotrichosis. A chronic crusting primary lesion involving the nail bed of the third finger, with multiple painless nodules along the lymphatic channels draining this lesion. By courtesy of Dr T. F. Sellers, Jr.

North American blastomycosis

This is a chronic granulomatous disease caused by the dimorphic fungus *Blastomyces dermatitidis*. The natural reservoir of this organism seems to be soil from wooded areas that is rich in organic material. Almost all the cases have been reported from North America, particularly the Mississippi, Ohio, and St. Lawrence river valleys. It is thought that the respiratory tract is the entry route into the body in nearly all cases. Although lung lesions are often inconspicuous, they are nearly always found if careful pathological examination is performed. The acute phase of infection is often asymptomatic but may cause influenza-like symptoms. Most patients, however, present with chronic blastomycosis and multiple skin lesions on exposed areas of the body, especially the face or arms.

These begin as subcutaneous papules or nodules that eventually ulcerate and develop into raised, proliferative granulomatous lesions with dark red or violet irregular outlines (Fig. 11.109). As the lesion spreads, central healing with scar formation occurs while the outer margin is still advancing. In long-standing untreated cases, fibrosis and atrophic changes may predominate (Fig. 11.110). Other organs frequently involved are lung (see Chapter 2), bone (see Chapter 8), genitourinary tract, liver, spleen and CNS (see Chapter 3). *B. dermatitidis* only rarely acts as an opportunistic pathogen.

Diagnosis is made by finding the characteristic yeast forms by direct examination of exudate after digestion with KOH (Fig. 11.111) or histological examination of tissue stained with PAS or Gomori-silver stains. The fungus can be cultured from clinical specimens (Fig. 11.112).

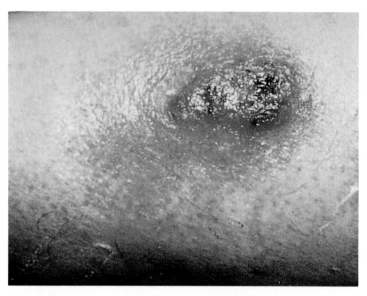

Fig. 11.109 Blastomycosis. Typical raised, crusting, proliferative, cutanenous lesion in a patient with chronic blastomycosis. By courtesy of Dr K. A. Riley.

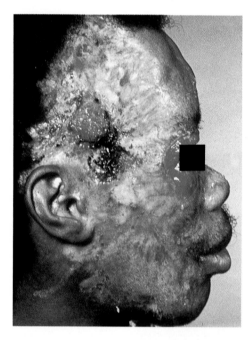

Fig. 11.110 Blastomycosis. This had been untreated for several years and the proliferative, ulcerating lesions were associated with pronounced fibrosis and atrophic changes in the skin. By courtesy of Dr K. A. Riley.

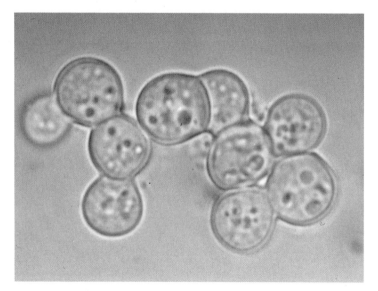

Fig. 11.111 Blastomycosis. Characteristic spherical budding yeast cells of *Blastomyces dermatitidis*. They are 8–15μm in diameter, have thick refractile walls and a single bud attached to the parent cell by a wide septum. KOH preparation. By courtesy of A. E. Provost.

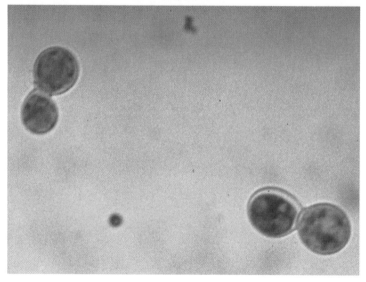

Fig. 11.112 Blastomycosis. Yeast form of *Blastomyces dermatitidis* from a culture incubated at 37°C. Cotton blue preparation. By courtesy of A. E. Provost.

Untreated chronic blastomycosis is usually slowly progressive, but all forms can be treated effectively with amphotericin B (a total dose of 1.5–2.0g). It now seems that ketoconazole (400–800 mg/day) or itraconazole are effective alternatives for those with non-life-threatening blastomycosis.

Cutaneous cryptococcosis

Although the lungs and central nervous system are the sites most commonly affected by *Cryptococcus neoformans* (Fig. 11.113), skin lesions occur in approximately 10% of patients. These cutaneous lesions are rarely sites of primary inoculation, but are almost always manifestations of disseminated disease in an immunocompromised individual (see Chapter 13). They may be papules, acneform pustules or subcutaneous abscesses which ulcerate, with relatively little surrounding reaction, or they may exhibit pronounced granulomatous inflammation and resemble lesions of blastomycosis, as in Fig. 11.114.

African histoplasmosis

This disease, caused by *Histoplama capsulatum* var. *duboisii* (a much larger yeast than the parent strain – Fig. 11.115) occurs in a belt across equatorial Africa. The disease may be localized, sometimes with only a single skin lesion, probably a result of inoculation. In the disseminated form, skin lesions may be numerous and scattered haphazardly over the body (Fig. 11.116), with prominent secondary lymphadenopathy and constitutional symptoms.

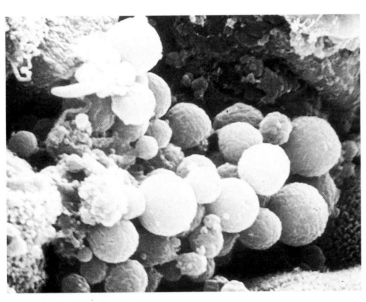

Fig. 11.113 Cryptococcosis. Scanning electron micrograph of spores of *Cryptococcus neoformans*.

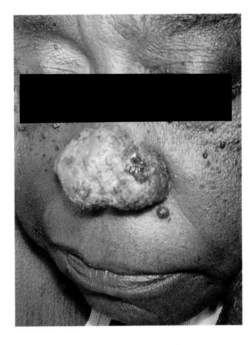

Fig. 11.114 Cutaneous cryptococcosis. Active granulomatous lesion on the nose of a 68-year-old woman with Hodgkin's disease. By courtesy of Dr T. F. Sellers, Jr.

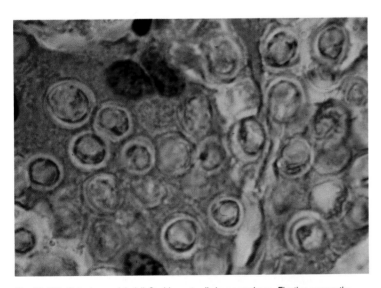

Fig. 11.115 *Histoplasma duboisii.* Ovoid yeast cells in macrophage. Fixation causes the cytoplasm to contract erroneously, suggesting the presence of a capsule. By courtesy of Prof. R. Y. Cartwright.

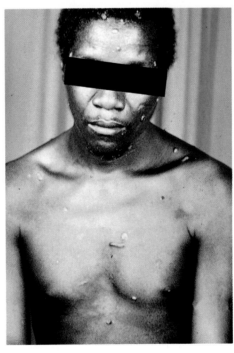

Fig. 11.116 African histoplasmosis. Multiple pale, nodular, granulomatous lesions of the skin in disseminated infection due to *Histoplasma duboisii*. By courtesy of Dr W. M. Rambo.

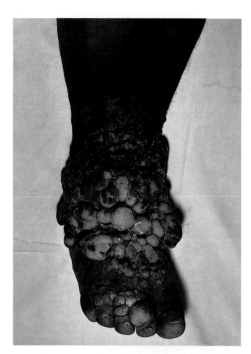

Fig. 11.117
Chromomycosis. Large verrucous mass on foot of African patient. By courtesy of Dr G. Griffin.

There may be multiple sites of osteomyelitis, with contiguous subcutaneous abscesses and chronically draining sinus tracts (see Chapter 8). The lungs are very rarely involved. The disease is usually extremely chronic but a more rapidly progressive, fatal form with fever, anaemia, weight loss and hepatosplenomegaly has been seen. Amphotericin B is still the drug of choice.

Chromomycosis

This chronic cutaneous and subcutaneous fungal infection occurs worldwide, but is more common in the tropics and in areas where people walk barefoot. A number of fungal species are responsible but all produce characteristic brown, thick walled, 'sclerotic bodies' in the tissues. The clinical appearance of chromomycosis characteristic of is groups of enlarging, warty purplish lesions that eventually look like cauliflowers (Fig. 11.117). There is as yet no satisfactory treatment.

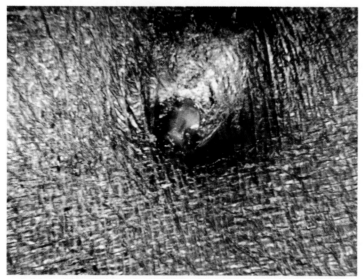

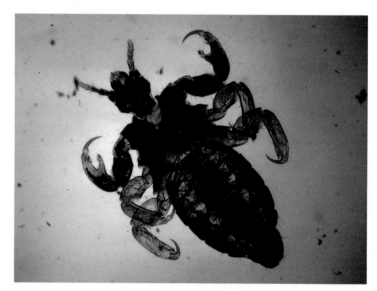

Fig. 11.119 *Pediculus corporis* – the body louse – is a small (up to 4mm), grey, flattened wingless insect with six legs ending in claws. By courtesy of Dr C. C. Kibbler.

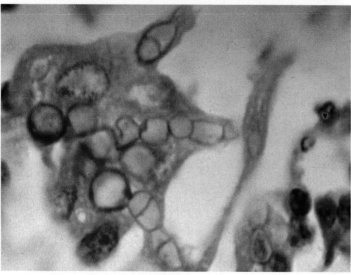

Fig. 11.120 *Phthirus pubis* (the pubic louse); its appearance has given it the nickname 'crab louse'. By courtesy of Dr C. C. Kibbler.

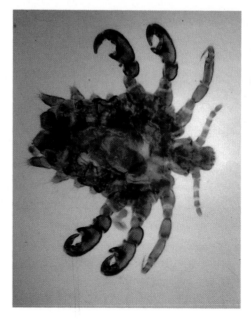

Fig. 11.118 Phaeohyphomycosis. Top: Subcutaneous abscess due to *Wangiella dermatitidis* in a diabetic patient who had several other fungal infections and who eventually died of tuberculous meningitis and *Escherichia coli* pneumonia. Bottom: Biopsy from the same lesion showing the characteristic brown septate mycelia of this fungus within a multinucleated giant cell. By courtesy of A. E. Prevost.

Other fungi

Several dematiaceous (dark-walled) saprophytic fungi can, on very rare occasions, produce cutaneous infection in man. These include species of *Phialophora* (Fig. 11.118).

ECTOPARASITES

Pediculosis (Lice)

There are three varieties of louse that infest humans: *Pediculus humanis* var. *corporis*, the human body louse; *P. humanis* var. *capitis*, the head louse; and *Phthirus pubis*, the pubic or crab louse. The body louse and head louse are almost identical (Fig. 11.119) but the pubic louse is distinctive (Fig. 11.20 – see also Chapter 7). Head lice are seen infrequently. In most cases, the eggs or nits are seen attached to the base of the hair in persons whose major complaint is itching of the scalp (Fig. 11.121). Body lice are usually seen in the seams of clothing. Infestation may be accompanied by papular excoriations on the body. A generalized eruption, often with secondary pigmenta-tion and lichenified skin, is sometimes seen in long-stand-ing infestation and is referred to as 'vagabonds' disease (Fig. 11.122).

Head lice are best treated with 0.5% malathion lotion, but this is not available in the USA. Less efficient reme-dies include lindane (gamma benzene hexachloride) or permethrin. Body lice need to be eradicated by ironing the seams of clothing laundered in hot water or by dusting the clothes with malathion or 10% DDT powder.

Myiasis

Myiasis is the invasion of human tissues by larvae of vari-ous species of fly. Sometimes this occurs when flies lay their eggs in necrotic tissue or open wounds and the mag-gots produce little damage (Fig. 11.123), the clinical conse-quences being merely revulsion. There are, however, sev-eral species of flies, usually found in tropical areas, where the life cycle specifically involves the invasion of living tis-sues. One such is the tumbu fly, the larvae of which cause a furuncular lesion after penetrating intact skin (Fig. 11.124). The spiracles (breathing tubes) of the larva can

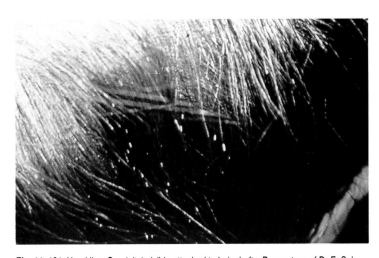

Fig. 11.121 Head lice. Ova (nits) visible attached to hair shafts. By courtesy of Dr E. Sahn.

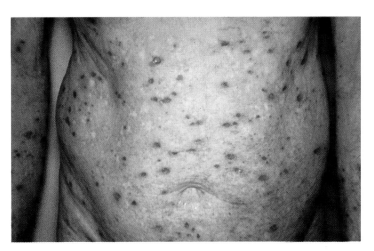

Fig. 11.122 Pediculosis. Massive infestation can, if it remains untreated, lead to a generalized hyperpigmentation and skin lichenification in association with numerous excoriations (vagabonds' disease). By courtesy of Dr S. Olansky.

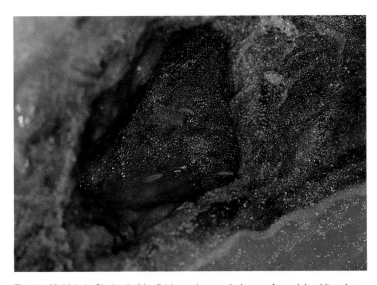

Fig. 11.123 Myiasis. Bluebottle (blowfly) larvae in necrotic tissues of sacral decubitus ulcer.

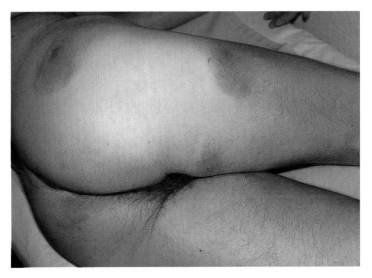

Fig. 11.124 Tumbu fly. Furuncular lesions over legs and buttock of a recent traveller to Africa.

usually be seen protruding through the surface of the lesion. Application of petroleum jelly to the lesion will suffocate the maggots and they often come wriggling out backwards (Fig. 11.125).

Chigoe flea

The chigoe flea (*Tunga penetrans*) is found in Africa and South America. The gravid adult burrows beneath the skin, particularly in the hands, feet and genitals. Painful swellings are produced, and these may become secondarily infected. Removal of the top of the lesion will reveal the egg-filled female flea (Fig. 11.126). If possible this should be removed intact.

Scabies

Scabies is caused by the mite *Sarcoptes scabiei* var. *hominis*, the female of which (Fig. 11.127) burrows into the skin of the host, laying its eggs in the base of the stratum corneum of the epidermis. The eruption and itch are caused by an immune reaction to the mite, its eggs or its faeces. Transmission is by personal contact, but this does not have to be intimate – hand holding is quite sufficient. The rash of scabies is most often found on the hands, especially in the interdigital webs and on the wrists (Fig. 11.128), in the anterior axillary folds, around the nipples, on the buttocks and penis (see Chapter 7), and sometimes on knees and feet. The head is spared, except in infancy

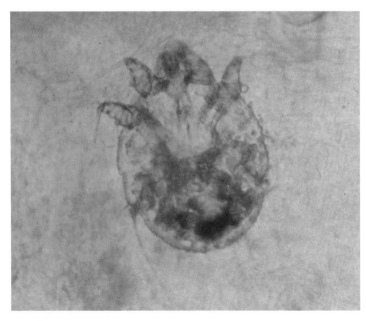

Fig. 11.125 Tumbu fly. Maggot on skin at side of lesion.

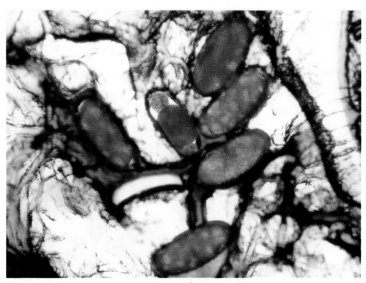

Fig. 11.126 Chigoe flea. Eggs and body parts of an adult in dermal tissues. By courtesy of Dr K. Nye.

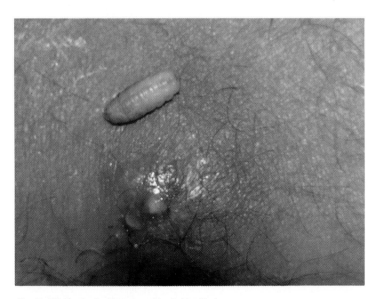

Fig. 11.127 Scabies. Female *Sarcoptes scabiei* mite.

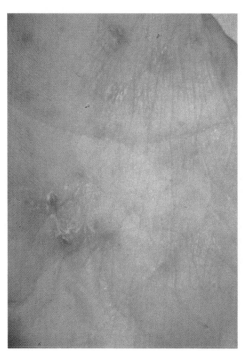

Fig. 11.128 Scabies. Minute burrows can be seen together with papules.

and childhood. The classic burrows are seen as short linear or wavy papules (Fig. 11.129). Ink applied to the skin is taken into the burrow by capillary action and aids visualisation if there is doubt. Alternatively the diagnosis can be confirmed by scraping the burrow with a scalpel blade covered with mineral oil. Microscopic examination of the result will demonstrate mites, mite eggs or characteristic black spiky faeces. A severe form of scabies, termed Norwegian scabies, is sometimes seen, especially in institutions for the mentally handicapped or in immunosuppressed persons. Widespread thickening and scaling of the skin is associated with myriad mites (Figs 11.130 & 11.131).

One of the most effective scabicides is lindane but this must be used carefully because of potential neurotoxicity in young infants and in pregnancy. Other effective lotions are cotamiton, malathion and monosulfiram. It is important to reapply the lotion to the hands after each washing and to treat the pruritus with a soothing skin preparation. The pruritus may last for several days after adequate antiscabetic therapy.

Necrotic spider bite

Bites by spiders of the genus *Loxosceles* (*L. reclusa*, the brown recluse spider, is the most common species in the USA) produce blistering followed by local ischaemia and necrosis. The resulting ulcer may continue to spread for weeks, with extensive tissue damage (Fig. 11.132). Systemic symptoms are common and include fever, rigors,

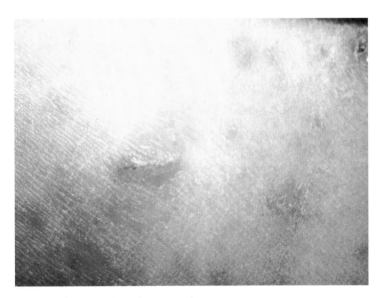

Fig. 11.129 Scabies. A diagnostic cutaneous burrow.

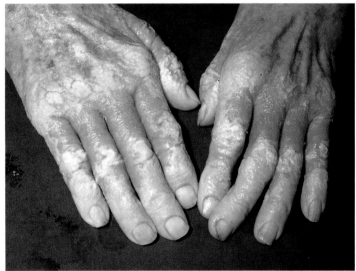

Fig. 11.130 Norwegian scabies. Hyperinfestation with *Sarcoptes scabiei* producing marked thickening and scaling of the skin of the hands. This condition is sometimes called Norwegian scabies.

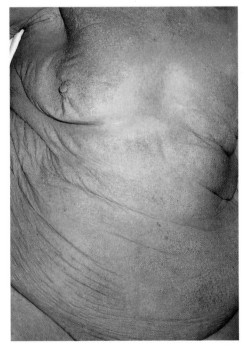

Fig. 11.131 Norwegian scabies, with thickening and scaling of the skin on the patient's trunk.

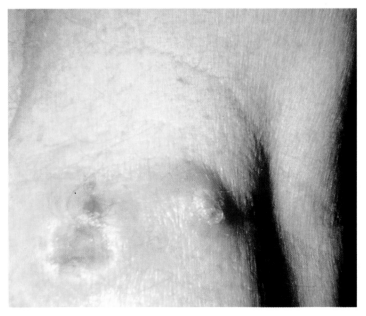

Fig. 11.132 Necrotic spider bite. Two lesions caused by a brown recluse spider; one of the lesions is beginning to ulcerate. By courtesy of Dr K. A. Riley.

vomiting and rashes. Acute haemolysis is an occasional complication.

Blister beetle

Contact with a number of different species of beetle causes local skin irritation with vesiculation or even large bullae (Fig. 11.133). The lesion is caused by a vesicant secretion produced when the beetle is crushed onto, or is brushed off the skin.

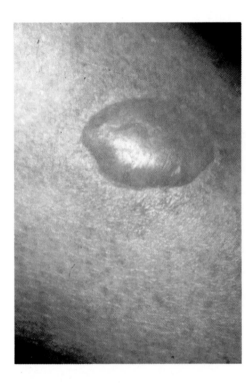

Fig. 11.133 Blister beetle. A large bulla caused by contact with the vesicant produced by a blister beetle. By courtesy of Dr K. A. Riley.

12

THE EYE

PERIOCULAR INFECTIONS

Infection of the eyelids is common, either in the form of local inflammation or abscesses, or as a diffuse blepharitis.

Abscesses of the eyelid

These are of two types: a stye (or external hordeolum) or an acute chalazion (or internal hordeolum). A stye is an acute infection of the glands of the eyelash follicle, and presents as a localized, painful abscess on the lid margin (Fig. 12.1). The abscess points and subsequently discharges. Recurrences are common. A chalazion is a granulomatous reaction that occurs when there is infection and plugging of one of the deeper Meibomian glands of the eyelid. This is more painful than a stye and generally remains as a localized tender swelling (Fig. 12.2). The cause of these abscesses is usually *Staphylococcus aureus*. Treatment is initially conservative, with warm compresses and topical antibiotics being administered. If there is no response, surgical incision and curettage may be needed.

Blepharitis

This is a common bilateral inflammation of the lid margins, usually of staphylococcal origin. It is characterized by hyperaemia of the lid margins, with crusts and scales, destruction of the lash follicles and, perhaps, ulceration (Fig. 12.3). Seborrhoea of the scalp commonly coexists and is treated with a combination of medicated shampoo and antibiotic ointment (for the infection).

Some viral infections, which mainly cause corneal disease (see below), may also affect the lids. Vaccinia with vesiculation of the lids (Fig. 12.4) was often caused by implantation from a site of vaccination before the smallpox eradication campaign made this a rare procedure: keratitis was a common complication. Herpes simplex can infect the lids and conjunctiva. Herpetic blepharoconjunctivitis is usually a primary infection resulting from inoculation of herpes simplex virus. The infection produces typical herpetic vesicles on and near the lids, and these lesions later become pustular (Fig. 12.5). There is often an associated conjunctival inflammation.

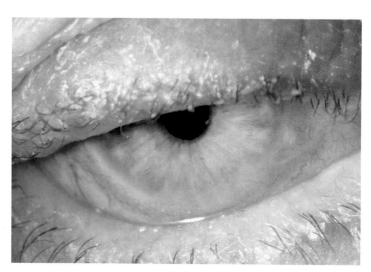

Fig. 12.1 Acute Stye. Acute inflammation of upper eyelid due to *Staphylococcus aureus*. By courtesy of Dr A. N. Carlson

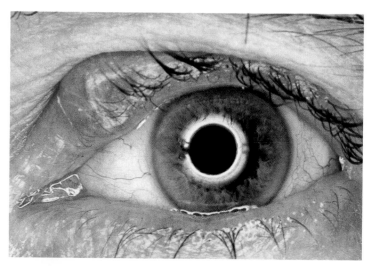

Fig. 12.2 Chalazion. Local redness and swelling due to granulomatous inflammation of the Meibomian gland. By courtesy of Mr R. J. Marsh.

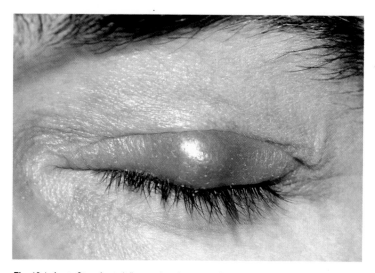

Fig 12.3 Blepharitis. Crusts and scales on the lid margin, which are erythematous and slightly swollen. The eyelashes are irregular and fewer in number than usual. By courtesy of Mr R. J. Marsh.

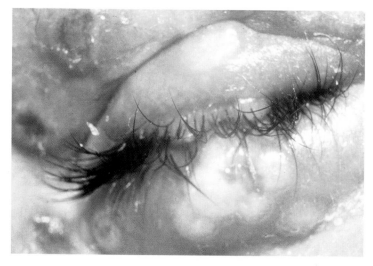

Fig 12.4 Vaccinia. Swelling and vesiculation of the lids following accidental implantation of vaccinia virus from a site of inoculation. By courtesy of Prof. A. M. Geddes.

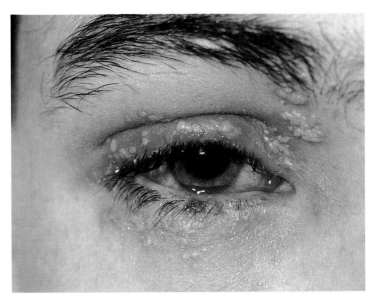

Fig. 12.5 Herpes simplex blepharitis. More often a cause of keratitis, herpes simplex infection of the eye may sometimes affect mainly the lids and conjunctiva. Apart from the presence of vesicles, which, as in this case, later become pustular, the appearances resemble other types of blepharoconjunctivitis.

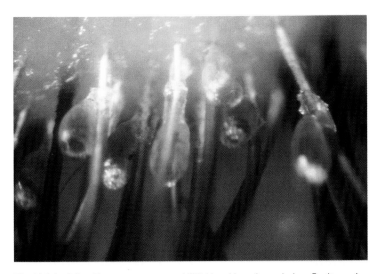

Fig. 12.6 Lash lice. The empty egg cases of *Phthiris pubis* on the eyelashes. Pruritus and chronic blepharitis may result. By courtesy of Mr S. Harding.

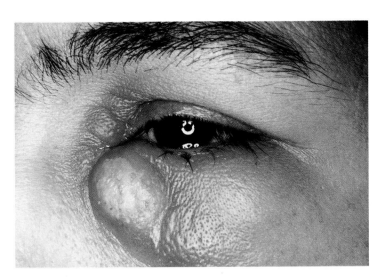

Fig. 12.7 Dacryocystitis. A localized swelling can be seen at the site of the lacrimal sac. Occasionally this identifying feature is obscured by surrounding inflammatory oedema. By courtesy of Mr R. J. Marsh.

Lash lice

Phthiris pubis (crab lice – see Chapter 7) are usually transmitted by sexual contact. The female louse attaches the egg cases (nits) to hair shafts. The pubic hair is most commonly affected but the eyebrow hair and eyelashes (Fig. 12.6) are sometimes infested.

Dacryocystitis

Acute or chronic inflammation of the lacrimal sac is usually associated with the unilateral obstruction of the nasolacrimal duct. Patients present with watering of the eye and an acutely painful and tender swelling in the medial corner of the eye (Fig. 12.7). The bacteria chiefly responsible for the acute cases are *S. aureus* and *Streptococcus pneumoniae,* although a large variety of pathogens can cause chronic dacryocystitis. Acute inflammation settles with systemic antibiotics and warm compresses, but surgical drainage of the nasolacrimal duct is needed once the acute episode is over.

Preseptal cellulitis

The upper and lower eyelids have similar structures: extending from the orbital rim is the orbital septum which separates the preseptal orbicularis muscle from the deeper contents of the bony orbit (Fig. 12.8). Infection anterior to

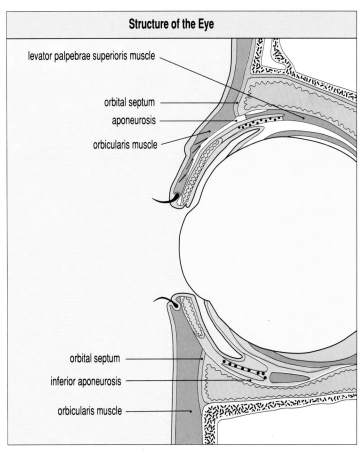

Structure of the Eye

levator palpebrae superioris muscle
orbital septum
aponeurosis
orbicularis muscle

orbital septum
inferior aponeurosis
orbicularis muscle

Fig. 12.8 Diagram of the anatomy of the upper and lower eyelids showing the position of the orbital septum separating the skin and orbicularis muscle from the pre-aponeurotic fat pad and the deeper orbital structures.

the septum must be distinguished from orbital cellulitis (see below). Preseptal cellulitis is usually secondary to small abrasions of the eyelids (when staphylococci and streptococci are the usual pathogens) or is caused by capsulated strains of *Haemophilus influenzae* in children under the age of 6 years. There is fever, pain, swelling and erythema of the eyelid (Fig. 12.9) but, unlike true orbital infection, proptosis and limitation of ocular mobility are not found. The septum usually prevents infection from spreading to the orbital tissues and the patient does not become desperately ill. Therapy lasts for 7–10 days using systemic antibiotics (a semisynthetic penicillin for older children and cefuroxime for possible haemophilus infections).

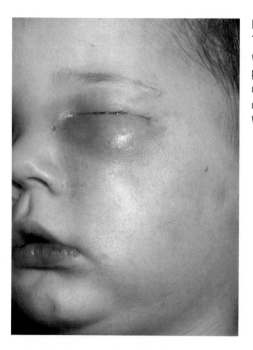

Fig. 12.9 Preseptal cellulitis. The cellulitis and lid oedema were not accompanied by any proptosis or limitations of ocular mobility in this young child. By courtesy of Dr M. J. Winterborn.

ORBITAL INFECTIONS

Acute infection of the orbital contents is potentially very serious because of the possibility of infection spreading posteriorly, leading to cavernous sinus thrombosis and death.

Most cases are caused by, and result from the spread of, bacteria from the paranasal sinuses, particularly the ethmoid or frontal sinuses. The orbit is surrounded by the paranasal sinuses and here the bones separating the structures are very thin so that infection spreads easily (Fig. 12.10). Other cases result from direct inoculation of bacteria following puncture wounds to the orbital septum (see Fig. 12.8) or from surgical or dental infections. The organisms most commonly implicated are the major sinus pathogens *S. aureus, Streptococcus pyogenes, H. influenzae* and *S. pneumoniae*. Anaerobes may also be responsible.

Five stages of orbital infection are recognised: inflammatory oedema; orbital cellulitis; subperiosteal abscess; orbital abscess; and cavernous sinus thrombosis. In the first stage there are no bacteria within the orbit but there is swelling of the eyelids secondary to suppurative sinusitis (particularly of the ethmoids in a child – Fig. 12.11). Once infection spreads within the orbit, the oedema is accompanied by the characteristic signs of fever, rhinorrhoea, headache, orbital pain and tenderness. Proptosis and chemosis follow and there is limitation of mobility of the eye. With development of a subperiosteal abscess there is lateral or vertical displacement of the globe (Fig. 12.12), and a decrease in visual acuity, due to vascular compromise, may occur at this or the orbital abscess stage. The patient with cavernous sinus thrombosis also has meningeal signs, retinal changes (engorged veins and papilloedema) and altered consciousness (Fig. 12.13).

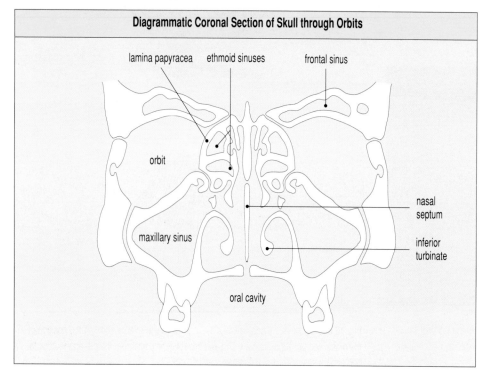

Diagrammatic Coronal Section of Skull through Orbits

lamina papyracea   ethmoid sinuses   frontal sinus

orbit

nasal septum

maxillary sinus

inferior turbinate

oral cavity

Fig. 12.10 Orbital infection. Diagram of the relationship between the orbit and the paranasal sinuses showing the lamina papyracea and other very thin bones through which sinus infection can track into the orbit.

All patients with suspected orbital infection should have an emergency ophthalmological assessment. Sinus and orbital x-rays may reveal the source of the infection (Fig. 12.14), and an otolaryngological consultation may be required for the aspiration of infected sinus contents. Ultrasonography and CT scanning techniques provide the most important information as to the appearance of an abscess (Fig. 12.15). Treatment is immediate with high dose parenteral antibiotics. Cefuroxime is a suitable choice as is a combination of ampicillin and a penicillinase-resistant penicillin, such as flucloxacillin or nafcillin. Sinus decongestion is essential and sinus drainage may be needed if there is no improvement within 24 hours. If there is a subperiosteal or orbital abscess it must be drained immediately.

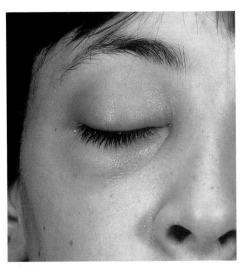

Fig. 12.11 Orbital cellulitis. Oedema and erythema of the eyelids in orbital cellulitis. This condition can be distinguished from preseptal cellulitis by pain and limitation of mobility when attempts are made to move the eye. By courtesy of the late Mr P. Shenoi.

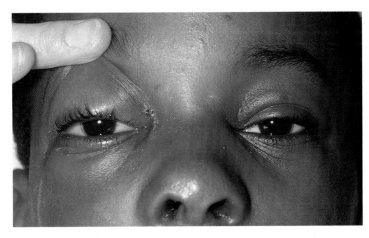

Fig. 12.12 Orbital cellulitis. Proptosis and lateral or vertical displacement of the globe (as in this boy) should suggest the development of a subperiosteal or orbital abscess.

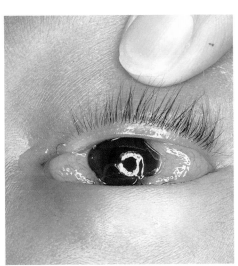

Fig. 12.13 Cavernous sinus thrombosis. This young child had severe chemosis, proptosis, external ophthalmoplegia, altered consciousness and meningism. By courtesy of Prof. A. M. Geddes.

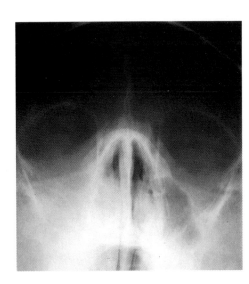

Fig. 12.14 Orbital cellulitis. Sinus x-ray in a 14-year-old with orbital cellulitis showing opacification of the right maxillary sinus.

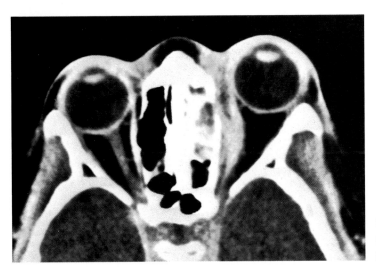

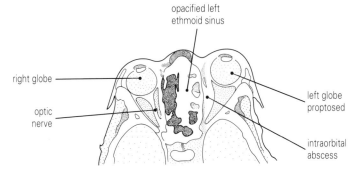

Fig. 12.15 Orbital abscess. CT scan showing opacification of the left ethmoid sinus, proptosis of the left globe and an intraorbital abscess. This should be an indication for immediate drainage.

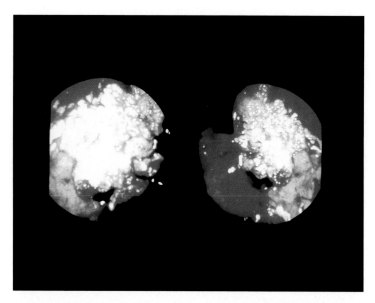

Fig. 12.16 Rhinocerebral mucormycosis. View through nasal speculum showing fungal material arising from nasal turbinates. By courtesy of Prof. R. Y. Cartwright.

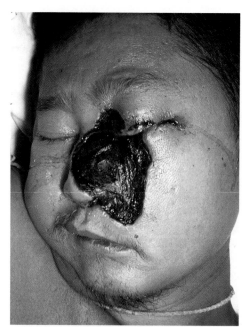

Fig. 12.17 Rhinocerebral mucormycosis. Advanced case with necrosis of nasal and maxillary tissue and black eschar. Note the periorbital oedema, and serosanguinous discharge from the eye. By courtesy of Prof. R. Y. Cartwright.

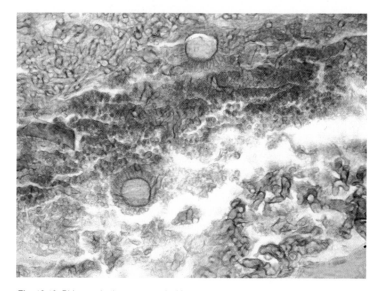

Fig. 12.18 Rhinocerebral mucormycosis. Mucor organisms visible in biopsy, showing irregular branching hyphae and sporangia. By courtesy of Prof. R. Y. Cartwright.

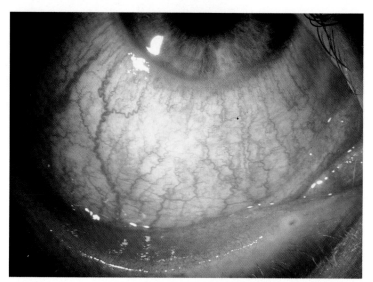

Fig. 12.19 Acute conjunctivitis. Typical distribution of hyperaemia, diminishing in severity towards the cornea. In iritis the hyperaemia is greatest at the limbus. By courtesy of Mr S. Harding.

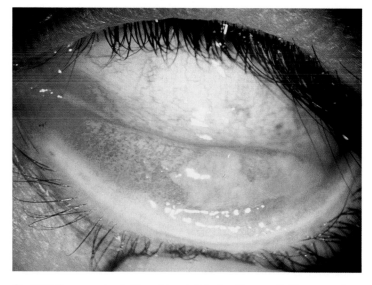

Fig. 12.20 Pharyngoconjunctival fever. Adenoviral infection of the eye with diffuse congestion of the palpebral and bulbar conjunctiva with formation of a patchy pseudomembrane.

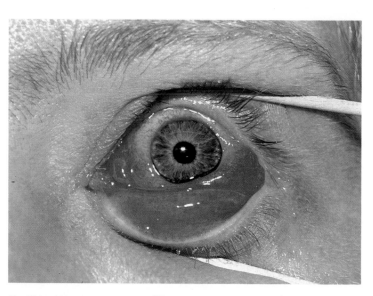

Fig. 12.21 Adenovirus conjunctivitis. Acute onset follicular conjunctivitis associated with preauricular lymphadenopathy and watery discharge. By courtesy of Dr. A. N. Carlson.

Rhinocerebral mucormycosis

This infection by fungi of the order Mucorales occurs in patients with diabetic ketoacidosis and in patients with prolonged neutropenia who have had broad spectrum antibacterial drugs (see Chapter 1). The hyphae invade from the nasal turbinates (Fig. 12.16) or paranasal sinuses and rapidly spread to the orbit and from there to the cranium. Blood vessel invasion and thrombosis occur early and cause infarction: necrosis of bone and contralateral hemiplegia (due to thrombosis of the internal carotid artery as it traverses the cavernous sinus) are common. The patient has signs of a rapidly progressive orbital cellulitis and a serosanguinous nasal discharge, with alteration of consciousness and cranial nerve palsies. Gangrenous lesions are common (Fig. 12.17). The Mucorales can be identified in a biopsy (Fig. 12.18). Treatment is extensive surgical debridement, correction of the underlying disorder and intravenous amphotericin B.

CONJUNCTIVITIS

Acute infection of the conjunctiva can be caused by numerous viruses, bacteria and chlamydia and more chronic infections can be caused by fungi and parasites. All forms cause discomfort (usually itching rather than pain), excessive lacrimation, and dilatation of the superficial conjunctival vessels, producing a red eye (Fig. 12.19). Secretions are produced which, in bacterial infections, are often purulent and may cloud vision. True visual impairment is, however, not present. The cornea is sometimes also involved in viral conjunctivitis and occasionally bacteria may also invade the cornea (see below).

Viral conjunctivitis

Of the viruses, the adenoviruses are the most important cause of conjunctivitis. Serotypes 3 and 7 are a common cause of swimming pool conjunctivitis and its associated fever and sore throat (pharyngoconjunctival fever) in the summer months (Fig. 12.20). Adenovirus conjunctivitis is often accompanied by enlargement of the preauricular lymph node and by follicle formation on the palpebral conjunctiva. This produces a greyish-white pebbly appearance to the conjunctiva. Adenoviruses types 8, 11 or 17 cause a more severe condition, epidemic keratoconjunctivitis (Fig. 12.21); this is often complicated a few days after its onset by punctate keratitis, which may result in persistent subepithelial corneal opacities (Fig. 12.22). These viruses are extremely contagious and may be spread nosocomially.

Acute haemorrhagic conjunctivitis (Fig. 12.23) is caused by a number of different viruses including enterovirus, type 70 and coxsackie virus, type A24, and is a disease of poor hygiene and overcrowding. Subconjunctival haemorrhages and lid oedema are seen in addition to the other signs of conjunctivitis. Neurological complications may follow. Conjunctivitis is also sometimes seen as part of other viral infections such as measles, rubella and influenza.

There is no specific therapy for viral conjunctivitis but symptomatic relief may be provided with eye drops.

Bacterial conjunctivitis

Many different bacteria have been described as causing conjunctivitis but the ones most commonly involved are *S. pneumoniae, S. aureus, S. pyogenes* and *H. influenzae*. Gonococcal infection is of particular importance in infants

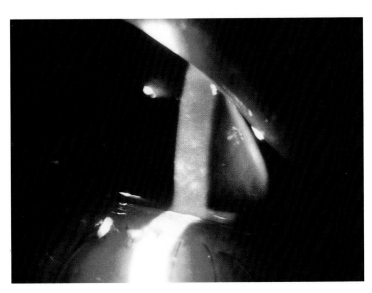

Fig. 12.22 Epidemic keratoconjunctivitis. Slit lamp photograph of the more severe form of adenoviral infection often accompanied by a subepithelial punctate keratitis.

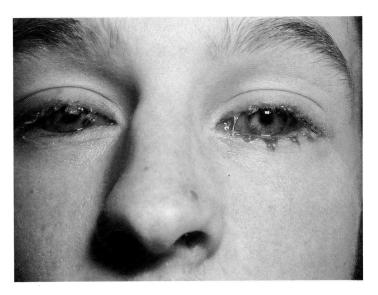

Fig. 12.23 Acute haemorrhagic conjunctivitis. Bilateral bulbar conjunctival haemorrhages in infection caused by coxsackievirus A24. By courtesy of Prof. A. M. Geddes.

(see below). The infection often begins unilaterally but spreads to cause a profuse, purulent discharge (Fig. 12.24) which may dry and stick the eyelids together. Treatment with topical antibiotics will reduce the duration of the illness. Eye drops should be used very frequently during the day and ophthalmic ointment (which is less easy to wash away) at night. The antibiotics commonly used are chloramphenicol, gentamicin, bacitracin or a combination of neomycin and polymyxin. It should be remembered that gentamicin is ineffective against streptococci. The use of eye patches should be avoided.

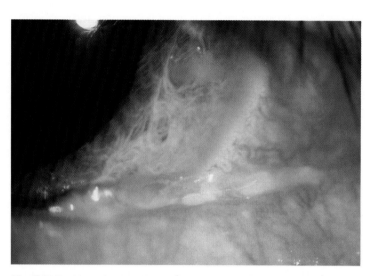

Fig. 12.24 Purulent conjunctivitis. Purulent fluid exuding from the eye. This is a common feature in bacterial conjunctivitis. By courtesy of Mr S. Harding.

Chlamydia trachomatis conjunctivitis

In adults, *C. trachomatis* causes two distinct eye infections: inclusion conjunctivitis (TRIC conjunctivitis) and trachoma.

Inclusion conjunctivitis

This is a form of follicular conjunctivitis that occurs in neonates or sexually active adults and is caused by the chlamydia of subgroups D–K (see Chapter 7). The organisms are transmitted sexually and inclusion conjunctivitis is associated with cervicitis in women and urethritis in men. In adults, it tends to be gradual in onset and the characteristic feature is the formation of large follicles, particularly in the lower palpebral conjunctiva (Fig. 12.25). The diagnosis can be made by demonstrating the basophilic inclusion bodies on Giemsa stain (see Fig. 7.8) and by direct immunofluorescence (see Fig. 7.11) of conjunctival scrapings. Treatment is with oral tetracycline or erythromycin given for 3 weeks.

Trachoma

Trachoma is a chronic follicular conjunctivitis, caused by infection with serotypes A–C of *C. trachomatis*. It is spread directly from eye to eye and is a major cause of blindness in areas of the world with poor standards of hygiene. There are four stages of the disease: Stage I (acute conjunctivitis) is very similar to inclusion conjunc-

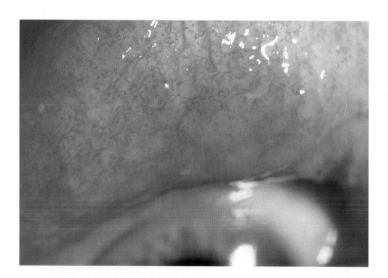

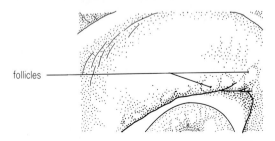

follicles

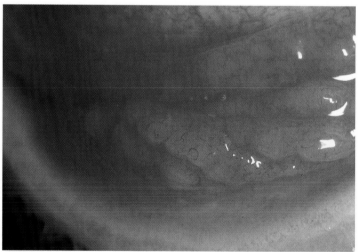

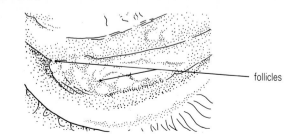

follicles

Fig. 12.25 TRIC conjunctivitis. A typical case with large follicles in the lower fornix. By courtesy of Mr P. A. Hunter.

tivitis; Stage II is characterized by corneal vascularization (Fig. 12.26); Stage III is typified by scarring of the palpebral conjunctiva (Fig. 12.27); and Stage IV, pannus formation invading the upper cornea (Fig. 12.28). The complications of trachoma result from scarring and contraction of the conjunctiva and corneal scarring secondary to drying and corneal vascularization. Treatment with oral tetracycline or erythromycin with or without rifampicin for 3–6 weeks will usually prevent such complications.

Ophthalmia neonatorum

Contamination of the neonate's eye during birth may lead to conjunctivitis. It is usually caused by *C. trachomatis*, gonococci or staphylococci (Fig. 12.29). The most serious form is that caused by *Neisseria gonorrhoeae*, which develops between the second and fifth day of life and produces a profuse bilateral purulent discharge. It may rapidly progress to damage the cornea and cause destruction of the eye. The finding of gram-negative diplococci on Gram staining should lead to immediate treatment with parenteral benzyl penicillin. For the b-lactamase-producing strains intramuscular cefuroxime or ceftriaxone is suitable. The mother must of course also be treated. In order to prevent neonatal gonococcal conjunctivitis, topical erythromycin, tetracycline or silver nitrate eye drops are routinely applied in many hospitals. Staphylococcal conjunctivitis in the neonate can usually be treated with topical antibiotics.

C. trachomatis has become the most common cause of conjunctivitis in neonates. Chlamydial conjunctivitis (Fig. 12.30) begins later than gonococcal infection, usually between days 5 and 10. It may be unilateral or bilateral. There is marked eyelid oedema and a purulent exudate but, since infants do not have lymphoid tissue, there is not the typical follicular conjunctivitis seen in adults (see above). This form of conjunctivitis cannot be prevented by the prophylactic use of topical silver nitrate, and recent studies suggest that topical erythromycin or tetracycline

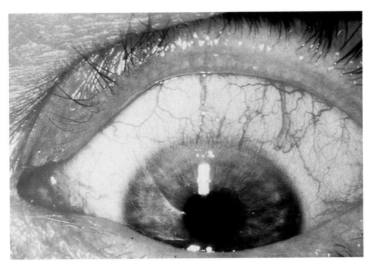

Fig. 12.26 Trachoma. Early involvement of the cornea with new vessel formation at the upper margin. By courtesy of Mr G. Gatford.

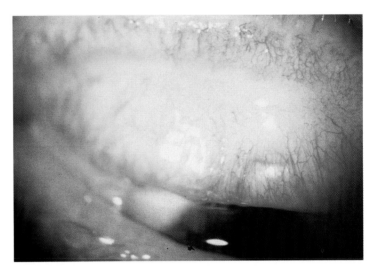

Fig. 12.27 Trachoma, with scarring of the palpebral conjunctiva of the upper lid.

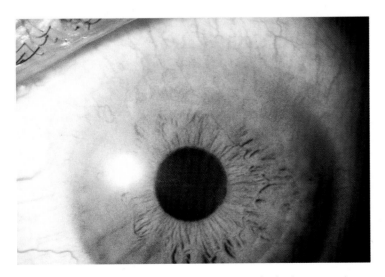

Fig. 12.28 Trachoma. The formation of trachomatous pannus showing the new vessel formation and hazy upper corneal margin.

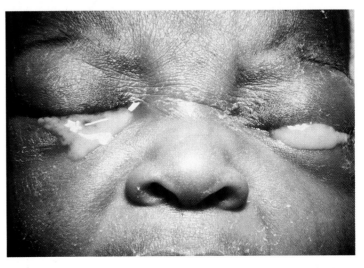

Fig. 12.29 Ophthalmia neonatorum. Marked bilateral purulent discharge in a neonate. This infection was subsequently shown to be caused by *S. aureus*. By courtesy of Dr P. Dobson.

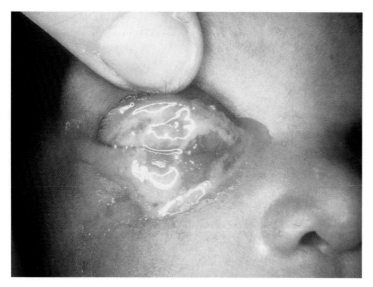

Fig. 12.30 *Chlamydia* ophthalmia neonatorum. This is now the most common form of neonatal conjunctivitis. By courtesy of Dr G. Ridgway.

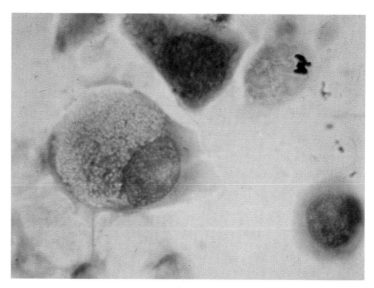

Fig. 12.31 *Chlamydia* conjunctivitis. Intracytoplasmic inclusion bodies in an epithelial cell from a neonate's eye. By courtesy of Dr G. Ridgway.

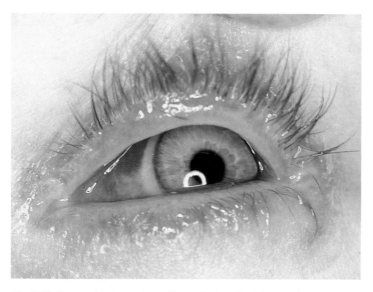

Fig. 12 32 Stevens–Johnson syndrome. Haemorrhagic conjunctivitis associated with skin lesions of erythema multiforme (lesions are just visible to left and right of illustration). This followed sulphonamide administration.

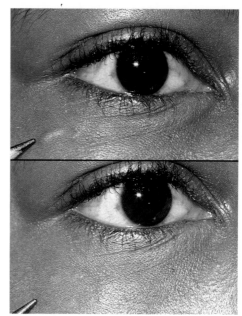

Fig 12.33 Loiasis. Top: subcutaneous worm involving the patients eyelid. Bottom: A few seconds later, the worm has disappeared. By courtesy of Dr. A. N. Carlson

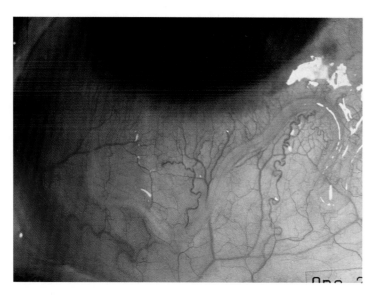

Fig. 12 34 Loiasis. Threadlike adult *L. loa* migrating in the subconjunctival tissues. By courtesy of Teaching Aids at Low Cost, Institute of Child Health, London.

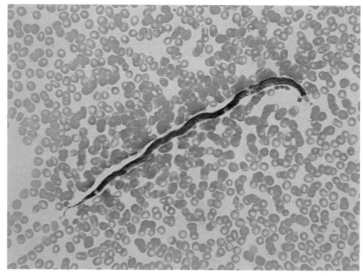

Fig. 12.35 Loiasis. A microfilaria of *L. loa* in the peripheral blood. The microfilaria measures about 300μm long.

drops at birth are equally ineffective. Diagnosis is made by Giemsa (Fig. 12.31) or immunofluorescence staining, and therapy is with oral erythromycin. Both parents need investigation and treatment for genital infection, even if they are asymptomatic.

Stevens–Johnson syndrome

A haemorrhagic conjunctivitis, this syndrome can occur as part of severe erythema multiforme (Fig. 12.32). Full details are given in Chapter 10.

Loiasis

Loa loa is a filarial nematode that is also known as the West African eyeworm. It is endemic in West and Central Africa. The life cycle is simple with man the sole host and the diurnally-biting banana fly (genus *Chrysops*) the vector. The larvae develop into adult worms which migrate through the subcutaneous tissues (Fig. 12.33) and sometimes beneath the conjunctiva (Fig. 12.34). Subcutaneous lumps known as Calabar swellings result from an immediate (Type I) hypersensitivity reaction to material released by a developing or adult worm. They usually arise singly and disappear spontaneously after a few days. Their appearance sometimes coincides with low grade pyrexia and headache. When the swellings arise over joints there is usually a painful sympathetic synovial reaction. Similar hypersensitivity reactions produce itching, pain and periorbital oedema when adult worms migrate through the conjunctiva. Visitors to endemic areas often develop prominent allergic symptoms and are much more ill than the local population when they contract loiasis.

The adults reproduce sexually releasing eggs from which larval microfilariae develop. During the day, these migrate to small blood vessels from which they are imbibed by the vector. Arthritis and meningoencephalitis have resulted from the migration of microfilariae. Diagnosis can be made by recognising Calabar swellings,

seeing the adult worms in the conjunctiva, or by finding microfilariae in the blood (Fig. 12.35) during the day. A high eosinophilia is common. Treatment, where necessary, is with diethylcarbamazine (DEC). DEC has also been shown to be of help in prophylaxis. The symptoms of conjunctival migration are best dealt with by the application of topical local anaesthetic rather than by attempting physical extraction.

KERATITIS

The infectious causes of keratitis (inflammation of the cornea) include a large number of bacteria, viruses, fungi and parasites. All causes are potentially serious; because of the risk of visual loss, the condition always needs urgent ophthalmic assessment. The cardinal clinical features of keratitis are pain, redness of the eye (due to the dilatation of the limbal vessels), decreased vision and photophobia. If there is a corneal ulcer, it may be recognized by the loss of corneal lustre and confirmed by the application of fluorescein stain. Associated intraocular infection is common.

Herpes simplex

Herpes simplex virus (HSV) is the most important viral cause of keratitis. It is always unilateral and may occur at any age. Corneal lesions may follow primary herpetic blepharoconjunctivitis (see above) but most ocular disease is associated with recurrences of HSV infection and repeated attacks are common. The symptoms of keratitis are less severe in the herpetic disease than in other forms of keratitis, as the condition is associated with corneal hypaesthesia. When the virus replicates in the corneal epithelium, the disease may have either a 'dendritic' or a geographic pattern. The typical dendritic ulcer may be seen more clearly with the use of fluorescein or bengal rose stains (Figs 12.36, 12.37 & 12.38). Amoeboid or geographical

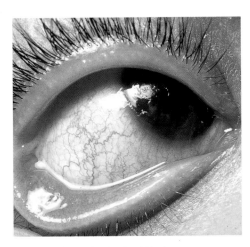

Fig. 12 36 Herpes simplex. Dendritic ulcers are a common manifestation of recurrent herpes simplex infection. Here a typical dendritic ulcer is seen on the cornea of an unstained eye. Note the associated circumlimbal vasodilatation.

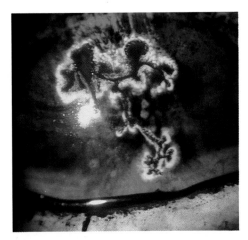

Fig. 12.37 Herpes simplex. A dendritic ulcer. Fluorescein stain.

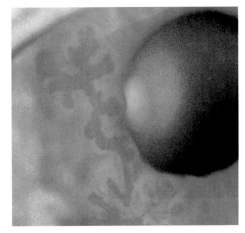

Fig. 12.38 Herpes simplex. Classical dendritic ulcer with no stromal involvement. Bengal rose stain. By courtesy of Mr P. A. Hunter.

ulcers (Figs 12.39 & 12.40) are noted for their prolonged duration. Some degree of stromal involvement is found in the more severe forms of recurrent herpetic keratitis: this is probably due to associated immune responses which may lead to corneal scarring and vascularization. Fig. 12.41 shows stromal involvement with slit-lamp photography.

The treatment of superficial herpes simplex keratitis is with topical antiviral preparations, with or without physical debridement of the affected area. Acyclovir ophthalmic ointment, or topical trifluridine, vidarabine or idoxuridine may be used. Topical weak steroid preparations may be combined with antiviral therapy to suppress the immune response in stromal disease.

Herpes zoster

Herpes zoster ophthalmicus (shingles) results from reactivation of latent varicella-zoster virus (VZV) in the part of the trigeminal ganglion associated with the first division of the trigeminal nerve (Fig. 12.42). The eye is involved in about three quarters of the cases, particularly, but not exclusively, when the nasociliary branch of the trigeminal

nerve is involved – this can be clinically diagnosed from the vesicles extending to the tip of the nose (Fig. 12.43). Ocular involvement can take several forms: most commonly it presents as iridocyclitis with punctate, segmental or disciform keratitis and visual clouding. Anterior uveitis occurs in about half the cases (Fig. 12.44). The disease may be prolonged and may lead to corneal scarring and vascularization (Fig. 12.45). Therapy of herpes zoster with oral acyclovir in high dosage (800mg, 5 times daily) for 7–10 days reduces the rate of ocular complications of trigeminal herpes zoster.

Once the complications occur, they can be treated with topical acyclovir, vidarabine or trifluridine.

Bacteria

Bacterial suppurative keratitis results from the organisms causing conjunctivitis invading the corneal stroma. The most common bacterial causes of keratitis are *S. pneumoniae*, *S. aureus* and various Gram-negative bacilli, particularly *Pseudomonas aeruginosa*, which produces rapid liquefaction of the ocular tissues. The increasing incidence of the latter is probably related to the use of soft contact

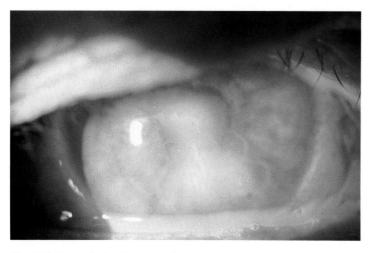

Fig. 12.39 Herpes simplex. More severe disease causes an amoeboid or geographic ulcer, here stained with fluorescein.

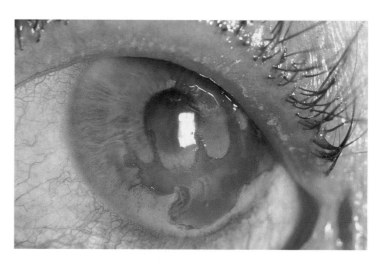

Fig. 12.40 Herpes simplex. Severe amoeboid ulcer resulting from topical steroid use. Bengal rose stain. By courtesy of Mr P. A. Hunter.

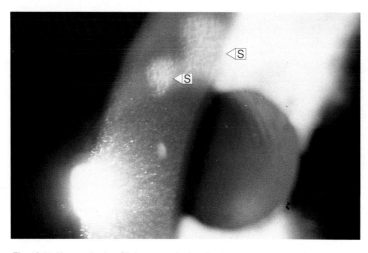

Fig. 12.41 Herpes simplex. Slit-lamp examination showing stromal scarring (S) resulting from a dendritic ulcer.

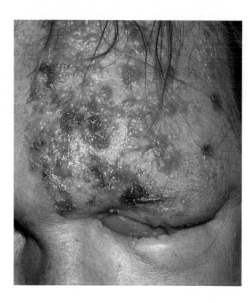

Fig. 12.42 Herpes zoster ophthalmicus. The skin supplied by the first division of the trigeminal nerve is the most frequent site for the rash of herpes zoster.

lenses. There is often acute pain in the eye, marked redness, especially at the limbus, and a well-defined grey corneal ulcer (Figs 12.46 & 12.47). The iritis associated with corneal ulceration may be severe and the resulting collection of leucocytes in the anterior chamber is known as a hypopyon (Figs 12.48 & 12.49).

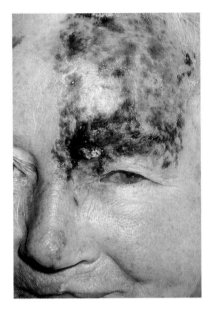

Fig. 12.43 Herpes zoster opthalmicus. Involvement of the nasociliary branch of the trigeminal nerve produces vesicles on the tip of the nose and is generally associated with corneal involvement. By courtesy of Mr. S. Harding

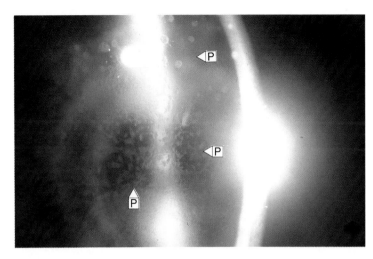

Fig. 12.44 Herpes zoster. In anterior uveitis, cells within the anterior chamber agglutinate into keratic precipitates (P) which become deposited in the corneal endothelium. By courtesy of Mr S. Harding.

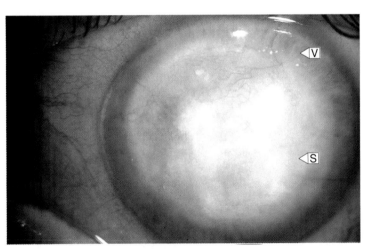

Fig. 12.45 Herpes zoster. The late result may be corneal vascularization (V) and scarring (S) and opacification. By courtesy of Mr S. Harding.

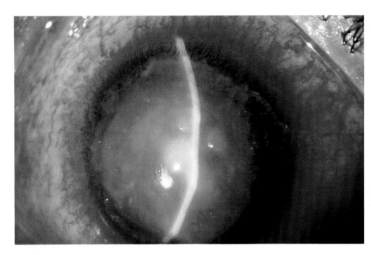

Fig. 12.46 Bacterial keratitis. Contact lens-associated keratitis due to *Pseudomonas aeruginosa*. By courtesy of Dr. A. N. Carlson

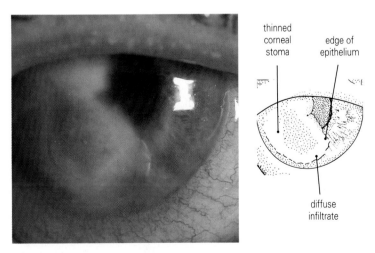

thinned corneal stoma
edge of epithelium
diffuse infiltrate

Fig. 12.47 Bacterial keratitis, in this case due to *P. aeruginosa*. An infiltrate is seen with central corneal thinning. By courtesy of Mr P. A. Hunter.

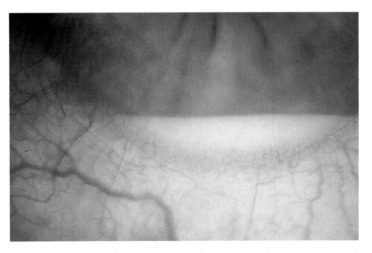

Fig. 12.48 Bacterial keratitis. A massive inflammatory response in anterior uveitis leads to precipitation of the cells as pus in the anterior chamber. This is called a hypopyon. By courtesy of Mr S. Harding.

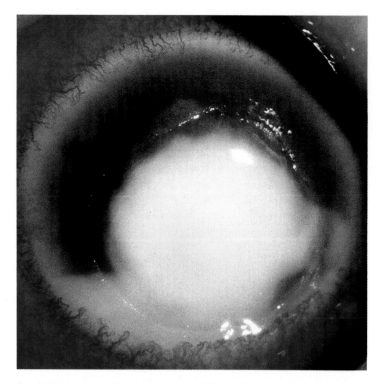

Fig. 12.49 Bacterial keratitis. *P. aeruginosa* eye infection showing corneal ulceration and hypopyon formation in this rapidly progressive eye infection.

If bacterial keratitis is suspected, patients need appropriate specimens taken from the cornea, conjunctiva and, sometimes, the anterior chamber for Gram's stain (Fig. 12.50) and culture. Appropriate antibiotic therapy can then be given. If the Gram's stain fails to show any organisms, then empirical therapy must include cover against *P. aeruginosa*, the most virulent infection.

Fungi

Fungal keratitis is uncommon but is increasing, particularly in the immunocompromised individual or in association with topical steroid usage. A number of fungi are responsible: *Fusarium solani*, *Aspergillus* and *Candida* species, *Pseudallescheria boydii* and *Curvularia* species are the most common. It may be difficult to distinguish clinically from bacterial infection (Figs 12.51 & 12.52). In all cases of suppurative keratitis, therefore, fungi should be sought in corneal scrapings (Fig. 12.53) and by culture. Prolonged therapy with topical and parenteral antifungal drugs is required.

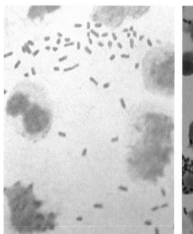 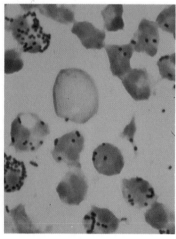

Fig. 12.50 Bacterial keratitis. Two corneal scrapings showing gram-negative bacilli (left) and gram-positive streptococci (right). By courtesy of Mr P. A. Hunter.

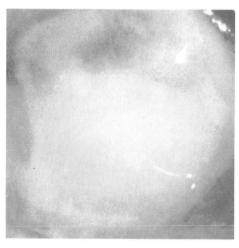 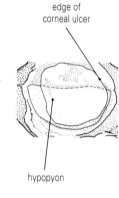

Fig. 12.51 Fungal keratitis. A large corneal ulcer with hypopyon occupying half the anterior chamber. By courtesy of Mr P. A. Hunter.

edge of corneal ulcer

hypopyon

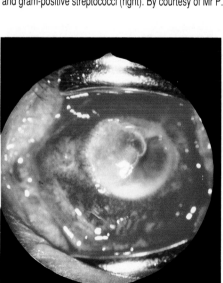

Fig. 12.52 Fungal keratitis. Corneal ulcer due to *Aspergillus flavus* infection. By courtesy of Prof. R. Y. Cartwright.

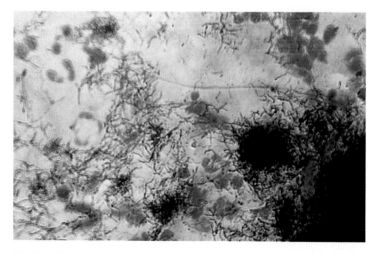

Fig. 12.53 Fungal keratitis. Fungal hyphae seen on corneal scraping. By courtesy of Mr P. A. Hunter.

Acanthamoeba

Free-living amoebas of the genus *Acanthamoeba* are now recognized as an uncommon cause of severe persistent keratitis, particularly after foreign body eye injuries or in association with soft contact lens usage. There is severe pain and examination of the eye reveals either a central corneal opacity and ulcer with pronounced surrounding inflammation or a distinctive paracentral annular corneal abscess. The diagnosis can be made by stained preparations (Fig 12.54) or axonic cultures (Fig 12.55) of corneal scrapings. Therapy with topical propamidine isethionate, clotrimidazole and neomycin may be successful but subsequent corneal transplantation is often still required.

Onchocerciasis

Onchocerciasis or 'river blindness' is caused by the nematode *Onchocerca volvulus* which is transmitted by the bite of black flies of the genus *Simulium*. It is widespread in tropical Africa, and is also found in parts of Central and South America. Infective larvae enter the wound when the fly bites, and develop over the next year or so into adult worms which lie coiled up in fibrous nodules within the subcutaneous tissues. These nodules may be felt over bony prominences (See Chapter 10). Female worms live for 15–20 years, producing several thousand larvae (microfilariae) each day. These microfilariae migrate into the skin, eyes and lymphatic tissues and are either taken up by biting black flies (and hence transmitted to infect other persons) or die after about one year.

Live microfilariae are tolerated remarkably well. It is the inflammatory reaction which surrounds the dead microfilariae that causes the serious pathology of onchocerciasis. The skin changes are described in Chapter 10. It is the microfilariae in the eye that produce the most serious effects. Patients with only a few microfilariae in the eye have a punctate keratitis with 'snowflake' opacities in the cornea (Fig. 12.56) but such patients rarely

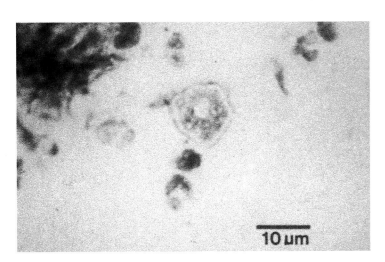

Fig. 12.54 Acanthamoeba keratitis. Corneal scraping showing a double-walled polygonal cyst. Giemsa–Wright stain. By courtesy of Dr G. S. Visvesvara. Reproduced with permission from *Reviews of Infectious Diseases* (1990) **12**, 490–513.

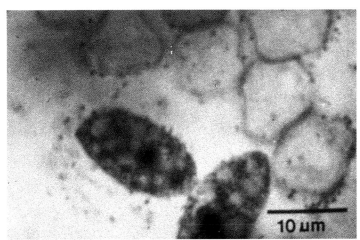

Fig. 12.55 Acanthamoebic keratitis. Two tophozoites and many polygonal cysts of *A. polyphaga* in 5-day old culture of a corneal scraping in 1.5% nonnutrient agar layered with *E. coli*. By courtesy of Dr. G. S. Visvesvera. Reproduced with permission from *Reviews of Infectious Diseases* (1990) **12**, 490–513.

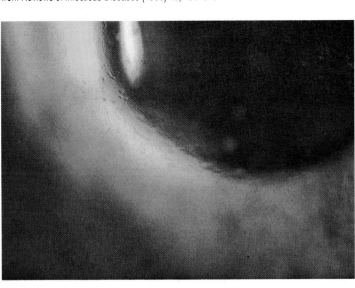

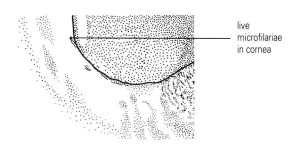

live microfilariae in cornea

Fig. 12.56 Onchocerciasis. Microfilariae in the cornea. By courtesy of Prof. B. R. Jones.

develop severe lesions. Those born in hyperendemic areas with large numbers of microfilariae have chronic eye disease including sclerosing keratitis with eventual corneal fibrosis (Fig. 12.57), iridocyclitis or optic atrophy. The diagnosis of onchocerciasis is made by demonstrating microfilariae in the skin or in the cornea or anterior chamber by slit lamp examination.

Therapy of onchocerciasis is with diethylcarbamazine and suramin (which may cause severe allergic reactions as the microfilariae are killed), or ivermectin (which is associated with a less severe host reaction and less serious adverse effects). Neither drug kills the adult worms, so surgical removal of those adults that can be discovered is necessary in order to limit the source of fresh microfilariae.

ENDOPHTHALMITIS

Endophthalmitis is the most serious of all ocular infections and is a suppurative infection of the intraocular tissues. The infection may affect only specific tissues within the eye or may involve the intraocular contents generally. It usually results as a complication of ocular surgery or other trauma but it may also develop as a metastatic manifestation of septicaemia or fungaemia, often in immunocompromised patients.

Bacteria

Following ocular surgery the most common bacteria involved are staphylococci and *P. aeruginosa*. When endophthalmitis occurs in an eye that has not recently been operated upon, haematogenous spread from a distant focus is likely. There are usually other signs of a septic focus and the most commonly implicated pathogens are *S. pneumoniae*, *S. aureus* and the meningococcus (Fig. 12.58).

The clinical features of endophthalmitis are the sudden onset of severe pain in the eye, marked chemosis and intense hyperaemia of the globe. The cornea is opaque and there is a hypopyon (Fig. 12.59). Rupture of the globe or panophthalmitis (involvement of the episcleral tissues) may occur and the progression may be very rapid. If the diagnosis of endophthalmitis is suspected urgent ophthalmological referral for vitreous aspiration and/or vitrectomy is mandatory. Antibiotic therapy is needed, using broad spectrum agents given systemically and by intravitreal injections.

Fungi

Fungal endophthalmitis may result from trauma (either surgical or non-surgical) or from endogenous sources. After trauma, the symptoms and signs are often delayed for much longer (often several weeks) than bacterial infections and the course is more indolent.

Candida albicans is the most common form of haematogenous fungal endophthalmitis, occurring in about 5% of patients with disseminated candidiasis. It is associated with the use of intravascular catheters, immunosuppression, the use of broad spectrum antibiotics and heroin addiction. Reduction of vision is the earliest symptom but many patients are too ill to report this. The first sign is a small preretinal white exudate with an over-

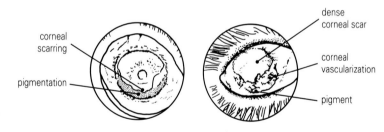

Fig. 12.57 Onchocerciasis. Advanced cases, with corneal scarring and pigment migration. By courtesy of Prof. B. R. Jones.

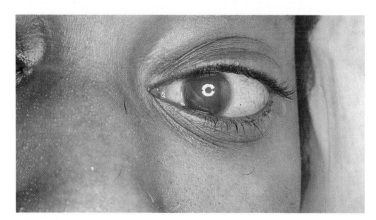

Fig. 12.58 Meningococcal endophthalmitis. There is a marked redness of the eye with corneal haziness. The patient had been admitted with meningococcal meningitis. By courtesy of Dr A. M. Geddes.

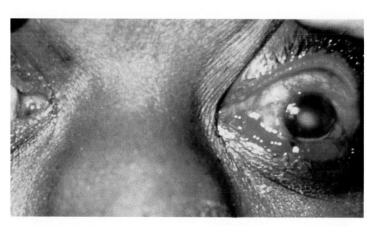

Fig. 12.59 Endophthalmitis. This was part of a pneumococcal septicaemia. There is general hyperaemia of the eye, opacification of the cornea and a hypopyon. By courtesy of Dr T. F. Sellers, Jr.

lying haze that enlarges to a fluffy white ball extending into the vitreous humour (Fig. 12.60). Progression to the anterior chamber may occur. Systemic antifungal therapy is required, and in view of the poor vitreal penetration of amphotericin B, 5-flucytosine is usually added: even so recovery of vision may not be complete.

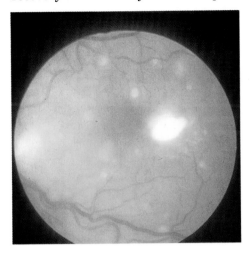

Fig. 12.60 Candida endophthalmitis. Fundus photograph showing patches of white fluffy exudate. These may be the only evidence of systemic candidiasis. By courtesy of Dr A. M. Geddes.

Other fungal infections that may develop endophthalmitis as part of disseminated disease include cryptococcosis, coccidiomycosis and histoplasmosis (this is distinct from the 'presumed ocular histoplasmosis syndrome' – see below).

Posterior Uveitis

Posterior uveitis is another term for chorioretinitis and may be purulent or granulomatous. The acute, purulent types are described as forms of bacterial or fungal endophthalmitis above. There are a number of other distinct causes of granulomatous chorioretinitis.

Toxocariasis

The common roundworms of dogs and cats are the most frequent parasitic cause of endophthalmitis. The life cycle of *Toxocara* species does not always follow the usual route of larval migration via the lungs, trachea, posterior pharynx, and thence to the bowel where the adults mature (Fig. 12.61). If the eggs are eaten by mature animals

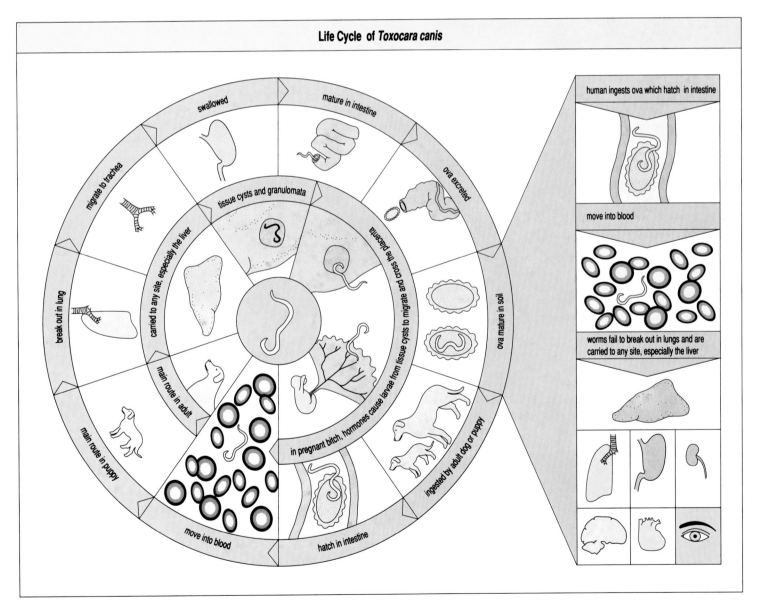

Fig. 12.61 Life cycle of *Toxocara canis*.

(including humans), the second stage larvae may migrate into various tissues, evoke a granulomatous response and become encysted. The process of migration in humans is called visceral larva migrans. The life cycle of *T. canis* is, however, unique. In the pregnant bitch, hormonal changes stimulate the transplacental migration of the encysted larvae to the fetal puppies, where they then mature within the bowel. Prenatal infection of cats with *T. catis* does not

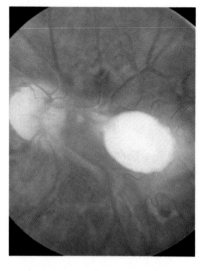

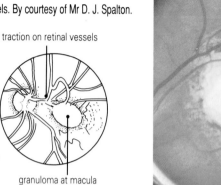

Fig. 12.62 Toxocariasis. Fundal photograph showing a large central granuloma and traction on the retinal vessels. By courtesy of Mr D. J. Spalton.

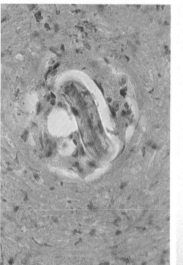

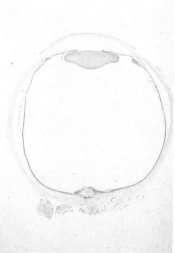

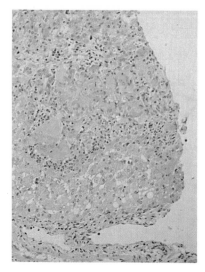

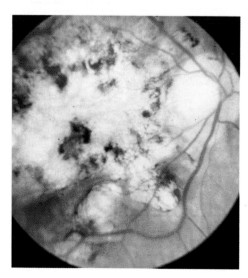

Fig. 12.63 Toxocariasis. Another fundus with a large white granuloma at the posterior pole. By courtesy of Dr P. Dobson.

Fig. 12.64 Toxocariasis. Histology shows a granuloma in the posterior pole of an eye. Higher power demonstrates the encysted nematode.

Fig. 12.65 Toxocariasis. Liver biopsy showing granuloma with numerous eosinophils. Remains of the nematode can sometimes be detected in the centre of the granuloma.

Fig. 12 66 Toxoplasmosis. Fundus photograph showing large areas of chorioretinitis with irregular scarring and pigmentation.

occur; cats become infected by ingesting larvae in the tissues of mice and other 'accidental' hosts.

Infective eggs of *T. canis* are usually ingested in soil by young children with pica. The larvae penetrate the bowel wall and migrate through the systemic circulation to the tissues, where they become dormant and are surrounded by an eosinophilic inflammatory response. Although most cases are asymptomatic, a variety of clinical symptoms (cough, fever, abdominal pain, etc.) may be produced. Other more specific features depend upon the organs involved in the granulomatous process. Hepatomegaly and pulmonary infiltrates are frequent and a peripheral blood eosinophilia is characteristic and often marked.

Eye involvement in toxocariasis unfortunately often occurs in the absence of any other visceral features and without an eosinophilia. It usually manifests as a single, large, white granulomatous lesion at the posterior pole of the eye causing unilateral non-progressive visual loss (Figs 12.62, 12.63 & 12.64). In other cases there are peripheral smaller white lesions in the retina. The diagnosis of visceral larva migrans can be attempted by direct visualization of larvae in liver biopsy specimens; this is only successful in a minority of cases, however, and most merely show granulomatous reactions containing large numbers of eosinophils (Fig. 12.65). The diagnosis is therefore usually dependent upon serology using the enzyme-linked immunosorbent assay. This is also the only diagnostic method of value in ocular toxocariasis.

Therapy of ocular toxocariasis is with thiabendazole given with an anti-inflammatory drug. The risks of infection be minimized by regular worming of dogs and reducing the pollution by dog excreta of environments frequented by young children.

Toxoplasmosis

The epidemiology and clinical features of acquired toxoplasmosis are described in more detail in Chapters 1 and 3; the features of congenital infection are also briefly mentioned in Chapter 3. Toxoplasmosis of the eye is usually the result of congenital infection and, although infected infants can appear normal at birth, reactivation of this disease can produce chorioretinitis in later childhood or early adult life. The appearances are diagnostic with a focal destructive chorioretinitis which leaves well-defined heavily pigmented scars (Figs 12.66 & 12.67). The foci tend to be in the macular region although any part of the fundus may be involved. Lesions may appear to be quiescent but have a tendency to become reactivated, producing a new fluffy white retinal lesion in an area of previous scarring.

Ocular toxoplasmosis, involving the macula or causing a vigorous vitreal reaction, is treated with sulphonamides and pyrimethamine, co-trimoxazole or clindamycin together with systemic steroids to damp down the inflammatory reaction.

Presumed Ocular Histoplasmosis Syndrome

This is the name given to ocular disease seen in the presence of a positive histoplasmin skin test but without evidence of either active histoplasmosis in other organs or *Histoplasma capsulatum* organisms in the ocular lesions. The small, multiple, yellow foci are in the choroid and are composed of inflammatory cells (Fig. 12.68): they may be reactivated at a later date to produce disciform scars and neovascularization (Fig. 12.69).

Cytomegalovirus

Acute infection with cytomegalovirus (CMV) beyond the neonatal period is either asymptomatic or causes an infectious mononucleosis-like syndrome (Chapter 1). The virus remains latently present, however, and if cell-mediated immunity is impaired then CMV may reactivate to produce a variety of clinical syndromes, including retinitis. Retinitis is particularly likely to occur in renal transplant recipients and patients with the acquired immune deficiency syndrome (AIDS). CMV retinitis presents with visual loss, often initially unilateral but later becoming

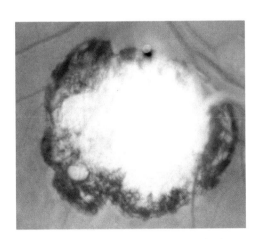

Fig. 12.67 Toxoplasmosis. Fundus photograph showing a well-defined yellow scar surrounded by pigment in healed congenital toxoplasmosis.

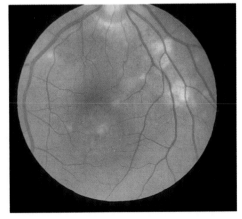

Fig. 12.68 Ocular histoplasmosis syndrome. Fundus photograph showing early discrete focal lesions of retinal histoplasmosis. By courtesy of Mr M. J. Gibson.

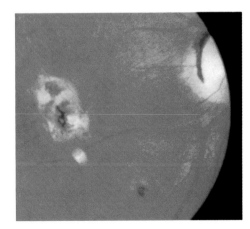

Fig. 12.69 Ocular histoplasmosis syndrome. Fundus photograph of later stage showing yellow well-defined scars and some pigmentation. By courtesy of Dr T. F. Sellers, Jr.

bilateral, severe and progressive. The fundal changes initially comprise small white granular lesions (Fig. 12.70) which later coalesce into fluffy white exudates with associated scattered haemorrhages and sheathing of vessels (Fig. 12.71). In severe forms the fundus has the so-called 'tomato sauce and salad dressing' appearance (Figs 12.72 & 12.73)). Histopathology reveals full thickness coagulation necrosis.

The atrophy and scarring that occurs with CMV retinitis may lead to retinal detachment, causing sudden and total loss of sight in the affected eye. This may occur even after the active retinitis appears to be healing.

The diagnosis of CMV retinitis is essentially a clinical one, as it is often impracticable to obtain tissue or fluid from the eye for CMV culture or DNA probing.

Concerning treatment, some success has been achieved with ganciclovir, an acyclic thymidine analogue that inhibits CMV replication. Because haemorrhages and exudates do not reverse therapy must be started early. Improvement occurs in about 80% of those treated, with a 14-day course of ganciclovir (Fig. 12.73) but this must be followed by maintenance therapy for the remainder of the period of immunosuppression. In AIDS patients, maintenance therapy is lifelong.

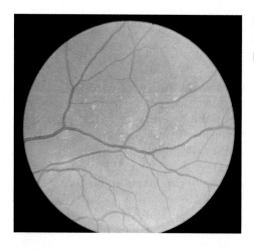

Fig. 12.70 Cytomegalovirus. Early granular lesions in a patient with AIDS.

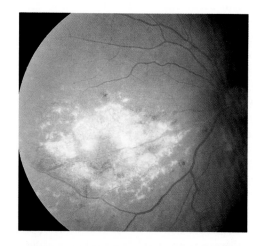

Fig. 12.71 Cytomegalovirus retinitis. Scattered exudates and haemorrhages with sheathing of vessels in a patient with AIDS. By courtesy of Dr C. J. Ellis.

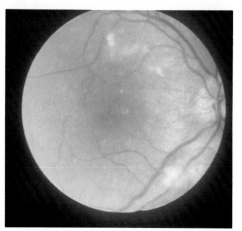

Fig. 12.72 Cytomegalovirus retinitis. Fundus photograph showing fluffy exudate and occasional haemorrhages. By courtesy of Dr C. J. Ellis.

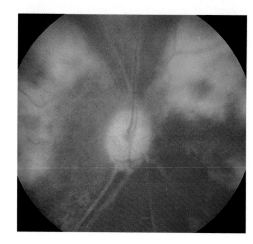

Fig. 12.73 Cytomegalovirus retinitis. Fundus photograph showing haemorrhages and white retinal infiltration producing the 'tomato sauce and salad dressing' appearance. By courtesy of Mr D. S. I. Taylor.

13

SYSTEMIC INFECTIONS

Normal body temperature is controlled within a narrow range by a thermoregulatory centre in the anterior hypothalamus. Stability of body temperature is achieved in the face of changing environmental conditions by adjusting the level of heat conservation via autonomic control of sweating, skin perfusion and involuntary muscular activity. There is feedback control involving temperature sensitive vessels in the periventricular regions. When environmental conditions exceed the capacity of these heat conserving or heat loosing autonomic mechanisms then hypothermia or hyperthermia may ensue. Damage to this feed-back inhibition by certain neuroleptics and the use of some anaesthetic agents in susceptible individuals results in a syndrome of malignant hyperthermia. In none of these circumstances is there any change in the hypothalamic set-point.

When fever occurs in the presence of infection and other inflammatory conditions, however, it is the result of shifting the temperature set-point. Microbial products and other extrinsic biological agents (exogenous pyrogens) stimulate the release of leucocyte cytokines (endogenous pyrogens), which act via chemical mediators upon the thermoregulatory centre in the hypothalamus to alter the set-point (Fig. 13.1).

Many microorganisms and microbial products are capable of acting as exogenous pyrogens. Such inducers include endotoxins from gram-negative bacteria, exotoxins such as the toxin-1 associated with toxic shock syndrome and other enterotoxins from *Staphylococcus aureus*, erythrogenic toxins from *Streptococcus pyogenes*, breakdown products of bacterial cell walls (peptidoglycans), tuberculin, polysaccharides (from fungi and yeasts), lymphocyte products (interferons provoked by virus infections and other mechanisms) and complement fragments (C3a, C5a provoked by antigen–antibody complex formation and other mechanisms).

Endogenous pyrogen is not one substance but several polypeptide cytokines with the ability to interact with the thermoregulatory mechanisms. Interleukin-1a (IL-1a) and IL-1b, interferon-α (IFNα), tumour necrosis factor (TNF) and IL-6 are all involved in changing the set-point. The mechanism appears to involve prostaglandins (especially PGE$_2$), arachidonic acid metabolites, catecholamines and cAMP. Fever provokes the local production of inhibitory neuropeptides (melanocyte stimulating factor and somatostatin) which limit the height of the fever to 41°C.

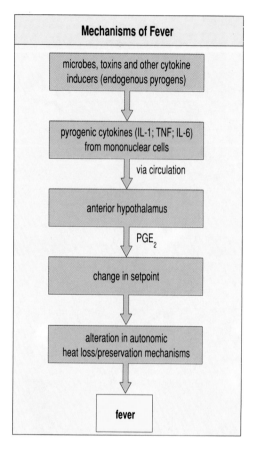

Fig. 13.1 Mechanisms of fever.

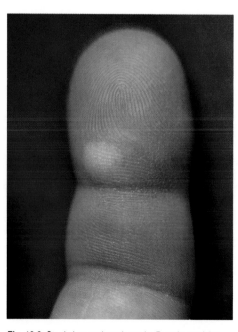

Fig. 13.2 Staphylococcal septicaemia. Pustule overlying site of osteomyelitis which was the source of infection.

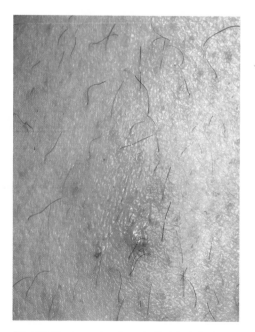

Fig. 13.3 Streptococcal septicaemia. Pustule similar to gonococcal septicaemia.

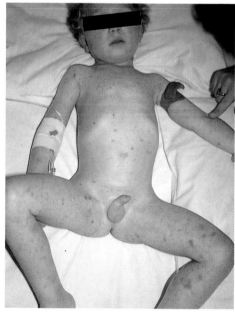

Fig. 13.4 Meningococcal septicaemia. Rash at the time of presentation.

Inhibition of the final pathway of fever induction at the hypothalamus may be achieved by blocking pyrogenic cytokine production (corticosteroids), cyclo-oxygenase inhibition and reduction in PGE_2 synthesis (paracetamol [acetaminophen]; aspirin; non-steroidal anti-inflammatory drugs), and interference with peripheral heat generation (phenothiazines blocking skin vasoconstriction).

There is good evidence from animal models that fever is a protective mechanism involved in combatting microbial invasion.

Experiments in cold blooded animals show that with induced bacterial infection they seek a warmer environment. This results in considerable reductions in bacteraemia. With humans it is more difficult to separate the precise role of fever from a large number of other acute-phase responses that may be induced by the same cytokines acting at different sites. Changes in immunological function (increased T and B cell responsiveness), the haematological system (stem-cell activation), iron sequestration (and interference with bacterial siderophore production, limiting iron availability to bacteria), hepatic production of acute-phase proteins (C-reactive protein, increased gluconeogenesis, haptoglobins, complement components), neurological (fatiguability and somnolence) and even endocrine alteration in thyroid and insulin production—all are part-dependent upon cytokine activity. The majority of these acute phase responses are protective but there may be a price to pay. For instance, muscle protein breakdown provides the substrate for these protein-rich responses.

BACTERAEMIA AND SEPTICAEMIA

Bacteraemia means the presence of viable bacteria in the blood, as demonstrated by a positive blood culture. Septicaemia is an imprecise term applied to a bacteraemia accompanied by symptoms suggesting that the bacteria are multiplying within the blood stream. Primary bacteraemia or septicaemia, again imprecisely, is blood-stream infection in which there is no obvious source of the infection elsewhere in the body whereas a secondary septicaemia occurs in the presence of a localized source of the sepsis.

The spectrum of organisms causing primary bacteraemia depends upon the age of the patient and the clinical setting. In those patients acquiring bacteraemia in hospital, the portal of entry is usually associated with either a site of instrumentation, surgery or a respiratory infection. The spectrum of organisms is influenced by the prior use of antibiotics, nosocomial colonization and the immune status of the patient. Gram-negative aerobic bacteria, especially those resistant to multiple antibiotics, are frequently isolated, particularly in the intensive care setting and in immunosuppressed patients.

Febrile symptoms with sweating, rigors, muscle pains, hyperventilation (and resultant respiratory alkalosis), headache, apprehension and change in mental state may be the only features of primary septicaemia. With secondary septicaemia these symptoms are superimposed upon those of the initiating infection, e.g. pneumonia, pyelonephritis, cellulitis or wound infection. Commonly there may be skin features that may suggest the primary focus of infection or give important clues to the aetiology. These include superficial pustular lesions from which organisms can be seen on Gram's stain to confirm a staphylococcal (Fig. 13.2), streptococcal (Fig. 13.3) or gonococcal (see Fig. 8.31) aetiology. Classical petechial and ecchymotic skin and mucous membrane manifestations may occur with meningococcal septicaemia (see Fig. 13.4 and Chapter 3) and occasionally also occur with other septicaemias and endocarditis. The rose spots of salmonella bacteraemia are sparse (see Fig. 13.5 and Chapter 4).

Pseudomonas aeruginosa characteristically causes lesions called ecthyma gangrenosum. These are round or oval, 1–5cm in diameter and have a rim of erythema or induration. The central area is necrotic or possibly ulcerated (Figs 13.6 & 13.7). They are particularly seen in neutropenic patients.

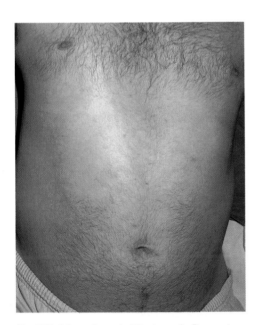

Fig. 13.5 *Salmonella paratyphi* bacteraemia. Rose spots on abdomen.

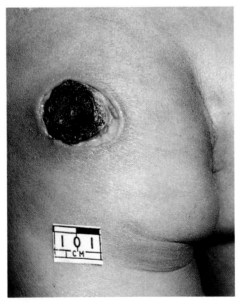

Fig. 13.6 Ecthyma gangrenosum. Necrotic round lesion on the buttock of a child with *Pseudomonas* septicaemia associated with immunodeficiency.

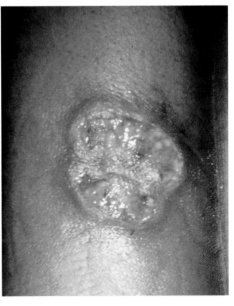

Fig. 13.7 Pyoderma gangrenosum. This florid and granulomatous lesion was thought at first to be a cutaneous mycosis. By courtesy of A. E. Prevost.

Septic shock

Some patients with septicaemia develop hypotension and diminished organ perfusion, a condition associated with a high mortality. It is caused by a complex series of enzymatic reactions triggered by microorganisms or microbial products in the bloodstream. The most important precipitant is endotoxin, a component present on the surface of the gram-negative cell wall. Endotoxins are lipopolysaccharides consisting of a polysaccharide attached to a lipid (lipid-A). The terminal part of the endotoxin molecule is the O-specific chain of oligosaccharides; these provide the diverse immunogenicity of the bacterium. This is attached to a core of hexose sugars of limited variation. The lipid-A component is similar in all gram-negative bacteria and is responsible for the toxic activity.

Endotoxin activates a series of physiological cascades in a pathological manner (Fig. 13.8). These include the systemic coagulation pathways, complement system, fibrinolysis and bradykinin. At a local level there is inappropriate stimulation of cytokines, particularly TNF.

TNF is a cytokine named after its ability to induce necrosis in certain tumours. It has many physiological roles including inflammation, wound healing and anti microbial activities. Endotoxin provokes TNF production and only small amounts of the two together are required for lethal shock to ensue.

Initially in sepsis the hypotension is accompanied by

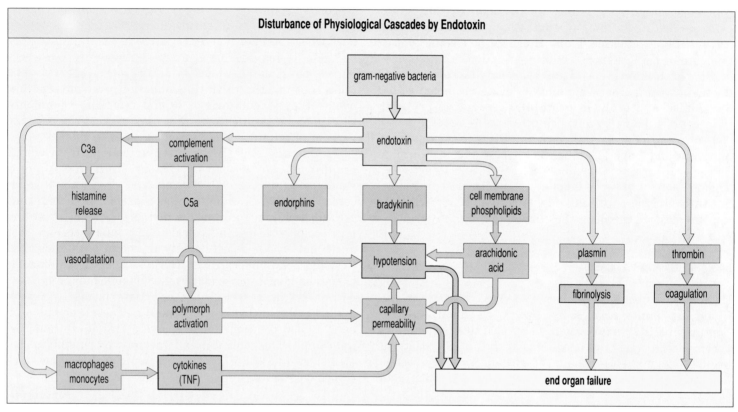

Fig. 13.8 Disturbance of physiological 'cascades' by endotoxin.

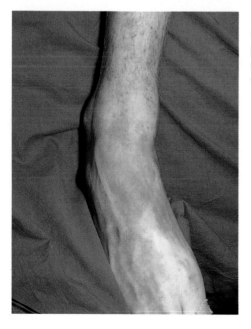

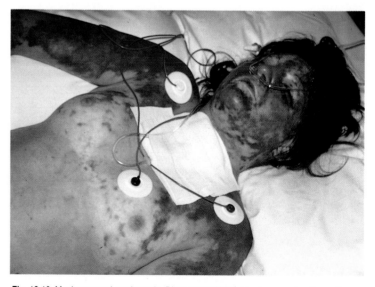

Fig. 13.9 Staphylococcal septicaemia. Lower leg of patient with irreversible septic shock showing intense vasoconstriction and pallor.

Fig. 13.10 Meningococcal septicaemia. Disseminated intravascular coagulopathy and purpura fulminans (Waterhouse–Friedrichsen syndrome). By courtesy of Dr Steve Wilkinson.

peripheral vasodilatation and the peripheries are well perfused (warm shock). Later the peripheral resistance rises and intense vasoconstriction, pallor, cold peripheries and oliguria occur (Fig. 13.9). Bacterial endotoxins also activate the coagulation and fibrinolytic systems (see Fig. 13.9). The clotting results in the consumption of platelets and coagulation factors in the syndrome of disseminated intravascular coagulation (DIC), which results in both thrombosis and clinical bleeding, the latter exacerbated by the fibrinolytic mechanisms. The clinical features are petechiae, ecchymoses (Fig. 13.10), peripheral gangrene (Fig. 13.11) and organ failure (Figs 13.12 & 13.13).

Dyspnoea and cyanosis herald the development of the adult respiratory distress syndrome, ARDS. It is believed that ARDS may be caused by the activation of neutrophils and other inflammatory cells by blood borne factors. The activated neutrophils release agents which injure the endothelial and epithelial linings of adjacent capillary and endothelial surfaces. This eventually causes interstitial oedema and stiff lungs, leading to permeability and alveolar oedema. There may be impairment of cardiac or hepatic function or an organic confusional state.

Secondary foci of sepsis may complicate septicaemias. Sites include the brain, endocardium, bones, joints, spleen, liver, urinary tract and lungs.

A wide range of laboratory abnormalities may be present in septicaemia. Leucocytosis is common but the white count may be normal or low. There may be thrombocytopenia with disturbed coagulation, impairment of renal function reflected in the plasma and urine electrolytes and a non-specific disturbance of liver functions. The chest x-ray in ARDS shows patchy opacification of alveoli with interstitial oedema (Fig. 13.14); the blood gases have a low pO_2 with lactic acidosis causing an anion gap.

Antibiotics must be given urgently to patients with suspected or proven septicaemia. The usual practice involves a very broad spectrum of activity but the choice of antibiotics must cover the most likely organisms in the particular clinical setting. In practice the aerobic gram-positive and gram-negative spectrum and anaerobes are usually covered as completely as possible. The possible presence of *Pseudomonas aeruginosa* in patients with neutropenia or burns must be considered. *Candida* septicaemia in

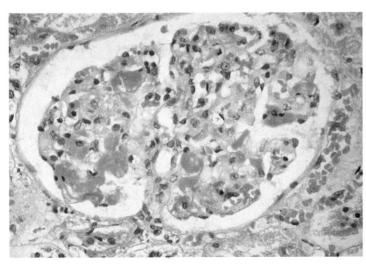

Fig. 13.11 *Vibrio vulnificans* septicaemia. Peripheral gangrene as a result of disseminated intravascular coagulation. By courtesy of Dr J. R. Cantey.

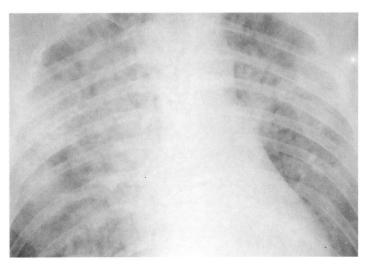

Fig. 13.12 Meningococcal septicaemia; haemorrhagic adrenal glands.

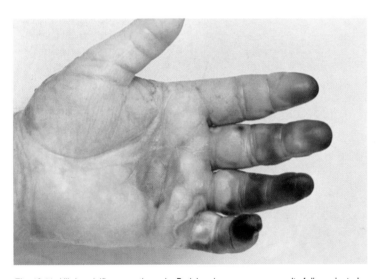

Fig. 13.13 Septicaemia. Renal histology in disseminated intravascular coagulation showing fibrin deposition within glomeruli. By courtesy of Dr C. Edwards.

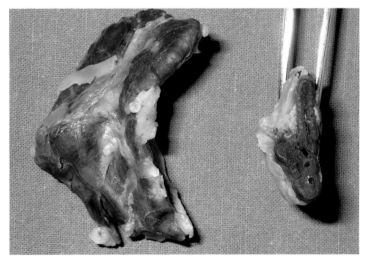

Fig. 13.14 Adult respiratory distress syndrome (ARDS). Chest x-ray showing diffuse, confluent opacity in both lung fields resulting from interstitial and alveolar oedema.

patients with indwelling cannulae, catheters and intravenous alimentation must not be overlooked.

Fluid replacement using colloid or crystalloid solutions (or fresh frozen plasma/blood where indicated) should be provided under scrupulous control using central venous pressure and left atrial (Swann–Ganz catheter) pressure monitoring. Sympathomimetic amines improve the cardiac output.

Having achieved improvement in the systemic blood pressure, maintenance of renal and tissue perfusion is important if renal failure and escalation of consumptive coagulopathy are to be avoided. The use of heparin in the prevention and control of DIC has not proved clinically useful despite favourable experimental evidence.

Although in animal experiments pre-treatment with steroids before induced septicaemia has improved the survival in septic shock, this has not been borne out in clinical practice. Opiate antagonists have not provided significant benefit in clinical use.

Mortality from septic shock has not improved in parallel with antibiotics and intensive care; this may well be because continued septicaemia is not necessary for perpetuation of a deteriorating downward spiral of the physiological cascades. Furthermore, antibiotics may release a bolus of endotoxin as they clear the bacteraemia and thus fuel the fire. Immunotherapeutic approaches to counter the effect of endotoxin released from organisms killed by initial antibiotic treatment have been tried. Prior immunization against endotoxin protects, as does the provision of anti-endotoxin immunoglobulin (IgM). These are intravenous immunoglobulin preparations containing high titres of antibodies produced using mutant organisms (strain J5, for instance, of *E. coli*) in which the outer O chain and core are deficient, revealing the lipid-A.

Common Causes of Pyrexia of Uncertain Origin
Infections (30–40%)
Tuberculosis
Endocarditis
Localized abscesses (particularly intra-abdominal)
Neoplasia (20–30%)
Lymphoma
Renal carcinoma
Gastrointestinal carcinoma
Ovarian carcinoma
Collagen-vascular diseases (15%)
SLE
Rheumatoid arthritis
Vasculitis
Others (15–20%)
Drugs
Pulmonary emboli
Inflammatory bowel disease
Factitious fever
Sarcoidosis

Fig. 13.15 Common causes of pyrexia of uncertain origin.

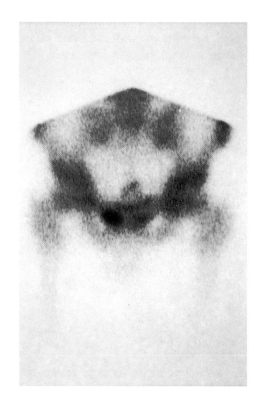

Fig. 13.16 Pyrexia of uncertain origin. Young male athlete presenting with fever, polymorph leucocytosis and low right ileac fossa pain. Bone scan shows abnormal radionuclide uptake in the right pubic ramus from a staphylococcal osteomyelitis.

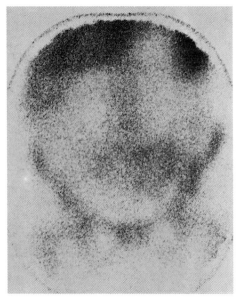

Fig. 13.17 Pyrexia of uncertain origin in a 28-year-old male with mild diarrhoea, leucocytosis and abnormal liver function tests. This [111]Indium leucocyte scan shows an area of abnormal radionuclide collection in the left ileac fossa. The final diagnosis was that of left pericolic inflammatory pathology complicated by portal vein thrombosis.

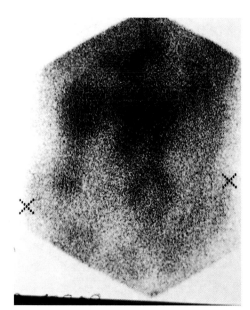

Fig. 13.18 Pyrexia of uncertain origin; 54-year-old male presenting with prolonged fever. [67]Gallium scan showing pathological radionuclide uptake in retroperitoneal lymphadenopathy of Hodgkin's disease.

Monoclonal antibodies to endotoxin and to TNF are currently being tested. Anti-TNF antibodies have the disadvantage that TNF is only transiently present in the blood stream and that it is only one of the many mediators of shock.

PYREXIA (FEVER) OF UNCERTAIN ORIGIN

In order to fulfil the strict criteria of PUO (FUO) the temperature must have exceeded 38.3°C on several occasions and the aetiology of the fever escaped detection after a week of investigation in hospital. The practical consequence of this definition is that the fever has persisted beyond the two or three weeks of self-limiting viral infections, post-operative fevers or fevers of obvious cause. The majority of PUO's are the results of infection, of collagen vascular disorders or of neoplastic disease (Fig. 13.15); most are relatively common disorders presenting with a paucity of other clinical features.

Osteomyelitis (Fig. 13.16), endocarditis, diverticulitis (Fig. 13.17), pelvic inflammatory disease and organ abscesses are the most common localized infections. Of the collagen vascular disorders, systemic lupus erythematosus (SLE), adult and juvenile Still's disease, polyarteritis nodosa and polymyalgia rheumatica are most often found. Lymphomata (Fig. 13.18) are the most frequent malignancy, primary or disseminated solid tumours, including renal and hepatic adenocarcinomata, are the next most frequently identified. In childhood neuroblastomata feature more frequently.

Rarities such as familial Mediterranean fever and such metabolic disorders such as Fabry's lysosomal storage disorder, hyper triglyceridaemia and amyloidosis, are outside the common experience.

The proportion of the three major diagnostic categories changes with age. Infection is most prominent amongst infants and children; collagen vascular disorders are most prominent in middle age; and neoplasia is most prominent in later life.

MALARIA

Four species of the genus *Plasmodium* (*P. vivax*, *P. ovale*, *P. malariae* and *P. falciparum*) infect humans. Infections due to *P. vivax* and *P. falciparum* are far more common than those due to *P. ovale* or *P. malariae*, although these two species are more important in some areas of Africa. *P. falciparum* is the most severe. The life cycle involves sexual multiplication within female *Anopheles* mosquitoes and an asexual multiplication in man (Fig. 13.19).

Sporozoites (Fig. 13.20) injected with the mosquito saliva circulate, enter parenchymal cells of the liver and multiply asexually (tissue schizogony) to form a tissue schizont full of merozoites. The merozoites are invasive forms. Rupture of these liver schizonts releases merozoites which then invade red cells. Released merozoites attach themselves to specific binding sites on red cells. With *P. vivax* this is associated with the Duffy blood group antigen (the absence of the Duffy gene in the West African population is responsible for the low incidence of *P. vivax* malaria). With *P. falciparum* a more ubiquitous surface glycoprotein, glycophorin, is involved. With *P. vivax* and *P. ovale* merozoites may also be released from long-term persisting liver forms called hypnozoites; these are responsible for late relapses.

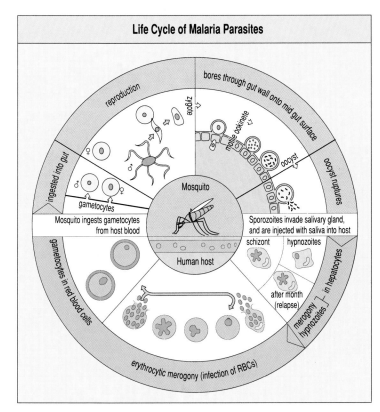

Fig. 13.19 Life cycle of malaria parasites in man.

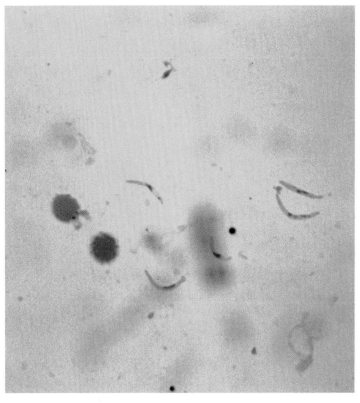

Fig. 13.20 Sporozoites, from an infected mosquito.

Within the red cell the invading merozoite divides asexually forming trophozoites (Figs 13.21, 13.22, 13.23, & 13.24) which then sub-divide into mature red cell schizont (Figs 13.25 & 13.26) containing many merozoites.

These are then released and re-invade red blood cells. After several cycles the re-invading merozoites form male or female gametocytes (Figs 13.27 & 13.28). With *P. malariae* the erythrocyte stages may continue as a low-grade infection for many years, causing late relapses.

Initially the red cell cycle is asynchronous and the fever is irregular. As a result of host immune responses the later cycles become more synchronous and the fever more regular (48 hours for *P. vivax*, *P. ovale* and *P. falciparum*, 72 hours for *P. malariae*).

Gametocytes are taken up into the mosquito stomach and the sexual part of the cycle takes place (sporogony). Ultimately sporozoites are formed which then move through the mosquito body cavity and enter the salivary glands, ready to be passed on to the next host.

Blood transfusion and trans-placental transmission are the only non-vector borne modes of infection.

The distribution of malaria is essentially worldwide in tropical and warm temperate regions. About 100 million people are infected annually. The most common presentation of malaria is with fever. This fever occurs 10–14 days after infection, although parasites may be found in the blood stream prior to this. The fever is variable in a primary infection: later on, the more classical periodicity may

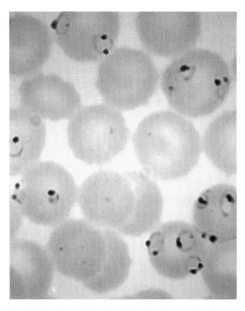

Fig. 13.21 Malaria. Thin blood film showing trophozoites (ring forms) of *P. falciparum*. Note two parasites within the same red cell and double chromatin knobs. Giemsa stain. By courtesy of Department of Tropical Medicine, Mahidol University, Bangkok.

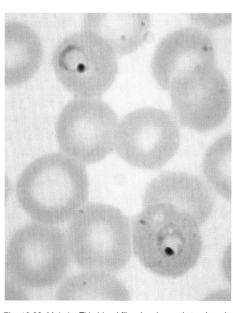

Fig. 13.22 Malaria. Thin blood film showing early trophozoite (ring form) of *P. vivax*. See fig 13.21 for source.

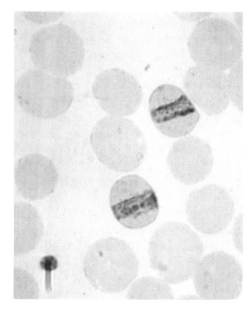

Fig. 13.23 Malaria. Thin blood film showing band forms (trophozoites) of *P. malariae*. This is a characteristic feature of *P. malariae*. Giemsa stain. See fig 13.21 for source.

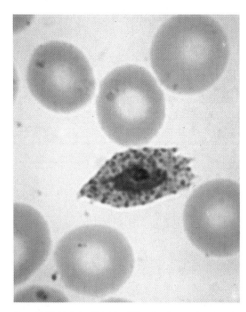

Fig. 13.24 Malaria. Thin blood film showing trophozoite of *P. ovale*. Note pronounced stippling of red cell and coarse pigment within parasite. Giemsa stain. See fig 13.21 for source.

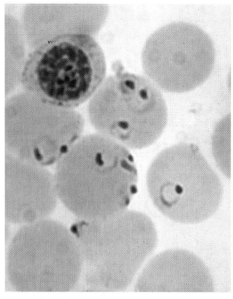

Fig. 13.25 Malaria. Thin blood film showing several ring forms and a schizont of *P. falciparum*. This is only seen in severe cases. Giemsa stain. See fig 13.21 for source.

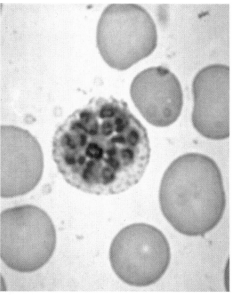

Fig. 13.26 Malaria. Thin blood film showing fully developed schizont of *P. vivax* with merozoites ready to burst out. Giemsa stain. See fig 13.21 for source.

develop. The paroxysms of fever in malaria start with rigors and headache, associated with pale, cold skin. An hour or two later there is a phase of delirium, tachypnoea and hot skin, lasting for several hours. The fever then settles and there is marked sweating and fatigue. Patients are often completely free of symptoms between paroxysms but hepatosplenomegaly is commonly detected, (the spleen is very fragile and can easily be ruptured by over-vigorous palpation).

The major clinical features of malaria are those of the complications. Apart from anaemia, the majority of these complications are associated with *P. falciparum* infections. Anaemia is present in most severe infections and parallels the parasitaemia. Haemolysis of infected erythrocytes, delayed release of reticulocytes from the marrow, and immune-mediated haemolysis of non-infected red cells each contribute to this anaemia. In the past haemoglobinuria and blackwater fever were recorded in expatriate Europeans with an exaggerated haemolytic response to quinine-sensitized erythrocytes; this is now rare. Mild unconjugated jaundice is common (Fig. 13.29) and parallels the haemolysis although hepatocellular dysfunction may also contribute to icterus.

A number of other complications are due to tissue hypoxia, which results from alterations in the microcirculation compounded by the anaemia. The maturation of erythrocyte schizonts in *P. falciparum* infections occurs within the tissue capillaries and venules. This 'deep tissue schizogony' is the reason why often in *P. falciparum* malaria only the early ring forms are seen in peripheral blood films. Sequestration of *P. falciparum* parasitized red cells in the microcirculation results from alterations in the deformability of parasitized red cells and from specific adhesion involving parasite-derived proteins within the red cell and glycoproteins on the vascular endothelium.

Cerebral malaria (see Chapter 3) is the most severe common complication in malaria. Renal failure as a result of acute tubular necrosis may be provoked by dehydration, hypotension and hyperviscosity resulting in diminished cortical renal blood flow.

Pulmonary oedema resembling ARDS may occur during the acute phase of severe malaria, when fluid overload may contribute.

Hypoglycaemia may mimic or compound cerebral malaria. Low blood sugars may occur in severe infections due to increased glucose consumption, and lactic acidosis is commonly present; insulin levels are low. Quinine and quinidine stimulate insulin secretion causing hypoglycaemia during treatment. Bleeding manifestations may follow thrombocytopenia or a consumptive coagulopathy.

Shock may occur as a result of endotoxaemia. Diarrhoea is a variable feature. Hyponatraemia is attributed to inappropriate secretion of anti-diuretic hormone (this is contentious).

With pregnant patients there is an increased mortality. Anaemia, hypoglycaemia and pulmonary oedema are all more frequent. Abortion, stillbirth, premature delivery and low birth weight contribute to the high infant mortality. The higher parasitaemia is more possibly the result of the placenta providing a privileged site for *P. falciparum*. Placental insufficiency results from microcirculatory obstruction.

Heterozygous children with the sickle cell trait are less likely to contract *P. falciparum* malaria. In those with sickle cell disease there is no such protection and the mor-

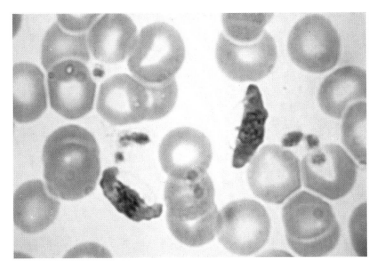

Fig. 13.27 Malaria. Thin blood film showing banana-shaped gametocyte of *P. falciparum*. Note the central mass of pigment. Giemsa stain. See fig 13.21 for source.

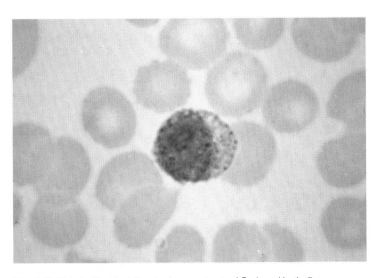

Fig. 13.28 Malaria. Thin blood film showing gametocyte of *P. vivax* with stippling (Schuffner's dots) in the cytoplasm. Giemsa stain. See fig 13.21 for source.

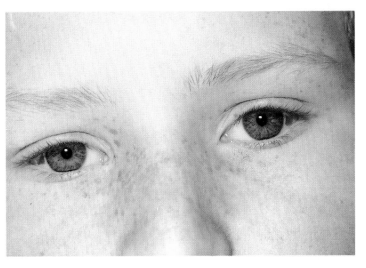

Fig. 13.29 Malaria. Child with mild jaundice, pallor and bilateral conjunctival haemorrhages associated with *P. falciparum* infection.

tality is much higher than with normal individuals. Similarly, the thalassaemic is partially protected and this may be due to persistence of fetal haemoglobin. Glucose-6-phosphatase-deficient red cells are less amenable to *P. falciparum* parasitization.

In highly endemic areas mortality from malaria is greatest during the first 4 years of life, beyond which individuals acquire a considerable degree of immunity. This immunity may wane quite quickly when they travel out of endemic areas.

Late complications include tropical splenomegaly (Fig. 13.30) in *P. falciparum* endemic areas; nephrotic syndrome with *P. malariae;* and Burkitt's lymphoma, where the mitogenic stimulation of chronic *P. falciparum* infection appears to act in concert with Epstein–Barr virus.

For practical purposes, diagnosis relies on detection and identification of the organisms in a properly stained blood film (see Figs 13.28–13.36). High *P. falciparum* counts (more than 5% of erythrocytes parasitized – Fig. 13.31) usually presage clinical severity. Severely ill patients occasionally have low levels of parasitaemia which are difficult to detect. Treatment of the clinical disease (Fig. 13.32) requires eradication of the red cell multiplication phase of the parasites, using red cell schizontocides. Chloroquine was the drug of choice for all species with uncomplicated malaria, until the recent prevalence of *P. falciparum* resistance. Quinine is required for complicated and resistant *P. falciparum* infections. Almost all endemic areas of *P. falciparum* now report the presence of some degree of chloroquine resistance. Quinine should always be given by a slow infusion rather than an IV bolus and

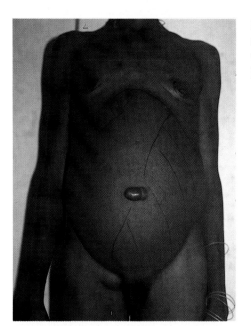

Fig. 13.30 Malaria. Tropical splenomegaly in a patient with evidence of hypersplenism living in a *P. falciparum* endemic area.

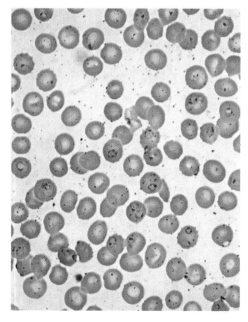

Fig. 13.31 Malaria. Very heavy parasitaemia in a patient with severe *P. falciparum* infection. Despite chemotherapy and exchange transfusion the patient died of cerebral malaria.

Antimalarial Treatments		
Stage in cycle	**Purpose of treatment**	**Agents used**
red cell schizont	treats acute infection	red cell schizonticides quinine chloroquine amodiaquine mefloquine quinhaosu proguanil pyrimethamine sulphonamides sulphones
hypnozoites (persistent tissue forms)	prevents relapse	tissue schizonticides primaquine proguanil pyrimethamine dapsone

Fig. 13.32 Antimalarial treatments.

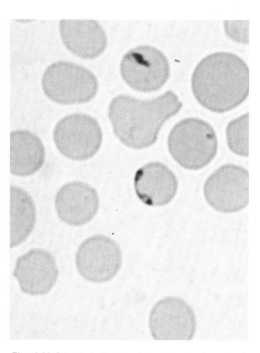

Fig. 13.33 Babesiosis. Peripheral blood film showing red cell infestation with the typical small coccoid and dumb-bell shaped *Babesia* organisms. By courtesy of Mr P. J. Humphries.

the patient should be monitored for evidence of cardiotoxicity.

Clearance of persistent tissue forms of *P. vivax* and *P. ovale* requires primaquine (a tissue schizontocide). Care must be taken to avoid giving primaquine to patients with glucose-6-phosphatase dehydrogenase deficiency.

Additional supportive measures include the following: blood transfusion (even exchange transfusion); the treatment and prophylaxis of hypoglycaemia, particularly in pregnant women; care with intravenous fluids to prevent overload; and dialysis in the event of renal failure. Steroids for cerebral malaria and heparin in the prophylaxis of consumptive coagulopathy have not proved helpful.

Indigenous pregnant women should receive prophylaxis, as should non-immune travellers. With travel to areas with *P. falciparum* resistance to chloroquine, a combination of proguanil and chloroquine is useful. Alternatives currently being used include mefloquine and halofantrine. The prophylactic use of dapsone-pyrimethamine and sulphadoxine-pyrimethamine combinations has been restricted as the result of uncommon but severe adverse reactions (agranulocytosis and Stevens–Johnson syndrome respectively). An effective vaccine is awaited.

BABESIOSIS

Babesiosis is caused by several species of intra-erythrocytic malaria-like protozoa of the genus *Babesia* which infect mammals of all sizes. Man is an uncommon and incidental host of the rodent strain *B. microti* and the cattle strains *B. bovis* and *B. divergens*.

B. bovis is present in most developing countries, but also in eastern Europe and the USSR. It is transmitted by cattle ticks (*Ixodes ricinus*). In North America *B. microti* has a wide host range, from mice to deer, and is transmitted by *Ixodes dammini*. Most human cases have occurred in the Northeastern coastal regions of the USA.

All three stages of tick development require a blood meal for further maturation to occur. Larvae, nymphs and adult ticks can all transmit the disease to humans. The sporozoites are transmitted from the salivary glands of the tick and infect red blood cells to form trophozoites. In man asexual division in red cells produces four merozoites and the blood film shows single or multiple rings rather similar to *P. falciparum* (Fig. 13.41).

The clinical features of babesiosis in the USA differ from those seen in Europe. In the USA the human illness is usually mild or subclinical. More severe infections occur in the elderly and in those without normal splenic function. In Europe, all cases of babesiosis have been in asplenic patients. In the USA, after an incubation period of 1–4 weeks there is fever, malaise, generalized myalgia, mild hepatosplenomegaly, haemolytic anaemia and renal dysfunction. In asplenic individuals severe haemolytic anaemia with jaundice, and renal failure (hepatorenal syndrome) may develop. Although *B. bovis* infections are very rare and only occur in patients with splenectomy, the haemolysis and its complications are usually fatal.

Diagnosis is made by microscopy of blood films and serology (which cross-reacts with *Plasmodium* species).

Most patients with *B. microti* infection recover without therapy: combinations of quinine and clindamycin have been used in serious disease but their efficacy is uncertain. Chloroquine is ineffective. Tick eradication is of importance in the control of bovine babesiosis for economic agricultural reasons. With *B. microti* the host reservoir range makes this more difficult.

BARTONELLOSIS (OROYA FEVER)

Bartonella bacilliformis, a gram-negative pleomorphic coccobacillus, is transmitted from person to person by night-biting sandflies in a restricted area to the west of the Andes. Bacilli adhere to red blood cells and invade endothelial cells causing a severe acute haemolytic anaemia.

Clinically the presentation is with acute fever, bone pain, rapidly progressing intravascular haemolysis and anaemia, with evidence of lymphadenopathy and hepatosplenomegaly. This acute stage (Oroya fever), which may be complicated by meningoencephalitis and myelitis, has a high death rate. Intercurrent infections with salmonellae and other enteric pathogens are particularly common.

The acute haemolysis of Oroya fever may be followed by a more chronic reticulo-endothelial disease involving liver, spleen, lymph nodes, bone marrow and endothelial linings of the blood vessels and lymphatic channels in skin. A widespread granulomatous vascular response in the skin produces miliary nodules (the verruga stage). A more chronic verruga stage may also occur *de novo*.

Diagnosis involves identifying *B. bacilliformis* on the red cells (Fig. 13.34) during the acute illness and by culture. Response to chloramphenicol is prompt. Penicillins, tetracyclines and aminoglycosides are also effective.

The vector is controlled by using DDT in human dwellings.

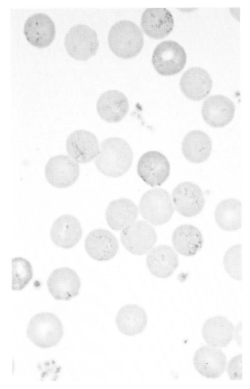

Fig. 13.34 Bartonellosis. Peripheral blood film showing rod-shaped coccobacilli of *Bartonella bacilliformis* on the red cells in Oroya fever. By courtesy of Mr H. Furze.

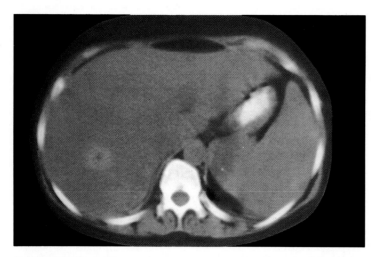

Fig. 13.35 Brucellosis. CT scan showing hepatosplenomegaly in *Brucella melitensis* infection.

BRUCELLOSIS

Three *Brucella* species, zoonotic gram-negative coccobacilli responsible for bacteraemia and abortion in animal hosts, are pathogenic for man. *B. abortus* is acquired by the ingestion of infected milk, milk products and aerosol inhalation. *B. melitensis*, causing disease in Mediterranean and African countries, comes from goats, milk products and organisms inhaled from placental contamination of the dust. *B. suis* requires direct contact with the infected carcasses of pigs.

Following entry to the body, brucellae are phagocytosed by polymorphs, but are capable of remaining viable (particularly *B. melitensis*). Organisms that are not killed localize in mononuclear cells of the reticulo-endothelial system. Again the organisms resist killing and this leads

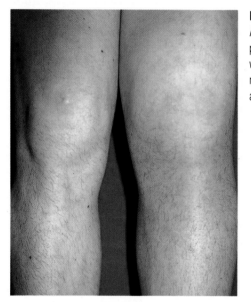

Fig. 13.36 Brucellosis. Arthritis of the left knee in a patient with brucellosis. This was accompanied by fever, malaise, generalized myalgia and depression.

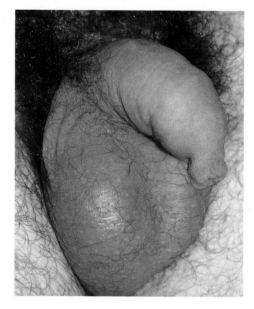

Fig. 13.37 Brucellosis. Orchitis in a patient with *Brucella abortus* infection.

Fig. 13.38 Serology in brucellosis.

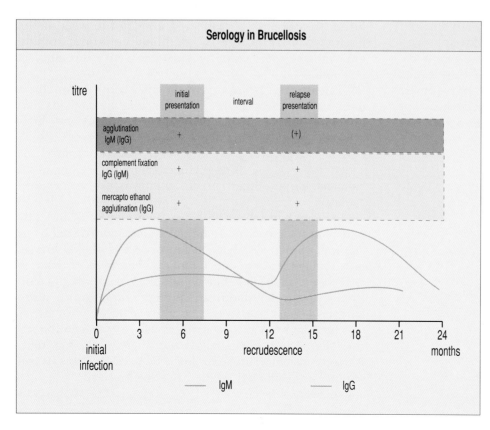

to lymphokine production and granuloma formation. Hence, giant cell granulomata develop in the bone marrow, spleen, liver and lymph nodes.

The clinical features of brucellosis are very variable and some are dealt with elsewhere (Chapter 8). The severity of the disease depends upon the individual host's immunity and the species involved; *B. melitensis* and *B. suis* cause more serious disease than *B. abortus*. After an incubation period (of at least 10 days and sometimes many weeks) the illness is acute or subacute in onset. Only one-third of patients have drenching sweats and high fever – in the remainder the fever, when present, is low-grade and the 'undulant' pattern is rare. A considerable range of non-specific symptoms occurs. These include anorexia, lethargy, and muscle and joint pain. The liver, spleen (Fig. 13.35) and lymph nodes may be enlarged. In a minority of patients acute brucellosis is complicated by problems affecting almost any organ system. The clinical features of skeletal involvement (see Figs 13.36, 8.52 & 8.53), endocarditis, hepatitis, haemolytic anaemia, epididymo-orchitis (Fig. 13.37), meningo-encephalitis, myelitis or depression may be present.

Re-exposure to *Brucella* species in seropositive persons (particularly in veterinarians or laboratory workers) may cause hypersensitivity reactions which mimic acute brucellosis.

Cultural isolation of *Brucella* species. from the blood and bone marrow can be achieved but serodiagnosis provides the usual confirmation. By the time of diagnosis in the acute phase both IgM and IgG antibodies are usually present: with adequate treatment IgG disappears or decreases to very low levels. In the chronic phase or with exacerbation or reinfection IgG antibodies rise again (Fig. 13.38). Agglutination techniques measure both IgG and IgM; pre-treatment with mercapto-ethanol removes the IgM antibodies. The complement fixation test measures IgG. Thus, in acute brucellosis there will be a rise in both IgG and IgM agglutination titres. In more persistent active infections the agglutination titre remains elevated and does not fall, mercapto-ethanol is usually positive and the compliment fixation titre is positive.

A combination of rifampicin (600–900mg/day) with doxycycline (200mg/day) for six weeks is the treatment of choice. Tetracycline and intramuscular streptomycin is cheaper but more difficult to administer. Endocarditis requires prolonged combination treatment with additional cotrimoxazole; valve replacement may be required.

Two controlling strategies have largely eliminated brucellosis in countries with organized agriculture: vaccination of cattle and goats to produce brucella-free herds; and pasteurization of milk and dairy products. Human vaccines are not widely available or reliably protective.

LEPTOSPIROSIS

Leptospires (genus *Leptospira*) are finely coiled, thread-like spirochaetes, 6–20mm long with typically hooked or bent ends. Free-living saprophytic strains are included in a separate species (*Leptospira biflexa*). Leptospirosis is due to a single species, *L. interrogans*. The pathogenic *L. interrogans* complex comprises nineteen serogroups and ten times that number of serotypes. Pathological serogroups included *L. icterohaemorrhagiae*, *L. hebdomadis*, *L. hardjo*, *L. canicola*, *L. pomona* and *L. grippotyphosa*.

Leptospirosis is a zoonosis; man is an incidental host who becomes infected through direct or indirect contact with the reservoir animal. Different serotypes tend to have different animal reservoirs. Thus infection with *L. canicola* relates to dogs, *L. hardjo* to cattle, *L. grippotyphosa* to voles and classical *L. icterohaemorrhagiae* to rats. Animals continue to excrete the organisms in the urine for a long time without any evidence of disease.

Transmission results from direct contact with the body fluids of reservoir animals or indirect contact with water contaminated by animal urine. The leptospires gain access through ingestion, mucous membranes or skin abrasion. A primary bacteraemia results in leptospires being delivered to all body tissues with multiplication at these sites, at least until the development of an immune response after 7–14 days. Thus the disease has initial features relating to bacterial multiplication in many organs and a second phase resulting from the interaction between the spirochaete and the immune response.

In the early phase the pronounced bacterial replication can result in organ failure, with renal glomerular injury and centrilobular hepatic necrosis being most prominent (see Fig. 5.22). Antibodies appear, the bacteraemia resolves and bacterial multiplication within organ parenchyma remits. Interestingly, despite leptospiral penetration of the brain and cerebrospinal fluid, meningeal inflammatory changes do not occur until relatively late and coincide with the presence of an immune response.

Subclinical infection is common in those exposed to infected animals and of those who are ill, only about 10% have severe disease with jaundice. The illness is often biphasic. The initial clinical symptoms occur from 1–2 weeks after infection and are heralded by fevers, headache, myalgia, rash and conjunctival injection. This initial phase of the illness lasts for 5–7 days and complete or partial defervescence then occurs. In some cases the second phase never occurs but, in most, a day or two later the immune phase of the illness is evident. In mild cases this consists of a severe headache with meningitis (see Chapter 3), myalgia, rash, splenomegaly and abdominal pain. Pulmonary (Fig. 13.39) or cardiac involvement with

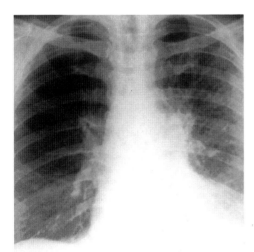

Fig. 13.39 Leptospirosis. Chest x-ray showing increased bronchopulmonary markings in a patient with leptospiral bronchopneumonitis.

cough and breathlessness may occur. In severe forms of the disease (Weil's syndrome) the immune phase is complicated by jaundice, renal failure, haemorrhage (Fig. 13.40) and vascular collapse.

The initial phase, if mild, is difficult to distinguish from influenza, atypical pneumonia, viral meningitis, or viral hepatitis but the combination of fever with renal, hepatic and neorological features is diagnostic.

The jaundice is not usually associated with marked hepatocellular damage. The urine contains blood and protein and the blood urea nitrogen may be raised in the second week. Thrombocytopenia is common.

Direct microscopy of body fluids and bacterial culture are the only ways of making the diagnosis early in the course of leptospirosis, but are hampered by the innocent presence of saprophytic leptospires. Serology is more helpful when the patient presents with the second phase of leptospirosis.

In severe infections treatment should be with 7 days of either intravenous penicillin or ampicillin. Less severely ill patients should be given oral doxycycline or amoxycillin. The contribution of antibiotics to the resolution of the second, immune phase presentation is less convincing than the bacteraemic early presentation. Vaccines are not available for human use but do exist for animals. Prevention therefore relies upon avoiding contamination.

RELAPSING FEVERS

Borrelia recurrentis and *B. duttoni* are helical spirochaetes spread by lice or ticks; they cause, respectively, epidemic louse-borne relapsing fever and endemic tick-borne relapsing fever. The spirochaetes are widely distributed in the body, multiply in the blood and are removed by macrophages within the reticulo-endothelial system.

A rising bacteraemia associated with fever is subsequently quelled by IgM antibodies to the organism. Such antibodies promote phagocytosis but do not achieve eradication. A fresh generation of borrelia are produced bearing different surface antigens causing symptomatic relapse, later to be controlled by further specific IgM antibodies. Natural resolution requires IgG antibodies.

Louse-borne relapsing fever

The borreliaa are not transmitted by louse bite; they are released from the louse after it is crushed, and then penetrate skin or mucous membranes. The initial features of fever, myalgia and headache, occur after an incubation period of up to 10 days. There may also be organic confusion, arthralgia, cough and dyspnoea, jaundice, petechial rash and conjunctivitis. The initial episode lasts for about 5 days and then, a week or so later, there is a relapse lasting for only 1–2 days. Generally only a single relapse occurs.

The investigations may include a mild anaemia, polymorph leucocytosis, mild to severe disturbance of coagulation, abnormal liver function tests (hepatocellular pattern), and cerebrospinal fluid pleocytosis.

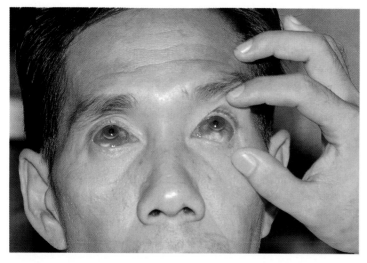

Fig. 13.40 Leptospirosis. Scleral haemorrhages in an icteric patient. By courtesy of Dr D. Lewis.

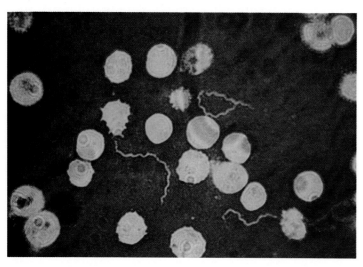

Fig. 13.41 Relapsing fever. *Borrelia recurrentis* shown on dark-ground microscopy.

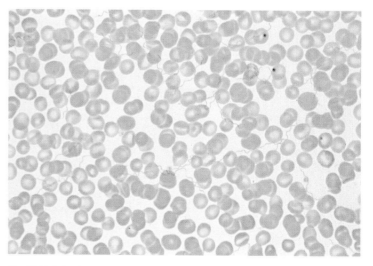

Fig. 13.42 Relapsing fever. Mouse inoculation test. *Borrelia recurrentis* identified in thin film.

Diagnosis is made by identifying spirochaetes in the blood (on thick and thin blood films or dark ground microscopy) from samples taken during the febrile period (Fig. 13.41). Mouse inoculation (Fig. 13.42) may be necessary in mild infections or during afebrile periods. Serological tests tend to cross-react.

Treatment with a single dose of tetracycline, penicillin, erythromycin and chloramphenicol are all effective. Jarisch–Herxheimer reactions are not uncommon. The disease is controlled by louse eradication.

Tick-borne relapsing fever

The nymph and adult stages of *Ornithodoros* species (soft ticks) transmit *B. duttoni* and other *Borrelia* species from the animal reservoir (monkeys, rats, squirrels etc.) to man, an incidental host, via their saliva or excrement. The spirochaetes can pass trans-ovarially to the next generation of ticks.

The overall pathology and presentation is very similar to louse-borne relapsing fever, although the febrile periods and afebrile intervals are shorter and there tend to be more relapses.

Diagnosis is by identification of borrelia in the blood (less numerous than with louse-borne disease), or by mouse inoculation.

Treatment is with a 5–10 day course of tetracycline or erythromycin. Jarisch–Herxheimer reactions are not a problem.

RICKETTSIAL INFECTION

Rickettsia organisms are obligatory intracellular coccobacilli. They have many features in common with other gram-negative bacilli, including the possession of endotoxins. Apart from louse-borne typhus, the major human rickettsial diseases are zoonoses (Fig. 13.43). Rickettsiae are able to multiply within their vectors as well as the mammalian host. With the exception of *Coxiella burnetii* (the cause of Q fever – see Chapter 2), they do not survive well outside their vector or host. Transmission occurs directly through bites or faecal contamination.

The predominant pathology of rickettsial diseases involves infection and damage to the vascular endothelial cells. This results in small vessel obstruction, microinfarcts and a local perivascular inflammatory response.

The clinical features of some rickettsial infections are dealt with in Chapter 10 (Rocky Mountain Spotted Fever) and Chapter 2 (Q fever).

EPIDEMIC LOUSE-BORNE TYPHUS

Epidemic louse-borne typhus is caused by *Richettsia prowazeki*. It is prominent in Europe and Asia during periods of war and social upheaval. There is no zoonotic reservoir and the body louse (*Pediculus humanis*) is infected for its lifetime with the organism. It is the louse faeces that are infectious (Fig. 13.44). Infection occurs by contamination of skin abrasions, or by inhalation.

Rickettsial Diseases					
Disease	**Organism**	**Reservoir**	**Vector**	**Distribution**	**Clinical**
Epidemic (Louse-Borne) Typhus	*R. prowazeki*	humans	body lice	Europe, Africa South and Central America	typhus
Endemic (Flea-Borne) Murine Typhus	*R. mooseri*	rats	fleas	Africa, Central America, South–East Asia	typhus
Rocky Mountain Spotted Fever	*R. rickettsiae*	wild animals, rodents, canines	ticks	North, Central and South America	spotted fever
African Tick Typhus, and *Fièvre Boutonneuse*	*R. conori*	rodents dogs	ticks	Africa, India, Mediterranean, Central Asia	eschar, fever, rash
Rickettsial pox	*R. akari*	mice	mites	Asia, Africa, North America	eschar, fever macular rash, then vesicular rash
Scrub Typhus	*R. tsutsugamushi*	rodents	mites	India and South–East Asia	eschar, fever, lymphadenopathy, papular rash
Q-fever	*Coxiella burnetii*	cattle	ingestion of milk, dust and ticks	Worldwide	fever, hepatitis, pneumonitis, endocarditis

Fig. 13.43 Details of the diseases caused by rickettsiae.

After an incubation period of 1–3 weeks there is fever, severe headache and myalgia. The fever remains high and unremitting, and a fine pink macular rash spreads from the axillae to the trunk and abdomen and then to the periphery (Fig. 13.45). The vasculitic lesions may affect the central nervous system, cardiovascular system, kidneys and skeletal muscle as well as the skin. Within a few days the rash involves the whole body and it may become petechial or frankly haemorrhagic.

Complications include organic confusion, meningitis, cranial nerve palsies, hepatitis, bronchitis and a poor cardiac output. Secondary infections may occur. Co-existing louse-borne relapsing fever (see p. 13.14) may be superimposed. The fever settles in 2 weeks or so but there is a considerable morbidity through post-infectious fatigue, which can last for months. Untreated the mortality may be 25% or more.

Diagnosis is usually made by serological identification. This includes the non-specific Weil–Felix reaction and more specific rickettsial serologies. The Weil–Felix reaction depends upon the agglutination of various strains of *Proteus vulgaris* by the serum of patients with rickettsial infections. In epidemic typhus the reaction is to the OX-19 and, to a lesser extent, OX-2 strains. OX-K is negative.

Unfortunately, serology takes several weeks to become positive and therapy has to be started on clinical grounds. Treatment is with tetracycline or chloramphenicol until defervescence. Control involves delousing measures. There is a typhus vaccine used for those at particular risk.

Late relapses of the original *R. prowazeki* infection may ensue; these are attributed to diminishing immunity and stress and are termed Brill–Zinsser disease.

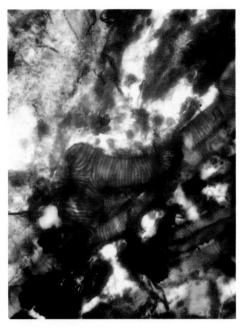

Fig. 13.44 Typhus. Smear from crushed louse showing rickettsiae. By courtesy of Dr J Newman.

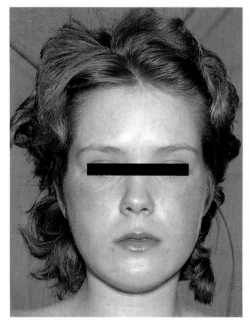

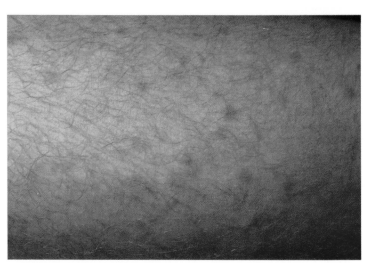

Fig. 13.45 Epidemic louse-borne typhus. Fine macular, erythematous, rash over face and periphery early in the infection.

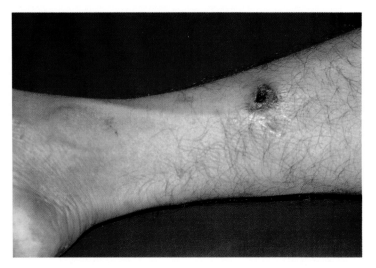

Fig. 13.46 Scrub typhus. Eschar at site of mite bite. By courtesy of Dr D. Lewis.

Fig. 13.47 Scrub typhus. Small discrete petechiae appearing about the fourth day of illness. By courtesy of Dr J. R. Cantey.

Endemic murine typhus

Murine typhus is caused by *R. typhi* and is found world-wide. It is spread by the faeces of the rat flea (*Xenopsylla cheopis*). The clinical illness is similar to louse-borne typhus but somewhat less severe. The serological reactions and treatment are identical to those given above. The two diseases can only be distinguished by isolation of organisms or special procedures at reference laboratories.

Scrub typhus

Scrub typhus is caused by *R. tsutsugamushi* transmitted by larval mites (chiggers) in the Far East. Following infection there is local multiplication and formation of an eschar (Fig. 13.46) with local lymphadenopathy. After 10–14 days there is fever, headache, myalgia, and often ocular pain and apathy. A rash appears on the trunk a few days later still (Fig. 13.47).

If untreated, the mortality is 5–20% and is usually due to cardiac failure. The serological response is to OX-K. Treatment with tetracycline or chloramphenicol is rapidly effective. Continuation of therapy for 2 weeks reduces the chances of relapse.

VIRAL HAEMORRHAGIC FEVERS

A number of zoonotic viruses, some arthropod-borne and some spread by direct contact, have haemorrhagic manifestations as well as causing specific organ damage. Haemorrhage results from damage to small vessels. This is exacerbated by pathological activation of the physiological cascades resulting in consumptive coagulopathy, loss of intravascular fluid volume and secondary organ pathology including renal failure and adult respiratory distress syndrome.

Lassa fever

This zoonotic arenavirus (Fig. 13.48) is carried in otherwise healthy multimammate rats (*Mastomys natalensis*). It was first described in West Africa, but the geographical

range of the host extends throughout Africa south of the Sahara, and foci of human disease have been described as far south as Mozambique.

Spread to man occurs when rodent urine contaminates household foodstuffs. Transmission from patients to hospital staff may occur by direct contact with body fluids, and by needle stick injury. Pathology includes widespread interstitial haemorrhages. There is a hepatitis with areas of hepatic necrosis, renal tubular necrosis, pneumonitis and a broad spectrum of other tissue pathologies.

Presentation occurs 4–14 days after exposure. The majority of indigenous human cases are mild. Pregnant women and expatriates are particularly likely to progress to severe disease. Fever, back and retrosternal chest pains and generalized myalgia are followed by an ulcerative pharyngitis, facial oedema and hypotension.

In severe cases a notable finding is elevated liver enzymes. The disease can be confirmed by serology or by virus isolation in special facilities.

Supportive treatment requires the correction of any hypovolaemia, anaemia and electrolyte disturbance, the appropriate management of renal failure and the consideration of specific therapy. The latter may include immune convalescent serum and intravenous ribavirin.

In West Africa normal barrier nursing procedures, the avoidance of needle stick injury and other body fluid contamination are enough to prevent spread of infection to staff and other patients. However, the possibility of nosocomial spread and the severity of the disease have led to the use of much more stringent precautions for cases imported into western nations. These include the use of isolation tents, chemical treatment of all body fluids and special arrangements for laboratory investigations.

In the absence of a vaccine, control depends upon reducing rodent exposure.

Argentinean and Bolivian haemorrhagic fevers

The Junin (AHF) and Machupo (BHF) viruses are arenaviruses restricted geographically to particular parts of South America which have the propensity to cause severe haemorrhagic fever. The spread is from rodent urine and

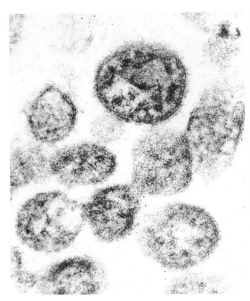
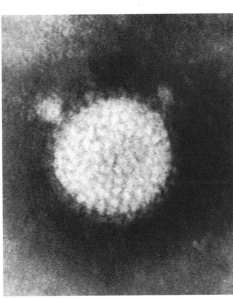

Fig. 13.48 Lassa fever. Left: Infected vero cells. The virions contain dense interior granules which are host ribosomes. Right: The virus particle. These vary in shape, have club-shaped projections on their surfaces and are about 80–150nm in diameter. By courtesy of Dr D. S. Ellis.

the incubation period 1–2 weeks. The onset is insidious with fever, myalgia, conjunctivitis and petechial rash. Capillary leakage and neurological disease cause most fatalities. Relapse may occur after recovery. Diagnosis is undertaken serologically and the treatment involves supportive management similar to that of Lassa fever. Control is that of the rodent host.

Ebola and Marburg fevers

The filoviruses that cause these diseases are endemic in Central and East Africa. The primary animal source of these infections is uncertain. Ebola occurs in explosive outbreaks in Sudan and Zaire and is spread from person to person, particularly nosocomially by contaminated syringes. Marburg virus has been spread from vervet monkeys and their organs used in tissue culture. Clinical disease in both infections involves an incubation period of one-two weeks, acute fever, myalgia and headaches and then gastrointestinal problems together with haemorrhagic features and shock. There is a high mortality.

Treatment requires supportive care in appropriate isolation facilities. Interferon and convalescent serum have been tried to little effect.

Rift Valley fever

Rift Valley fever is a zoonosis occurring in the Rift Valley of Central, East and South Africa. Transmission of the virus from the rodent hosts to humans and their domestic animals involves a variety of mosquitoes. Human outbreaks and epizootics occur.

After an incubation period of less than one week, there is usually a short febrile illness with headache and muscle pains. Some progress to haemorrhagic, encephalitic, ocular and hepatitic complications. Diagnosis is confirmed serologically and the treatment is supportive. Both human and veterinary vaccines are available.

Omsk haemorrhagic fever

This flavivirus is transmitted between small rodents by *Dermacentor* ticks. Usually it is a minor febrile illness but occasionally this is complicated by intestinal and skin

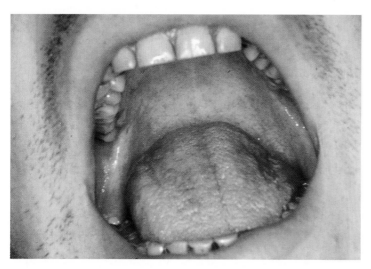

Fig. 13.49 Omsk haemorrhagic fever. A laboratory-acquired infection showing a petechial enanthem on the palate. By courtesy of Dr T.F. Sellers, Jr.

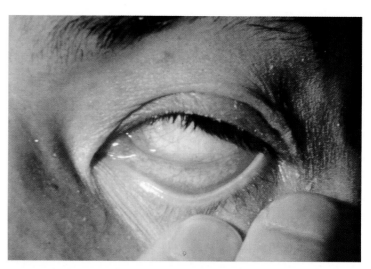

Fig. 13.50 Omsk haemorrhagic fever. The same patient as in Fig. 13.49 showing conjunctivitis of moderate severity. By courtesy of Dr T.F. Sellers, Jr.

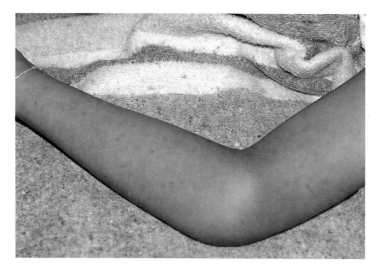

Fig. 13.51 Dengue. Convalescent macular rash. By courtesy of Dr D. Lewis.

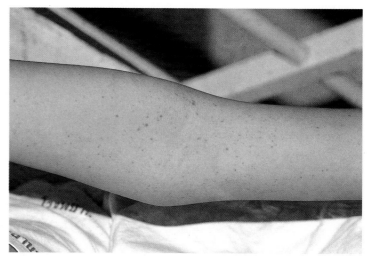

Fig. 13.52 Dengue haemorrhagic fever. Positive Hess' test, showing petechiae developing distal to the site of an inflated sphygmomanometer cuff. By courtesy of Dr D. Lewis.

haemorrhages (Fig. 13.49 & 13.50). Diagnosis is serological and the treatment supportive. The major source of infection is the musk-rat trapped for its fur. Control involves avoidance, but a vaccine is available.

Congo–Crimean haemorrhagic fever

Ticks spread this Bunyavirus from domestic animals to man in Asia and Africa. There is a brief febrile illness then variably severe haemorrhagic features including jaundice, disseminated intravascular coagulation and thrombocytopenia. Diagnosis is serological, treatment supportive. Spread can occur to medical staff and extended isolation procedures are therefore necessary.

Hantaan virus infection

Four strains of the Hantaan virus, a Bunyavirus, are involved in human disease. These rodent viruses are geographically widespread, with varying epidemiologies and clinical presentations. The transmission is from rodent urine, faeces, respiratory aerosols and bites. Presentation occurs after 2–3 weeks of incubation with a febrile illness, followed by a hypotensive phase in which there may be haemorrhagic features and renal failure (hence Haemorrhagic Fever with Renal Syndrome). Patients often have blurred vision and an erythematous blanching rash. Other presentations involve acute nephritis. There may be person-to-person spread and isolation is therefore necessary. Treatment is supportive.

DENGUE FEVERS

There are four serotypes of this flavivirus that are transmitted by *Aedes* mosquitoes in tropical Central America, the Caribbean, Asia, South East Asia, the Pacific and to a lesser extent in Africa.

Epidemics occur with high attack rates. The virus multiplies in the reticulo-endothelial system and later involves the endothelial linings of small blood vessels in the skin and other organs.

Classic dengue fever

Classic dengue fever has an incubation period of 3–7 days, followed by a prominent fever, myalgia, headache and retro-orbital pain. There is an erythematous blanching flush and a generalized transient macular rash spreading centrally from the extremities. Hepatomegaly and lymphadenopathy may be present. After the fever settles there is a short-lived macular rash (Fig. 13.59) that may be followed by desquamation. Convalescence is often prolonged.

The diagnosis is confirmed serologically. There is no specific treatment. Dengue haemorrhagic fever is the major complication.

Dengue haemorrhagic fever

Dengue haemorrhagic fever is relatively common in Southeast Asia and the Caribbean. A suggested pathomechanism is a primary uncomplicated dengue infection with one serotype and later exposure to a second infection with a different serotype. It is proposed that the previous exposure results in immune enhancement as a result of non-neutralizing antibodies enhancing the entry of virus into mononuclear cells via the Fc receptor. Such enhancement results in promotion of viral replication with the second infection rather than the expected inhibition of viral growth.

Immune complex vascular damage occurs and this results in increased capillary permeability, hypovolaemia and disseminated intravascular coagulation (with haemorrhagic features).

Clinically the initial fever, headaches and myalgia of dengue are superseded by hypotension, positive tourniquet test (Fig. 13.52) and haemorrhagic features in the skin, gums, and gastrointestinal tract (Figs 13.53 & 13.54). Circulatory failure may follow and the mortality in untreated cases may be as high as 50%.

Laboratory changes include an increased haematocrit from haemoconcentration, leucopenia, thrombocytopenia and later serological confirmation.

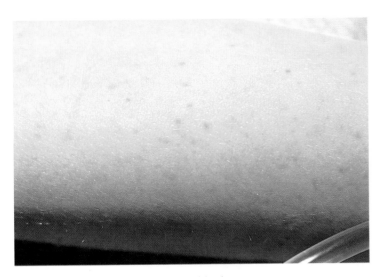

Fig. 13.53 Dengue haemorrhagic fever. Petechial rash.

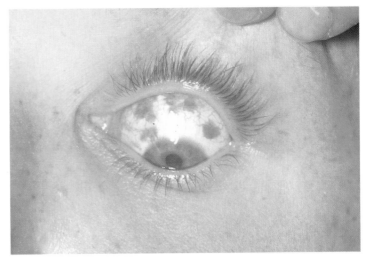

Fig. 13.54 Dengue haemorrhagic fever. Scleral haemorrhage.

The treatment is supportive and requires prompt plasma expansion, correction of hyponatraemia and acidosis and the provision of platelets or fresh blood transfusions in the event of haemorrhage. *Aedes* mosquito control is important, as vaccine prophylaxis is not yet reliably available.

PLAGUE

Yersinia pestis is a gram-negative bacillus that causes a zoonosis of wild rodents and is endemic in many parts of the world. Transmission is through fleas, droplet inhalation and direct contact with laboratory or infected animal material.

The principal rat flea (*Xenopsylla cheopis*) transmits the organism from rat to rat; as an epizootic builds up amongst rats the rat fleas may leave their dying hosts and bite man. In the historic pandemics of plague the spread from man to man was through the human flea (*Pulex irritans*) and also via aerosols from pulmonary infections. The disease is maintained in endemic rodent areas, as the bacillus can remain dormant in burrow-soil for prolonged periods.

Y. pestis passes from the flea bite to the local and central lymphatics. Bacteraemia involves many organs. Much of the pathology is due to endotoxins and exotoxins which cause inappropriate activation of the complement and coagulation pathways, resulting in disseminated intravascular coagulation (DIC) and shock.

There are a number of different syndromes caused by *Y. pestis*. The most common is bubonic plague. In this, after an incubation period of less than a week, there is sudden onset of fever and painful local suppurative lymphadenitis, usually in the groin, axilla or neck. These buboes are very tender and are surrounded by oedema (Figs 13.55 & 13.56). The disease progresses to septicaemia with DIC.

Another form of septicaemic plague is manifest by massive bacteraemia and DIC without the development of a bubo. A further severe and often fatal form of plague is pneumonic infection with cough, dyspnoea, blood-flecked sputum and respiratory failure (see Fig. 2.28). Meningitis may also occur.

In severe plague there is usually a high neutrophil count with features of DIC. Lymph node aspirate, blood and splenic puncture aspirate are cultured; animal inoculation of these materials increases the yield.

Untreated plague has a mortality of almost 50%. Treatment may be with intramuscular streptomycin or oral tetracycline for less ill patients, with chloramphenicol in cases complicated by meningitis. Outbreaks require control of rodents and their fleas. Those involved in such work may be given tetracycline prophylaxis. The vaccines available give incomplete protection.

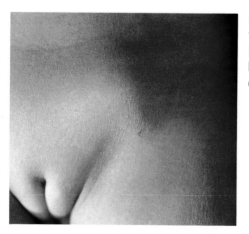

Fig. 13.55 Plague. Enlarged, tender inguinal lymph nodes in a Vietnamese child with bubonic plague. By courtesy of Dr J.R. Cantey.

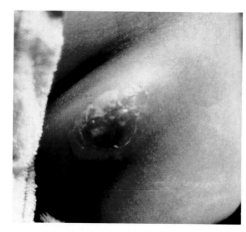

Fig. 13.56 Plague. Advanced stage of inguinal lymphadenitis in bubonic plague. The nodes have undergone suppuration and the lesion has drained spontaneously. By courtesy of Dr J.R. Cantey.

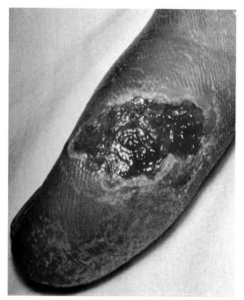

Fig. 13.57 Tularaemia. Irregular ulcer at the site of the initial lesion. By courtesy of Dr T.F. Sellers, Jr.

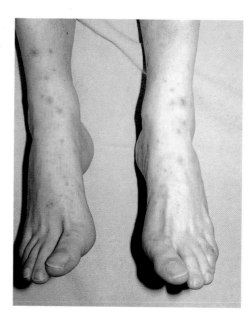

Fig. 13.58 *Streptobacillus moniliformis* infection. Rat-bite fever occurring in a man bitten by a rat. Maculopapular rash on the legs (and arms). *S. moniliformis* was isolated from the blood.

TULARAEMIA

Francisella tularensis is a zoonotic gram-negative coccobacillus infection occuring predominantly in the USSR, Europe, North America and Japan.

Transmission occurs by direct contact with wild rodents and small mammals, by contact with water contaminated by their excreta or corpses, by ingestion of infected tissue and by insect vectors (ticks, flies and mosquitoes). Infection by ingestion involves the tonsils and bowel. Transcutaneous access is through vector bites or direct contact.

In addition to fever and fatigue, patients may develop either an ulceroglandular or a typhoidal form of tularaemia . In the former, there is an infected nodule at the site of a tick or rodent contact, which later ulcerates (Fig. 13.57) with local lymph node enlargement. This may then progress to a bacteraemic (typhoidal) form. Fever, myalgia, headaches and, later, pleomorphic rashes occur with the bacteraemia. Ingestion of infected tissues may result in pharyngeal and intestinal involvement with ulceration. Pulmonary infection causes pneumonitis features with mediastinal lymph node enlargement (see Fig. 2.41).

The diagnosis is made serologically as the organism is difficult to culture. Treatment is with streptomycin. Tetracycline and chloramphenicol are alternatives. Prevention involves tick avoidance and using protective clothing when handling animals, particularly rodents and wild mammals.

RAT-BITE FEVER

Streptobacillus moniliformis is commensal to the rodent oropharynx but responsible for 'Haverhill fever' in humans. The infection occurs after a rat-bite or after ingesting food or fluids contaminated by rodent urine. The incubation period is 3–10 days. Fever, myalgia, arthralgia, headache and then a distal maculopapular erythematous rash occur (Fig. 13.58); the latter occasionally becomes pustular. Rarely there are direct infective complications involving the spleen, pericardium and endocardium, as well as a glomerulonephritis.

The diagnosis may be confirmed by cultural isolation of *S. moniliformis* or by serology. Benzylpenicillin is the antibiotic of choice.

Spirillum minor is another rodent commensal that may be transmitted from rats or domestic cats or dogs. When man is bitten the incubation (1–3 weeks) is longer than with *S. moniliformis*. Clinically the disease is similar but more severe. Local reaction to the rat bite is greater and there is local lymphadenopathy. Penicillin is again the most effective treatment.

VISCERAL LEISHMANIASIS (KALA-AZAR)

Of the numerous leishmanial protozoan parasites capable of causing infection in man, it is those of the *Leishmania donovani* complex that are responsible for visceral leishmaniasis. This complex involves *Leishmania d. infantum* in the Mediterranean and Middle East, *L. d. donovani* in India and Africa and *L. d. chagasi* in South America. Other species are responsible for cutaneous and mucocutaneous disease (see Chapter 10).

In the Mediterranean and Middle East *L. d. infantum* infections are a zoonosis, the reservoir being domestic and wild canines. Transmission is by the *Phlebotomus* sandfly (Fig. 13.59).

In India *L. d. donovani* is anthroponotic; humans are the reservoir and the infection may be endemic, sporadic or epidemic, again transmitted by *Phlebotomus* species.

There are two phases to the Leishmania life cycle. Within the sandfly vector the sexual multiplication in the gut produces flagellate forms (leptomonads) which are injected as promastigotes (Fig. 13.60) into the host when the sandfly next feeds. In the reservoir animal, or man, these flagellate forms are taken up by macrophages and spread to the reticulo-endothelial system. They multiply asexually within the macrophages producing non-flagellate amastigote forms (the Leishman–Donovan bodies

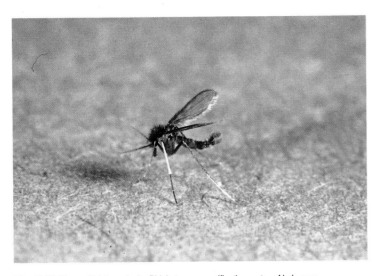

Fig. 13.59 Visceral leishmaniasis. Phlebotomus sandfly, the vector of kala-azar.

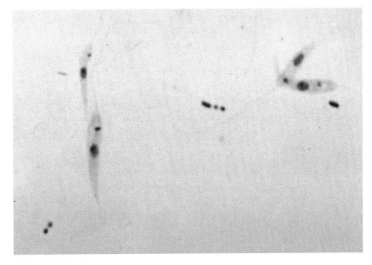

Fig. 13.60 Visceral leishmaniasis (kala-azar). Promastigote forms of *L. donovani* from culture. Note the anterior kinetoplast and flagellum. Giemsa stain. By courtesy of the Department of Medical Protozoology, London Schoool of Hygiene and Tropical Medicine.

seen in reticulo-endothelial tissue within the spleen (Fig. 13.61), bone marrow, gastrointestinal tract, lymphatics and to a lesser extent lungs and other organs. Schistocytes and sinusoidal lining cells of the spleen contain parasites as do Kupffer cells within the liver (see Fig. 5.35) and histiocytes within the bone marrow.

After an incubation period of 2–12 months, fever and weight loss associated with hepatosplenomegaly are the most common features. Skin lesions may occur early at the site of infection. Early lymphatic involvement is relatively rare. Later there may be generalized lymphadenopathy, increased pigmentation (kala-azar is the Hindi for 'black fever') and cachectic wasting. As the disease progresses the spleen may become truly enormous and the anaemia and wasting worsens. Involvement of other organs may provide additional symptoms.

Visceral leishmaniasis is a recognised problem amongst immunocompromised patients. This is now proving true of patients with AIDS (Fig. 13.62).

Where there has been spontaneous recovery of the initial systemic infection there may be a form of relapse involving the skin known as post-kala-azar dermal leishmaniasis

(PKDL). This is most common in India (up to 20% of those infected). The organism infects histiocytes within the dermis causing depigmentation followed by granulomatous infiltration.

Tests show the following: normocytic anaemia in the absence of reticulocytosis; neutropenia; mild abnormalities of liver function; hypoalbuminaemia; and a prominent rise in IgG and, to a lesser extent IgM antibodies. Specimens from splenic aspiration, bone marrow, liver, palpable lymph node or Buffy coat may yield leishmanial intra-cellular amastigote forms (Leishman–Donovan bodies) or prove culture positive (in 3N medium). Detection of leishmanial antibodies has become equally sensitive (greater than 90%).

Pentavalent antimony preparations (sodium stibogluconate) are the drug of choice and these may be used with allopurinol which has a direct inhibitory effect on amastigotes. Pentamadine and amphotericin B are less effective and more toxic. Prevention requires the control of reservoir hosts, control of the vectors and the human endemic areas, case finding and treatment.

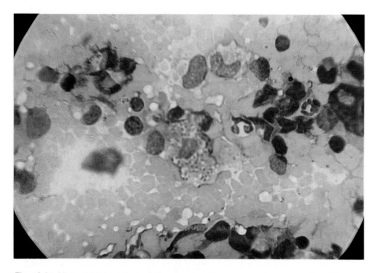

Fig. 13.61 Visceral leishmaniasis. Spleen smear with an excess of plasma cells and the presence of the amastigote Leishman–Donovan bodies.

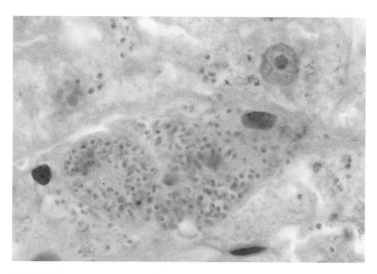

Fig. 13.62 Visceral leishmaniasis in AIDS. Profuse amastigote Leishman–Donovan bodies can be seen in macrophages. H & E stain. By courtesy of Dr B. Peters.

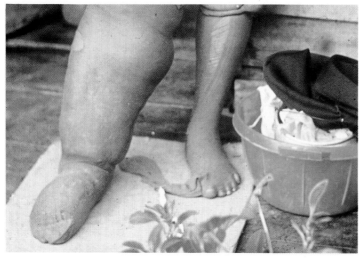

Fig. 13.63 Bancroftian filariasis. Pronounced oedema of the right leg in a woman in Porto Limon, Costa Rica. By courtesy of Dr R. Muller.

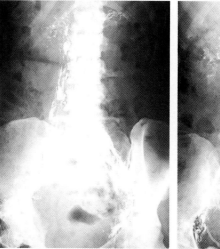
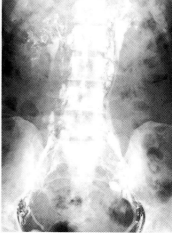

Fig. 13.64 Filariasis presenting with chyluria. Left: Lymphangiogram showing contrast within the lymphatics passing in a retrograde manner within the kidneys. Right: Concurrent IVP, showing contrast within the renal pelvis and ureters.

FILARIASIS

There are two major groups of filarial diseases. Lymphatic filariasis results from infections with *Wuchereria bancrofti* and *Brugia malayi*. Subcutaneous filariasis due to *Onchocerca volvulus*, *Loa loa* and the Guinea-worm *Dracunculus medinensis*, is dealt with in Chapter 10.

Lymphatic filariasis

Wuchereria bancrofti is distributed throughout the tropical regions, and is transmitted by several species of mosquitoes including *Culex*, *Aedes* and *Anopheles* species. With the exception of *Aedes* species (which transmit filariasis in the Pacific) these mosquitoes are all night-biting. *Brugia malayi* is restricted to the Pacific and *Mansonia* mosquitoes are the vectors.

The adult filarial worms exist in the lymphatics and produce large numbers of larval microfilariae. These microfilaria are found within the blood stream. The microfilaria of *W. bancrofti* retreat into the arterioles of the lung by day and are present in the peripheral blood at night (nocturnal periodicity), when they are available to the night-biting mosquitoes.

Microfilariae develop through several larval stages within the female mosquito until an infective larval form is produced. These are transmitted with the next mosquito bite, pass from the skin to the lymphatics and mature over the course of a year. The adult forms are long-lived (10–20 years).

The early immunological response to adult worms results in a low-grade lymphadenitis and lymphangitis. As the lymphatic inflammatory changes become more chronic with granuloma formation, fibrosis and lymphatic obstruction. A non-lymphatic inflammatory response to microfilariae in the pulmonary vessels results in tropical pulmonary eosinophilia.

After an incubation period of 12–24 months, painful lymphadenitis sometimes accompanied by epididymo-orchitis occurs, and may be associated with fever. There may be peripheral lymphangitis. Secondary infection may result from streptococcal lymphatic infection and accelerate the progression of lymphatic obstruction with peripheral oedema. Filarial abscesses may occur. Later on the chronic pathology results in persistent lymphadenopathy, scrotal lymphoedema, hydrocele, gross peripheral oedema (elephantiasis – Fig 13.63) and involvement of renal and intestinal lymphatics to produce chyluria (Figs 13.64 & 13.65) and chylous diarrhoea. Involvement of the central nervous system, joints, eye and myocardium are rare.

Confirmation of the clinical diagnosis requires the identification of microfilariae in the blood (Figs 13.66 & 13.67). Nocturnal samples should be taken; alternatively, a small dose of diethylcarbamazine (DEC) can be used to provoke peripheral microfilaraemia during the day.

Serology will give evidence of filarial exposure but species specificity is poor. A prominent eosinophilia is usually present and lymphatic radiography shows dilated lymphatics with abnormal lymphatic flow.

Microfilaria respond to the use of DEC. This drug has some activity upon the adult worms but suramin, the most effective adult worm treatment, has considerable toxicity. As the microfilariae are rendered susceptible to the immune responses by the action of (DEC) there is often very prominent local inflammation. Swelling of the lymph nodes and lymphangitis occur; to a lesser extent there may be generalized symptoms with fever, asthma, urticaria, abdominal pain and diarrhoea.

Control of the disease requires elimination of the reservoir of human infection using mass chemotherapy. Vector control is made difficult by the differing habits of the various mosquito species.

Asthma, cough, breathlessness, fever, splenomegaly and some lymphadenopathy may occur. Cardiomyopathy is

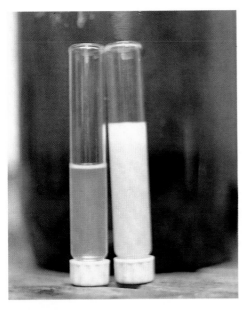

Fig. 13.65 Filariasis. Chyluria. The milky urine (right) clears with the addition of chloroform (left). Milky-looking lymph draining from the lower limbs (chyle) passes into the urine as a result of a reverse flow in the kidney, from cortex to pelvis. This reversal is occasioned by proximal lymphatic obstruction higher in the abdomen or thorax.

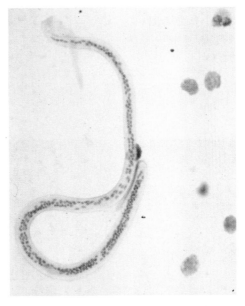

Fig. 13.66 Bancroftian filariasis. Blood smear showing sheathed microfilaria of *Wuchereria bancrofti*. Haematoxylin stain. By courtesy of Dr R. Muller.

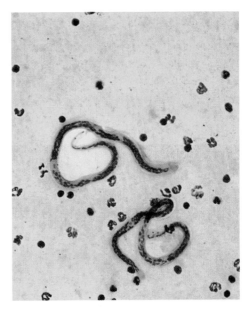

Fig. 13.67 Filariasis. Microfilaria of *Brugia malayi.*

well described and there is an epidemiological link with endomyocardial fibrosis. Neurological features are uncommon. Chest x-rays are abnormal in 25% patients with miliary, nodular and linear shadowing (Fig. 13.68). Lung functions are reduced in the majority of patients. As this disease is the result of an effective immune response, microfilariae are not found in the blood, and the diagnosis depends upon serology. The complement fixation test is sensitive although poorly specific within the filarial group.

DISSEMINATED FUNGAL INFECTIONS

Although several of the major pathogenic fungi show a strong predilection for certain organ systems (for example, the lung in histoplasmosis and coccidioidomycosis, skin and bone in blastomycosis, meninges and brain in cryptococcosis – all of which are dealt with in the relevant chapters) widespread disseminated infection may also occur, with production of characteristic clinical syndromes. These syndromes are particularly common in patients with defects in immune function.

Disseminated candidiasis

Many of the most important factors predisposing to life-threatening disseminated candidiasis are iatrogenic.

These include administration of multiple antibiotics, corticosteroids and antineoplastic agents, heroin addiction, parenteral hyperalimentation, indwelling intravascular catheters, prosthetic implants (especially heart valves), renal transplantation and severe burns. The organisms reach the bloodstream via burn or surgical wounds, infected thrombophlebitis around intravascular foreign bodies or erosive lesions of the gastrointestinal tract.

When *Candida* disseminates, there is usually involvement of many organs with cerebral microabscesses and meningitis, renal lesions (see Figs 6.27, 6.28 & 13.69), pneumonia, endocarditis and endophthalmitis (Fig. 13.70). The gut (Fig. 13.71) and skin (Fig. 13.72) are also often involved. An increasingly recognized syndrome in immunocompromised patients is a marked fever associated with hepatosplenic abscesses (Fig. 13.73) and, sometimes, ocular lesions. Its recognition often depends upon CT scan appearances.

Diagnosis of disseminated candidiasis is difficult since, particularly in neutropenic patients, blood cultures are usually negative and the finding of organisms at superficial sites is not infrequent in non-infected individuals. Serological methods are of little help; in the immunocompetent host the presence of antibodies cannot distinguish colonization from infection and in the immunocompromised patient there is often an inability to mount an

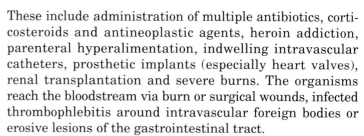

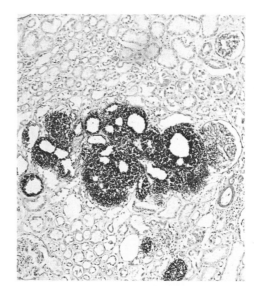

Fig. 13.68 Tropical pulmonary eosinophilia. A 48-year-old Indian male presented with 3 months of cough, sputum, wheeze and dyspnoea: widespread crepitations were audible at presentation. $10.3 \times 10^9/l$ eosinophils were present, and the filarial complement fixation test was positive. His symptoms and eosinophilia resolved after treatment with diethylcarbamazine. The chest x-ray shows diffuse mottling and increased bronchial marking.

Fig. 13.69 Disseminated candidiasis. Histological appearance of Candida in kidney. By courtesy of Dr M. J. Leyland

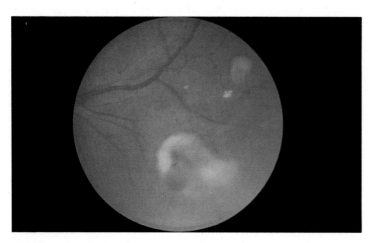

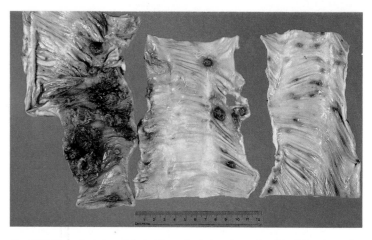

Fig. 13.70 Disseminated candidiasis. Fundal examination may reveal the typical lesions of disseminated candidiasis.

Fig. 13.71 Disseminated candidiasis. Ulceractive lesions due to *Candida albicans* in small bowel. By courtesy of Dr D. Milligan.

cannot be given simultaneously with AZT because both agents are myelosuppressive.

Cerebral toxoplasmosis

Toxoplasmosis is the commonest cause of mass lesions in the brain in patients with AIDS; 50–70% of mass lesions seen on CT scanning in these patients are due to *Toxoplasma gondii*. The disease usually presents clinically as a diffuse encephalitis with headache and focal neurological deficits, developing gradually over a period of several weeks. The typical finding on CT scanning is of multiple ring-enhancing lesions, distributed bilaterally with a predilection for the basal ganglia (see Fig. 3.106). The immunoperoxidase stain is the most sensitive and specific technique for diagnosing toxoplasmosis in a brain biopsy specimen (see Fig. 3.103). The serum antibody test for *T. gondii* is not helpful unless the result is negative; 97% of patients with CNS toxoplasmosis have serum antibody. A CSF:serum ratio of specific toxoplasma IgG antibody greater than 1 suggests the diagnosis of cerebral toxoplasmosis. Response to antimicrobial treatment is often prompt, with rapid improvement in the level of conscious-ness and return of neurological function, but relapse is very common unless suppressive therapy is continued.

Other opportunistic infections

Cryptosporidium parvum, a protozoan parasite which commonly produces a mild self-limited diarrhoeal illness, especially in children, often causes a severe, chronic, relentless diarrhoea in patients with AIDS (Fig. 14.18). Although the infection responds to treatment with spiramycin in immunocompetent individuals, no therapy has been found to be consistently effective in cases of cryptosporidiosis occurring in association with AIDS. Both *Cryptosporidium* and CMV have been associated with acalculous cholecystitis in a few instances (Fig. 14.19).

Tuberculosis may occur early or late in the course of HIV infection. It is most common in population groups in whom the incidence of tuberculosis and tuberculous infection is already high. In some cities in the USA up to 30% of new cases of tuberculosis are associated with HIV infection. When tuberculosis occurs early in HIV infection, when the patient is asymptomatic and the CD4 count is normal, the disease usually affects primarily the lungs, and upper lobe

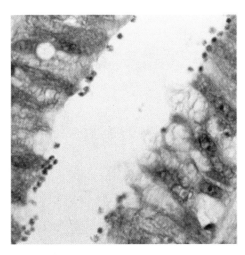

Fig. 14.18 Cryptosporidiosis. Colonic crypt with numerous cryptosporidial sporozoites attached to goblet cells and epithelial cells. Giemsa stain.

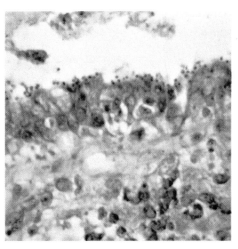

Fig. 14.19 Cryptosporidiosis. Gall bladder mucosa with numerous organisms attached to columnar epithelial cells. Lymphocytes and plasma cells have infiltrated the submucosa. Giemsa stain.

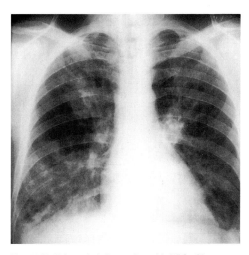

Fig. 14.20 Tuberculosis in a patient with AIDS. Chest x-ray showing multiple pulmonary infiltrates and prominent involvement of the lower lung fields.

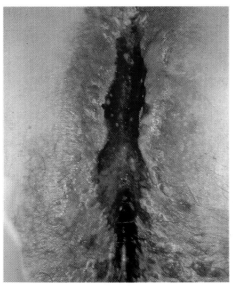

Fig. 14.21 Herpes simplex virus type 2 infection. Progressive, deeply-eroding perianal lesion in a homosexual man with AIDS. By courtesy of Dr E. Sahn.

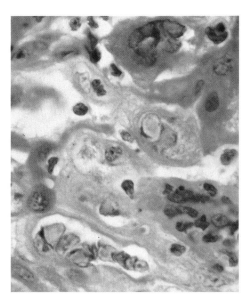

Fig. 14.22 Herpes simplex virus infection. Ground-glass lilac-stained early inclusions and eosinophilic haloed inclusions in nuclei of enlarged squamous cells. A multinucleated giant cell is also present. Haematoxylin–phloxin–saffranin stain.

patients in whom cell-mediated immunity is severely depressed; the incidence is highest in those in whom the CD4+ count has fallen below 200. The commonest manifestation is oral thrush, whitish patches on the tongue and buccal mucosa which may be scraped off to reveal an erythematous base (Fig. 14.12). Occasionally the white exudate may be absent. Candida oesophagitis, manifested by dysphagia, odynophagia and substernal pain, may coexist with oral thrush, especially if immunosuppression is severe (see Fig. 4.2). The disease often responds dramatically to topical or oral treatment with antifungal agents but may recur soon after treatment is discontinued.

Cryptococcosis

Extrapulmonary cryptococcosis occurs in up to 10% of patients with AIDS in the USA; the incidence is even higher in certain areas where cryptococcal infection is especially common. The most common manifestation is cryptococcal meningitis (see Chapter 3). In patients with AIDS this disease is characterized by minimal signs of inflammation and abundant organisms in the CSF. The India Ink preparation reveals cryptococci in 50–90% (see Fig. 3.31), the CSF cryptococcal antigen test is positive in approximately 90%, and culture yields the organism in virtually all patients. Treatment is with amphotericin B plus 5-fluorocytosine, as in the non-AIDS patient, but the incidence of relapse, often heralded by a rising CSF antigen titre after apparently successful treatment, is high unless post-treatment prophylaxis with fluconazole is continued indefinitely.

Mycobacterium avium–intracellulare infection

Disseminated infection with organisms of the *Mycobacterium avium–intracellulare* (MAI) complex is very rare except in patients with AIDS, and in whom this infection may occur at some time during the course in up to 30%. At least half of the cases are diagnosed only at autopsy. The clinical picture is usually of a constitutional illness with fever, night sweats, severe fatigue, weight loss and persistent diarrhoea. Hepatosplenomegaly, anaemia and leucopenia are common. CT scanning often reveals abdominal lymphadenopathy and a thickened bowel wall suggesting an inflammatory colitis. Gallium scanning may reveal intense uptake in the wall of the colon. Most patients exhibit a continuous bacteraemia with large numbers (10^4–10^5) of organisms per ml of blood. Sputum culture is positive in 75%, but there is usually no evidence of pneumonia on x-ray. Stool culture is often positive. Biopsy of involved organs reveals a blunted inflammatory response, with poorly formed granulomata (Fig. 14.13) containing many macrophages packed with acid-fast organisms (Figs 14.14 & 14.15). The prognosis of this infection has been extremely poor with most patients dying within six months in spite of anti-mycobacterial therapy.

Cytomegalovirus infection

Cytomegalovirus is often isolated from various tissues and body fluids in patients with advanced HIV infection. Common sites of involvement are the gastrointestinal tract, especially stomach and colon (Fig. 14.16), lung (Fig. 14.17), liver, brain and eye (see p. 12.20). This virus is often isolated along with other pathogenic microorganisms, and its role in the patient's illness may be difficult to ascertain. Isolation of CMV from blood, urine or respiratory secretions does not prove that the patient's illness is due to CMV infection; it must be isolated from a biopsy specimen of the involved tissue, or the characteristic histopathological features of CMV infection must be observed. The only effective antiviral agent available at present is ganciclovir, which has been useful in the treatment of all types of CMV infection except pneumonia. A serious problem in many AIDS patients is CMV retinitis, which produces a characteristic funduscopic picture of white exudates with surrounding oedema and haemorrhage. Ganciclovir therapy may produce significant resolution of retinitis in many patients, but often ganciclovir

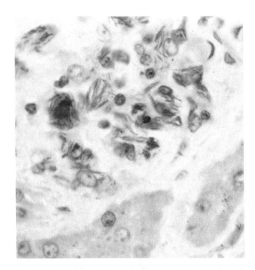

Fig. 14.15 *Mycobacterium avium–intracellulare* infection of liver. A granuloma with foamy histiocytes filled with large numbers of acid-fast bacilli. Kinyoun's stain.

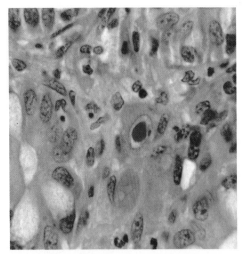

Fig. 14.16 Cytomegalovirus colitis. Large intranuclear CMV inclusions and surrounding clear halos in histiocytes of inflamed colonic lamina propria, with lymphocytes, plasma cells and neutrophils. Haematoxylin–phloxin–saffranin stain.

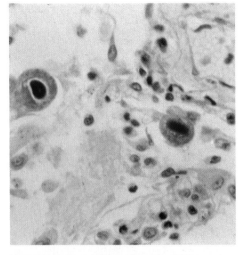

Fig. 14.17 Cytomegalovirus pneumonitis. CMV intranuclear inclusion bodies within alveolar cells. Small amounts of alveolar exudate and interstitial lymphocytic infiltrate are also present. Haematoxylin–phloxin–saffranin stain.

cavitary disease, cough, fever and weight loss are common. Most patients (60–80%) have a positive reaction to the PPD skin test. When tuberculosis occurs in a patient with AIDS, the disease is often disseminated by the time the diagnosis is made, with diffuse pulmonary infiltrates (Fig. 14.20) (or a normal chest x-ray), intrathoracic adenopathy (with or without pleural effusion) and extrapulmonary lesions. Only 30–40% will have a positive PPD reaction. Histopathologically there may be typical granuloma formation or none, depending on the degree of underlying immunosuppression. The prognosis in patients who have concomitant tuberculosis and AIDS is poor; although the tuberculosis responds to antimycobacterial therapy, the median survival is only six months.

Herpes simplex virus infection due to HSV-2 occurs in more than 90% of homosexual men with HIV infection and is usually manifested by lesions in the genital and perianal areas (Figs 14.21 & 14.22). The lesions are often chronic, lasting for many weeks or months, and may be progressive and produce much local destruction of tissue. Although the lesions usually respond to treatment with acyclovir, recurrence is common after treatment is discontinued and resistant variants of HSV-2 may appear.

Progressive multifocal leucoencephalopathy is a demyelinating disease of cerebral white matter due to the JC virus, a papovavirus. Patients usually present with headache, hemiparesis, ataxia, confusion and other mental changes. CT scanning reveals many low-density, non-enhancing lesions; MRI may be an even more sensitive way to detect these lesions (see Fig. 3.65). Diagnosis is made by brain biopsy. Deterioration is usually rapid, with death often occurring within three months after onset of symptoms.

Herpes zoster is a common initial manifestation of HIV infection even in young individuals who are otherwise asymptomatic. It may occur long before any other clinical signs of the HIV infection, and recurrence, which is relatively rare in the absence of HIV infection, is sometimes observed. Herpes zoster is not associated with early progression to AIDS. The distribution of lesions is usually dermatomal (see pp 11.13-16) and although the disease may be chronic, dissemination is uncommon.

Other cutaneous lesions which appear to be of increased frequency and/or severity in patients with HIV infection include perianal and genital condyloma acuminata (Fig. 14.23), seborrhoeic dermatitis, pruritic folliculitis, psoriasis staphylococcal and streptococcal ecthyma and molluscum contagiosum (Figs 14.24 & 14.25). Cutaneous lesions of disseminated cryptococcosis may resemble those of molluscum contagiosum (Fig. 14.26).

Symptomatic neurosyphilis, rarely seen in early syphilis in patients without HIV infection, appears to be much more common in patients with concurrent HIV infection. Clinical manifestations include aseptic meningitis, neuroretinitis (Fig. 14.27), deafness and stroke. The CSF

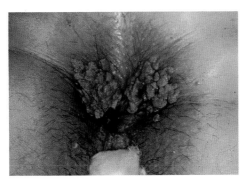

Fig. 14.23 Severe and extensive perianal condyloma acuminata in a patient with AIDS. By courtesy of Dr E. Sahn.

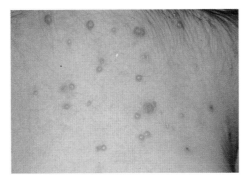

Fig. 14.24 Molluscum contagiosum. Multiple fleshy lesions on the neck.

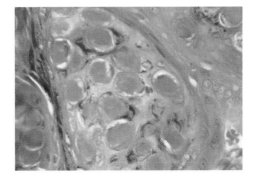

Fig. 14.25 Molluscum contagiosum. Molluscum bodies within enlarged keratinocytes of epidermis. The involved cells form distinct lobules. Haematoxylin–phloxin–saffranin stain.

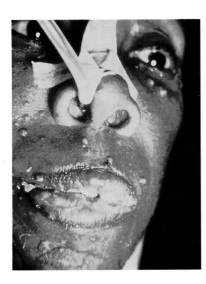

Fig. 14.26 Disseminated cryptococcosis. Many cutaneous lesions of cryptococcosis resembling those of molluscum contagiosum in a patient with AIDS. By courtesy of Dr E. Sahn.

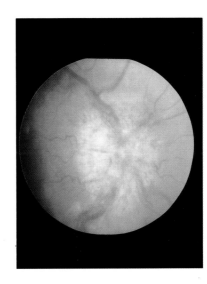

Fig. 14.27 Syphilitic papillitis. Fundus photograph showing severe oedema of the optic disk. By courtesy of Dr C. J. Ellis.

should be examined in all patients with early syphilis and HIV infection, and if evidence of neurosyphilis is found it should be treated promptly and aggressively. There is also evidence that other syphilitic lesions and the VDRL antibody titre in HIV-infected patients with secondary syphilis respond more slowly to conventional penicillin therapy.

Other infections which may be increased in frequency and/or severity in HIV-infected patients include disseminated histoplasmosis (Figs 14.28 & 14.29), disseminated coccidioidomycosis (Fig. 14.30), chronic isosporiasis, microsporidiosis, recurrent salmonella bacteraemia, severe or fatal shigellosis, listeriosis, nocardiosis, bacillary angiomatosis (Figs 14.31 & 14.32) and *Rhodococcus equi* infection.

Neoplasms associated with HIV infection

Kaposi's sarcoma

Kaposi's sarcoma (KS) is by far the commonest neoplasm associated with HIV infection. KS is an initial manifestation of AIDS in 11% of patients, and many more develop it later in the course of the illness. It is disproportionately common in homosexual men and in heterosexual black

Africans. KS is decreasing in incidence in the USA but its biological behaviour appears to be becoming more aggressive. KS is an endothelial neoplasm of either capillary or lymphatic origin. Histopathologically there is proliferation of vascular structures including large malignant-appearing endothelial cells and benign-appearing spindle cells. Inoculation of cells from human KS tumours into immunodeficient mice results in tumours in the mice composed of spindle cells of murine origin. This finding and the peculiar distribution among population groups suggests that KS may be due to a distinct virus. Most patients present with multiple, nodular pigmented lesions, which may be reddish, violaceous or nearly black. Initial lesions are usually found on the skin (Figs 14.33, 14.34, 14.35 & 14.36) and in the oral cavity (Fig. 14.37), but visceral lesions often appear in patients who have extensive cutaneous involvement. The lung (Fig. 14.38) and gastrointestinal tract (Figs 14.39 & 14.40) are common sites of visceral lesions. Pulmonary involvement is associated with a poor prognosis – most patients die within three months of this diagnosis being made. Definitive diagnosis of cutaneous KS is made by biopsy; visceral lesions seen at endoscopy may be difficult or dangerous to biopsy, but the clinical appearance is often characteristic.

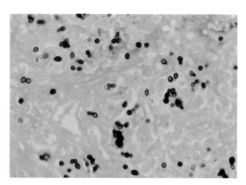

Fig. 14.28 Disseminated histoplasmosis. Non-necrotizing granuloma of liver containing numerous organisms. Fatty change of hepatocytes is also observed.

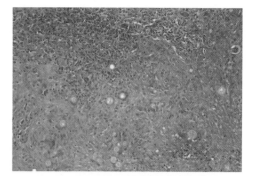

Fig. 14.29 Disseminated histoplasmosis. High power of the same section showing numerous yeast cells. Gomori–methenamine silver stain.

Fig. 14.30 Disseminated coccidioidomycosis. Section of lymph node showing chronic inflammatory reaction and numerous organisms. H & E stain. By courtesy of Dr M. B. Cohen.

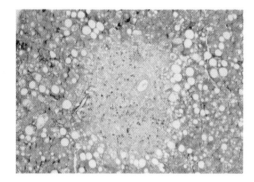

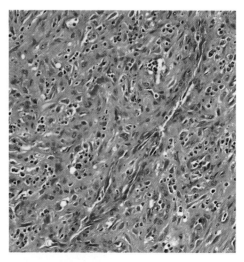

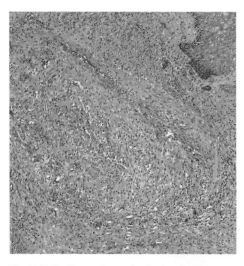

Fig. 14.31 Bacillary angiomatosis. Section of cutaneous lesion showing proliferation of small blood vessels and inflammatory response. H & E stain. By courtesy of Dr M. B. Cohen.

Fig. 14.32 Bacillary angiomatosis. Higher power view showing prominent infiltration by polymorphonuclear leucocytes. H & E stain. By courtesy of Dr M. B. Cohen.

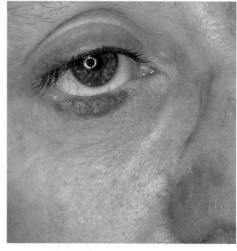

Fig. 14.33 Kaposi's sarcoma. A single lesion on the eyelid. By courtesy of Dr B. K. Fisher.

Non-Hodgkin's lymphoma

The other malignant neoplasm that has been specifically associated with HIV infection is non-Hodgkin's lymphoma (NHL). Although this tumour is much less frequent than KS, the incidence appears to be increasing rapidly, perhaps because of longer survival of patients treated with AZT. Recent studies indicate that nearly half of patients with symptomatic HIV infection who survive for three years on AZT therapy may develop NHL. NHL seen in AIDS patients is usually a high-grade B cell malignancy which exhibits aggressive biological behaviour. Histopathologically it may be large-cell, undifferentiated or immunoblastic in type (Figs 14.41 & 14.42). Epstein–Barr virus DNA sequences can be found in some but not all of these tumors. Presence of malignant B cells

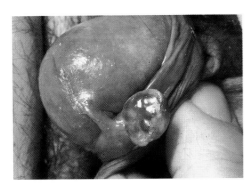

Fig. 14.34 Kaposi's sarcoma. Localized lesion on the penis. By courtesy of Dr B. K. Fisher.

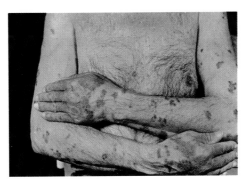

Fig. 14.35 Kaposi's sarcoma. Extensive brownish pigmented lesions on the upper extremities. By courtesy of Dr E. Sahn.

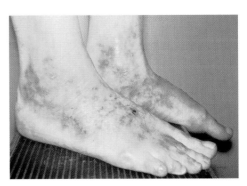

Fig. 14.36 Kaposi's sarcoma. Multiple violaceous lesions on the feet. By courtesy of Dr E. Sahn.

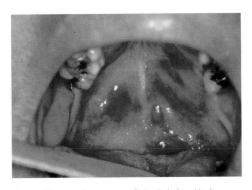

Fig. 14.37 Kaposi's sarcoma. Raised, dark-red lesions on the hard palate.

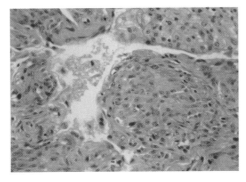

Fig. 14.38 Kaposi's sarcoma. Nodule of Kaposi's sarcoma cells, with palisading spindle-shaped nuclei and rare mitoses, pushing into an alveolar space. Haematoxylin–phloxin–saffranin stain.

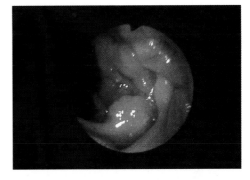

Fig. 14.39 Kaposi's sarcoma. Endoscopic view of lesion in the duodenum. By courtesy of Dr G. Griffin.

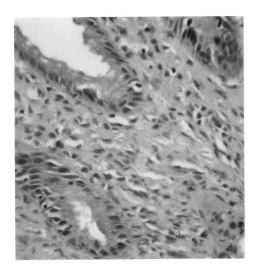

Fig. 14.40 Kaposi's sarcoma. Section of the same lesion showing small anastomotic slit-like vascular channels, extravasation of red blood cells and many spindle cells typical of this neoplasm. H & E stain. By courtesy of Dr M. B. Cohen.

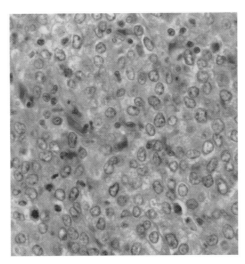

Fig. 14.41 Non-Hodgkin's lymphoma. Diffuse, undifferentiated Burkitt's cell type. Starry-sky pattern, round nuclei with fine nucleoli, and numerous mitoses are seen. Haematoxylin–phloxin–saffranin stain.

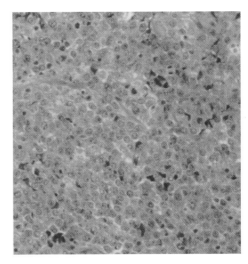

Fig. 14.42 Non-Hodgkin's lymphoma. Diffuse large non-cleaved cell type. Uniform large round nuclei with multiple small nucleoli and numerous mitoses are seen. Haematoxylin–phloxin–saffranin stain.

in the peripheral blood is common. NHL involving the central nervous system (Figs 14.43 & 14.44) is strongly associated with AIDS. It usually presents as a single mass lesion in the brain; biopsy is necessary for definitive diagnosis. In peripheral NHL associated with AIDS, extranodal disease is common, occurring in approximately two-thirds of patients. The prognosis is poor, with a median survival of less than 12 months even with aggressive treatment.

Other conditions associated with HIV infection

Neurological disease occurs at some time during the course of HIV infection in nearly all individuals. Aseptic meningitis is seen in approximately 25% of cases of acute retroviral syndrome, and various cranial neuropathies without meningeal signs occur less frequently. HIV encephalopathy (Fig. 14.45), due to involvement of the white matter of the CNS by the human immunodeficiency virus, is very common, and the incidence increases with progression of the HIV infection. More than 90% of patients with AIDS have cognitive, affective or psychomotor abnormalities. Early in the course of HIV encephalopathy there may be loss of memory, decreased ability to concentrate, mental slowing, affective symptoms, apathy, change in behaviour, motor complaints, increased deep tender reflexes, hypertonia, frontal-release signs and ataxia. CT scanning reveals generalized atrophy in 70-90%, and MRI is even more sensitive, revealing abnormalities in the white matter and multifocal areas of increased signal intensity. As the disease progresses the dementia becomes more severe with marked abnormalities in cognition, profound memory loss, changes in behaviour, psychosis, weakness, tremors and occasionally seizures. CT scanning and MRI reveal extreme atrophy and progressive changes in the white matter. Histopathologically there is gliosis, focal necrosis, microgleal nodules, demyelination and occasional multinucleated giant cells. Vacuolar myelopathy (Fig. 14.46 & 14.47) may occur and result in spastic paralysis of the extremities and faecal and urinary incontinence.

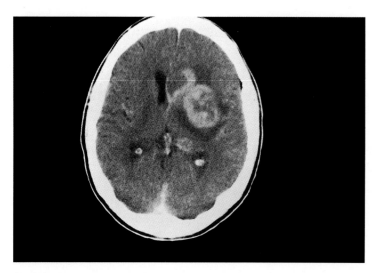

Fig. 14.43 Cerebral lymphoma. CT scan showing multiple enhancing lesions of the right side of the brain due to non-Hodgkin's lymphoma in a patient with AIDS. By courtesy of Dr G. Griffin.

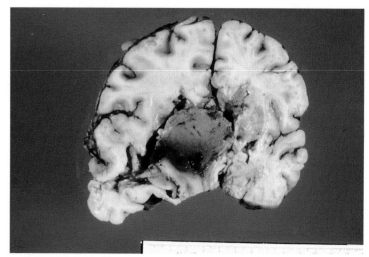

Fig. 14.44 Cerebral lymphoma. Coronal section of brain showing a firm, focally necrotic and haemorrhagic tumor mass, extending from the anterior putamen to the posterior portion of the thalamus, occupying the third ventricle and protruding laterally into the left parietal and temporal lobes.

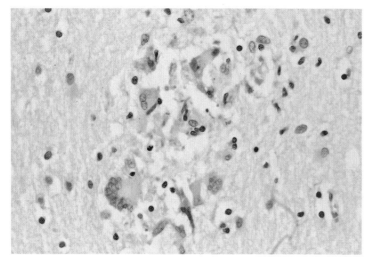

Fig. 14.45 HIV encephalopathy. Histological section of brain showing accumulation of multinucleated giant cells in a perivascular location. H & E stain. By courtesy of Dr P. Garen.

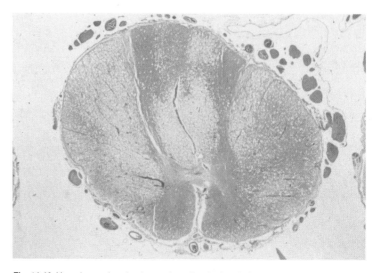

Fig. 14.46 Vacuolar myelopathy. Lower thoracic spinal cord showing marked confluent vacuolation in posterior and lateral columns and mild-to-moderate vacuolation in anterior columns. H & E stain. By courtesy of Dr C. K. Petito.

Peripheral neuropathies are also common during the course of HIV infection. Acute inflammatory demyelinating polyneuropathy (Guillain–Barré Syndrome) is usually seen at an early stage, but a more chronic inflammatory demyelinating polyneuropathy may be seen at any stage of the infection. A multiple mononeuropathy may be seen in advanced ARC and AIDS. The most common type of peripheral neuropathy in patients with AIDS is a distal, predominantly sensory polyneuropathy, with chronic symmetric painful dysaesthesias in a stocking distribution, most severe on the soles of the feet, sometimes accompanied by numbness and motor weakness. Electromyography shows evidence of demyelination and nerve biopsy often reveals degeneration of axons (Fig. 14.48).

Rheumatological complications of HIV infection are frequent. A painful, non-symmetric, non-destructive arthropathy may be seen early or late in the course of the infection. Severe reactive arthritis (Reiter's syndrome) is seen with increased frequency in patients with HIV infection. Polymyositis, with involvement primarily of proximal muscles, has also been reported.

Renal disease in patients with AIDS is often be due to intravenous drug abuse, but a specific AIDS-associated focal and segmental glomerulosclerosis (Fig. 14.49) probably exists. The patients usually present with proteinuria without hypertension. The renal disease progresses rapidly, and these patients respond poorly to maintenance haemodialysis; most die within four months of diagnosis. Activation of the cellular immune system by chronic haemodialysis may accelerate progression of the HIV infection.

Dilated cardiomyopathy and myocarditis (see Fig. 14.50) may be clinically apparent or may be found at autopsy. Some cases are undoubtedly due to opportunistic viral infections but cardiac involvement by HIV may also occur.

Prevention and treatment of HIV infection

The only sure ways to prevent sexual transmission of HIV are abstinence and a completely monogamous relationship between two uninfected partners. Transmission can be reduced by reducing the number of sexual partners and minimizing exposure of oral and genital mucous membranes to blood, semen, saliva and cervical and vaginal secretions during intercourse. Latex condoms are an effective mechanical barrier to HIV and epidemiological data suggest that correct condom use reduces the risk of acquisition of infection by a seronegative partner. Transmission by blood and blood products can be prevented by serological testing of blood and plasma and by heat treatment of clotting factors. Transmission among intravenous drug abusers can be reduced by appropriate educational efforts and addiction treatment programs. Perinatal transmission can be reduced by serological screening of high risk women of childbearing age (those with risk factors or residence in high-prevalence areas) and avoidance of pregnancy and breast feeding in seropositive women.

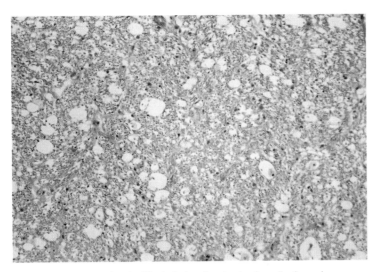

Fig. 14.47 Vacuolar myelopathy. Histological section showing demyelination and vacuolation. Luxol-fast blue stain. By courtesy of Dr M. B. Cohen.

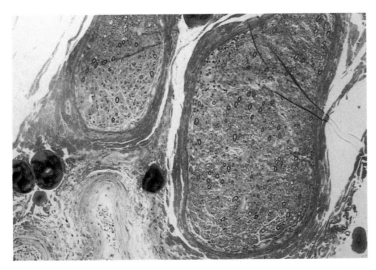

Fig. 14.48 Peripheral polyneuropathy. High power view of section of sural nerve showing severe loss of myelinated fibres and minimal inflammatory reaction. Toluidine blue stain. By courtesy of Dr H. V. Vinters.

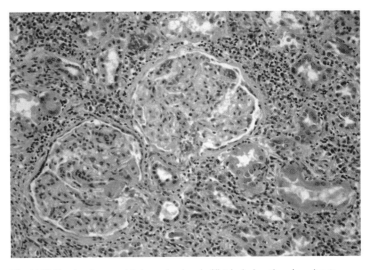

Fig. 14.49 Focal and segmental glomerulosclerosis. Histological section of renal cortex with focal interstitial inflammatory infiltrates, tubular degeneration and segmental glomerulosclerosis. Haematoxylin-phloxin-saffranin stain.

The only antiviral agent which has been used extensively in the treatment of HIV infection at the time of this writing (January 1991) is 3'-azido-2',3'-dideoxythymidine (AZT, azidothymidine, zidovudine). This drug, like other 2',3'-dideoxynucleosides such as 2',3'-dideoxycytidine (ddC) and 2',3'-dideoxyinosine (ddI), exerts its antiviral effect by inhibiting the DNA polymerase of HIV (reverse transcriptase). AZT is converted by cellular kinases into the triphosphate which inhibits HIV reverse transcriptase approximately 100 times more effectively than the mammalian DNA polymerases. AZT triphosphate and other 2',3'-dideoxynucleoside triphosphates are also incorporated into the growing DNA chain and cause termination of viral DNA synthesis because the normal 5' to 3' phosphodiester linkage cannot be completed. Clinical studies have demonstrated that AZT therapy delays progression of HIV infection, reduces the incidence of opportunistic infection and results in prolonged survival. Karnovsky performance status is often increased and significant improvement in cognitive functions is observed in many patients with HIV-related dementia. CD4$^+$ cell count often increases during therapy with AZT, and p24 antigen may disappear from the blood. In thrombocytopenic patients the platelet count may be restored toward normal. Enlarged lymph nodes, liver and spleen may decrease in size during treatment. Recent studies suggest that AZT therapy is more effective and less toxic if given early in the course of HIV infection, and most authorities now recommend initiation of treatment when the CD4$^+$ count falls to 500/mm^3 or less, or when the patient develops an AIDS-defining opportunistic infection. A dose of 500mg/day, divided into 5 doses, appears to be as effective as higher dosage and is associated with fewer adverse effects. Nausea, headache, myalgias, insomnia, anxiety and confusion are experienced by many patients during the first few weeks after initiation of AZT therapy, but these symptoms often abate as therapy is continued. Bluish discolouration of the nails may be seen in black patients (Fig. 14.51). Macrocytosis with elevation in the mean corpuscular volume is observed in many patients; it is rarely associated with anaemia and serum folate and B$_{12}$ levels are normal. A dose-dependent anaemia may develop after prolonged AZT therapy and may be treated by reduction in dosage, recombinant human erythropoietin (if serum erythropoietin levels are low) or transfusions. The most common dose-limiting toxic effect of AZT is neutropenia; the drug must be discontinued, at least temporarily, if the neutrophil count falls below 500–750/mm^3. Myelotoxicity of AZT is often increased when the drug is combined with other myelosuppressive agents such as ganciclovir, trimethoprim/sulphamethoxazole, pentamidine, flucytosine or cyclophosphamide.

Since integration of HIV DNA into the host cell genome results in a permanent latent infection it is unlikely that antiviral chemotherapy will ever be capable of completely eradicating HIV from an infected individual. This situation, plus the fact that most or all HIV-infected individuals undergo progression to AIDS and death, makes development of a vaccine which prevents infection, or at least prevents or retards progression to AIDS, a major priority in the effort to control this disease.

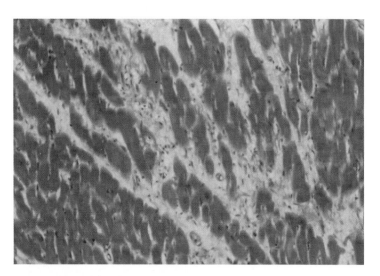

Fig. 14.50 Myocarditis in AIDS. Histological section showing multiple foci of myocardial necrosis, inflammation and fibrosis. Haematoxylin-phloxin-saffranin stain.

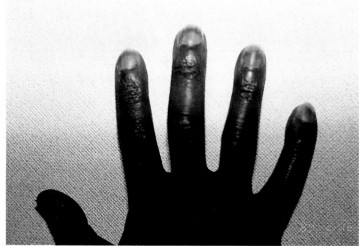

Fig. 14.51 Bluish discolouration of nail beds in a patient receiving AZT. By courtesy of Dr H. P. Holley.

INDEX